T0251329

Crohn's Disease

Gastroenterology and Hepatology

Executive Editor

J. Thomas LaMont, M.D.

Chief, Division of Gastroenterology
Beth Israel Hospital
Boston, Massachusetts
and
Irving W. Rabb Professor of Medicine
Harvard Medical School
Boston, Massachusetts

Crohn's Disease

edited by

Cosimo Prantera
Ospedale Nuovo Regina Margherita
Rome, Italy

Burton I. Korelitz
Lenox Hill Hospital and
New York University School of Medicine
New York, New York

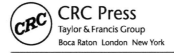

CRC Press
Taylor & Francis Group
Boca Raton London New York

CRC Press is an imprint of the
Taylor & Francis Group, an **informa** business

CRC Press
Taylor & Francis Group
6000 Broken Sound Parkway NW, Suite 300
Boca Raton, FL 33487-2742

© 2008 by Taylor & Francis Group, LLC
CRC Press is an imprint of Taylor & Francis Group, an Informa business

No claim to original U.S. Government works

This book contains information obtained from authentic and highly regarded sources. Reasonable efforts have been made to publish reliable data and information, but the author and publisher cannot assume responsibility for the validity of all materials or the consequences of their use. The authors and publishers have attempted to trace the copyright holders of all material reproduced in this publication and apologize to copyright holders if permission to publish in this form has not been obtained. If any copyright material has not been acknowledged please write and let us know so we may rectify in any future reprint.

Except as permitted under U.S. Copyright Law, no part of this book may be reprinted, reproduced, transmitted, or utilized in any form by any electronic, mechanical, or other means, now known or hereafter invented, including photocopying, microfilming, and recording, or in any information storage or retrieval system, without written permission from the publishers.

For permission to photocopy or use material electronically from this work, please access www.copyright.com (http://www.copyright.com/) or contact the Copyright Clearance Center, Inc. (CCC), 222 Rosewood Drive, Danvers, MA 01923, 978-750-8400. CCC is a not-for-profit organization that provides licenses and registration for a variety of users. For organizations that have been granted a photocopy license by the CCC, a separate system of payment has been arranged.

Trademark Notice: Product or corporate names may be trademarks or registered trademarks, and are used only for identification and explanation without intent to infringe.

Visit the Taylor & Francis Web site at
http://www.taylorandfrancis.com

and the CRC Press Web site at
http://www.crcpress.com

Preface

This book takes us on a journey through the labyrinth of Crohn's disease. It covers most, if not all, of the aspects of this enigmatic and painful disease, and provides the reader with different points of view on every topic treated.

The journey begins with an imaginary nostalgic conversation among Henry Janowitz, Burrill Crohn, Gordon Oppenheimer, and Leon Ginzburg, who exchange questions and answers about how the approaches to etiology and therapeutics have changed with the passing of time. In the next chapter, causes and mechanisms are treated by Jeffry A. Katz and Claudio Fiocchi, with a commentary by Derek Jewell; this gives us the benefit of a Latin outlook tempered by Anglo-Saxon pragmatism. We all know how particularly useful the Scandinavian Registry of IBD is, and it is therefore fitting that the chapter on epidemiology has been written by Anders Ekbom, with a comment by Robert S. Sandler.

As a practicing gastroenterologist, I have often wondered why it did not occur to me sooner that there is a considerable difference, as far as smoking is concerned, between patients with ulcerative colitis and patients with Crohn's disease. Bret A. Lashner has written an interesting chapter on this topic.

Chapter 5 introduces the field of clinical practice. The pathophysiology of symptoms is an aspect that is often neglected in the treatment of patients and, not infrequently, is the source of therapeutic errors. William J. Tremaine is the author of this chapter, with a comment by Sidney Phillips, an expert on the subject. X-rays and endoscopy are two complementary techniques; Geert D'Haens, Paul Rutgeerts, and Burt Korelitz, with a comment by Robert Modigliani, show us where one surrenders arms to the other and vice versa. Radiologists come into their own when using the newer imaging techniques in Crohn's disease; Richard M. Gore et al. outline the results, and Daniel Maklansky gives his view on the subject.

By now, we are all aware of the fact that physical examination of the patient, in terms of palpation and ausculation, is increasingly being replaced by new methods of investigation. Today, diagnostic skills can also be measured by a doctor's ability in interpreting laboratory tests. I have written about this with Anna Kohn in the chapter entitled "Proposed Measures of Disease Activity," and the informed comment is by John W. Singleton. We have known for some time that Crohn's disease is heterogeneous; in his chapter, Lloyd R.

Sutherland distinguishes among the different subgroups and explains the utility of this distinction in clinical practice. The commentary is by David B. Sachar, who is the author of a recent Crohn's disease classification.

The editors of the present volume have taken responsibility for a section on general therapeutic approaches (Chapters 11–13) in which the usefulness and results of treatment with steroids, salazopyrine, and 5-ASA derivatives are evaluated; Burt Korelitz, who is one of the first to use immunosuppressors in the treatment of Crohn's disease, outlines the history of these drugs in a separate section. However, the main difficulty of a general therapeutic approach to Crohn's disease lies in the enormous differences that exist among patients according to the different localizations of the lesions. Adrian Greenstein and James Aisenberg, in Chapter 14, and Norman Sohn, in Chapter 15, deal with this problem, with John Alexander-Williams providing commentary to Chapter 15.

In Chapters 16–30, the book enters into the specific situations that the treatment of Crohn's disease can present. First, there is the prevention of relapse and recurrence after surgery, which has been my concern. This is followed by a chapter in which John E. Lennard-Jones analyzes some of the nutritional problems faced by patients requiring special diets in the treatment of the disease; Arthur D. Heller adds his comment. We all know that Crohn's disease affects young people, and today it seems likely that the disease can be present very early in life. The many cases of young and elderly patients are dealt with respectively by Richard J. Grand and Jay A. Barth, with a comment by Frederic Daum, and by Geetanjali A. Akerkar and Mark A. Peppercorn, with commentary by Nadir Arber and Peter R. Holt. Steven B. Hanauer then writes about the treatment of cases that are refractory to therapy, and Theodore M. Bayless gives his point of view based on his long experience in this field. Now that bacteria and viruses are suspected of being if not the direct cause, then at least close accomplices of Crohn's disease and its complications, long-term treatment with antibiotics is much more common today than it was yesterday. Peter S. Margolis and Walter R. Thayer, Jr., outline the advantages and limitations of this therapy, and I have given my own comment.

In Chapter 22, Daniel H. Present gives us the benefit of his considerable experience and reassures us that Crohn's disease and its treatment do not have much effect on the pregnancy or fertility of those who suffer from it. Douglas A. Drossman, Susan Levenstein, and Marvin Kaplan write respectively about quality of life, the psychological impact of the disease on the patient, and the possibilities for psychological and pharmacological therapy. Barbara S. Kirschner comments on all three chapters. Sometimes, the only serious symptoms from which Crohn's disease patients suffer are the extraintestinal manifestations; Andrew S. Warner and Richard P. MacDermott deal with this in their chapter, with a comment by Lloyd Mayer. Involvement of the liver in this disease is unexpectedly frequent; Harvey M. Lieberman writes on this aspect and Nicholas F. LaRusso gives his comment.

For many years, gastroenterologists have been concerned about the risk of cancer in ulcerative colitis. Paul M. Choi reports on the data demonstrating that Crohn's disease patients also run this risk with increasing frequency; Burt Korelitz adds a brief comment. A surgeon, R. John Nicholls, deals with what happens when a Crohn's disease patient is fitted with an ileo-anal pouch—not such a dire disaster as it would appear to be. The further the endoscope penetrates, the more it discloses the damage to the digestive tract caused by NSAIDs, particularly in cases of patients with Crohn's disease, as Joseph B. Felder explains in his chapter.

In Chapter 31, Samuel Meyers lists the various therapies that over the years, and on the strength of anecdotal reports, have laid claim to relief of symptoms and miraculous cures. How many of them have maintained their promises? What is the psychological reaction of physicians suffering from Crohn's disease? Howard M. Spiro gives an account of the reactions of some patients who are medical doctors. Finally, as the first chapter was dedicated to the past history of this disease, the last chapter by Stephan R. Targan outlines the many "possible futures."

Thus structured, the book is designed to fulfill two main purposes: first, to provide general practitioners with a good basic knowledge of the disease, and second, to furnish specialists with more detailed information and to act as a stimulant for new research in the field. If such research is successful and we achieve the major breakthrough that we are all striving for, then this book could suddenly look as outdated as a blueprint for the trireme and fulfill no purpose at all; but this is a development that all of us—publisher, editors, and contributors included—would like to see.

In conclusion, the editors would like to thank all those people who have made its publication possible: the authors of the various chapters and the commentators; and by no means less important, Tanja Noren at Marcel Dekker, Inc., who has acted as a go-between for the editors, authors, and commentators; and Jill Whitelaw-Cucco, who has assisted me in the difficult duties of reviewing all the manuscripts.

For a long time, Crohn's disease was considered an Anglo-Saxon disease, or at least a disease that affected mainly these populations and those of Northern Europe and the United States. The fact that one of the editors of this book is an Italian—whose experience has been with Italian patients—shows that the gap between Southern Europe on the one hand and Northern Europe and the United States on the other has closed.

Cosimo Prantera

No collection of information on etiology, pathogenesis, clinical manifestations, and treatment of Crohn's disease, in contrast to IBD or ulcerative colitis, has been published since the second edition of *Regional Ileitis* by Burrill Crohn. In order to recognize the progress that has occurred in the field, one need only examine the contents of Crohn's book, where one will find tables of clinical features and personal observations from a time when laboratory investigation and drug therapy were in their infancy.

The sophisticated chapters presented in the current volume represent the keen observations of subsequent clinicians, many clinical serendipitous revelations, and the adaptation of basic scientists, each in his or her own area of interest, to those clinical contributions, and the continued cooperation and productivity of both disciplines.

It has been a great pleasure for me to coedit this volume on Crohn's disease with my friend Cosimo Prantera; together we have perfected the art of international communication.

Burton I. Korelitz

Contents

Contributors

Maria T. Abreu Cedars–Sinai Medical Center, Los Angeles, California

James Aisenberg, M.D. Instructor, Department of Medicine, Mount Sinai Hospital, New York, New York

Geetanjali A. Akerkar, M.D. Senior Medical Resident, Department of Medicine, Beth Israel Hospital and Harvard Medical School, Boston, Massachusetts

John Alexander-Williams, M.D. Professor of Gastrointestinal Surgery, Edgbaston, Birmingham, England

Arnaldo Andreoli, M.D. Assistant Chief, Department of Gastroenterology, Ospedale Nuovo Regina Margherita, Rome, Italy

Nadir Arber, M.D. Visiting Research Fellow, St. Luke's–Roosevelt Hospital Center and Columbia University College of Physicians and Surgeons, New York, New York

Jay A. Barth, M.D. Fellow, Pediatric Gastroenterology and Nutrition, New England Medical Center, Tufts University School of Medicine, Boston, Massachusetts

Theodore M. Bayless, M.D. Professor of Medicine, Department of Gastroenterology, The Johns Hopkins University School of Medicine, Baltimore, Maryland

Eva Berto, M.D. Assistant, Department of Gastroenterology, Ospedale Nuovo Regina Margherita, Rome, Italy

Robert Burakoff, M.D., F.A.C.P., F.A.C.G. Division of Gastroenterology, Hepatology, and Nutrition, Winthrop–University Hospital, Mineola, New York and Professor of Medicine, Health Sciences Center, State University of New York at Stony Brook, Stony Brook, New York

Paul M. Choi, M.D. Clinical Assistant Professor, Department of Medicine, UCLA School of Medicine, Los Angeles, California

Frederic Daum, M.D. Co-Chief, Division of Pediatric Gastroenterology and Nutrition,

Director, The Center for Pediatric Ileitis and Colitis, and Professor of Pediatrics, North Shore University Hospital–Cornell University Medical College, Manhasset, New York; and Director, Pediatric Gastroenterology, New York University–Bellevue Hospital, New York, New York

Geert D'Haens, M.D.   Assistant Professor of Medicine, Department of Gastroenterology, University of Leuven, Leuven, Belgium

Douglas A. Drossman, M.D.   Professor of Medicine and Psychiatry, Department of Medicine, University of North Carolina at Chapel Hill, Chapel Hill, North Carolina

Anders Ekbom, M.D., Ph.D.   Associate Professor, Department of Cancer Epidemiology, Uppsala University, Uppsala, Sweden

Joseph B. Felder, M.D.   Lenox Hill Hospital, New York, New York

Claudio Fiocchi, M.D.   Professor of Medicine, Division of Gastroenterology, University Hospitals of Cleveland, Case Western Reserve University School of Medicine, Cleveland, Ohio

Gary G. Ghahremani, M.D., F.A.C.R.   Professor and Chairman, Department of Diagnostic Radiology, Evanston Hospital–McGaw Medical Center of Northwestern University, Evanston, Illinois

Richard M. Gore, M.D., F.A.C.R., F.A.C.G.   Professor of Radiology and Vice Chairman, Chief of Gastrointestinal Radiology, Evanston Hospital–McGaw Medical Center of Northwestern University, Evanston, Illinois

Richard J. Grand, M.D.   Chief, Division of Pediatric Gastroenterology and Nutrition, and Professor, Department of Pediatrics, New England Medical Center, Tufts University School of Medicine, Boston, Massachusetts

Adrian Greenstein, M.D., F.A.C.S., F.R.C.S.   Professor of Surgery, Department of Surgery, Mount Sinai Hospital, New York, New York

Stephen B. Hanauer, M.D.   Professor of Medicine and Clinical Pharmacology, Department of Medicine/Gastroenterology, University of Chicago Medical Center, Chicago, Illinois

Arthur D. Heller, M.D., F.A.C.P.   Clinical Assistant Professor of Medicine, Department of Medicine, New York Hospital–Cornell Medical Center, New York, New York

Peter R. Holt, M.D.   Professor of Medicine, Columbia University College of Physicians and Surgeons; and Chief, Gastroenterology Division, St. Luke's–Roosevelt Hospital Center, New York, New York

Henry D. Janowitz, M.D.   Clinical Professor of Medicine Emeritus, The Henry D. Janowitz Division of Gastroenterology, Department of Medicine, Mount Sinai School of Medicine, New York, New York

Derek P. Jewell, D. Phil., F.R.C.P.   Gastroenterology Unit, Radcliffe Infirmary, Oxford, England

Marvin Kaplan, M.D.   Attending Psychiatrist, Department of Psychiatry, Lenox Hill Hospital, New York, New York

Jeffry A. Katz, M.D. Assistant Professor of Medicine, Division of Gastroenterology, University Hospitals of Cleveland, Case Western Reserve University School of Medicine, Cleveland, Ohio

Barbara S. Kirschner, M.D. Professor, Department of Pediatrics and Medicine, Wyler Children's Hospital, The University of Chicago, Chicago, Illinois

Anna Kohn, M.D. Assistant Chief, Department of Gastroenterology, Ospedale Nuovo Regina Margherita, Rome, Italy

Burton I. Korelitz, M.D. Chief, Section of Gastroenterology, Lenox Hill Hospital, and Clinical Professor of Medicine, New York University School of Medicine, New York, New York

Nicholas F. LaRusso, M.D. Professor and Chairman, Division of Gastroenterology, Mayo Clinic, Rochester, Minnesota

Bret A. Lashner, M.D. Director, Center for Inflammatory Bowel Disease, Department of Gastroenterology, Cleveland Clinic Foundation, Cleveland, Ohio

John E. Lennard-Jones, M.D., F.R.C.P., F.R.C.S. Emeritus Professor of Gastroenterology, University of London, and Emeritus Consultant, St. Mark's Hospital, London, England

Susan Levenstein, M.D. Adjunct Research Physician, Gastroenterology Division, Ospedale Nuovo Regina Margherita, Rome, Italy

Harvey M. Lieberman, M.D. Assistant Chief, Section of Gastroenterology, Lenox Hill Hospital, and Clinical Associate Professor, Department of Medicine, New York University School of Medicine, New York, New York

Richard P. MacDermott, M.D. Chief, Section of Gastroenterology, Lahey Hitchcock Clinic, Burlington, Massachusetts

Daniel Maklansky, M.D. Associate Clinical Professor, Radiology, Mount Sinai School of Medicine, and Attending Radiologist, Mount Sinai Hospital, New York, New York

Peter S. Margolis, M.D. Clinical Instructor, Department of Medicine and Division of Gastroenterology, Rhode Island Hospital and Brown University, Providence, Rhode Island

Lloyd Mayer, M.D. David and Dorothy Merksamer Professor of Medicine, Department of Medicine, and Professor of Microbiology, Division of Clinical Immunology, Mount Sinai Medical Center, New York, New York

Samuel Meyers, M.D. Clinical Professor of Medicine, Division of Gastroenterology, Mount Sinai School of Medicine and Mount Sinai Hospital, New York, New York

Frank H. Miller, M.D. Assistant Professor of Radiology, Northwestern University Medical School, and Chief of Gastrointestinal Radiology, Northwestern Memorial Hospital, Chicago, Illinois

Robert Modigliani, M.D. Professor, Department of Gastroenterology, Saint-Louis Hospital, Paris, France

R. John Nicholls, M.Chir., F.R.C.S. Dean, St. Mark's Academic Institute, St. Mark's Hospital, Harrow, England

Mark A. Peppercorn, M.D.   Associate Professor of Medicine and Director, Center for Inflammatory Disease, Department of Medicine, Beth Israel Hospital and Harvard Medical School, Boston, Massachusetts

Sidney F. Phillips, M.D.   Professor of Medicine, Mayo Medical School, and Division of Gastroenterology, Mayo Clinic, Rochester, Minnesota

Cosimo Prantera, M.D.   Chief, Department of Gastroenterology, Ospedale Nuovo Regina Margherita, Rome, Italy

Daniel H. Present, M.D.   Clinical Professor of Medicine, Department of Gastroenterology, Mount Sinai School of Medicine, New York, New York

Paul Rutgeerts, M.D.   Professor of Medicine, Department of Medicine, University of Leuven, Leuven, Belgium

David B. Sachar, M.D.   The Dr. Burrill B. Crohn Professor of Medicine and Director, The Henry D. Janowitz Division of Gastroenterology, Mount Sinai Medical Center, New York, New York

Robert S. Sandler, M.D., M.P.H.   Professor of Medicine, Department of Medicine, University of North Carolina, Chapel Hill, North Carolina

Maria Lia Scribano, M.D.   Assistant, Department of Gastroenterology, Ospedale Nuovo Regina Margherita, Rome, Italy

John W. Singleton, M.D.   Professor, Department of Medicine, University of Colorado School of Medicine, Denver, Colorado

Norman Sohn, M.D.   Clinical Assistant Professor, Department of Surgery, New York University School of Medicine, New York, New York

Howard M. Spiro, M.D.   Professor of Medicine, Department of Internal Medicine, Yale University School of Medicine, New Haven, Connecticut

Lloyd R. Sutherland, M.D.C.M., M.Sc., F.R.C.P.C., F.A.C.P.   Professor and Head, Community Health Sciences, Foothills Hospital and University of Calgary, Calgary, Alberta, Canada

Stephan R. Targan, M.D.   Director of IBD Center, Cedars–Sinai Medical Center, and Professor of Medicine, UCLA School of Medicine, Los Angeles, California

Walter R. Thayer, Jr., M.D.   Professor, Department of Medicine and Division of Gastroenterology, Rhode Island Hospital and Brown University, Providence, Rhode Island

William J. Tremaine, M.D.   Director, IBD Clinic, and Associate Professor of Medicine, Division of Gastroenterology, Mayo Foundation, Rochester, Minnesota

Andrew S. Warner, M.D.   Director, IBD Center, Section of Gastroenterology, Lahey Hitchcock Clinic, Burlington, Massachusetts

1

Conversation with Burrill B. Crohn, Leon Ginzburg, and Gordon Oppenheimer 63 Years After the Discovery of Crohn's Disease

Henry D. Janowitz   *Mount Sinai School of Medicine, New York, New York*

Through the good offices of Drs. Korelitz and Prantera, this unusual dialogue with these three physicians "on the other side" allowed me to discuss some aspects of "regional ileitis" with its original describers.

> HDJ: Good evening, Burrill, Leon, and Gordon. It has been a long time since I had the pleasure of seeing you all at a meeting, nearly a quarter of a century ago in 1968 at a meeting of the National Foundation for Ileitis and Colitis, of which you all were honorary chairmen.

> GO: Someone joked that this would be the first time we were together again since we wrote the original paper.

> LG: Like most jokes, it is probably true, but, like a lot of other things, we don't worry any more about that over here.

> HDJ: So I can call it Crohn's disease without stepping on anyone's toes?

> BBC: Now, Henry, you know I never referred to Crohn's disease. It was Brian Brooke in his editorials in the *Lancet* who popularized the term.

> HDJ: Yes, Burrill. When I got to know you better in the 1950s, you always seemed almost embarrassed by the term. Yes, Leon, although you are smiling, that's true.
>
> Now that I have got you all here together, there are several things I want to get straight. It was early in 1960 that Lockhart-Mummery and Morson put regional enteritis of the colon definitively into the literature and on the map.
>
> Now Leon and Gordon, you had described the colonic involvement of granulomatous disease in your first independent paper in the surgical world in 1933 after the joint paper at the American Medical Association meeting in New Orleans in 1932. Why didn't you follow that up?

> LG: The idea seemed clear enough to me. Gordon was interested in urology and I was born to be a surgeon. Pathologists and other medical men could worry that bone.

> HDJ: Well Burrill, I can remember when I, as a newcomer on the scene, had almost daily conversations with you and Dick Marshak, a great radiologist, about the fact that the same process that occurred in the ileum could occur in the colon. I still

recall how exasperated Dick was with you and how you were reluctant to accept the concept.

BBC: Yes, Dick Marshak was easily exasperated. But you remember I did come around to accept the fact, although a bit slowly.

HDJ: I always blamed that delay on the tight hold that the Department of Pathology under Paul Klemperer had on medical conceptual thinking at Mount Sinai.

BBC: You are right. Dr. Otani was also a great pathologist, but he clung firmly to the belief that the ileocecal valve separated ileitis from ulcerative colitis. Ileitis north, ulcerative colitis south of the valve. Others, like Wells, had been writing about granulomatous colitis for some years before Dick Marshak and, finally, Lockhart-Mummery and Morson published their paper.

HDJ: Now something else has bothered me for years. You published your original paper from the Departments of Surgery and Pathology. Why didn't it have a single photograph of a gross specimen, or a single photomicrograph?

LG: My hazy recollection is that Gordon and I published quite a few gross anatomical pictures in our own paper and, I suppose, the Department of Pathology was planning to publish the histology for the disciples of that field.

HDJ: So the emphasis on the granuloma system became important only after Hadfield's paper 7 years later.

I know that according to the rules I am supposed to ask the questions, but surely there is one all of you are burning to ask.

BBC: "Burning?" That's something we try not to think about up here.

LG and GO (simultaneously): Of course! Have you found out either the cause or the cure by now?

HDJ: Unfortunately, we still do not know the cause or have a cure.

LG: I may be less cynical and also less sarcastic on this side, but I have not lost my wits. I always felt that if we didn't find out right away that it would take a long time.

HDJ: It has taken a long time, but perhaps more that 60 years is not so long after all. Besides we have learned a lot about the natural history and the manifestations of the disease and its pathophysiology. We have accumulated a lot of information regarding the intricate steps of the inflammatory process in the bowel. Also, we have found quite a few medicines that help, and we have come to appreciate better the gains and losses of surgery.

What I want to do now is to compare what you thought then with what we have added or subtracted since your clinical description of this disorder.

I always thought that there were two pleasures of growing old in medicine. I didn't say pleasures of growing old, but growing old in medicine. First, one learns what happens to one's former patients. Second, the outmoded theories of our youth are revived again.

In this context, Burrill, you told me when you first met me in 1939, 7 years after the seminal paper, that Emanuel Libman, distinguished clinician whose name is attached to Libman-Sachs disease, or verrucous endocarditis, had proposed, rather facetiously, that ileitis was a new disease attributable to the widespread use of toothpaste containing silica particle matter.

BBC: But I don't think that this was taken very seriously.

HDJ: No, but the Chesses did, and so they fed silica containing mixtures to animals and produced lesions of the small bowel. Now, you may be interested that during the last year or two, a series of letters in the *Lancet* have revived the theory and redirected attention to the possibility of submicroscopic material in the intestinal lesions. But I, too, feel that this will not lead us very far.

Anyhow, in a more serious vein, what did you three or perhaps the paper's original surgeon, A. A. Berg, think about this disease when you first began to study it and recognize its distinction from other small bowel conditions?

LG: At the operating table, it looked different from our preoperative expectations of either cancer or tuberculosis and it was certainly different when we opened the specimen. One couldn't help thinking that it might be a variant of tuberculosis in these relatively young people.

BBC: One couldn't help thinking of other granulomatous diseases of the area— tuberculosis, actinomycosis—or some chronic infection.

GO: It was soon obvious that the lesions did not contain acid-fast organisms. But we were all hipped on an infectious etiology. So we injected lots of material from lots of specimens into lots of animals, but never produced anything resembling regional ileitis.

HDJ: This idea of an infectious cause has never disappeared; it has been pursued vigorously and is revived from time to time. The search in recent years has been for a mycobacterium, because the veterinary world has recognized the similarity of regional enteritis and Johne's disease of cattle, that is due to *Mycobacterium paratuberculosis.*

The literature on the possible mycobacterial origin of Crohn's disease is tremendous. Many clinical trials of treatment with combinations of up to four or five antituberculosis drugs have had varying results, but, I think it is fair to say that the case is still not proven.

Workers are using more refined technology to demonstrate biochemical residuals of mycobacterial organisms in the tissues. Incidentally, the organism producing Whipple's disease that was seen by light microscopy and by staining techniques in 1902 has finally been identified by these newer techniques.

LG: We have also heard that this was accomplished just as Whipple's disease began to disappear as an intestinal disorder.

HDJ: But as more workers devoted themselves to this search for the infectious agent and none was forthcoming, what did you think, Burrill?

BBC: I still thought it was caused by an infectious agent. Some patients got better on the sulfa-containing drug, sulfathaladine, which was used widely by the profession before the introduction of steroids, but we never had the use of antibiotics directed against intestinal organisms. Then the introduction of steroids, which seemed to be so useful for inflammatory bowel disease, turned our thinking in other directions.

HDJ: Even in the late 1950s, you kept thinking in terms of "a viral etiology."

BBC: Yes. I always preferred a simple to a complex answer to a problem. I thought it might turn out to be a virus.

HDJ: Well, in fact, Wakefield and Pounder and their colleagues are pretty hot about the idea that it's essentially a granulomatous endothelial vasculitis caused by the measles virus.

BBC: Measles? You're kidding!

HDJ: Well, they make a strong case for it, but it's got a long way to go. I clearly remember your responding to my question as to whether Crohn's disease and ulcerative colitis, which you clearly separated, could occur in the same individual.

BBC: Don't laugh. I said yes. If the agent is a viral one, why couldn't a patient with one virus have been infected by another virus and have both diseases?

HDJ: Another early concept that Leon stressed is having a renewal. I mean the idea that the fecal stream plays a role in the pathogenesis of Crohn's disease. You came to this concept from your observations on the results of diversionary operations in regional enteritis.

LG: Thanks for reminding me. The observations were made so long ago that I have almost forgotten them. In the 1930s, operations for regional ileitis were not risk-free. We had no pre- or postoperative access to antibiotics, so removal of disease was done in two stages. In the first operation, the ileum was divided proximal to the disease and then closed. The proximal end was then implanted in the colon—the usual ileocolostomy. Several months later, in the second operation, the diseased ileum and cecal tip were removed. I was impressed at the time of the second operation how often the bypassed ileum had become a shrunken fibrotic cord and how much less inflamed it was. I had never seen this in the disconnected rectum of ulcerative colitis following subtotal colectomy, and it impressed me.

HDJ: I never forgot your telling me this, and I tried to explain the ileal and anal location in Crohn's disease as being related to the pile-up of the fecal stream at the valvular areas. So you may be interested that recent studies once again suggest a role for the fecal stream. One set of workers have temporarily protected an ileo-ascending colostomy for regional enteritis by a proximal ileostomy for up to 6 months and have not seen the endoscopic inflammation that usually takes place. Another group has once again studied the reparative process of the colon in Crohn's disease, with evidence of healing, after temporarily diverting the fecal stream.

LG: Of course I am delighted to hear about this finding. The healing of granulomatous disease of the colon does not last very long. By 6 months, patients were ready to have their colons removed.

BBC: But, even in the days when we didn't separate the two causes of colonic inflammation, occasionally, an ileostomy led to temporary improvement.

HDJ: Didn't you sense that it was no accident that regional enteritis was frequently seen at a hospital like Mount Sinai, recorded by doctors with names like Ginzburg, Oppenheimer, and Crohn, and patients with names related to Jewish descent?

GO: At first we blamed it on the fact that we were a Jewish hospital, but later, we sensed that this was not the basis of this congregation of patients.

BBC: We knew that Bargen at the Mayo Clinic was seeing similar patients and collecting cases.

LG: Probably patients from New York seeking a second opinion.

HDJ: By 1939 to 1941, during my internship, we all recognized that it was a Jewish disease and joked whether to blame the Jewish mother, Jewish food, or Jewish genes.

GO: It is our turn to ask questions again. What did you learn about this congregation of patients?

HDJ: We are no longer the chosen people but many of us are called. Crohn's disease is a worldwide disease of all social classes and of all races. There is much good data from cohort studies and twin studies on the familial susceptibility to inflammatory bowel disease. If you have Crohn's disease, then there is a good chance that others in your family will too, and, if you and your wife have the disease, a large proportion of your children will too. But the problem still remains of how to identify the genetic markers. Some exciting recent studies indicate that ulcerative colitis and Crohns's disease have different HLA typing, but not all fit into two distinct patterns. Equally exciting is the finding that half or more of ulcerative colitis patients have a marker in the blood known as pANCA—peripheral antinuclear cytoplasmic antibody—that patients with Crohn's disease do not. Don't ask me to define this further. I'll have trouble doing so.

BBC: I am delighted to hear how the search thrives. You will remember, Henry, that in 1961 you introduced me to a session of the New York Academy of Sciences devoted to granulomatous disease. The next day, I had to confess to you that I really understood very little of what was presented.

HDJ: The important point about the pANCA is that it reopened the question of the unity of each disease. We spent the last 30 years separating nonspecific inflammatory bowel disease into two separate containers—ulcerative colitis and Crohn's disease—and distinguishing them from infections and ischemia. But it appears that there is heterogeneity within each group.

And, even with the specimen in their hands, expert pathologists have trouble classifying 10%, maybe 15%, "the indeterminate group." Some patients may lack both markers—HLA type and ANCA marker. So Burrill and Sidney Truelove might be right. Patients might have both diseases.

HDJ: Furthermore, the two diseases might be more than two. But now I want to ask all of you a question from an evolutionary point of view. When you identified regional enteritis, did you think it was a new disease or one that had been overlooked?

LG: I thought it was relatively new. We couldn't believe that the great pathologists from the 19th century, Virchow, Connheim, etc., who did routine examinations of the entire small bowel in every autopsy, would have missed it. They knew tuberculosis very well and wouldn't have confused it.

HDJ: Even if it is only relatively new, not many observers have recognized it, but one had. Dalziel, a prominent Scottish surgeon, published a paper in the *British Journal of Surgery* in 1912 that clearly distinguished a group of patients with fibrosing lesions in the small and large bowel that had all the earmarks of regional enteritis and Crohn's disease.

I asked you once before, Burrill, whether you and Leon had ever heard of this paper, because Brooke specifically raised the question.

BBC: Paul Klemperer's Department of Pathology had long been interested in fibrotic lesions of the bowel. We had a very good library in those days but never came across Dalziel's paper.

HDJ: To me, the most unusual question is why didn't the British surgeons pick up this report and pay more attention to it? It was not published in an obscure journal.

LG: Part of the answer, I believe, is that there were no further follow-up papers to create the appropriate receptive climate as there were for the original JAMA paper by us three and the surgical paper by Gordon and myself in 1933. The Mount Sinai group, especially Burrill, kept on collecting and writing about the entity. Except for the paper on cancer of the jejunum in regional enteritis, I don't think I wrote any more and I am pretty sure that Gordon didn't.

HDJ: Which brings me to the following question. How important did you think your original observations were or might turn out to be?

GO: I thought it was an interesting finding, but I went on to fry other fish.

LG: It was new, interesting, even curious. It might turn out to be important, but I didn't give it that much thought. Remember, in those days at Mount Sinai we were supposed to find new diseases or at least new signs. Koplik had his spots, Tay and Sachs had their disease, Brill described his disease, and there were a bunch of others.

BBC: It was new to us and exciting because of that. We didn't know whether it would be important. Others like Bargen were collecting their own cases. We thought we should keep on looking for new cases and keep those records separate, so I segregated the charts in my office. I didn't think the disease would take on such worldwide clinical importance. I was astounded after the floodgates opened with the identification of involvement of the large bowel by Lockhart-Mummery and Morson.

LG: I was gratified by the confirmation of Gordon's and my observation that the colon was involved in this disease, but it was old hat to us by then.

HDJ: There was another observation that you, Leon, made fairly early on and that has blossomed into an important point for the future.

LG: I didn't write much about regional enteritis but you reminded me a moment ago that I did report the first case of carcinoma of the small bowel in the jejunum in a patient with longstanding ileojejunitis.

HDJ: Yes, in 1955, 22 years after the original description of regional enteritis, you presented a paper on a cancer of the small bowel in a patient with regional enteritis. You obviously were aware of the propensity of patients with ulcerative colitis to develop cancer and you explained the rarity of your case on the basis of the fact that cancer rarely occurs in the small bowel. You were right about the rarity, but, since then, almost all the cancers of the small bowel have occurred in patients with Crohn's disease. For a while, we thought they had a particular predilection for the bypassed loop and that the bypass played a major role, but it is clearer now that small bowel cancer takes a long time to develop, even longer than colon cancer does in ulcerative colitis. It has little to do with the bypass. Just as you, Leon, published the first paper on cancer in regional ileitis, so Burrill published the first case of cancer of the colon in ulcerative colitis in 1925.

LG: What is the story with Crohn's disease in the colon?

HDJ: It is far from settled, but the likelihood of cancer in the colon is increased several-fold over the normal expected rate in the general population, but perhaps not as much as in ulcerative colitis in the colon.

Our belief is that few patients tolerate regional enteritis of the colon for long periods of time, without colectomy. Most observers think that cancer is more likely to develop in Crohn's disease of the colon and that it takes a decade longer to develop than in ulcerative colitis.

BBC: Do you keep all the patients with Crohn's disease of the colon under surveillance with colonoscopy as you do with patients with ulcerative colitis?

HDJ: The consensus has not been reached yet, although many of us do.

LG: The one case I reported seems to have started up something.

HDJ: But not as much as the 14 original patients with regional enteritis. Did the problem of cancer in regional enteritis, either of small or large bowel, occupy much of your concern?

LG: We really didn't give the cancer problem much thought. My case just seemed an oddball.

HDJ: As we close this interview, I want to direct comments to each of you that would indicate that we have made some progress in understanding the entity you so clearly described over 60 years ago.

Gordon, the urological aspects of this intestinal disease have ramified widely. We understand the nature and therapy of uric acid calculi, oxalate metabolism, and the role of hyperoxaluria in relation to the formation of oxalate stones. Obstructive uropathy and bladder fistulas have given an important place to the urologist in the management of enteritis of the large and small bowel.

GO: Had I but known . . .

HDJ: Leon, we understand now why your ileitis patients had gallstones; they are secondary to the reduction of the bile salt pool. But, saving bowel is the watchword of small bowel surgery today, with the use of stricturoplasties whenever resection would be too drastic.

LG: I await the long-term follow-up.

HDJ: Burrill, as the colonic involvement of the basic disease became clearer, a whole host of extraintestinal manifestations became obvious. They included iritis, stomatitis, axial and peripheral arthritis, erythema nodosum, pyoderma gangrenosum, amyloidosis, even pancreatitis. The spectrum has widened and each manifestation is more puzzling, making more interesting the whole range of this disorder.

BBC: So Crohn's disease has replaced the lues of my medical student days.

HDJ: While the whole world has paid tribute to your joint papers, miracle of miracles, you have not been forgotten at your own hospital. Burrill, you have been honored by a medical professorship and a research foundation, both linked to gastroenterology, and, Gordon and Leon, you are honored each year by an annual lectureship at your medical school that was established by your friends and colleagues and is given by distinguished members of the profession.

And, oh yes, the National Foundation for Ileitis and Colitis, now renamed the Crohn's and Colitis Foundation of America, of which you were the honorary chairmen, thrives, having raised and spent about $27 million of funds for teaching, education, and research. It serves as the model for similar foundations throughout the world.

I do hope the next time we meet I can bring the news that we have found the cause or, at least, a cure for this disorder.

COMMENTARY

Burton I. Korelitz   *Lenox Hill Hospital and New York University School of Medicine, New York, New York*

I was thrilled with the "conversation" and found it realistic and accurate. One of my own observations, which Dr. Janowitz did not bring into the conversation, was the heritage not only from Crohn, Ginsberg, and Oppenheimer but also from Mount Sinai Hospital, where this challenging disease we now call Crohn's disease has served to stimulate and motivate us, through the work of a series of investigators including Aufses, Korelitz, Greenstein, Sachar, Present, Gelernt, Meyers, Kornbluth, Mayer, Itzkowitz, and others, as well as those who still followed. The leader of these has been Dr. Janowitz himself, who has been a motivating force for those who followed as well as being the foremost disciple of the past.

2
Causes and Mechanisms
of Crohn's Disease

Jeffry A. Katz and Claudio Fiocchi   *University Hospitals of Cleveland,
Case Western Reserve University School of Medicine, Cleveland, Ohio*

I. PRELIMINARY CONSIDERATIONS

There are many chronic diseases of unknown etiology that continue to resist all efforts to
reveal their specific cause and unveil the mechanisms of tissue injury. Crohn's disease is
a prototype of such diseases. After being identified as a distinct clinical entity well over
half a century ago, Crohn's disease remains a true enigma despite having its clinical
heterogeneity recognized and classified, increasing worldwide incidence documented,
genetic and epidemiological aspects explored, plausible causes investigated, and every
conceivable therapy tested. The fact that so many attempts have been made to understand
this illness and that relatively few answers have been obtained may be telling about the
true nature of this disease. Perhaps the clinical manifestations are broad and unpredictable
because Crohn's disease represents many different illnesses. The fact that no clear and
undisputed causative microorganism has been found may be because such an agent does
not exist, or, on the contrary, a number of them cause Crohn's disease. Maybe its rapidly
increasing incidence around the globe is due to various environmental factors that simply
modulate a very common response of the bowel to nonspecific insults. Moreover, an
almost endless armamentarium of drugs and diets have been experimented with, often
giving less than desirable results, indicating that almost every approach is justified,
because we are treating different patients with different illnesses having nothing in
common except the name (Crohn's disease) used to diagnose and classify them. These
somewhat extreme but not unrealistic perspectives can be translated into two polarized
points of view: Crohn's disease is a single and unique clinical entity whose complexity is
beyond our present comprehension or Crohn's disease does not exist as a distinct entity
but represents a syndrome with multiple etiologies that are lumped under one heading for
lack of sufficient knowledge (1). Whatever the case, investigators and clinicians are left
with the unresolved challenge of finding the cause, understanding the mechanisms of
relentless bowel inflammation, and improving the forms of treatment. In this chapter,
possible causes and potential mechanisms of Crohn's disease are discussed. Information,
studies and concepts whose value and reliability are uncertain are included; however, this
is justifiable given the many unanswered questions surrounding the disease. Some import-

ant components of the pathogenesis of Crohn's disease, such as epidemiology, immuno-genetics, and smoking, are discussed in detail elsewhere in this book. Other forms of gut inflammation, such as ulcerative colitis, celiac disease, or infections, are discussed to point out differences between various forms of inflammatory bowel disease and to underline aspects unique to Crohn's disease.

II. INFECTIOUS AGENTS

Ever since Crohn's disease was recognized as a distinct condition, attempts have been made to link its cause to a variety of microorganisms. The same has happened for ulcerative colitis. When the two entities are considered together, the list of bacteria, bacterial products, viruses, and fungi implicated as potential etiological agents is astonish-ingly long (Table 1).

A. Bacteria

The intestinal mucosa normally functions to provide an effective barrier between the many challenges from the external environment and the carefully regulated internal milieu of the host. This barrier is not completely efficient, and immune reactivity directed against the

TABLE 1 Bacteria, Bacterial Products, Viruses, and Fungi Investigated in the Etiology of Inflammatory Bowel Disease

Bacteroides
Brucella
Citrobacter
Coprococcus
Candida albicans
C. colinum
Campylobacter fetus
Campylobacter jejuni
Chlamydia psittaci
Chlamydia trachomatis
Campylobacter sputorum
Eubacterium
Escherichia coli
Lipid A
Listeria
Mycobacterium avium
Mycobacterium kansasii
Mycobacterium paratuberculosis
Paramyxovirus
Peptostreptococcus
Pseudomonas
Rotavirus
S. cerevisiae
Streptococcus faecalis
Y. enterocolitica
Y. paratuberculosis

ubiquitous microorganisms of the gut or their metabolic and degradation products could trigger inflammation or contribute to the chronicity of a local immune response. This section reviews the evidence linking bacteria to the etiopathogenesis of Crohn's disease.

1. Bacterial Flora

Since Crohn's disease was first described, investigators have searched for an etiologic infectious agent. Although no single microorganism has been identified, several abnormalities of the enteric flora have been documented. Cultures of the obligate anaerobic flora have demonstrated greater numbers of gram-positive coccoid rods and gram-negative rods in Crohn's disease patients than in healthy control patients (2). This was related to genetic factors, and similar findings were detected in healthy relatives of Crohn's disease patients (3). Although conventional microbiological techniques have failed to identify any unique or specific bacteria associated with Crohn's disease, mucosal cultures have demonstrated a slight predominance of *Enterobacteriae* (4). Several studies have demonstrated a high (up to 50%) recovery of unusual bacterial L-forms from filtrates of homogenized Crohn's disease tissue (5–8). In contrast, such cell-wall–deficient bacteria were found in only a small fraction (1%–6%) of control homogenates (7,8). L-forms have been cultured from involved and uninvolved bowel and from lymph node from Crohn's disease patients, but they have also been cultured from ulcerative colitis patients, strongly suggesting that their presence is probably secondary to inflammation and mucosal damage (7,8). Revertants to parental bacterial forms have revealed *Pseudomonas*-like species, *Escherichia coli*, and *Streptococcus faecalis*. The role of L-forms in the etiopathogenesis of Crohn's disease continues to be debated, but there are no studies in which they have been used for successful transmission of the disease. Additional bacterial agents have been sought as an etiology for Crohn's disease, but equally without success (9–11).

2. Immune Reactivity to Bacterial Antigens

If bacteria are not directly pathogenic to intestinal tissue in Crohn's disease, perhaps inflammation could be caused by an immune response mounted against local microbes. In a classical study, Broberger and Perlmann first demonstrated in 1959 the presence of antibodies in ulcerative colitis sera which reacted with a component of the human colon (12). This raised the possibility that antigens derived from intestinal bacteria could instigate a damaging immune response in the host which would result in clinical inflammation. Early studies in ulcerative colitis focused on *E. coli* 0:14, which carries an antigen shared with the human colonic mucosa (13) and is capable of inducing a lymphocyte-mediated cytotoxic response (14). High titers of antibodies against *E. coli* antigens were also found in the sera of patients with Crohn's disease, but no specific serotype was predominant (15). In addition, *E. coli* antibodies are commonly found in a variety of other clinical entities of infectious and inflammatory nature, as well as in some normal subjects. Further studies of bacterial antibodies in Crohn's disease have looked for specific agglutination responses to *Clostridium sp.*, *Campylobacter sp.*, *Bacteroides sp.*, *Eubacterium*, *Peptostreptococcus*, *Brucella sp.*, and *Listeria sp.*, but all failed to find any significant difference from ulcerative colitis or control populations (16–19). Blaser et al. did find a significantly elevated response to *Yersinia paratuberculosis*, but also to several other bacterial pathogens, and concluded that this probably represented a nonspecific sensitization to cross-reacting antigens (17). This conclusion is supported by subsequent studies of Pirzer et al. who evaluated the proliferation of Crohn's disease intestinal T-cells in response to a panel of bacterial antigens (20). Lymphocytes from inflamed mucosa exhibited a heightened proliferation compared with cells from uninvolved mucosa, but this result was generalized to all antigens tested. Taken together, studies of bacterial immune reactivity suggest that the response to enteric bacteria in Crohn's disease is not a primary pathogenic phenomenon, but rather an event secondary to chronic inflammation and an impaired mucosal barrier.

3. Bacterial Products

Although little evidence from culture and antibody studies supports the possibility that any one particular bacterium causes Crohn's disease, there is good evidence that the bacterial flora and products play a role in the pathophysiology of the illness. This concept has been recently bolstered by reports of several experimental models of intestinal inflammation, in which animals kept in a germ-free or specific pathogen-free environment fail to develop intestinal inflammation or only present an attenuated inflammatory response (21–23). Clearly, without the intestinal microflora, chronic inflammation is absent or limited. Given the lack of histological evidence, it is unlikely that direct tissue invasion of an abnormally permeable or damaged mucosa by whole bacteria is involved in the inflammatory process of Crohn's disease. Rather, it is now established that soluble products of bacteria can reproduce the histological and immunological responses of the intact organism. In a rat model, Sartor et al. have convincingly shown that peptidoglycan-polysaccharide complex (PG-PS), a component of the bacterial cell wall, induces a chronic granulomatous enterocolitis when injected into the intestinal wall (24). This model is attractive because it has both an acute and a subacute reactivation phase, somewhat resembling human disease and suggesting that sensitization to PG-PS has occurred (25). Endotoxin injected intravenously into PG-PS–treated animals causes an exacerbation of enterocolitis analogous to flares of human inflammatory bowel disease (26). In addition to lipopolysaccharide (endotoxin), other microbial products with proinflammatory activity include N-formylmethionyl-leucyl-phenylalanine and muramyl peptides (27). These bacterial products can activate macrophages to release cytokines, stimulate endothelial adhesion molecule expression, modulate T- and B-cell responses, and trigger the kinin and complement systems (28). Although there is no firm evidence that abnormal acquired or genetic responses to microbial products are responsible for the etiology of Crohn's disease, the potent biological activities of these products can explain many pathophysiologic components of inflammatory bowel disease.

4. Mycobacteria

Ever since the first patients with Crohn's disease were reported, the similarity to intestinal tuberculosis has been appreciated (29,30). Dalziel noted, "The cases gave the impression that they were probably tuberculosis . . . ," but he could find no evidence of mycobacteria on histological examination (29). Crohn et al. remarked that the similarity to ileocecal tuberculosis probably accounted for past failures to recognize what they described as regional ileitis (30). They too searched carefully for, but could not find, proof of mycobacterial infection. Historically, the key feature that distinguishes Crohn's disease from any known mycobacterial infection is the inability to identify or culture mycobacteria from diseased tissue (31).

a. Mycobacterial Cultures. In 1913, Dalziel commented on the pathologic similarity between Crohn's disease and Johne's disease, a chronic mycobacterial enteritis of ruminants due to infection with *Mycobacterium paratuberculosis* (29). In 1972, Patterson and Allen revived the idea that Crohn's disease could be mycobacterial in origin (32). A few years later, Burnham and Lennard-Jones reported the isolation of *Mycobacterium kansasii* from a lymph node of a patient with Crohn's disease (33). They also recovered pleomorphic organisms suggestive of cell-wall–deficient forms in 22 of 27 patients with Crohn's disease, 7 of 13 patients with ulcerative colitis, and 1 of 11 control subjects. These authors proposed that cell-wall–deficient forms of *M. kansasii* played a role in the etiopathogenesis of Crohn's disease; however, they never definitively identified the cell-wall–deficient forms as *M. kansasii*. Subsequently, other groups have attempted to culture mycobacteria from Crohn's disease and some have been successful, although the total number of isolates by any one investigator is small.

In 1984, Chiodini et al. raised a new wave of interest in a mycobacterial etiology for Crohn's disease when they cultured an unidentified mycobacterium from 2 of 11 patients (34). The isolates belonged to the Runyon group III, which includes the *Mycobacterium avium* complex, but most closely resembles *M. paratuberculosis*, the organism responsible for Johne's disease. The isolates were called strain *Linda* from the name of the patients from whom the cultures were derived. Mice that were inoculated intravenously or intraperitoneally with the organism developed noncaseating granulomas in the liver, spleen, and lymph nodes; however, no effects were seen in rabbits, chickens, rats, or guinea pigs. When the unidentified mycobacterium was inoculated into infant goats, the animals developed segmental granulomatous disease of the ileum, proximal small intestine, and regional lymph nodes (35). The organism could be recovered from the intestinal tissue of the infected animals, although acid-fast bacteria were detected in only half of the animals. The *Mycobacterium* sp. took up to 18 months to culture and was characterized by fastidious growth requirements and mycobactin dependence (34). Slow-growing spheroplastic forms of the organism were identified in 12 additional patients with Crohn's disease, but not in tissue from patients with ulcerative colitis or in control tissues (36). Some of these spheroplasts eventually transformed into the acid-fast *M. paratuberculosis*-like organism.

Since these reports were made, several other research groups have attempted to culture mycobacteria from Crohn's disease intestinal tissues. Graham et al. cultivated both rapid-and slow-growing mycobacteria from Crohn's disease, ulcerative colitis, and control tissues, but could find no relationship between the presence or the species of mycobacteria and Crohn's disease (37). They suggested that chronic inflammatory bowel disease might be the result of an abnormal host response to commensally occurring mycobacteria. The stringency of the culture conditions in this study has been questioned (38). Another group cultured, *M. paratuberculosis* similar to the organism isolated by Chiodini et al. from Crohn's disease tissue, but the organism failed to elicit an inflammatory response when inoculated into neonatal goats (39).

b. DNA Hybridization Studies. Given the great difficulty in culturing mycobacteria and the scant results obtained using classical microbiological approaches, the sophisticated methods of molecular biology have been invoked to search for mycobacteria. The techniques of DNA hybridization, restriction fragment length polymorphism (RFLP), genomic cloning, and polymerase chain reaction (PCR) have provided new powerful tools to investigate the presence of mycobacteria in Crohn's disease (40–43). Yoshimura et al. used DNA–DNA hybridization to specifically define the *M. paratuberculosis*-like strain (*Linda*) of Chiodini and colleagues (40). *Linda* was identified as a strain of *M. paratuberculosis*. Further hybridization studies detected strain *Linda* in some, but not all, Crohn's disease specimens studied. The authors commented that the inability to consistently detect specific DNA hybridizing sequences in all specimens could possibly reflect a limitation in the sensitivity of the techniques used. In other experiments, Butcher et al. failed to detect mycobacterial DNA in 17 specimens from Crohn's disease patients using Southern blotting (42). Their assay was estimated to be capable of detecting *M. paratuberculosis* at a level of one mycobacterial cell per 100 human cells.

In an effort to develop even more sensitive detection systems, McFadden et al. cloned the *M. paratuberculosis* genome and used RFLP to obtain probes capable of distinguishing between the closely related commensal mycobacterium, *M. avium* and the potentially pathogenic mycobacterium *M. paratuberculosis*. (41,44–47). They isolated a clone (pMB22) that contained a single copy of a mycobacterial insertion sequence, IS900, found in multiple copies in the genome of *M. paratuberculosis*, but not in *M. avium*. This probe was then used in hybridization studies to unambiguously match the mycobacteria isolated by Chiodini et al. with *M. paratuberculosis* (44). These authors have since identified *M. paratuberculosis* in 6 of 206 Crohn's disease specimens, but none from 63 ulcerative colitis or 43 control specimens (45). Using the IS900 insertion element and even more sensitive PCR techniques, *M. paratuberculosis* has been identified in 26 of 40 (65%) specimens of Crohn's disease tissue in one study (48). However, in a subsequent double-blind control study using PCR and the IS900 probe, only 4 of 31 Crohn's disease specimens were positive for *M. paratuberculosis* (49). In this investigation, Crohn's disease specimens containing granuloma were more likely to amplify *M. paratuberculosis* DNA than specimens without granuloma. This raises the possibility that only a specifically susceptible subset of Crohn's disease patients might have a mycobacterial etiology for their illness.

c. Immune Reactivity to Mycobacterial Antigens.   Even the most difficult to isolate or culture infectious agents invariably elicit a host immune response, and several investigators have used serologic and cellular markers to look for evidence of mycobacterial infection in Crohn's disease. Thayer et al. (50) used an enzyme-linked immunosorbent assay (ELISA) to link their *Mycobacterium* sp. isolate with Crohn's disease. Antibodies to the then unclassified mycobacteria cross-reacted with *M. paratuberculosis*, and an ELISA for *M. paratuberculosis* was positive in 23% of 56 patients with Crohn's disease; whereas, an ELISA in all 34 patients with ulcerative colitis was negative. Other laboratories have been unable to duplicate these findings using a variety of different *M. paratuberculosis* antigens (51–55). Stainsby et al. recently evaluated by ELISA eight mycobacterial preparations from Crohn's disease and control subjects (52). Although there was strong evidence of serologic response to environmental mycobacteria, especially *M. avium*, *M. tuberculosis*, and *M. kansasii*, there were no differences between Crohn's disease patients and control subjects including in their response to *M. paratuberculosis*. One-fourth of Crohn's disease patients did have IgG concentrations to *M. paratuberculosis* greater than two standard deviations above the control group, but this response was not specific and was also observed in 20% of celiac disease patients. Immunohistochemical examination of Crohn's disease tissue by one group did not detect any mycobacteria in 67 specimens from 20 patients (56).

In addition to studies of humoral immunity, an abnormal host response to mycobacterial antigens in Crohn's disease was sought by investigating specific cellular immunity to mycobacteria. Markesich et al. studied the in vitro interaction of peripheral blood monocytes with *M. paratuberculosis* to verify whether cells from patients with Crohn's disease reacted differently from those of controls (57). They found that the survival of

M. paratuberculosis in Crohn's disease monocytes was less than in control monocytes and that macrophages from patients with Crohn's disease inhibited mycobacterial growth more effectively than control macrophages. This response, however, was nonspecific and probably due to a generalized immune activation in Crohn's disease. Seldenrijk and colleagues investigated the T-cell mediated response of Crohn's disease, ulcerative colitis, and control peripheral lymphocytes to a variety of mycobacterial species using a macrophage inhibition assay (58). No significant difference in the prevalence of responders and non-responders was observed among the three groups. Other researchers looking at the cellular immune responses of isolated mesenteric lymph node mononuclear cells, also found no evidence of specific sensitization to mycobacteria in Crohn's disease (59).

d. *Antituberculous Therapy.* If Crohn's disease is the result of an active mycobacterial infection, then treatment specifically directed at the infecting organism should result in clinical improvement. Indeed, there are many case reports and small uncontrolled series of patients that have improved on antimycobacterial regimens (60–62). However, when carefully executed controlled trials were performed, results were less encouraging. Shaffer et al. treated 27 patients with Crohn's disease using ethambutol and rifampicin compared with placebo (63). In the group of 14 patients who completed the course of antibiotics, there was no difference between active drug treatment and placebo treatment with regard to the Crohn's Disease Activity Index (CDAI), need for surgery, number of relapses, or prednisolone or sulfasalazine dose. In 1992, Afdahl et al. randomized 49 patients to receive clofazimine plus steroids or placebo plus steroids (64). Again, there was no significant difference in response between the clofazimine-treated patients and the placebo group. Other researchers have found no benefit from triple therapy with isoniazid, rifampicin, and ethambutol compared with placebo (65). Recently, Prantera et al. conducted a randomized, double-blind, placebo-controlled trial using steroids and four drugs (ethambutol, rifampicin, clofazimine, and dapsone) in patients with Crohn's disease (66). Forty patients were enrolled and followed up for nine months. In three of 19 patients who completed the study and who received the drugs, relapse occurred during the treatment period (relapse being a recurring need for steroids); relapse occurred in 11 of 17 patients treated with placebo. This difference was statistically significant. Nine patients on placebo with persistent disease were crossed over to the four-drug treatment; of these, five achieved remission, two continued with active disease, and two were taken off of therapy because of drug side effects. There was no significant difference in the radiologic or endoscopic assessment of Crohn's disease between the two groups. The authors concluded that treatment with the four-drug regimen relieves symptoms in some patients with Crohn's disease (66). However, the study did not address the issue of whether the beneficial effects of therapy were related to specific antimycobacterial activity of the drugs or to generalized changes of the enteric flora.

Overall, the clinical and histologic similarity between Crohn's disease and intestinal tuberculosis, the relationship between Johne's disease and *M. paratuberculosis,* and the steady growth of scientific and clinical data linking Crohn's disease and infection with *M. paratuberculosis* make a persuasive argument for an etiological role of mycobacteria in Crohn's disease. However, despite extensive study, only a small portion of Crohn's disease cases can be associated with mycobacterial infection. Still, even if only a few cases are proved to be due to mycobacterial infection, what can be learned from studying such patients may be invaluable in advancing our understanding of Crohn's disease pathogenesis.

B. Viruses and Other Transmissible Agents

In illnesses of unknown etiology, like Crohn's disease, it is common for investigators to search for viruses as possible culprits. There is epidemiological evidence suggesting that perinatal viral infections are one of the strongest identifiable risk factors for the subsequent development of inflammatory bowel disease (67). Early investigations focused on well-defined viruses known to be associated with chronic infections. However, initial serologic studies of the herpes group of viruses did not support an association with Crohn's disease (68,69). Increased serum antibody titers to cytomegalovirus (CMV) was documented in patients with ulcerative colitis, but this was considered a secondary phenomenon (69,70).

In addition to these reports, a series of studies, using a variety of innovative approaches, sought to identify new or less common viruses. In 1970, Mitchell and Rees reported that granulomas could be induced in the foot pads of mice injected with homogenates of lymph node and intestinal tissue from Crohn's disease (71). These findings suggested that a small transmissible agent could be responsible for Crohn's disease and the search to identify a specific virus was underway. A few years later, Aronson et al. reported on the isolation of a small RNA agent from 16 of 24 patients with Crohn's disease using a modified cocultivation technique (72). The agent was cultured from both lymphoid and intestinal tissue and had characteristics of an enterovirus. Although it was isolated from Crohn's disease tissue, it could not be etiologically linked to the illness because it was also cultivated from 14 of 20 specimens with other gastrointestinal diseases. Using an original and sensitive rabbit ileum tissue culture system, Gitnick et al. cultured cytopathic agents from all of four Crohn's disease ileal specimens, but from none of the control specimens (73). The cytopathic effect of this agent could be passed repeatedly in chick and duck embryo cell cultures and was inhibited by low dilutions of serum from Crohn's disease patients. Electron microscopic evaluation of these agents revealed particles with an electron dense central core, spiculated coat, and 30-nm mean diameter (73). The physical, chemical, and electron microscopic qualities were consistent with the appearance of a picornavirus (73). Riemann was also able to demonstrate viruslike particles in 7 of 9 patients with Crohn's disease, and other researchers have isolated reoviruslike agents from gut homogenates of Crohn's disease tissue and found ultrastructural evidence of paramyxovirus (74–76).

Despite the potentially exciting results, several other investigators were unable to reproduce or confirm them. Dvorak et al. used electron microscopy to examine surgically resected specimens from 12 patients with Crohn's disease, but could not detect any viral particles after a careful search (31). Electron microscopic examination of Crohn's disease tissue by other groups did not provide evidence of a persistent retroviral infection (77,78). Phillpotts et al. examined fresh or frozen extracts of diseased intestine and lymph nodes from 16 patients with active Crohn's disease using eight different types of cell culture under a variety of conditions (79). Although a cytopathic effect similar to the one commonly seen with viral infection could be produced, no definitive virus could be isolated or clearly identified. Furthermore, the cytopathic effect was also induced by extracts from ulcerative colitis and acutely inflamed, noninflammatory bowel disease appendixes, an effect possibly due to toxic constituents of the homogenates (79). At least three other groups have looked at tissue-culture cytopathic effects using biopsy homogenates, fecal samples, or leukocyte-rich plasma from patients with Crohn's disease and failed to identify viruses (78,80,81).

A different approach to the search of transmissible agents in Crohn's disease was adopted by Das et al. who reported the induction of lymphomas in immunodeficient athymic mice injected with lymph node homogenates from Crohn's disease tissue (82). Using indirect immunofluorescence, these lymphomas showed cytoplasmic staining with most sera from Crohn's disease patients, but only occasionally with sera from ulcerative colitis patients and other control subjects. Subsequent studies demonstrated that the lymphoma could be passed through successive generations of mice, again supporting the existence of live, replicating particles (83). Although no agent could be identified, a virus was hypothesized to be the responsible agent. Later, this same group reported that sera from household contacts of patients with Crohn's disease, both blood relatives and spouses, also reacted with the Crohn's disease-induced murine lymphomas, providing further support for a factor that could be transmitted in a restricted environment (84). Further investigation suggested a cross-reacting antigen between Crohn's disease tissue and the murine lymphomas, and characterization of this antigen revealed two Crohn's disease tissue-specific glycoproteins (85,86). Whether these proteins are unique to Crohn's disease, represent byproducts of inflammatory tissue injury, or are remnants of an environmental agent remains unclear.

As in the case of *M. paratuberculosis*, in which investigators used molecular biological techniques to demonstrate the presence of specific DNA sequences in Crohn's disease, PCR methodology has also been applied to study viruses. Wakefield et al. have used the highly sensitive technique of nested PCR to search for herpesvirus DNA in the colon of patients with inflammatory bowel disease (87). In this study, primer pairs specific for CMV, human herpesvirus 6 (HHV6), varicella zoster virus, or Epstein-Barr virus (EBV) were used. Although there was a statistically significant association of ulcerative colitis with the simultaneous presence of HHV6, CMV, or EBV DNA, the same was not true for Crohn's disease (87). The same investigators have also reported on an intriguing series of studies linking the measles virus to Crohn's disease, which is discussed further under Miscellaneous Factors.

There is presently no evidence supporting a viral etiology for Crohn's disease. However, new methods of identifying and detecting viruses are constantly being devised; a few years ago, we could not detect the hepatitis C or the human immunodeficiency viruses. Clusters of Crohn's disease in time and place, such as the one reported by VanKruiningen et al. still suggest a live environmental agent as the culprit of the disease (88). Until the cause is found, viral infections remain an etiological possibility for Crohn's disease.

C. Yeast

Although a classical fungal infection has never been considered of primary etiological importance, several groups have recently proposed that *Saccharomyces cerevisiae* (baker's and brewer's yeast) may be important in Crohn's disease (89,90). McKenzie et al. found raised serum levels of IgG antibody to *S. cerevisiae* in patients with Crohn's disease, but not in patients with ulcerative colitis or control subjects (90). This was not simply a nonspecific finding, because the antibody response to *Candida albicans* did not differ significantly among the three groups. The authors raised the issue of whether hypersensitivity to common dietary antigens (e.g., yeast) was playing a role in the pathogenesis of Crohn's disease. Their serological study was supported by in vitro work showing an increased peripheral lymphocyte response to *S. cerevisiae* by isolated lymphocytes from patients with Crohn's disease (91). Another group evaluated the specificity of the response to *S. cerevisiae* by looking at the antibody response to multiple common dietary proteins in twins with inflammatory bowel disease (89). In twins discordant for inflammatory bowel disease, the one with Crohn's disease displayed higher IgG, IgA, and IgM responses to yeast cell-wall mannan and to whole yeast than the unaffected twin. In contrast, the response to gliadin, ovalbumin, and β-lactoglobulin was comparable between the healthy and affected twin. The researchers therefore argued that yeast cell-wall material may selectively activate the local and systemic immune system and be an etiological factor in Crohn's disease. Other researchers have suggested that the immune response to *S. cerevisiae* is characteristic of but not specific for Crohn's disease, because it can also be found in celiac disease (92).

III. ANIMAL MODELS

A detailed investigation of the intimate mechanisms of inflammation and tissue damage often requires methodological approaches, tissue samples, specific cell types, or other materials that are not readily obtained from patient sources. For this reason, the availability of a good animal model can be of paramount importance, allowing studies that cannot be performed in humans. For example, in experiments with autoimmune encephalomyelitis, mice are sensitized to myelin basic protein. The animals develop an illness that is remarkably similar to multiple sclerosis, a disease whose immunopathogenesis has benefitted considerably from this model. For many years, only few and rudimentary models of inflammatory bowel disease have been available, but during the last decade a large number of them have been developed (93–95). Tables 2 and 3 list a variety of agents and manipulations that can be used to induce inflammation in the bowel of several different species. Although most of them represent acute models and none closely resembles Crohn's disease or even ulcerative colitis, their study has permitted major advances in the pathophysiology of bowel inflammation (96). Some models potentially relevant to Crohn's disease are discussed in the following paragraphs to highlight specific aspects and stress their value to selected aspects of human disease.

A. Spontaneous Inflammation

Truly spontaneous forms of inflammatory bowel disease exist, but they tend to be rare. One example is the colitis that appears in the cotton-top tamarin (*Saguinus oedipus*), a

TABLE 2 Animal Models of Inflammatory Bowel Disease, Exogenous Induction

Irritants	Ethanol, acetic acid
Drugs	Nonsteroidal anti-inflammatory drugs
Immunologic	Immune complexes, trinitrobenzene sulfonic acid
Bacterial products	Peptidoglycan-polysaccharide
Feeding	Dextran sulfate
Nitric oxide–related	Peroxynitrite
Surgery	Infarction
	Ileopouchitis

Consult references 94 and 95 for details.

TABLE 3 Animal Models of Inflammatory Bowel Disease,
Endogenous Induction

Spontaneous	Cotton-top tamarin, C3H/HeJ Bir mouse
Clonal deletion	Cyclosporine A in neonatal mice
Cell reconstitution	CD45RB^{high}, CD4-positive T cells in SCID mice
Transgenic	HLA-B27 gene in rats
Gene targeting	IL-2, IL-10, TGF-β1, TCRαβ, Giα "knock out" mice

Consult references 94 and 95 for details.

South American monkey that develops diffuse and severe colonic inflammation complicated by carcinoma when kept in captivity for prolonged periods of time (97). Another type of spontaneous colitis has been created by continuous inbreeding of C3H/HeJ mice resulting in right sided colitis (98). Both models can be valuable to study inflammatory bowel disease, but they bear no resemblance to Crohn's disease.

B. Granulomatous Inflammation

Animals in which a granulomatous type of inflammatory bowel disease can be induced are particularly attractive as models, because granulomas are a salient feature of Crohn's disease. When mycobacterial antigens contained in live BCG and *Mycobacterium leprae* are injected directly into the bowel of guinea pigs, the animals develop a granulomatous inflammation in the colon and terminal ileum, a typical histological characteristic of Crohn's disease (99). This, however, represents a response to known infectious agents, which may or may not be the case in Crohn's disease. Thus, other types of granulomatous bowel inflammation independent of live agents might be more relevant and better recapitulate Crohn's disease pathogenesis. This has been achieved by Sartor et al., who induced a form of granulomatous enterocolitis by injecting the bowel of rats with streptococcal bacterial cell-wall fragments (24). Particularly attractive features of this model are a granulomatous inflammatory response that can be systemic and the display of acute and chronic phases. The latter occurrence is highly suggestive of a local immune sensitization that may be responsible for recurrence of inflammation as observed in humans. Another important feature of the bacterial cell-wall injection model is that the severity of inflammation is strain-dependent, recalling the widely diverse clinical manifestations seen in patients with Crohn's disease (100).

C. Genetic and Immune Manipulation

Novel approaches to the development of inflammatory bowel disease animal models take advantage of advances in molecular biological and genetic manipulations (101). Transfection of the human HLA-B27 and β2-microglobulin in rats induces generalized inflammation in multiple organs, including the small and large bowel (102). This is reminiscent of possible effects of primarily systemic disease with secondary bowel involvement. Reconstitution of SCID (severe combined immunodeficiency) mice with naive (CD45RB^{high} CD4$^+$) but not mature T cells results in a severe form of colitis, an excellent example of how imbalances of distinctive immune cell subpopulations powerfully control inflammatory responses (103). Similarly, abnormalities of several immunoregulatory molecules can also lead to inflammation, as seen in mice mutant for the T-cell receptor (TCR) α chain, TCR β chain, TCR β × δ chains, and class II major histocompatibility, all of which develop chronic colitis (104). Finally, mice in which cytokine genes have been selectively targeted and rendered functionally deficient for production of interleukin (IL)-2 and IL-10 unexpectedly develop colitis and colitis plus enteritis, respectively (21,22). All the above models, although disparate as far as pathogenic mechanisms, share in common some type of bowel inflammation that results from various forms of altered immune reactivity, a phenomenon likely to be of central importance in Crohn's disease.

D. Additional Models

Feeding of selected substances may cause inflammatory bowel disease, as seen in Swiss-Webster mice receiving oral administration of dextran sulfate sodium (105). The animals develop an acute and chronic form of colitis in which an initial insult at the epithelial cell level is postulated to induce secondary changes leading to inflammation. Antigen-specific immune responses can also cause an inflammatory bowel disease–like picture. Mice subjected to graft-versus-host disease develop florid gut lesions secondary to local immune-mediated injury (106). These lesions can be almost entirely prevented by treatment with antibodies to tumor necrosis factor α (TNF-α), emphasizing the importance of immunomodulation in the development and treatment of intestinal inflammation. Evidence exists for the protective function of extrinsic sensory neurons in a rabbit model of formalin–immune complex–induced colitis, because capsaicin pretreatment induces worsening of inflammation accompanied by loss of immunoreactive substance P and calcitonin gene-related peptide (107). This model highlights how specific pathogenic events, such as neuropeptide-mediated stress responses, might also be relevant to gut inflammation.

IV. IMMUNOLOGIC FACTORS

Alterations of the immune system are frequently involved in diseases manifested by chronic inflammation, especially when a specific cause is not obvious or an etiological agent has yet to be identified. This is certainly the case in Crohn's disease, wherein continuous research has failed to discover the exact factors responsible for the disease. Despite whether such factors exist, there is overwhelming evidence pointing to immune abnormalities as an intrinsic component of the mechanisms of inflammation and tissue injury. An in-depth review of immunological factors potentially implicated in Crohn's disease is discussed in several reviews (108–112). This section discusses selected cellular, soluble, and other immune components, emphasizing findings derived from the mucosal immune system and those most recently implicated in the pathogenesis of inflammatory bowel disease in general and in Crohn's disease in particular.

A. Cellular Components

1. Immune Cells

Any acute or chronic inflammatory response is mediated by the specific and nonspecific activation of a variety of leukocytes that either circulate systematically or accumulate preferentially at the site of injury. Thus, the evaluation of the type and number of T cells, B cells, macrophages, eosinophils, mast cells, and other cells in the peripheral blood or the intestinal mucosa of Crohn's disease patients holds the potential for yielding information on the type of immune response elicited by the disease process and indirectly generates clues to its pathogenesis. This approach has yielded results that have been less informative than hoped for.

a. Peripheral Blood. Studies of T- and B-cell numbers in the peripheral blood of Crohn's disease patients have not shown any major or consistent alterations in the relative proportions of these two cell populations (113,114). A trend toward a decrease in the number of T cells and increase of B cells has been reported by some investigators, but usually only in subjects with clinically active disease, suggesting that these changes represent secondary events (115,116). Evidence of an enhanced state of T-cell activation was documented by a significant increase of cells expressing cell surface activation markers, such as 4F2 and 5E9 (116). Raedler et al. found a strong positive correlation between the number of circulating T cells displaying the T9 (transferrin receptor) marker as an indicator of enhanced immune activation and the degree of clinical activity, as measure by the CDAI (117). In this study, as Crohn's disease patients improved clinically using standard anti-inflammatory therapy, the number of activated T-cells in their blood decreased proportionally. Furthermore, the same authors found that the number of activated T cells in the circulation correlated significantly with those infiltrating the gut (118). These results point out that a cause-and-effect relationship may exist between immune system stimulation and clinical manifestations and that assessment of activated immune cells may be used as an indicator of disease activity or degree of bowel inflammation.

b. Intestinal Mucosa. During the last decade, most studies regarding immunological factors in Crohn's disease have been focused on the mononuclear cells forming the inflammatory infiltrate present in actively diseased bowel (119). Although the absolute number of lymphocytes is increased in a manner roughly proportional to the local degree of inflammation, the relative proportions of some of the infiltrating cells, such as T-cell subsets, are not dramatically different from those present in the normal intestinal mucosa (120,121). Other cell types, on the contrary, are altered in both number and type. The most dramatic example is a decrease in the normally predominant IgA plasma cells accompanied by a striking increase in the relative proportion of IgG immunocytes that usually make up no more than 5% of local plasma cells (122). Expectedly, the state of activation of the mucosal cells is also substantially enhanced, as reflected by an increase in the percentage of cells expressing cell surface activation markers such as CD25 (IL-2Rα), transferrin receptor (T9), 4F2, and others or high levels of immune activation genes (123–125).

T cells.   T lymphocytes, key mediators of cellular immunity, have received special attention because of their dominant regulatory function in normal mucosal immunity and importance in gastrointestinal disease (126,127). Many of the morphological and destructive changes observed in the inflamed human gut, including Crohn's disease, can be mediated through activation of mucosal T cells, strongly suggesting that cell-mediated events play a critical role in inflammatory tissue damage (128,129). What remains undetermined is the direct cause of mucosal T-cell activation in Crohn's disease. Possible candidates are specific antigens of dietary and bacterial origin, bacterial superantigens, and nonspecific stimuli secondary to local inflammation (130,131).

In an attempt to better define the types of T cells involved in intestinal inflammation, detailed analyses of their TCR's were carried out. In the normal human gut mucosa, T cells expressing the TCR αβ are far more numerous than those expressing the TCR γδ both in the intraepithelial and lamina propria compartments. In Crohn's disease, the increase in T cells during active inflammation is almost entirely due to TCR αβ-positive cells, but differences exist in the relative changes of intraepithelial and lamina propria TCR γδ-positive cells (132,133). Compared with that of control subjects, the ratio of colonic TCR γδ-positive intraepithelial lymphocytes to CD3-positive cells is decreased in Crohn's disease and ulcerative colitis patients, particularly in the lamina propria of ileal Crohn's disease, suggesting unique changes in each type of inflammatory bowel disease. Using a series of monoclonal antibodies recognizing different variable (V) regions of the TCR β chain, Posnett et al. detected increased numbers of Vβ8-positive T lymphocytes in cell isolates of mesenteric lymph nodes of a subset of Crohn's disease patients (134). A similar enrichment was not present among the intraepithelial or lamina propria T cells. In contrast, an immunohistochemical study comparing normal, Crohn's disease, and celiac disease mucosal T cells failed to detect any difference in TCR Vβ usage (135). A recent flow cytometric analysis comparing the TCR Vβ repertoire between peripheral blood and lamina propria CD4- and CD8-positive T lymphocytes found alterations in the lamina propria repertoire of Crohn's disease but not in the control or ulcerative colitis mucosa (136). The same group of investigators also reported no differences in the TCR Vβ repertoire between monozygotic twins discordant for Crohn's disease using a sensitive quantitative PCR methodology (137). Taken together, these studies still support the concept that T cells are important to the mechanism of Crohn's disease, but the crucial question of whether pathogenic T cells are stimulated and respond to disease-specific antigens remains to be answered.

B cells. The previously mentioned increase in IgG plasma cells probably is not a random event due to the nonspecific effect of mucosal inflammation. In fact, the subclass distribution of IgG-producing cells is quite different between Crohn's disease and ulcerative colitis. In the latter condition, IgG1 immunocytes are disproportionately increased in comparison with those secreting other IgG subclasses, whereas, in Crohn's disease, IgG2 plasma cells predominate (138). The exact reason for this discrepancy is not apparent, but it suggests that local immunoregulation, inciting antigens, or cells recruited to the inflammatory sites differ in the two forms of inflammatory bowel disease. In one recent study analyzing the state of differentiation of CD19-positive B cells in the blood and gut of Crohn's disease patients, an unexpectedly high proportion of the CD45RO phenotype was found, reflecting an enhanced state of B-cell stimulation (139). This finding was supported by the additional observation that patients with a high CDAI tended to have elevated numbers of CD45RO-positive B cells, suggesting a relationship between degree of disease activity and stimulation of humoral immunity. To explore this possibility, the same investigators correlated the expression of the CD45RO marker on circulating CD19-positive B cells with intestinal lactulose and mannitol permeability in Crohn's disease patients and their healthy first-degree relatives (140). They found that the fraction of the CD45RO isoform was significantly increased not only in the patients but also in normal relatives who had an increased intestinal permeability. These findings are provocative and point to heightened antigen absorption through an exceedingly leaky mucosal barrier leading to enhancement of systemic immunity reflected by high numbers of mature B cells. Whether increased intestinal permeability is primary or secondary is not resolved by these observations, but they reinforce the close link between the immune system and the pathogenesis of Crohn's disease.

Other cells. In addition to T and B cells that are numerically predominant in both the blood and the mucosa of normal and Crohn's disease subjects, several other types of immunocytes are found, including monocytes, macrophages, eosinophils, mast cells, and basophils. During inflammation, such cells are expected to express an enhanced proportion of activation markers suggestive of their involvement in the inflammatory response. However, phenotypic analysis of cell surface markers does not appear to be a particularly sensitive indicator of the immune status of these cells.

Peripheral blood monocytes of Crohn's disease patients express the same percentage of major histocompatibility complex (MHC) class II antigens (HLA-DR and DQ) found in control and ulcerative colitis patients (141). In Crohn's disease–involved gut mucosa, a high proportion of CD68-, LI-positive macrophages can be detected by immuno-fluorescence, suggesting recent recruitment from peripheral blood monocytes, but again without any significant differences from ulcerative colitis (142). More subtle differences can be detected by exploring monocyte function. For instance, Crohn's disease blood monocytes are primed for accentuated release of toxic oxygen metabolites after in vitro stimulation (143,144). This, however, is not unique to Crohn's disease; the same phenomenon is seen in other inflammatory conditions. Thus, monocytes/macrophages do not display any unique abnormality in Crohn's disease, and they may be nonspecific contributors to the immune reactivity accompanying chronic inflammatory conditions.

Additional evidence of immune activation in Crohn's disease is provided by studies measuring mast cell responses. Jejunal secretions of patients with active Crohn's disease contain significantly enhanced concentrations of histamine compared with those found in patients with inactive disease and controls (145). Whereas this most likely reflects a nonspecific phenomenon, there is some evidence that antigen-specific responses may contribute to mast cell activation in Crohn's disease. Augmented histamine release is observed in culture supernatants of human mucosal mast cell suspension stimulated by gut epithelial proteins such as epithelial cell–associated components (ECAC) (146). Similar results were also seen with mast cells from ulcerative colitis mucosa.

2. Nonimmune Cells

a. Epithelium. A possible involvement of enterocytes and colonocytes in intestinal immunity and inflammation was initially suggested by early reports of an abnormally high expression of class II (HLA-DR) antigens by inflamed intestinal mucosa (147). This was confirmed by subsequent studies showing that epithelial cells can actually function as atypical antigen-presenting cells, an activity critical to mucosal immune homeostasis (148). Epithelial cells from normal mucosa preferentially activate CD8-positive suppressor T cells rather than CD4-positive helper T cells as classical antigen-presenting cells (macrophages and dendritic cells) do. This is important for two reasons: first, it indicates that intestinal immune responses are geared toward local suppression of a possibly excessive reactivity induced by dietary or enteric antigens; second, this capacity is lost in inflammatory bowel disease, because gut epithelial cells preferentially activate CD4-positive helper T cells, thus favoring an undesirable or prolonged immune stimulation that might contribute to chronic inflammatory reaction (149). In regard to the latter observation, no functional differences were detected between Crohn's disease or ulcerative colitis, and both generally express similar levels of HLA-DR antigens in similarly inflamed tissues. However, an anomalous expression of HLA-DR antigens in Crohn's disease has been reported by one group of investigators examining the epithelium surrounding colonic lymphoid nodules in Crohn's disease (150). This group claimed that the degree of expression was significantly higher and stronger in Crohn's disease–involved areas compared with inflammatory and noninflammatory control areas. Such an increase, however, is probably secondary to local immune reactivity, because aberrant expression of class II antigens is also encountered on nerve, endothelial, and vascular muscle cells in association with infiltrating T cells in small bowel Crohn's disease (151).

b. Fibroblasts and Muscle Cells. It is becoming increasingly recognized that the chronicity of the leukocytic infiltrate in the mucosa of inflammatory bowel disease patients results from complex interactions between the immune cells described above with other structural components in the surrounding microenvironment. Such "structural cells" of mesenchymal origin play an active role in inflammation and exert many activities that, until recently, were thought to be the exclusive domain of classical immune cells. This concept has already been proven and accepted in other types of chronic inflammation (152). The participation of fibroblasts and muscle cells is particularly evident in Crohn's disease, in that their activation and secretion are largely responsible for stricture formation (153). Muscularis propria cells from Crohn's disease–strictured intestine produce increased amounts of collagen, as do fibroblasts from the same location (154,155). Although increased collagen formation is also a feature of ulcerative colitis, expression of procollagen genes is more abundant, more diffuse, and deeper in the intestinal layers in Crohn's disease than in ulcerative colitis (156). These differences are more likely to depend on the type and distribution of the inflammatory infiltrates surrounding mucosal mesenchymal cells than on an intrinsically abnormal capacity for collagen formation in the various types of gut inflammation (157).

B. Soluble Mediators

Among the many immunological factors implicated in the pathogenesis of Crohn's disease, none has attracted more attention nor been investigated to a greater extent than the soluble mediators of immunity. These include a large number of molecules released by activated immune cells (e.g., T cells, B cells, macrophages) as well as nonimmune cells (e.g., epithelial, endothelial, muscle and nerve cells, fibroblasts). In this section, the definition of soluble mediators includes not only immunocyte-derived cytokines but also eicosanoids (prostanoids and leukotrienes), neuropeptides, and reactive oxygen metabolites. All together, these molecules display a broad spectrum of activities and influence all aspects of systemic and local immunity. Although this is one of the main reasons for being so important, the number and multiple and overlapping functions of these substances make their evaluation difficult. In addition, confusing or contradictory results are often observed, largely due to diverse experimental conditions.

Despite these pitfalls, there is general agreement that abnormalities found in all forms of intestinal inflammation are largely mediated by cytokines or are direct manifestations of abnormal cytokine production or function. In addition, cytokines are implicated not only in the mechanism of inflammatory bowel disease but also in intestinal immunoregulation, clinical manifestations, differential diagnosis, and potential therapies. In-depth examination of this topic can be found in several excellent reviews (158–163). Most of the following discussion on the role of soluble mediators in Crohn's disease is on selected cytokines (lymphocyte- and monocyte/macrophage-derived; i.e., lymphokines and monokines, respectively). Due to the extensive and complex nature of the subject, comments are focused on Crohn's disease–related findings and differences from other types of intestinal inflammation. Cytokines are divided into two main categories, immunoregulatory and proinflammatory: the former are preferentially produced by T lymphocytes and exert an immunomodulatory function, whereas the latter are the predominant products of monocytes/macrophages and are more directly responsible for tissue injury.

1. Immunoregulatory Cytokines

a. Interleukin-2 and Soluble Interleukin-2 Receptor. Interleukin-2 is a prototypical immunoregulatory cytokine produced by T lymphocytes. Being secreted in small quantities, it is not usually detectable in the circulation of patients with Crohn's disease, but it can be readily measured in vitro in cultures of activated intestinal mucosal mononuclear cells. Using the latter approach, the production of IL-2 was initially found to be decreased in Crohn's disease (as well as in ulcerative colitis) compared with control subjects (164,165). In addition, the response of lamina propria mononuclear cells (LPMC) to IL-2 was found to be markedly different between Crohn's disease and ulcerative colitis cells. When IL-2 was used to induce cytotoxicity, Crohn's disease cells exhibited an enhanced response as evidenced by a significantly greater degree of killing than that of control LPMC, whereas ulcerative colitis cells showed a markedly decreased response under the same experimental conditions (166). This dichotomy in IL-2 responsiveness between Crohn's disease and ulcerative colitis was confirmed in a study of IL-2 production in a pediatric population (167). These data suggest that, despite similar clinical manifestations, the two forms of inflammatory bowel disease have diverse or even opposite immune mechanisms: in Crohn's disease, T-cell–mediated responses may be excessive and, in ulcerative colitis, abnormally low.

In addition to measuring production and release of the IL-2 protein, studies have evaluated the quantity of mRNA (messenger RNA) in endoscopic biopsy samples of whole mucosa and extracts of cultured LPMC. The results of these studies have been inconsistent, in that the relative amounts of IL-2 mRNA were higher than control in the biopsy-based studies but lower than control when cultured cells were evaluated (125,168). However, both reports agreed that IL-2 mRNA is less abundant in ulcerative colitis regardless of the tissue source, further supporting the existence of major differences in the role of this cytokine in the pathogenesis of Crohn's disease versus ulcerative colitis. Finally, additional reports demonstrate the involvement of IL-2 in Crohn's disease. James makes a strong point for a key role of this mediator in Crohn's disease in a case report of a patient who entered complete clinical remission when he developed CD4-positive T-cell (the cell responsible for most IL-2 production) lymphocytopenia secondary to advanced acquired immunodeficiency syndrome (AIDS) (169). In contrast, another case report describes patients with Crohn's disease in remission who become symptomatic while receiving IL-2 as an adjuvant chemotherapeutic agent for renal cell carcinoma (170).

A component of the IL-2 receptor on the surface of activated T cells, B cells, and macrophages can be released, diffuse into interstitial fluids, and circulate systemically. This component, named soluble IL-2 receptor (sIL-2R), can be measured and used as an index of T-cell stimulation, thus providing an indirect assessment of immune activation in patients with inflammatory, autoimmune, and neoplastic diseases (171). In Crohn's disease patients, levels of sIL-2R are significantly elevated in the serum and supernatants of stimulated peripheral blood mononuclear cells (172). Such levels generally correlate with the degree of clinical activity and decrease significantly when patients receive drugs that suppress T cells, such as cyclosporine A (173,174). These findings have led to the suggestion that monitoring sIL-2R levels in Crohn's disease could be a reliable way to assess severity of disease. Unfortunately, this does not appear to be a very sensitive method, because the association of plasma levels or spontaneous sIL-2R production by LPMC with the degree of intestinal inflammation is weak and there is a wide overlap with control values (175).

b. Interferon. Interferon (IFN) represents a large family of related molecules with antiviral and immunomodulatory functions. Interferon-α and -β display mainly antiviral activity, whereas IFN-γ is a potent regulator of cellular and humoral immunity. Various investigators have measured IFN in the circulation of patients with Crohn's disease, but concentrations tend to be low or absent, generating inconsistent and contradictory results (176). The first report on the production of IFN-γ by in vitro activated LPMC found this cytokine to be decreased in Crohn's disease and ulcerative colitis culture supernatants (177). However, subsequent studies using different experimental conditions arrived at different conclusions. One study detected spontaneous release of IFN-γ by intestinal LPMC in Crohn's disease, and, in another, the activity of IFN-α was also enhanced in the same cells (178,179). In agreement with these findings, Northern blot analysis or dot blot hybridization detects mRNA for both IFN-γ and IFN-α more abundantly and frequently in Crohn's disease than ulcerative colitis or control intestinal cells (180,181).

c. Interleukin-4 and Interleukin-10. Among cytokines, immunoregulatory properties are not limited to IL-2 and IFN-γ but there is little information about other factors with similar modulatory properties in Crohn's disease or inflammatory bowel disease in general. Schreiber et al. have recently published two studies on the function of IL-4 and IL-10 with possible functional implications (182,183). This group of investigators reported that inflammatory bowel disease peripheral blood and intestinal mucosa mononuclear cells are relatively resistant to the immunosuppressive activity of IL-4 in vitro, showing that downregulation of IL-1β or TNF-α and up regulation of IL-1 receptor antagonist (IL-1ra) production by these cells is not inhibited by IL-4 as much as disease specificity or control cells are (182). Generally comparable results were observed in regard to IL-10 down regulatory function on the same cells (183). In both studies, no obvious differences were noticed between the response of Crohn's disease and ulcerative colitis cells to either IL-4 or IL-10. These data are relevant when considered in the light of the previously discussed response to IL-2; this cytokine induces a differential reactivity between Crohn's disease and ulcerative colitis cells, but other modulatory cytokines apparently do not, indicating that distinctive rather than generalized defects of immunoregulation are present in each form of inflammatory bowel disease.

2. Proinflammatory Cytokines

a. Interleukin-1 and Interleukin-1 Receptor Antagonist. Interleukin-1 is probably the most potent of the proinflammatory cytokines and its systemic or localized elevation is synonymous with acute or chronic inflammation in a variety of disease states. In Crohn's disease, circulating levels of IL-1 are found only in a minority of patients with active disease, but some of these patients' circulating cells can release measurable amounts of this cytokine under unstimulated culture conditions (184,185). In contrast, IL-1 is consistently detected in large quantities in supernatants of mucosal biopsy organ cultures or isolated LPMC from Crohn's disease and ulcerative colitis patients (186,187). Within the inflamed intestinal mucosa, both forms of IL-1, IL-β and IL-1α, are produced, and their source of protein, immunoreactivity, and bioactivity is restricted to the local mononuclear cells (188). Although IL-1 is elevated in both forms of inflammatory bowel disease and values overlap broadly, all reports agree that higher concentrations are found in ulcerative colitis than in Crohn's disease. Enhanced IL-1 production in the gut is not exclusive of either form of inflammatory bowel disease, and enhanced tissue levels are found in other forms of local inflammation, including ileal pouchitis and infectious diseases (189,190).

A novel concept that has recently emerged from the study of cytokines in general, and of proinflammatory cytokines in particular, is that of the balance between proinflammatory and anti-inflammatory activities. The best example of this key concept is offered by IL-1 and its natural antagonist, the IL-1ra (191). The IL-1ra is a cytokine structurally similar to both forms of IL-1 that binds to the same receptors used by IL-1β and IL-1α, but receptor occupation by IL-1ra fails to trigger a cascade of immune or inflammatory events. Normally, the body produces substantially larger amounts of IL-1ra than IL-1, so that the balance between the two is physiologically tilted toward an anti-inflammatory state (192). Therefore, an excessive production of IL-1 not accompanied by a parallel increase of its natural antagonist could turn the balance in the opposite direction and eventually result in inflammation. This has been shown in other chronic inflammatory states and has recently been reported in inflammatory bowel disease (190,193). In both Crohn's disease and ulcerative colitis, the ratio of IL-1ra to IL-1 production by LPMC or mucosal biopsy cells is significantly reduced when compared with the ratio found in control mucosa. Furthermore, the ratio is normal in tissues involved by spontaneously resolving inflammatory processes such as infections. This suggests that the relative impairment of IL-1ra production may be a mechanism predisposing the patient to chronicity of gut inflammation, a hypothesis that is potentially important for Crohn's disease pathogenesis as well as treatment.

Further information relevant to the IL-1ra/IL-1 balance relates to the concept of genetic polymorphism, that is, the ability of any individual to produce different amounts of agonist or antagonist products. Depending on the frequency of use of each genetic allele involved in the production of a given substance, more or less of a particular product is generated, with obvious implications on its ultimate biological effects. A recent study has shown that allele 2 of the IL-1ra gene is significantly overrepresented in ulcerative colitis patients and is associated with more extensive or severe colitis (194). This is not the case in Crohn's disease, again demonstrating significant differences between the two diseases in regard to their genetic makeup or modulatory elements. This is important because it may help explain not only differences between Crohn's disease and ulcerative colitis but also why some individuals with inflammatory bowel disease have a clinically serious or recurrent disease while others only have mild disease. Studies in animal models support this hypothesis (100). Lewis rats, which are prone to severe and chronic colitis, have higher IL-1 and IL-1ra tissue levels than Fisher or Buffalo rats, which are more resistant to colitis and do not develop chronic inflammation.

b. Interleukin-6. Interleukin-6 is a cytokine produced by a large variety of cell types, and it shares many of the same functional activities with IL-1 and TNF-α, hence its discussion under the proinflammatory grouping. In contrast to IL-1, IL-6 is easily measurable in the peripheral blood of Crohn's disease and ulcerative colitis patients, in whom differentially expressed amounts can be displayed. Two studies investigating adult subjects initially reported high circulating concentrations of IL-6 in active Crohn's disease but not in ulcerative colitis (195,196). This was later confirmed in a pediatric population, in whom colonic Crohn's disease had higher serum IL-6 levels than disease limited to the small bowel, and worsening clinical severity was accompanied by increasing concentrations of IL-6 (197). An additional study, however, arrived at different results, detecting similarly elevated IL-6 serum levels in both Crohn's disease and ulcerative colitis patients compared with control subjects (198). All these data are important because they indicate that systemic levels of certain cytokines, namely IL-6, could be useful as markers of clinical activity or even help in the differential diagnosis of Crohn's disease versus ulcerative colitis.

However, this suggestion must be interpreted with care, because subsequent investigations of IL-6 levels in the intestinal mucosa failed to find changes comparable to those observed in the periphery. In these studies, IL-6 protein and mRNA levels were measured in biopsy extracts and organ cultures as well as in whole or purified subpopulations of mucosal cells (199–200). In all reports, IL-6 was elevated in inflammatory bowel disease, but in no case was a significantly different concentration observed between Crohn's disease and ulcerative colitis. Thus, systemic cytokine measurement apparently does not closely reflect cytokine activity at the site of active disease. This is a fundamental concept because it strongly suggests that an understanding of the pathogenesis of Crohn's disease or ulcerative colitis requires the direct examination of events as they occur in the involved gut.

c. *Interleukin-8.* Interleukin-8 is a potent neutrophil chemoattractant produced mostly by monocytes/macrophages in addition to neutrophils, endothelial and epithelial cells, fibroblasts, and hepatocytes. Because of its ability to recruit neutrophils, IL-8 is relevant to a variety of inflammatory processes. As in the case of IL-6, the first report that measured IL-8 levels in the circulation and the mucosa of inflammatory bowel disease patients suggested a differential pattern of expression. Compared with plasma of control subjects, significantly elevated levels of IL-8 antibodies were noticed in plasma of ulcerative colitis but not in Crohn's disease patients, with similar results in mucosal tissue homogenates (203). However, subsequent studies found considerably, but equally, elevated levels of IL-8 protein in both Crohn's disease and ulcerative colitis biopsy material (204–206). When mRNA levels were investigated, those of IL-8 and the related monocyte-chemoattractant protein-1 (MCP-1) were also enhanced in both Crohn's disease and ulcerative colitis (207,208). Again, this underscores the importance of measuring local as well as systemic cytokine concentrations to obtain a realistic assessment of mechanisms of cytokine-mediated responses in Crohn's disease.

d. *Tumor Necrosis Factor-α.* Tumor necrosis factor-α is another cytokine with potent proinflammatory activity similar to that of IL-1 and IL-6, but, in addition, it displays some direct cytotoxic potential that may be relevant to tissue damage in conditions such as bowel inflammation. Serum concentrations of TNF-α were initially reported to be elevated in children with Crohn's disease and ulcerative colitis in one study, but not in another, when compared with a control pediatric population (209,210). The investigators who reported elevated serum levels also claimed that TNF-α could be detected in large quantities in the stools of patients with active inflammatory bowel disease and that they could serve as markers of intestinal inflammation (211). By immunohistochemical staining, the number of TNF-α–positive cells in the involved mucosa is significantly elevated, with a diffuse distribution in the lamina propria in Crohn's disease; whereas, in ulcerative colitis, TNF-α–positive cells are present mostly in the subepithelial space (212,213). In studies of cells isolated from the inflamed mucosa of children, TNF-α–secreting cells were more abundant in Crohn's disease patients than in ulcerative colitis patients (214,215). In additional investigations, TNF-α protein production and mRNA levels were comparably elevated in Crohn's disease and ulcerative colitis patients (200,201), except in one report in which TNF-α mRNA did not significantly vary between control and inflammatory bowel disease specimens (199–201).

2. Eicosanoids

Eicosanoids represent products of the metabolism of arachidonic acid through the activity of the enzyme phospholipase A2 on membrane phospholipids (216). There are two major pathways of arachidonic acid metabolism: one is mediated by cyclooxygenase and results in formation of prostaglandins and thromboxanes; the other is mediated by neutrophil lipoxygenase, leading to the formation of leukotrienes. Because elevation of prostaglandins, thromboxanes, and leukotrienes is almost invariably associated with inflammatory responses, these substances have received considerable attention as possible mediators of inflammatory bowel disease (217). Initially, because marked elevation of prostaglandin E_2 and leukotriene B_4 was reported in active ulcerative colitis tissue, the involvement of these mediators was considered less important in Crohn's disease (218,219). However, even though the in vivo greatest elevations of prostaglandin E_2, thromboxane E_2, and leukotriene B_4 occur in active ulcerative colitis, increased synthesis and secretion of eicosanoids are found in all types of gut inflammation, including Crohn's disease (220). Crohn's disease patients have an elevated synthesis of eicosanoids even in the absence of clinical activity as shown by the abnormal release of leukotriene C_4 in rectal mucosal biopsy samples from patients with quiescent disease and in perfusates of unaffected jejunal segments (221,222). This is also true for proinflammatory cytokines and points to an abnormally high baseline of intestinal immune activation in Crohn's disease (223). Downregulation of eicosanoid production by the administration of omega fatty acids such as those contained in fish oil has been tried with moderate success in ulcerative colitis (224). Because eicosanoid modulation may also be a factor contributing to the pathogenesis of Crohn's disease, supplementation with fish oil may have a place in this condition.

3. Neuropeptides

Neuropeptides are substances released by nerve cells and include a variety of molecules (e.g., substance P, vasoactive intestinal peptide, somatostatin) exerting a broad range of functions. Two reasons justify the inclusion of neuropeptides in a discussion on Crohn's disease pathogenesis: first, a close functional interaction exists between the immune and neuroendocrine systems, each modulating the other during physiological and pathological conditions; second, neuropeptides are key mediators of the stress response modulating inflammatory diseases such as rheumatoid arthritis, systemic lupus erythematosus, and probably inflammatory bowel disease (225–227). Some patients suffering from Crohn's disease are susceptible to stressful life events, and these not infrequently accompany clinical disease flares. The explanation for these observations is unclear, but mounting evidence suggests that the modulation of immune cells and functions by neuropeptides plays an important role as a complementary function (228).

Several abnormalities of neuropeptide level and distribution have been described in Crohn's disease. Peripheral blood mononuclear leukocytes from patients with Crohn's disease contain about half the amount of β-endorphin as that found in the cells of healthy control subjects, ulcerative colitis patients, and in other inflammatory and infectious disorders (229). Furthermore, an inverse relationship between leukocyte β-endorphin concentrations and various parameters of inflammatory activity was detected, suggesting a functional relationship of the neuropeptide with clinical activity. Even more compelling is the finding of major abnormalities of vasoactive intestinal peptides, substance P, and somatostatin or their receptors in the intestine of patients with inflammatory bowel disease (230–233). Data are controversial regarding the concentration of specific neuropeptides in Crohn's disease and ulcerative colitis and at present it is impossible to accurately speculate on the potential role of any specific peptides in inflammatory bowel disease (234,235).

4. Reactive Oxygen Metabolites

Whatever the etiology of Crohn's disease might be and regardless of whatever immune events are involved in its mechanism, it is likely that the ultimate pathway to tissue damage is mediated by nonspecific factors. Among these, nonspecific effector cells, including macrophages and neutrophils, and their secretory products, such as reactive oxygen metabolites, are indicated by substantial evidence (236). Such evidence is found at the systemic as well as the tissue level. In a study in which phorbol ester was used to stimulate circulating monocyte and polymorphonuclear leukocyte production of active oxygen species in vitro, peak chemiluminescence was significantly higher with active Crohn's disease than with control cells (143). In contrast, two other reports found an impaired respiratory burst and superoxide production by neutrophils from Crohn's disease patients with active or inactive disease (237,238). The reasons for this difference are not apparent but all results confirm the existence of important abnormalities of oxygen metabolism in Crohn's disease leukocytes. Most likely, such abnormalities are secondary to bowel inflammation leading to an altered intestinal barrier, allowing the massive uptake and systemic circulation of proinflammatory products such as bacterial peptide formyl-methionyl-leucylphenylalanine and lipopolysaccharide (144,239). In the inflamed bowel, chemiluminescence assays also show a significantly enhanced production of neutrophil- and macrophage-derived oxidants, directly implicating these toxic molecules in local tissue destruction (240). These findings are not restricted to Crohn's disease, and elevated levels of free-oxygen radicals are also found in ulcerative colitis. Polymorphonuclear leukocyte–dependent free-radical mediated inflammation and tissue damage are eminently nonspecific events. Excessive neutrophil function is amenable to modulation and can be used for therapy of inflammatory bowel disease (241). Preliminary results with superoxide dismutase have shown promising results in Crohn's disease (242).

C. Autoimmunity

Autoimmunity is traditionally defined as the specific sensitization of immune cells to the body's own components, resulting in injury and, eventually, clinical manifestations. For decades, investigators have speculated on whether inflammatory bowel disease might be a true autoimmune disease (243), and a number of abnormalities classically thought to be autoimmune in origin have been associated with Crohn's disease. An early theory proposed that intestinal inflammation occurs as a consequence of epithelial injury caused by an autoimmune reaction to a colonic epithelial antigen (244). The increased mucosal permeability and sensitization to luminal antigens caused by an antibody- or lymphocyte-mediated attack could then lead to bacterial or food antigens amplifying and perpetuating the inflammatory process.

In the late 1950s and early 1960s, initial search for evidence of autoimmune phenomena led a group of Swedish investigators to the identification of autoantibodies to colonic epithelial antigens in ulcerative colitis, but also in Crohn's disease (12,245,246). When these antibodies were also found to react with certain strains of *E. coli*, speculation arose that inflammatory bowel disease could result from a cross-reactivity with antigens shared between intestinal bacteria and colonic epithelial cells (247). Further investigation, however, revealed that these antibodies were not specific for inflammatory bowel disease, bore no correlation with disease activity, and did not cause tissue damage in an animal model of inflammatory bowel disease (248). Furthermore, these anticolon antibodies could not bind complement or mediate antibody-dependent cell-mediated cytotoxicity (ADCC); they presently are considered of no pathogenic relevance (249). Nevertheless, the concept of antibody-mediated autoimmunity has been recently revived by Takahashi and Das who have described circulating and tissue-bound antibodies to a specific colonic epithelial cell surface protein (250). This as yet not fully characterized antigen, has been localized to colonic, biliary, and skin epithelium, raising an interest in its possible role as a true autoantigen, and as a culprit for some of the extraintestinal manifestations characteristic of inflammatory bowel disease (251). These findings have been derived only from studies using ulcerative colitis not Crohn's disease tissues. Other potential gut-derived auto-antigens have been described, but reactivity against ECAC was present in both Crohn's disease and ulcerative colitis patients, as well as their healthy relatives (252,253).

Several investigators have reported lymphocyte-mediated cytotoxicity against colonic, but not small bowel, epithelial cells in both ulcerative colitis and Crohn's disease (244,254–256). In these studies, the killing mechanism was characterized as ADCC, with attacking lymphocytes carrying an epithelial antibody. The true significance of these findings has been questioned, and a subsequent study using colonic epithelial cells as targets failed to show any cytotoxicity by peripheral mononuclear cells or even very potent lymphokine-activated killer cells (257,258). The results of the original cytotoxicity experiments cannot explain every feature of Crohn's disease. For instance, the described cytotoxic reaction against epithelium is limited to colonocytes and does not occur against enterocytes. Finally, multiple questions have been raised about the technical limitations of the earlier studies (257).

In addition to reactivity against cells of intestinal origin, autoimmune responses to nonepithelial cells have also been described in inflammatory bowel disease, although their pathogenic significance remains doubtful (112). Serum antibodies against lymphocytes (lymphocytotoxic antibodies) have consistently been detected in inflammatory bowel disease (259). These cold reactive lymphocytotoxins are typically of the IgM class and are found in a variety of typical autoimmune diseases, including rheumatoid arthritis and pernicious anemia, and in up to 40% of patients with Crohn's disease (260,261). An interesting associated finding is that lymphocytotoxins have also been detected in up to one-third of relatives of patients with inflammatory bowel disease and even in 40% of household contacts (consanguineous and nonconsanguineous), raising questions about genetic predisposition versus environmental exposure (262). The true relevance of these findings is uncertain, but they likely represent one of the many nonspecific abnormalities of immune regulation in Crohn's disease, rather than a central point of its pathogenesis.

1. Immune Reactivity to Heat Shock Proteins

One aspect of autoimmunity relates to reactivity against heat shock proteins (HSP). These are substances produced by most cells submitted to "stress" induced by fever, oxygen-free radicals, nutritional deficiencies, and infection (263,264). Mycobacteria produce several antigens of various molecular weight that are HSP (HSP 48, 65, 70) (265). In view of the postulated mycobacterial etiology, evidence of a broad immune reactivity to multiple bacterial antigens, and the persistence of a chronic inflammatory process, immune cross-reactivity with HSP could play a role in Crohn's disease pathogenesis.

Several investigators have suggested that mycobacterial proteins could trigger an autoimmune response in susceptible individuals, leading to the clinical manifestations of Crohn's disease (266–268). Markesich et al., using an immunoblotting technique, compared antibody responses to mycobacterial and human HSP in patients with Crohn's disease and ulcerative colitis and in control subjects (267). No statistically significant enhanced antibody response to mycobacterial or human stress proteins was observed. Another group looked at antibody levels to human and mycobacterial recombinant HSP 70, human HSP 60, and mycobacterial HSP 65 in patients with Crohn's disease and in control subjects (268). Approximately one-half of Crohn's disease patients had elevated titers to mycobacterial HSP 65 without elevation of antihuman HSP 60 titers; by contrast human and mycobacterial HSP 70 titers were comparable to those of controls. A different pattern was seen in ulcerative colitis. In addition, tissue immunohistochemical staining fails to detect any major difference in the pattern of expression of HSP 60 between Crohn's disease and control or ulcerative colitis specimens (269). Finally, although there is some evidence for T-lymphocyte reactivity to HSP 65 in active Crohn's disease, proliferative responses of peripheral blood and gut mucosal lymphocytes to HSP 60 are generally comparable in Crohn's disease and control subjects (266,269). Taken together, the above data do not suggest that specific sensitization to HSP is a major event leading to a pathogenically relevant autoimmune response in Crohn's disease. Nevertheless, a role for these protective substances cannot be completely ruled out, because lack of a more vigorous immune response against HSP in the setting of a chronically active inflammatory disease could be considered a defect in itself and may deserve further investigation.

D. Adhesion Molecules

The physical and functional interactions among various types of immunocytes, and immune and nonimmune cells are mediated by a variety of molecules expressed on their cell surface. These molecules come under the general designation of cell adhesion molecules (CAM), and are classified in various categories (selectins, integrins, immunoglobulin superfamily and others) based on their molecular structure and restriction of expression to certain cell types (270). Interactions involving CAM occur under physiological conditions, but they become even more important under inflammatory conditions because they contribute not only to cell–cell communication but also to cell activation, migration, and the final outcome of an inflammatory process (217). Given these important functions, an investigation of the role of CAM in inflammatory bowel disease and Crohn's disease in particular should generate highly relevant data. A limited number of studies have been carried out, but most support the concept that CAM have a role in systemic and mucosal immunity in Crohn's disease.

An early study measuring the expression of the integrin CD11/CD18 on circulating leukocytes by fluorocytemetric analysis failed to find any significant differences between Crohn's disease, ulcerative colitis, and healthy control subjects (272). In contrast, a detailed in vitro study on cell aggregation and adhesion molecule expression by Mishra et al. detected important differences using peripheral blood mononuclear cells from Crohn's disease patients (273). By culturing these cells with polyacrylamide beads, these investigators found that the size of aggregates correlated significantly with clinical activity and that monoclonal antibodies against LFA-2, LFA-3, and Mac-1 adhesion molecules inhibited aggregation. These results imply a key role for several CAM in cell activation as well as granuloma formation in Crohn's disease. Another in vitro study showed quantitative differences in the ability of organ culture supernatants from Crohn's disease and ulcerative colitis specimens to modulate CAM expression: Crohn's disease supernatants were considerably more potent in upregulating the expression of E-selectin and ICAM-1 by human umbilical vein endothelial cells than those from ulcerative colitis, pointing to different cell communication pathways in each form of inflammatory bowel disease (274). This greater capacity for upregulation of CAM in Crohn's disease than ulcerative colitis is also supported by higher levels of soluble ICAM-1 in the circulation of Crohn's disease patients compared with ulcerative colitis patients (275).

Even more relevant and direct are observations on the expression and localization of CAM in the intestinal mucosa. A quantitative analysis using an immunofluorescence technique showed a dramatic increase of ICAM-1 on mucosal macrophages that closely correlated with histological activity in both Crohn's disease and ulcerative colitis specimens (276). Similar although not as dramatic alterations can be detected in uninvolved inflammatory bowel disease mucosa, suggesting that abnormal expression of CAM may be an early event in local inflammation (277). There is also evidence that this expression may be different among T and B cells present in Crohn's disease, ulcerative colitis, and normal mucosa (140). A recent study using a three-color immunofluorescence technique and isolated LPMC shows that β1, β7, α2, α4, α5, α6 integrins display unique patterns depending on the type and presence or absence of inflammatory process. Abnormal CAM expression is not restricted to mononuclear cells, because VCAM-1 and especially E-selectin are also expressed at high levels in vessels of human and animal forms of inflammatory bowel disease (278). The functional importance of these phenotypic and histological observations is that the binding and circulation of inflammatory leukocytes is profoundly affected by CAM, with implications for the mechanisms and outcome of inflammatory bowel disease. Furthermore, knowledge of which and where certain adhesion molecules are expressed may allow specific modulation of leukocyte accumulation and interfere with the progress or degree of intestinal inflammation. The validity of such an experimental approach is supported by a study in the cotton-top tamarin in which histological attenuation of colitis was achieved by administration of anti-α4 integrin monoclonal antibodies (279).

E. Complement

Activation of the complement cascade is a classical pathway leading to cell damage, and it participates in a number of inflammatory disorders. Thus, the possibility that complement components are produced in abnormal amounts or locations in the gut involved by inflammatory bowel disease has been investigated. Immunohistochemical staining of vessels in the normal intestinal mucosa is positive for C3d, C5, C9, terminal complement complex, and S-protein, but the intensity is much greater in Crohn's disease and ulcerative colitis, demonstrating that complement activation does not take place in actively inflamed mucosa (280,281). Complement deposition is also found on epithelial cells, and codeposition of IgG1 and C3b is marked in ulcerative colitis but absent in Crohn's disease (282,283). This difference does not necessarily mean a less relevant role of the complement cascade in the pathogenesis of the latter condition, since jejunal perfusates of mucosa apparently uninvolved by Crohn's disease contain significantly elevated concentrations of C4 compared with control subjects (284).

V. MISCELLANEOUS FACTORS

A. Intestinal Permeability

As discussed, one of the primary functions of the intestinal mucosa is to separate the carefully regulated internal environment from the potentially hostile external environment. In any intestinal inflammatory disorder, inflammation and ulceration lead to a loss of mucosal integrity. This breakdown results in an increased intestinal permeability, probably accounting for the findings of increased bacterial translocation in Crohn's disease, and may contribute to elevation of serum antibodies against bacteria (17,285). Several studies have shown that intestinal permeability is greater in patients with Crohn's disease than in patients with ulcerative colitis or in normal control subjects (286–289). These conclusions are based on studies of urinary excretion of poorly absorbed, water-soluble compounds that cannot be metabolized (polyethylene glycol 400, mannitol, rhamnose, lactulose) or markers such as 51-chromium-labeled ethylenediaminetetraacetate (^{51}Cr-EDTA) (287, 289). The rate at which these probes cross the mucosal barrier is a reflection of their molecular size, and the rate of permeability is directly proportional to the probes cross-sectional diameter (290). The above findings are not surprising in that the bowel of the subjects studied was diseased, and increased permeability was interpreted as being secondary to chronic inflammation.

A study by Hollander et al., however, unexpectedly found increased intestinal permeability in a number of healthy relatives of patients with Crohn's disease, suggesting that the defect might be genetically determined (288). This led to the hypothesis that a defect in intestinal permeability could be a primary phenomenon and therefore be of etiologic importance in the disease pathogenesis (244,288,290). The number of subjects studied by Hollander et al. was small and the techniques for measuring urinary polyethylene glycol 400 concentrations complex, raising questions about the broad applicability of their findings (288). When further studies examining larger groups of patients and testing several different absorption probes were performed, no statistically significant differences in permeability between the relatives of Crohn's disease patients and healthy control subjects could be demonstrated (291–294).

The issue of increased intestinal permeability in healthy relatives of Crohn's disease patients has been critically reevaluated by May et al. (295). These investigators argued that, if only a small percentage (3%–10%) of relatives are statistically likely to develop active Crohn's disease, then the group of relatives analyzed as a whole would be unlikely to show abnormal permeability, and no more than 10% of them should be expected to have such a defect. In agreement with this rationale, these investigators found that approximately 10% of first-degree relatives indeed had abnormally high permeability when tested by a lactulose/mannitol ratio (295). Using the same logic to reassess the raw data from a previous study by Katz et al. led to a similar conclusion (296). There is a growing consensus for the idea that a small subgroup of relatives of Crohn's disease patients do have increased intestinal permeability in the absence of any obvious clinical symptoms. However, it is impossible to state whether these relatives have subclinical Crohn's disease with abnormal permeability secondary to silent intestinal inflammation or a true, genetically determined abnormality of intestinal permeability as a factor predisposing to Crohn's disease. A preliminary report by Peeters et al. favors the former hypothesis (297). These investigators, studying relatives of families with and without a family history of Crohn's disease, found no evidence of a genetic pattern of increased permeability, which was even detected in 31% of healthy spouses, and concluded that the abnormality is likely due to environmental factors.

B. Vasculitis and the Measles Virus

A state of hypercoagulability can be found in Crohn's disease, which is compatible with the occasional finding of cutaneous, ocular, mesenteric, and systemic vasculitis in this condition (298). These observations and a series of reports by the group of Wakefield et al. have led to the hypothesis that Crohn's disease results from multifocal gastrointestinal infarctions due to chronic mesenteric vasculitis (299). Several findings tend to support this hypothesis. Resected surgical specimens from Crohn's disease patients and controls were perfused and resin-fixed to preserve the vascular morphology for histological and electron microscopic examination. On visual inspection, casts of macroscopically affected Crohn's disease tissue were notable for intense neovascularization, whereas uninvolved tissue was similar to that of normal control subjects. Electron micrograph studies showed fibrin plugs, often associated with mononuclear inflammatory cells, in many vessels within the muscularis propria and submucosa. Abnormal blood vessels were frequently seen in continuity with morphologically normal vasculature, especially in early lesions. The mechanism of vasculitis is hypothesized to be thrombosis related to the interaction of immune cells with the vascular endothelium and activation of the coagulation cascade (299). Follow-up studies by the same investigators showed that a majority of granulomas in Crohn's disease specimens form within the walls of blood vessels (300). Many of these lesions were found distant from sites of active mucosal ulceration and macroscopic disease, suggesting that they may represent an early lesion. Granulomatous inflammation was associated with the adherence of chronic inflammatory cells to vessel wall and fibrin deposition, similar to the intestinal vasculitis discussed previously (299,300).

To further generate evidence for a role of the intestinal microcirculation in the etiology of Crohn's disease, an animal model of acute multifocal gastrointestinal infection was developed (301). After an intra-arterial injection of occluding styrene microspheres, focal mucosal inflammation, necrosis, and ulceration were induced in ferrets. Fibrinous and acute inflammatory exudation and glandular disruption could be seen adjacent to histologically normal tissue after infarction (301). Although the acute lesion was histologically quite different from the chronic inflammatory lesions of Crohn's disease, the authors succeeded in demonstrating that discrete intramural arterial occlusion can cause multifocal infarctions, giving additional credibility to their previous hypothesis regarding a vascular etiology for Crohn's disease. Intriguing, yet indirect, evidence also favoring this hypothesis comes from the clinical and epidemiological observation that both smoking and oral contraceptive use are associated with vascular thrombosis as well as Crohn's disease (302).

A clue to the possible etiology of the proposed vasculitis emerged from transmission electron microscopy by Wakefield et al. who identified Paramyxovirus-like inclusions in foci of microvascular inflammation in Crohn's disease tissue (303). This raised the possibility that Crohn's disease was caused by a persistent measles virus infection in the intestinal microvascular endothelium. Positive in situ hybridization for measles virus genomic RNA and positive immunohistochemical staining with measles-specific monoclonal and polyclonal antibodies further support that possibility. Additionally, there is epidemiological correlation between early childhood infections and the later appearance of Crohn's disease in selected populations (304–307). The measles virus–mesenteric vasculitis hypothesis is both unexpected and puzzling, but this is no reason to discard it a priori. Its proponents have recently argued that most of the typical features of Crohn's disease can be explained by this hypothesis, including the presence of granulomas, the proximal anastomotic recurrence after resection, the beneficial effect of fecal stream diversion, and the epidemiologic findings (308). Additional studies by independent investigators using different study populations are needed to confirm or dismiss the measles virus as a relevant etiological agent.

C. Luminal and Dietary Factors

Several lines of evidence suggest that, in Crohn's disease, the continuous stimulation of the mucosal immune system by enteric bacterial and dietary antigens is a factor contributing to the inflammatory response. This concept, which until recently was solely based on indirect or anecdotal evidence, has been considerably strengthened by a recently developed animal model of inflammatory bowel disease. Mice whose IL-2 and IL-10 genes have been functionally incapacitated (IL-2 and IL-10 "knock-out" mice) show histological and clinical evidence of colitis when raised in a routine laboratory environment, whereas littermates raised under germ-free conditions have no gut inflammation or only an attenuated illness (21,22). Therefore, at least in some animals, chronic intestinal inflammation cannot occur in the absence of intestinal flora. If the same happens in Crohn's disease can not be tested in humans. However, the known beneficial effects of antibiotics, metronidazole, and even sulfasalazine are likely to depend, at least in part, on their ability to modify the quantity or quality of intestinal bacteria. The same may be true in those patients who sporadically improve on antituberculous therapy. The exact role of the luminal flora in mucosal inflammation is unclear, but it probably involves some degree of immune sensitization as suggested by the elevated serum antibody titers and mucosal lymphocyte proliferation to several microbial antigens seen in Crohn's disease patients (17,20).

The critical importance of luminal antigenic load in mucosal inflammation has been further highlighted by an interesting study on the fecal stream diversion by Rutgeerts et al. (309). These investigators found no endoscopic evidence of disease recurrence in five patients who underwent ileal resection and ileocolic anastomosis followed by a diverting ileostomy, as opposed to clear endoscopic recurrence in 53 of 75 patients who underwent one-step surgery without ileostomy. The importance of the fecal stream and composition in intestinal inflammation is further emphasized by studies on pouchitis. Several groups have provided evidence that fecal stasis, luminal contents, and microbial imbalance are crucial to the development of this condition (310–312).

Bacterial flora is probably not the only factor contributing to chronic intestinal inflammation in a nonspecific manner, and a similar situation may exist in relationship to food antigens (89). Extensive evidence from clinical studies supports this hypothesis, even though there is no direct evidence linking a particular dietary component to the development or perpetuation of Crohn's disease. The success of the food elimination diets of Hunter et al. in the maintenance of remission suggests that certain foodstuffs contribute to the maintenance of intestinal inflammation (313–315). However, these results have not been reproduced by other groups. Many different types of dietary manipulations such as elemental diets, polymeric diets, and enteral nutrition have also been shown to have beneficial effects on intestinal inflammation and permeability, again supporting a role for dietary antigens in the pathogenesis of Crohn's disease (316–320). The mechanism for the beneficial effect of these diets remains unclear. Some investigators argue that the very low fat content of the diets reduces the available precursors for arachidonate derived eicosanoid synthesis (320). Others suggest that these diets improve total body protein stores and thus help maintain clinical remission (319). An additional possibility is that, by altering the diet, there is less "antigenic pressure" on the local immune system as there might be in the case of reducing the bacterial antigenic load discussed above.

We do not currently understand the relative importance of dietary antigens versus intestinal microbial factors or how the two interact, but the available data leave little doubt that these two factors play more than an incidental role in the pathogenesis of inflammation in Crohn's disease.

D. Mucus

Because the mucus layer covering the intestinal epithelium is the first line of defense that separates the luminal content rich in food and bacterial antigens from the mucosal immune compartment, the possibility that some abnormality of mucin composition contributes to inflammatory bowel disease pathogenesis has been suspected for a long time. This concept has been investigated more intensely in ulcerative colitis, and early reports suggested that a specific defect represented by the selective depletion of mucin fraction IV was present in this condition but not in Crohn's disease (321,322). Later studies using ion exchange chromatography failed to confirm this observation and purified mucus glycoproteins were found to be qualitatively normal not only in ulcerative colitis but also in Crohn's disease and other inflammatory control subjects (323). Despite the lack of a biochemically defined defect in mucus composition, lectin binding to colonic mucin is altered in both Crohn's disease and ulcerative colitis, indicating that the attachment of microorganisms or other substances to epithelial cells may be altered in inflammatory bowel disease (324). This almost certainly represents a secondary and nonspecific phenomenon. Nevertheless, it could still have relevance to Crohn's disease in that luminal antigens and persistent stimulation of the mucosal immune system are likely contributors to intestinal inflammation.

VI. CONCLUSION

At the end of this chapter the reader may feel that enough information has been provided to allow him or her to judge the relative importance of each factor presented, and thus create a personal state of mind about the possible causes and mechanisms of Crohn's disease. On the other hand, the reader may be overwhelmed with the amount of data available in the literature and be as, or even more, perplexed than he or she was at the beginning of the chapter. In either case, a few final considerations are offered with as much objectivity as possible, and as little bias as allowed by the authors' own experience and personal views.

No infectious agent has been convincingly proven to cause Crohn's disease. From time to time candidate microorganisms will burst onto the scene to claim that honor. Perhaps many of them are involved, alone or in combination, each masking the other, or perhaps a single agent is responsible, hidden by the myriad of microbes that normally inhabit the gut. The history lesson provided by *Helicobacter pylori* is still unfolding, and it should be exploited by those courageous investigators ready to tackle the challenge of the enteric flora.

The field of animal models has exploded in less than a decade, and the number of experimental colitides now available is far greater than the resources available to the research community to explore each one in detail. It is highly unlikely that "Crohn's disease" will ever be faithfully reproduced in an animal. However, even those models whose disease does not mimic that of the human have something to offer in regard to the cellular and molecular mechanisms of gut inflammation. Should the precise cause of Crohn's disease continue to elude us, at least one day we may be able to understand how it happens, if not why it happens.

The science of immunology has created hopes of uncovering the cause of several puzzling illnesses. The promise has been fulfilled in some, but not all diseases, and, unfortunately, Crohn's disease falls in the latter category. At the same time, a growing body of knowledge of how immune cells communicate with each other is providing a solid understanding of "physiological" and pathological intestinal inflammation. From this understanding, novel and rational forms of therapy are emerging that will benefit those individuals to whom we cannot say what causes their illness.

Finally, if an aspect of Crohn's disease deserves any sympathy or has the slightest positive angle, it is that the mysteries of the disease motivate researchers to use their inquisitive minds, develop innovative theories, and test new hypotheses. Without these, hopes for the final answer may go unfulfilled forever.

With these considerations in mind and regarding the information contained in the next two chapters, one could formulate a reasonable pathogenic hypothesis: under the influence of environmental, genetic, and dietary factors, the enteric flora, and perhaps a yet undiscovered microbiological agent, the intestinal mucosal immune system is inappropriately and continuously stimulated. This results in the activation of T cells, B cells, macrophages, and other immune and nonimmune cells that secrete antibodies, cytokines, reactive oxygen metabolites, and other factors that together mediate a nonspecific form of tissue damage. Much is known about each of these components, but much remains to be learned. Knowledge of the mechanisms is expanding faster than knowledge of the causes of Crohn's disease. If the cause is destined to remain obscure, it will still be possible to conquer the disease by effectively manipulating its mechanisms.

ACKNOWLEDGMENTS

The authors wish to thank the following organizations for supporting some of the studies reported in this chapter: The National Institute of Diabetes, Digestive and Kidney Diseases, National Institutes of Health, Bethesda, Maryland; the Crohn's & Colitis Foundation of America, Inc., New York, New York; Case Western Reserve University and University Hospitals of Cleveland, Cleveland, Ohio; The Cleveland Clinic Foundation, Cleveland, Ohio. In addition, the authors thank Kim Katusha and Alessandro Musso for help in preparing and reviewing the manuscript.

REFERENCES

1. Walvoort HC, Pena AS. Crohn's disease: entity and aetiopathogenic concepts. J Clin Nutr Gastroenterol 1987; 2:194–200.
2. Wensinck R. The fecal flora in patients with Crohn's disease. Antonie Van Leeuwenhoek 1975; 41:214–215.
3. Van de Merwe JP, Schroder AM, Wensinck F, Hazenberg MP. The obligate anaerobic faecal flora of patient's with Crohn's disease and their first-degree relatives. Scand J Gastroenterol 1988; 23:1125–1131.
4. Peach S, Lock MR, Katz D, Todd IP, Tabaqchali S. Mucosal-associated bacterial flora of the intestine in patients with Crohn's disease and in a control group. Gut 1978; 19:1034–1042.
5. Parent K, Mitchell PD. Bacterial variants: etiologic agents in Crohn's disease? Gastroenterology 1976; 71:365–368.
6. Parent K, Mitchell P. Cell wall–defective variants of *Pseudomonas*-like (group Va) bacteria in Crohn's disease. Gastroenterology 1978; 75:368–372.

7. Ibbotson JP, Pease PE, Allan RN. Cell-wall deficient bacteria in inflammatory bowel disease. Eur J Clin Microbiol 1987; 6:429–431.

8. Belsheim MR, Darwish RZ, Watson WC, Schieven B. Bacterial L-form isolation from inflammatory bowel disease patients. Gastroenterology 1983; 85:364–369.

9. McGarity BH, Robertson DA, Clarke IN, Wright R. Deoxyribonucleic acid amplification and hybridisation in Crohn's disease using a chlamydial plasmid probe. Gut 1991; 32:1011–1015.

10. Dorman SA, Liggoria E, Winn WC, Beeken WL. Isolation of *Clostridium difficile* from patients with inactive Crohn's disease. Gastroenterology 1982; 82:1348–1351.

11. VanDyke TE, Dowell VR, Offenbacher S, Snyder W, Hersch T. Potential role of microorganisms isolated from periodontal lesions in the pathogenesis of inflammatory bowel disease. Infect Immun 1987; 53:671–677.

12. Broberger O, Perlmann P. Autoantibodies in human ulcerative colitis. J Exp Med 1959; 110:657–674.

13. Perlmann P, Hammarstrom S, Lagercrantz R, Gustafsson BE. Antigen from colon of germfree rats and antibodies in human ulcerative colitis. Ann N Y Acad Sci 1965; 124:377–394.

14. Bull DM, Ignaczack TF. Enterobacterial common antigen-induced lymphocyte reactivity in inflammatory bowel disease. Gastroenterology 1973; 64:43–50.

15. Tabaqchali S, O'Donague DP, Bettelheim KA. *Escherichia coli* antibodies in patients with inflammatory bowel disease. Gut 1978; 19:108–113.

16. Tvede M, Bondesen S, Nielsen OH, Rasmussen SN. Serum antibodies to *Bacteroides* species in chronic inflammatory bowel disease. Scand J Gastroenterol 1983; 18:783–789.

17. Blaser MJ, Miller RA, Lacher J, Singleton JW. Patients with active Crohn's disease have elevated serum antibodies to antigens of seven enteric bacterial pathogens. Gastroenterology 1984; 87:888–894.

18. Auer IO, Roder A, Wensinck F, Van de Merwe JP. Selected bacterial antibodies in Crohn's disease and ulcerative colitis. Scand J Gastroenterol 1983; 18:217–223.

19. Matthews N, Mayberry JF, Rhodes J, Neale L, Munro J, Wensick F, Lawson GH, Rowland AC, Berkhoff GA, Barthold SW. Agglutinins to bacteria in Crohn's disease. Gut 1980; 21:376–380.

20. Pirzer U, Schonhaar A, Fleischer B, Hermann E, Buschenfelde K-HM. Reactivity of infiltrating T lymphocytes with microbial antigens in Crohn's disease. Lancet 1991; 338:1239–1239.

21. Sadlack B, Mertz H, Schorle H, Schimpl A, Feller AC, Horak I. Ulcerative colitis-like disease in mice with a disrupted interleukin-2 gene. Cell 1993; 75:253–261.

22. Kuhn R, Lohler J, Rennick D, Rajewsky K, Muller W. Interleukin-10–deficient mice develop chronic enterocolitis. Cell 1993; 75:263–274.

23. Onderdonk AB, Franklin ML, Cisneros RL. Production of experimental ulcerative colitis in gnotobiotic guinea pigs with simplified microflora. Infect Immun 1981; 32:225–231.

24. Sartor RB, Cromartie WJ, Powell DW, Schwab JH. Granulomatous enterocolitis induced in rats by purified bacterial cell wall fragments. Gastroenterology 1985; 89:587–595.

25. Yamada T, Sartor RB, Marshall S, Specian RD, Grisham MB. Mucosal injury and inflammation in a model of chronic granulomatous colitis in rats. Gastroenterology 1993; 104:759–771.

26. Green KD, Sartor RB. Systemic lipopolysaccharide reactivates peptidoglycan-polysaccharide-induced intestinal inflammation in rats. Gastroenterology 1988; 94:A154.

27. Chadwick VS, Anderson RP. Microorganisms and their products in inflammatory bowel disease. In: MacDermott RP, Stenson WF, eds. Inflammatory Bowel Disease. Current Topics in Gastroenterology. New York: Elsevier, 1992:241–258.

28. Sartor RB. Role of intestinal microflora in initiation and perpetuation of inflammatory bowel disease. Can J Gastroenterol 1990; 4:271–277.

29. Dalziel TK. Chronic interstitial enteritis. BMJ 1913; 2:1068–1070.

30. Crohn BB, Ginzburg L, Oppenheimer GD. Regional ileitis: a pathologic and clinical entity. JAMA 1932; 99(16):1323–1329.

31. Dvorak AM, Dickersin GR, Osage JE, Monahan RA. Absence of virus structure in Crohn's disease tissues studied by electron microscopy (letter). Lancet 1978; 1:328.

32. Patterson DS, Allen W. Chronic mycobacterial enteritis in ruminants as a model of Crohn's disease. Proc R Soc Med 1972; 65:998–1001.

33. Burnham WR, Lenneard-Jones JE. Mycobacteria as a possible cause of inflammatory bowel disease. Lancet 1978; 2:693–696.

34. Chiodini RJ, Kruiningen HJV, Thayer WR, Merkal RS, Coutu JA. Possible role of mycobacteria in inflammatory bowel disease. I. An unclassified *Mycobacterium* species isolated from patients with Crohn's disease. Dig Dis Sci 1984; 29:1073–1079.

35. VanKruiningen HJ, Chiodini RJ, Thayer WR, Coutu JA, Merkal RS, Runnels PL. Experimental disease in infant goats induced by a Mycobacterium isolated from a patient with Crohn's disease. Dig Dis Sci 1986; 31:1351–1360.

36. Chiodini RJ, Kruiningen HJv, Thayer WR, Coutu JA. Spheroplastic phase of Mycobacteria isolated from patients with Crohn's disease. J Clin Microbiol 1986; 24:357–363.

37. Graham DY, Markesich DC, Yoshimura HH. Mycobacteria and inflammatory bowel disease. Results of culture. Gastroenterology 1987; 92:436–442.

38. Chiodini RJ. Crohn's disease and the mycobacterioses: a review and comparison of two disease entities. Clin Microbiol Rev 1989; 2:90–117.

39. Gitnick G, Collins J, Beaman B, Brooks D, Arthur M, Imaeda T, Palieschesky M. Preliminary report on isolation of Mycobacteria from patients with Crohn's disease. Dig Dis Sci 1989; 34:925–932.

40. Yoshimura HH, Graham DY, Estes MK, Merkal RS. Investigation of association of Mycobacteria with inflammatory bowel disease by nucleic acid hybridization. J Clin Microbiol 1987; 25:45–51.

41. McFadden JJ, Butcher PD, Thompson J, Chiodini RJ, Hermon-Taylor J. The use of DNA probes identifying restriction fragment-length polymorphisms to examine the *Mycobacterium avium* complex. Mol Microbiol 1987; 283:–291.

42. Butcher PD, McFadden JJ, Hermon-Taylor J. Investigation of mycobacteria in Crohn's disease tissue by Southern blotting and DNA hybridization with cloned mycobacterial genomic DNA probes from a Crohn's disease isolated mycobacteria. Gut 1988; 29:1222–1228.

43. Moss MT, Sanderson JD, Tizard ML, Hermon-Taylor J, El-Zaatari FA, Markesich DC, Graham DY. Polymerase chain reaction detection of *Mycobacterium paratuberculosis* and *Mycobacterium avium* subsp *silvaticum* in long term cultures from Crohn's disease and control tissues. Gut 1992; 33:1209–1213.

44. McFadden JJ, Thompson J, Hull E, Hampson S, Stanford J, Hermon-Taylor J. The use of cloned DNA probes to examine organisms isolated from Crohn's disease tissue. In: MacDermott RP, ed. Inflammatory Bowel Disease: Current Status and Future Applications. Amsterdam: Elsevier, 1988:515–520.

45. McFadden JJ, Seechurn P. Mycobacteria and Crohn's disease. A molecular approach. In: MacDermott RP, Stenson WF, ed. Inflammatory Bowel Disease. New York: Elsevier, 1992:259–271.

46. Hermon-Taylor J, Moss MT, Tizard ML, Malik Z, Sanderson JD. Molecular biology of Crohn's disease mycobacteria. Baillieres Clin Gastroenterol 1990; 4:23–42.

47. Green E, Tizard ML, Thompson J, Winterbourne D, McFadden JJ, Hermon-Taylor J. Sequence and characteristics of IS900, an insertion sequence identified in a human Crohn's disease isolate of *Mycobacterium paratuberculosis*. Nucleic Acids Res 1989; 17:9063–9073.

48. Sanderson JD, Moss MT, Tizard MLV, Hermon-Taylor J. *Mycobacterium paratuberculosis* DNA in Crohn's disease tissue. Gut 1992; 33:890–896.

49. Fidler HM, Thurrell W, Johnson NM, Rook GA, McFadden JJ. Specific detection of *Mycobacterium paratuberculosis* DNA associated with granulomatous tissue in Crohn's disease. Gut 1994; 35:506–510.

50. Thayer WR, Coutu JA, Chiodini RJ, Kruiningen HJV, Merkal RS. Possible role of myco-

bacteria in inflammatory bowel disease. II. Mycobacterial antibodies in Crohn's disease. Dig Dis Sci 1984; 29:1080–1085.

51. Tanaka K, Wilks M, Coates PJ, Farthing MJ, Walker-Smith JA, Tabaqchali S. *Mycobacterium paratuberculosis* and Crohn's disease. Gut 1991; 32:43–45.

52. Stainby KJ, Lowes JR, Allan RN, Ibbotson JP. Antibodies to *Mycobacterium paratuberculosis* and nine species of environmental mycobacteria in Crohn's disease and control subjects. Gut 1993; 34:371–374.

53. Kobayashi K, Brown WR, Brennan PL, Blaser MJ. Serum antibodies to mycobacterial antigens in active Crohn's disease. Gastroenterology 1988; 94:1404–1411.

54. Cho SN, Brennan PJ, Yoshimura HH, Korelitz BI, Graham DY. Mycobacterial aetiology of Crohn's disease: serologic study using common mycobacterial antigens and a species-specific glycolipid antigen from *Mycobacterium paratuberculosis*. Gut 1986; 27:1353–1356.

55. Brunello F, Pera A, Martini S, Marino L, Astegiano M, Barletti C, Gastaldi P, Verme G, Emmanuelli G. Antibodies to *Mycobacterium paratuberculosis* in patients with Crohn's disease. Dig Dis Sci 1991; 36:1741–1745.

56. Kobayashi K, Blaser MJ, Brown WR. Immunohistochemical examination for mycobacteria in intestinal tissues from patients with Crohn's disease. Gastroenterology 1989; 96:1009–1015.

57. Markesich DC, Graham DY, Yoshimura HH. Interaction of human monocytes and mycobacteria: studies comparing Crohn's disease to controls. In: Macdermott R, ed. Inflammatory Bowel Disease. Current Status and Future Approach. Amsterdam: Elsevier, 1988:553–558.

58. Seldenrijk CA, Drexhage HA, Meuwissen SGM, Meijer CJLM. T-Cellular immune reactions (in macrophage inhibitor factor assay) against *Mycobacterium paratuberculosis*, *Mycobacterium kansasii*, *Mycobacterium tuberculosis*, *Mycobacterium avium* in patients with chronic inflammatory bowel disease. Gut 1990; 31:529–535.

59. Ibbotsdon JP, Lowes JR, Chahal H, Gaston JSH, Life P, Kumararatne DS, Sharif H, Alexander-Williams J, Allan RN. Mucosal cell-mediated immunity to mycobacterial, enterobacterial and other microbial antigens iin inflammatory bowel disease. Clin Exp Immunol 1992; 87:224–230.

60. Prantera C, Bothamley G, Levenstein G, Mangiarotti R, Argnetieri R. Crohn's disease and mycobacteria: two cases of Crohn's disease with high anti-mycobacterial antibody levels cured by dapsone therapy. Biomed Pharmacother 1989; 43:295–299.

61. Thayer WJ, Coutu R, Chiodini RJ, VanKruiningen HJ. Use of rifabutin and streptomycin in the therapy of Crohn's disease—preliminary results. In: MacDermott RP, ed. Inflammatory Bowel Disease. Current Status and Future Approach. Amsterdam: Elsevier, 1988:565–568.

62. Warren JB, Rees HC, Cox TM. Remission of Crohn's disease with tuberculosis therapy. N Engl J Med 1986; 314:182.

63. Shaffer JL, Hughes S, Linaker BD, Baker RD, Turnberg LA. Controlled trial of rifampicine and ethambutol in Crohn's disease. Gut 1984; 25:203–205.

64. Afdhal NH, Long A, Lennon J, Crowe J, O'Donoghue DP. Controlled trial of antimycobacterial therapy in Crohn's disease: clofazimine versus placebo. Dig Dis Sci 1991; 36:449–453.

65. Swift GL, Srivastava ED, Stone R, Pullan RD, Newcombe RG, Rhodes J, Wilkinson S, Rhodes P, Roberts G, Lawrie BW, Evans KT, Williams GT, Strohmeyer G, Kreutzpainter G. A controlled trial of 2 years' antituberculous chemotherapy in Crohn's disease. Gastroenterology 1993; 104:A787.

66. Prantera C, Kohn A, Mangiarotti R, Andreoli A, Luzi C. Antimycobacterial therapy in Crohn's disease: results of a controlled, double-blind trial with a multiple antibiotic regimen. Am J Gastroenterol 1994; 89:513–518.

67. Ekbom A, Adami HO, Hernick CG, Jonzon A, Zack MM. Perinatal risk factors of inflammatory bowel disease: a case control study. Am J Epidemiol 1990; 132:1111–1119.

68. Jarnerot G, Lantorp K. Antibodies to EB virus in cases of Crohn's disease. N Engl J Med 1972; 286:1215–1216.

69. Farmer GW, Vincent MM, Fuccillo DA, Horta-Barbosa L, Ritman S, Sever JL, Gitnick GL. Viral investigations in ulcerative colitis and regional enteritis. Gastroenterology 1973; 65:8–18.

70. Tamura H. Acute ulcerative colitis associated with cytomegalic inclusion virus. Arch pathol 1973; 96:164–167.

71. Mitchell DN, Rees RJ. Agent transmissable from Crohn's disease tissue. Lancet 1970; 2:168–171.

72. Aronson MD, Phillips CA, Beeken WL, Forsyth BE. Isolation and characterizartion of a viral agent from intestinal tissue of patients with Crohn's disease and other intestinal disorders. Prog Med Virol 1975; 21:165–176.

73. Gitnick GL, Arthur MH, Shibata I. Cultivation of viral agents from Crohn's disease. Lancet 1976; 2:215–217.

74. Riemann JF. Further electron microscopic evidence of virus-like particles in Crohn's disease. Acta Hepatogastroenterol 1977; 24:116–118.

75. Whorwell PJ, Phillips CA, Beeken WL, Little PK, Roessner KD. Isolation of reovirus-like agents from patients with Crohn's disese. Lancet 1977; 1:1169–1171.

76. Knibbs DR, VanKruiningen HJ, Colombel JF, Cortot A. Ultrastructural evidence of paramyxovirus in two French families with Crohn's disease. Gastroenterology 1993; 104:A726.

77. Philpotts RJ, Hermon-Taylor J, Teich NM, Brooke BN. A search for persistent virus infection in Crohn's disease. Gut 1980; 21:202–207.

78. Yoshimura HH, Estes MK, Graham DY. Search for evidence of a viral aetiology for inflammatory bowel disease. Gut 1984; 25:347–355.

79. Phillpotts RJ, Hermon-Taylor J, Brooke BN. Virus isolation studies in Crohn's disease: a negative report. Gut 1979; 20:1057–1062.

80. O'Morain C, Prestage H, Harrison P, Levi AJ, Tyrrell DA. Cytopathic effects in cultures inoculated with material from Crohn's disease. Gut 1981; 22:823–826.

81. Chiba M, McLaren LC, Strickland RG. Immunity to cytopathic agents associated with Crohn's disease: a negative study. Gut 1982; 23:333–339.

82. Das KM, Valenzuela I, Morecki R. Crohn disease lymph node homogenates produce murine lymphoma in athymic mice. Proc Natl Acad Sci U S A 1980; 77:588–592.

83. Zuckerman MJ, Valenzuela I, Williams SE, Kadish AS, Das KM. Persistence of an antigen recognized by Crohn's disease sera during in vivo passage of a Crohn's disease–induced lymphoma in athymic nude mice. J Clin Lab Med 1984; 104:69–76.

84. Das KM, Simon MR, Valenzuela I, Weinstock JV, Marcuard SM. Serum antibodies from patients with Crohn's disease and from their household members react with murine lymphomas induced by Crohn's disease tissue filtrates. J Clin Lab Med 1986; 107:95–100.

85. Bagchi S, Baral B, Das KM. Isolation and characterization of Crohn's disease tissue-specific glycoproteins. Gastroenterology 1986; 91:326–332.

86. Manzione NC, Bagchi S, Das KM. Demonstration of Crohn's disease tissue-specific proteins by enzyme-linked immunosorbent assay (ELISA). Dig Dis Sci 1987; 32:593–597.

87. Wakefield AJ, Fox JD, Sawyerr AM, Taylor JE, Sweenie CH, Smith M, Emery VC, Hudson M, Tedder RS, Pounder RE. Detection of herpesvirus DNA in the large intestine of patients with ulcerative colitis and Crohn's disease using the nested polymerase chain reaction. J Med Virol 1992; 38:183–190.

88. VanKruiningen HJ, Colombel JF, Cartun RW, Whitlock RH, Koopmans M, Kangro HD, Hoogkamp-Korstanje AA, Lecomte-Houcke M, Devred M, Paris JC, Cortot A. An in-depth study of Crohn's disease in two French families. Gastroenterology 1993; 104:351–360.

89. Lindberg E, Magnusson K-E, Tysk C, Jarnerot G. Antibody (IgG, IgA, and IgM) to baker's yeast (*Saccharomyces cerevisiae*), yeast mannan, gliadin, ovalbumin and betalactoglobulin in monozygotic twins with inflammatory bowel disease. Gut 1992; 33:909–913.

90. McKenzie H, Main J, Pennington CR, Parratt D. Antibody to selected strains of *Saccharomyces cerevisiae* (baker's and brewer's yeast) and *Candida albicans* in Crohn's disease. Gut 1990; 31:536–538.

91. Young CA, Sonnenberg A, Burns EA. Lymphocyte proliferation to baker's yeast in Crohn's disease. Digestion 1994; 55:40–43.
92. Giaffer MH, Clark A, Holdsworth CD. Antibodies to *Saccharomyces cerevisiae* in patients with Crohn's disease and their possible pathogenic importance. Gut 1992; 33:1071–1075.
93. Kirsner JB. Experimental "colitis" with particular reference to hypersensitivity reactions in the colon. Gastroenterology 1961; 40:307–312.
94. Stenson WF. Animal models of inflammatory bowel disease. In: Targan SR, Shanahan F, eds. Inflammatory Bowel Disease. From Bench to Bedside. Baltimore: Williams & Wilkins, 1994:180–192.
95. Sartor RB. Insights into the pathogenesis of inflammatory bowel diseases provided by new rodent models of spontaneous colitis. Inflammatory Bowel Diseases 1995; 1:64–75.
96. Fiocchi C. Cytokines and animal models: a combined path to inflammatory bowel disease pathogenesis. Gastroenterology 1993; 104:1202–1219.
97. Madara JL, Podolsky DK, King NW, Seghal PK, Moore R, Winter HS. Characterization of spontaneous colitis in cotton-top tamarins (*Saguinus oedipus*) and its response to sulfa-salazine. Gastroenterology 1985; 88:13–19.
98. Sundberg JP, Elson CO, Bedigian H, Berkenmeier EH. Spontaneous, heritable colitis in a new substrain of C3H/HeJ mice. Gastroenterology 1994; 107:1726–1735.
99. Mitchell IC, Turk JL. An experimental model of granulomatous bowel disease. Gut 1989; 30:1371–1378.
100. McCall RD, Haskill S, Zimmermann EM, Lund PK, Thompson CR, Sartor RB. Tissue interleukin-1 and interleukin-1 receptor antagonist expression in enterocolitis in resistant and susceptible rats. Gastroenterology 1994; 106:960–972.
101. Bhan AK, Mizoguchi E, Mizogushi A. New models of chronic intestinal inflammation. Curr Opin Gastroenterol 1994; 10:633–638.
102. Hammer RE, Maika SD, Richardson JA, Tang J-P, Taurog JD. Spontaneous inflammatory disease in transgenic rats expressing HLA-B27 and human b2m: an animal model of HLA-B27–associated human disorders. Cell 1990; 1099–1112.
103. Powrie F, Leach MW, Mauze S, Cadde LB, Coffman RL. Phenotypically distinct subsets of CD4+ T cells induce or protect from chronic intestinal inflammation in C. B-17 SCID mice. Int Immunol 1993; 5:1461–1471.
104. Mombaerts P, Mizoguchi E, Grusby MG, Glimcher LH, Bhan AK, Tonegawa S. Spontaneous development of inflammatory bowel disease in T cell receptor mutant mice. Cell 1993; 75:275–282.
105. Cooper HS, Murthy SNS, Shah RS, Sedergran DJ. Clinocopathologic study of dextran sulfate sodium experimental murine colitis. Lab Invest 1993; 69:238–249.
106. Piguet P-F, Grau GE, Allet B, Vassalli P. Tumor necrosis factor–cachectin is an effector of skin and gut lesions of the acute phase of graft-vs-host disease. J Exp Med 1987; 166:1280–1289.
107. Reinshagen M, Patel A, Sottili M, Nst C, Davis W, Mueller K, Eysselein VE. Protective function of extrinsic neurons in acute rabbit experimental colitis. Gastroenterology 1994; 106:1208–1214.
108. MacDermott RP, Stenson WF. Alterations of the immune system in ulcerative colitis and Crohn's disease. Adv Immunol 1988; 42:285–328.
109. Brandtzaeg P, Kett K, Halstensen TS, Helgeland L. Pathogenesis of ulcerative colitis and Crohn's disease: humoral immune mechanisms. Eur J Gastroenterol Hepatol 1990; 2:256–265.
110. Mayer L. Mucosal immune system in inflammatory bowel disease. In: MacDermott RP, Stenson WF, eds. Inflammatory Bowel Disease. New York: Elsevier, 1992:53–75.
111. Fiocchi C. New Concepts of pathogenesis in inflammatory bowel disease. In: Collins SM, Martin F, McLeod RS, Targan SR, Wallace JL, Williams CN, eds. Inflammatory Bowel Disease. Basic Research, Clinical Implications and Trends in Therapy. Lancaster: Kluwer Academic Publishers, 1994:243–261.

112. Elson CO, McCabe RP. The immunology of inflammatory bowel disease. In: Kirsner JB, Shorter RG, eds. Inflammatory Bowel Disease. Baltimore: Williams & Wilkins, 1995:203–251.

113. Selby WS, Jewell DP. T Lymphocytes subsets in inflammatory bowel disease: peripheral blood. Gut 1983; 24:99–105.

114. Yuan S-Z, Hanauer SB, Kluskens LS, Draft SC. Circulating lymphocyte subpopulations in Crohn's disease. Gastroenterology 1983; 85:1313–1318.

115. Strickland RG, Korsmeyer S, Soltis RD, Wilson ID, Williams RC. Peripheral blood T and B cells in chronic inflammatory bowel disease. Gastroenterology 1974; 67:569–577.

116. Pallone F, Montano S, Fais S, Boirivant M, Signore A, Pozzilli P. Studies of peripheral blood lymphocytes in Crohn's disease. Scand J Gastroenterol 1983; 18:1003–1008.

117. Raedler A, Fraenkel S, Klose G, Seyfarth K, Thiele HG. Involvement of the immune system in the pathogenesis of Crohn's disease. Gastroenterology. 1985; 88:978–983.

118. Raedler A, Schreiber S, Weerth Ad, Voss A, Peters S, Greten H. Assessment of in vivo activated T cells in patients with Crohn's disease. Hepatogastroenterology 1990; 37:67–71.

119. Fiocchi C. Mucosal cellular immunity. In: Targan SR, Shanahan F, eds. Immunology and Immunopathology of the liver and Gastrointestinal Tract. New York: Igaku-Shoin, 1990:107–138.

120. Meuwissen SGM, Feltkamp-Vroom TM, DelaRiviere AB, VondemBorne AEG, Tytgat GN. Analysis of the lympho-plasmacytic infiltrate in Crohn's disease with special reference to identification of lymphocyte-subpopulations. Gut 1976; 17:770–780.

121. Selby WS, Janossy G, Bofill M, Jewell DP. Intestinal lymphocyte subpopulations in inflammatory bowel disease: an anlysis by immunohistological and cell isolation technique. Gut 1984; 25:32–40.

122. Brandtzaeg P, Valnes K, Scott H, Rognum TO, Bjerke K, Baklien K. The human gastrointestinal secretory immune system in health and disease. Scand J Gastroenterol 1985; 20(suppl 114):17–38.

123. Pallone F, Fais S, Squarcia O, Biancone L, Pozzilli P, Boirivant M. Activation of peripheral blood and intestinal lamina propria lymphocytes in Crohn's disease. In vivo state of activation and in vitro response to stimulation as defined by the expression of early activation antigens. Gut 1987; 28:745–753.

124. Schreiber S, MacDermott RP, Raedler A, Pinnau R, Bertovich MJ, Nash GS. Increased activation of isolated intestinal lamina propria mononuclear cells in inflammatory bowel disease. Gastroenterology 1991; 101:1020–1030.

125. Matsuura T, West GA, Youngman KR, Klein JS, Fiocchi C. Immune activation genes in inflammatory bowel disease. Gastroenterology 1993; 104:448–458.

126. Kanof ME, James SP, Strober W. The phenotype and function of T cells in the lamina propria of the human intestine. Reg Immunol 1988; 1:190–195.

127. MacDonald TT. The role of activated T lymphocytes in gastrointestinal disease. Clin Exp Allergy 1990; 20:247–252.

128. Ferreira RDC, Forsyth LE, Richman PI, Wells C, Spencer J, MacDonald TT. Change in the rate of crypt epithelial cell proliferation and mucosal morphology induced by a T-cell–mediated response in human small intestine. Gastroenterology 1990; 98:1255–1263.

129. Lionetti P, Breese E, Braegger CP, Murch SH, Taylor J, MacDonald TT. T-cell activation can induce either mucosal destruction or adaptation in cultured human fetal small intestine. Gastroenterology 1993; 105:373–381.

130. Aisenberg J, Ebert EC, Mayer L. T-cell activation in human intestinal mucosa: the role of superantigens. Gastroenterology 1993; 105:1421–1430.

131. Kay RA. The potential role of superantigens in inflammatory bowel disease. Clin Exp Immunol 1995; 100:4–6.

132. Cuvelier CA, DeWever N, Meliants H, DeVos M, Veys EM, Roles H. Expression of T cell receptor $\alpha\beta$ and $\gamma\delta$ in the ileal mucosa of patients with Crohn's disease and with spondyloarthropathy. Clin Exp Immunol 1992; 90:275–279.

133. Fukushima K, Masuda T, Ohtani H, Sasaki I, Funayama Y, Matsuno S, Nagura H. Immuno-histochemical characterization, distribution, and ultrastructure of lymphocytes bearing T-cell receptor γδ in inflammatory bowel disease. Gastroenterology 1991; 101:670–678.

134. Posnett DN, Schmelkin I, Burton DA, August A, McGrath H, Mayer LF. T cell antigen receptor V gene usage. Increases in Vβ8+ T cells in Crohn's disease. J Clin Invest 1990; 85:1770–1776.

135. Spencer J, Choy MY, MacDonald TT. T cell receptor Vβ expression by mucosal T cells. J Clin Pathol 1991; 44:915–918.

136. Shalon L, Gulwani-Akolkar B, Fisher SE, Akolkar PN, Panja A, Mayer L, Silver J. Evidence for an altered T-cell receptor repertoire in Crohn's disease. Autoimmunity 1994; 17:301–307.

137. Gulwani-Akolkar B, Shalon L, Akolkar PN, Fisher SE, Silver J. Analysis of the peripheral blood T-cell receptor (TCR) repertoire in monozygotic twins discordant for Crohn's disease. Autoimmunity 1994; 17:241–248.

138. Kett K, Rognum TO, Brandtzaeg P. Mucosal subclass distribution of immunoglobulin G–producing cells is different in ulcerative colitis and Crohn's disease of the colon. Gastro-enterology 1987; 93:919–924.

139. Yacyshyn BR, Pilarski LM. Expression of CD45RO on circulating CD19+ B-cells in Crohn's disease. Gut 1993; 34:1698–1704.

140. Yacyshyn BR, Lazarovits A, Tsai V, Matejko K. Crohn's disease, ulcerative colitis, and normal intestinal lymphocytes express integrins in dissimar patterns. Gastroenterology 1994; 107:1364–1371.

141. Gardiner KR, Crockard AD, Halliday MI, Rowlands BJ. Class II major histocompatibility complex antigen expression on peripheral blood monocytes in patients with inflammatory bowel disease. Gut 1994; 35:511–516.

142. Rugtveit J, Brandtzaeg P, Halstensen TS, Fausa O, Scott H. Increased macrophage subsets in inflammatory bowel disease: apparent recruitment from peripheral blood monocytes. Gut 1994; 35:669–674.

143. Kitahora T, Suzuki K, Asakura H, Yoshida T, Suematsu M, Watanabe M, Aiso S, Tsuchiya M. Active oxygen species generated by monocytes and polymorphonuclear cells in Crohn's disease. Dig Dis Sci 1988; 33:951–955.

144. Baldassano RN, Schreiber S, Johnston RB, Fu RD, Muraki T, MacDermott RP. Crohn's disease monocytes are primed for accentuated release of toxic oxygen metabolites. Gastro-enterology 1993; 105:60–66.

145. Knutson L, Ahrenstedt O, Odlind B, Hallgren R. The jejunal secretion of histamine is increased in active Crohn's disease. Gastroenterology 1990; 98:849–854.

146. Fox CC, Lichtenstein LM, Roche JK. Intestinal mast cell responses in idiopathic inflammatory bowel disease. Dig Dis Sci 1993; 38:1105–1112.

147. Selby WS, Janossy G, Mason DY, Jewell DP. Expression of HLA-DR antigens by colonic epithelium in inflammatory bowel disease. Clin Exp Immunol 1983; 53:614–618.

148. Mayer L, Shlien R. Evidence for function of Ia molecules on gut epithelial cells in man. J Exp Med 1987; 166:1471–1483.

149. Mayer L, Eisenhardt D. Lack of induction of suppressor T cells by intestinal epithelial cells from patients with inflammatory bowel disease. J Clin Invest 1990; 86:1255–1260.

150. Chiba M, Iizuka M, Horie Y, Ishii N, Masamune O. Expression of HLA-DR antigens on colonic epithelium around lymph follicles. An anomalous expression in Crohn's disease. Dig Dis Sci 1994; 39:83–90.

151. Geboes K, Rutgeerts P, Ectors N, Mebis J, Penninckx F, Vantrappen G, Desmet VJ. Major histocompatibility class II expression on the small intestinal nervous system in Crohn's disease. Gastroenterology 1992; 103:439–447.

152. Gauldie J, Jordana M, Cox G, Ohtoshi T, Dolovich J, Denburg J. Fibroblasts and other structural cells in airway inflammation. Am Rev Respir Dis 1992; 145:S14–S17.

153. Graham MF. Stricture formation. In: MacDermott RP, Stenson W, Eds. Inflammatory Bowel Disease. New York: Elsevier, 1992:323–335.

154. Graham MF, Drucker DEM, Diegelmann RF, ElsonCO. Collagen synthesis by human intestinal smooth muscle cells in culture. Gastroenterology 1987; 92:400–405.

155. Stallmach A, Schuppan D, Riese HH, Matthes H, Rieken EO. Increased collagen type III synthesis by fibroblasts isolated from strictures of patients with Crohn's disease. Gastroenterology 1992; 102:1920–1929.

156. Matthes H, Herbst H, Schuppan D, Stallmach A, Milani S, Stein H, Riecken E-O. Cellular localization of procollagen gene transcripts in inflammatory bowel disease. Gastorenterology 1992; 102:431–442.

157. Strong SA, Klein JS, West GA, Fiocchi C. Activation of intestinal mesenchymal cells by IL1b induces inflammatory cytokine and procollagen gene expression. Gastroenterology 1993; 104:A784.

158. Fiocchi C. IBD: progress in pathogenesis. Can J Gastroenterol 1993; 7:110–114.

159. Fiocchi C. Cytokines. In: Targan SR, Shanahan F, Eds. Inflammatory Bowel Disease. From Bench to Bedside. Baltimore: Williams & Wilkins, 1994:106–122.

160. Fiocchi C, Binion DG, Katz JA. Cytokine production in the human gastrointestinal tract during inflammation. Curr Opin Gastroenterol 1994; 2:639–644.

161. Sartor RB. Cytokines in intestinal inflammation: pathophysiological and clinical considerations. Gastroenterology 1994; 106:533–539.

162. Herfarth HH, Sartor RB. Cytokine regulation of experimental intestinal inflammation. Curr Opin Gastroenterol 1994; 10:625–632.

163. Fiocchi C, Podolsky DK. Cytokines and growth factors in inflammatory bowel disease. In: Kirsner JB, Shorter RG, eds. Inflammatory Bowel Disease. Baltimore: Williams & Wilkins, 1995:252–280.

164. Fiocchi C, Hilfiker ML, Youngman KR, Doerder NC, Finke JH. Interleukin 2 activity of human intestinal mucosal mononuclear cells. Decreased levels in inflammatory bowel disease. Gastroenterology 1984; 86:734–742.

165. Kusugami K, Matsuura T, West GA, Youngman KR, Rachmilewitz D, Fiocchi C. Loss of interleukin-2-producing intestinal CD4$^+$ T cells in inflammatory bowel disease. Gastroenterology 1991; 101:1594–1605.

166. Kusugami K, Youngman KR, West GA, Fiocchi C. Intestinal immune reactivity to interleukin 2 differs among Crohn's disease, ulcerative colitis and control. Gastroenterology 1989; 97:1–9.

167. Gurbindo C, Sabbah S, Menezes J, Justinich C, Marchand R, Seidman EG. Interleukin-2 production in pediatric inflammatory bowel disease: evidence for dissimilar mononuclear cell function in Crohn's disease and ulcerative colitis. J Pediatr Gastroenterol Nutr 1993; 17:247–254.

168. Mullin GE, Lazenby AJ, Harris ML, Bayless TM, James SP. Increased interleukin-2 messenger RNA in the intestinal mucosal lesions of Crohn's disease but not ulcerative colitis. Gastroenterology 1992; 102:1620–1627.

169. James SP. Remission of Crohn's disease after human immunodeficiency virus infection. Gastroenterology 1988; 95:1667–1669.

170. Sparano JA, Brandt LJ, Dutcher JP, DuBois JS, Atkins MB. Symptomatic exacerbation of Crohn disease after treatment with high-dose interleukin-2. Ann Intern Med 1993; 118:617–618.

171. Rubin LA, Nelson DL. The soluble interleukin-2 receptor: biology, function, and clinical application. Ann Intern Med 1990; 113:619–627.

172. Mueller C, Knoflach P, Zielinski CC. T-cell activation in Crohn's disease. Increased levels of soluble interleukin-2 receptor in serum and supernatants of stimulated peripheral blood mononuclear cells. Gastroneterology 1990; 98:639–646.

173. Crabtree JE, Juby LD, Heatley RV, Lobo AJ, Bullimore DW, Axon ATR. Soluble interleukin-2

receptor in Crohn's disease: relation of serum concentrations to disease activity. Gut 1990; 31:1033–1036.

174. Brynskov J, Tvede N. Plasma interleukin-2 and soluble/shed interleukin-2 receptor in serum of patients with Crohn's disease. Effect of cyclosporin. Gut 1990; 31:795–799.

175. Matsuura T, West GA, Klein JS, Ferraris L, Fiocchi C. Soluble interleukin 2, CD8 and CD4 receptors in inflammatory bowel disease. A comparative study of peripheral blood and intestinal mucosal levels. Gastroenterology 1992; 102:2006–2014.

176. Capobianchi MR, Fais S, diPaolo MC, Agostini D, Paoluzi P, Pallone F, Dianzani F. Absence of circulating interferon in patients with inflammatory bowel disease. Suggestion against an autoimmune etiology. Clin Exp Immunol 1992; 90:85–87.

177. Lieberman BY, Fiocchi C, Youngman KR, Sapatnekar WK, Proffitt MR. Interferon γ production by human intestinal mucosal mononuclear cells. Decreased levels in inflammatory bowel disease. Dig Dis Sci 1988; 33:1528–1536.

178. Fais S, Capobianchi MR, Pallone F, DiMarco P, Boirivant M, Dianzani F, Torsoli A. Spontaneous release of interferon γ by intestinal lamina propria lymphocytes in Crohn's disease. Kinetics of in vitro response to interferon γ inducers. Gut 1991; 32:403–407.

179. Capobianchi MR, Fais S, Mercuri F, Boirivant M, Dianzani F, Pallone F. Interferon-alpha (IFN-α) production by human intestinal mononuclear cells. Response to virus in control subjects and in Crohn's disease. Gut 1992; 33:897–901.

180. Breese E, Braegger CP, Corrigan CJ, Walker-Smith JA, MacDonald TT. Interleukin-2– and interferon-γ–secreting T cells in normal and diseased human intestinal mucosa. Immunology 1993; 78:127–131.

181. Fais S, Capobianchi MR, Silvestri M, Mercuri F, Pallone F, Dianzani F. Interferon expression in Crohn's disease patients: increased interferon-γ and -α mRNA in the intestinal lamina propria mononuclear cells. J Interferon Research 1994; 14:235–238.

182. Schreiber S, Heinig T, Panzer U, Reinking R, Bouchard A, Stahl PD, Raedler A. Impaired response of activated mononuclear phagocytes to interleukin 4 in inflammatory bowel disease. Gastroenterolgoy 1995; 108:21–33.

183. Schreiber S, Heinig T, Thiele H-G, Raedler A. Immunoregulatory role of interleukin 10 in patients with inflammatory bowel disease. Gastroenterology 1995; 108:1434–1444.

184. Satsangi J, Wolstencroft RA, Cason J, Ainly CC, Dumonde DC, Thompson RPH. Interleukin 1 in Crohn's disease. Clin Exp Immunol 1987; 67:594–605.

185. Brynskov J, Hansen MB, Reimert C, Bendtzen K. Inhibitor of interleukin-1α and interleukin-1β–induced T-cell activation in serum of patients with active Crohn's disease. Dig Dis Sci 1991; 36:737–742.

186. Ligumsky M, Simon PL, Karmeli F, Rachmilewitz D. Role of interleukin 1 in inflammatory bowel disease–enhanced production during active disease. Gut 1990; 31:686–689.

187. Mahida YR, Wu K, Jewell DP. Enhanced production of interleukin 1-β by mononuclear cells isolated from mucosa with active ulcerative colitis and Crohn's disease. Gut 1989; 30:835–838.

188. Youngman KR, Simon PL, West GA, Cominelli F, Rachmilewitz D, Klein JS, Fiocchi C. Localization of intestinal interleukin 1 activity, protein and gene expression to lamina propria cells. Gastroenterology 1993; 104:749–758.

189. Gionchetti P, Campieri M, Belluzzi A, Paganelli GM, Bertinelli E, Ferretti M, Lauri A, Biasco G, Poggioli G, Miglioli M, Barbara L. Macrophage subpopulations and interleukin-1β tissue levels in pelvic ileal pouches. Eur J Gastroenterol Hepatol 1994; 6:217–222.

190. Casini-Raggi V, Kam L, Chong YJT, Fiocchi C, Pizarro TT, Cominelli, F. Mucosal imbalance of interleukin-1 and interleukin-1 receptor antagonist in inflammatory bowel disease: a novel mechanism of chronic imflammation. J Immunol 1995; 154:2434–2440.

191. Arend WP. Interleukin-1 receptor antagonism. J Clin Invest 1991; 88:1445–1451.

192. Dinarello CA, Thompson RC. Blocking IL-1: interleukin 1 receptor antagonist in vivo and in vitro. Immunol Today 1991; 12:404–410.

193. Chomarat P, Vannier E, Dechanet J, Rissoan MC, Banchereau J, Dinarello CA, Miossec P. Balance of IL-1 receptor antaganost/IL-1β in rheumatoid synovium and its regulation by IL-4 and IL-10. J. Immunol 1995; 154:1432–1439.

194. Mansfield JC, Holden H, Tarlow JK, DiGiovane FS, McDowell TL, Wilson AG, Holdsworth CD, Duff GW. Novel genetic association between ulcerative colitis and the anti-inflammatory cytokine interleukin-1 receptor antagonist. Gastroenterology 1994; 106:637–642.

195. Mahida YR, Kurlak L, Gallager A, Hawkey CJ. High circulating levels of interleukin 6 in active Crohn's disease but not ulcerative colitis. Gut. 1991; 32:1531–1534.

196. Gross V, Andus T, Caesar I, Roth M, Scholmerich J. Evidence for continuous stimulation of interleukin-6 production in Crohn's disese. Gastroenterology 1992; 102:514–519.

197. Hymas JS, Fitzgerald JE, Treem WR, Wyzga N, Kreutzer DL. Relationship of functional antigenic interleukin 6 to disease activity in inflammatory bowel disease. Gastroenterology 1993; 104:1285–1292.

198. Schurmann G, Betzler M, Post S, Herfarth C, Meuer S. Soluble interleukin-2 receptor, interleukin-6 and interleukin-1β in patients with Crohn's disease and ulcerative colitis: preoperative levels and postoperative changes of serum concentrations. Digestion 1992; 51:51–59.

199. Stevens C, Walz G, Singaram C, Lipman ML, Zanker B, Muggia A, Antonioli D, Peppercorn MA, Strom TB. Tumor necrosis factor-α, interleukin-1β, and interleukin-6 expression in inflammatory bowel disease. Dig Dis Sci 1992; 37:818–826.

200. Isaacs KL, Sarotr RB, Haskill S. Cytokine messenger RNA profiles in inflammatory bowel disease mucosa detected by polymerase chain reaction amplification. Gastroenterology 1992; 103:1587–1595.

201. Reinecker H-C, Steffen M, Witthoeft T, Pflueger I, Schreiber S, MacDermott RP, Raedler A. Enhanced secretion of tumour necrosis factor-alpha, IL-6, and IL-1β by isolated lamina propria mononuclear cells from patients with ulcerative colitis and Crohn's disease. Clin Exp Immunol 1993; 94:174–181.

202. Kusugami K, Fukatsu A, Tanimoto M, Shinoda M, Haruta J-I, Kuroiwa A, Ina K, Kanayama K, Ando T, Matsuura T, Yamaguchi T, Morise K, Ieda M, Iokawa H, Ishihara A, Sarai S. Elevation of interleukin-6 in inflammatory bowel disease is macrophage-and epithelial cell-dependent. Dig Dis Sci In press.

203. Mahida YR, Ceska M, Effenberger F, Kurlak L, Lindley I, Hawkey CJ. Enhanced synthesis of neutrophil-activating peptide-I/interleukin-8 in active ulcerative colitis. Clin Sci 1992; 82:273–275.

204. Izzo RS, Witkon K, Chen AI, Hadjiyane C, Weinstein MI, Pellecchia C. Interleukin-8 and neutrophil markers in colonic mucosa from patients with ulcerative colitis. Am J Gastroenterol 1992; 87:1447–1452.

205. Izzo RS, Witkon K, Chen AI, Hadjiyane C, Weinstein MI, Pellecchia C. Neutrophil-activating peptide (interleukin-8) in colonic mucosa from patients with Crohn's disease. Scand J Gastroenterol 1993; 28:296–300.

206. Mitsuyama K, Toyonaga A, Sasaki E, Watanabe K, Tateishi H, Nishiyama T, Saiki T, Ikeda H, Tsuruta O, Tanikawa K. IL-8 as an important chemoattractant for neutrophils in ulcerative colitis and Crohn's disease. Clin Exp Immunol 1994; 96:432–436.

207. Reinecker H-C, Loh EY, Ringler DJ, Metha A, Rombeau JL, MacDermott RP. Monocyte-chemoattractant protein 1 gene expression in intestinal epithelial cells and inflammatory bowel disease mucosa. Gastroenterology 1995; 108:40–50.

208. Izutani R, Loh EY, Reinecker H-C, Ohno Y, Fusunyan RD, Lichtenstein GR, Rombeau JL, MacDermott RP. Increased expression of interleukin-8 mRNA in ulcerative colitis and Crohn's disease mucosa and epithelial cells. Inflammatory Bowel Diseases 1995; 1:37–47.

209. Murch SH, Lamkin VA, Savage MO, Walker-Smith JA, MacDonald TT. Serum concentrations of tumour necrosis factor α in childhood chronic inflammatory bowel disease. Gut 1991; 32:913–917.

210. Hymas JS, Treem WR, Eddy E, Wyzga N, Moore RE. Tumor necrosis factor-α is not elevated in children with inflammatory bowel disease. J Pediatr Gastroenterol Nutr 1991; 12:233–236.

211. Braegger CP, Nicholls S, Murch SH, Stephens S, MacDonald TT. Tumour necrosis factor alpha in stool as a marker of intestinal inflammation. Lancet 1992; 339:89–91.

212. Murch SH, Braegger CP, Walker-Smith JA, MacDonald TT. Location of tumor necrosis factor α by immunohistochemistry in chronic inflammatory bowel disease. Gut 1993; 34:1705–1709.

213. Olson AD, Ayass M, Chensue S. Tumor necrosis factor and IL-1β expression in pediatric patients with inflammatory bowel disease. J Pediatr Gastroenterol Nutr 1993; 16:241–246.

214. MacDonald TT, Hutchings P, Choy M-Y, Murch S, Cooke A. Tumour necrosis factor-alpha and interferon-gamma production measured at the single cell level in normal and inflamed human intestine. Clin Exp Immunol 1990; 81:301–305.

215. Breese EJ, Michie CA, Nicholls SW, Murch SH, Williams CB, Domizio P, Walker-Smith JA, MacDonald TT. Tumor necrosis factor α–producing cells in the intestinal mucosa of children with inflammatory bowel disease. Gastroenterology 1994; 106:1455–1466.

216. Boughton-Smith N, Pettipher R. Lipid mediators and cytokines in inflammatory bowel disease. Eur J Gastroenterol Hepatol 1990; 2:241–245.

217. Stenson WF. Role of eicosanoids as mediators of inflammation in inflammatory bowel disease. Scand J Gastroenterol 1990; 25(suppl 172):13–18.

218. Sharon P, Ligumsky M, Rachmilewitz D, Zor U. Role of prostaglandins in ulcerative colitis, enhanced production during active disease and inhibition by sulfasalazine. Gastroenterology 1978; 75:638–640.

219. Sharon P, Stenson WF. Enhanced synthesis of leukotriene B4 by colonic mucosa in inflammatory bowel disease. Gastroenterology 1984; 86:453–460.

220. Lauritsen K, Laursen LS, Bukhave K, Rask-Madsen J. In vivo profiles of eicosanoids in ulcerative colitis, Crohn's colitis, and *Clostridium difficile* colitis. Gastroenterology 1988; 95:11–17.

221. Wardle TD, Hall L, Turnberg LA. Use of coculture of colonic mucosal biopsies to investigate the release of eicosanoids by inflamed and uninflamed mucosa from patients with inflammatory bowel disease. Gut 1992; 33:1644–1651.

222. Casellas F, Guarnier F, Antolin M, Rodriguez R, Salas A, Malagelada J-R. Abnormal leukotriene C4 release by unaffected jejunal mucosa in patients with inactive Crohn's disease. Gut 1994; 35:517–522.

223. Peeters M, D'Haens G, Ceuppens J, Peetermans W, Geboes K, Rutgeerts P. Increased proinflammatory cytokine production in macroscopically normal ileum and colon in Crohn's disease. Gastroenterology 1995; 108:A891.

224. Stenson WF, Cort D, Rodgers J, Bukaroff R, DeSchryver-Kecskemeti K, Gramlich TL, Beeken W. Dietary supplementation with fish oil in ulcerative colitis. Ann Intern Med 1992; 116:609–614.

225. Reichlin S. Neurondocrine-immune interactions. N Engl J Med 1993; 329:1245–1253.

226. Sternberg EM, Chrousos GP, Wilder RL, Gold PW. The stress response and the regulation of inflammatory disease. Ann Intern Med 1992; 117:854–866.

227. Ottaway CA. Vasoactive intestinal peptide as a modulator of lymphocyte and immune function. Ann N Y Acad Sci 1988; 527:486–500.

228. Boirivant M, Fais S, Annibale B, Agostini D, Fave GD, Pallone F. Vasoactive intestinal polypeptide modulates the in vitro immunoglobulin A production by intestinal lamina propria lymphocytes. Gastroenterology 1994; 106:576–582.

229. Wiedermann CJ, Sacerdote P, Propst A, Propst T, Judmaier G, Kathrein H, Vogel W, Panerai A. Decreased β-endorphin content in peripheral blood mononuclear leukocytes from patients with Crohn's disease. Brain Behav Immun 1994; 8:261–269.

230. Bishop AE, Polak JM, Bryant MG, Bloom SR, Hamilton S. Abnormalities of vaso-

active intestinal polypeptide-containing nerves in Crohn's disease. Gastroenterology 1980; 79:853–860.

231. Manyth CR, Gates TS, Zimmerman RP, Welton ML, Passaro EP, Vigna SR, Maggio JE, Kruger L, Manyth PW. Receptor binding sites for substance P, but not substance K or neuromedin K, are expressed in high concentrations by arterioles, venules, and lymph nodes in surgical specimens obtained from patients with ulcerative colitis and Crohn disease. Proc Natl Acad Sci U S A 1988; 85:3235–3239.

232. Kubota Y, Petras RE, Ottaway CA, Tubbs RR, Farmer RG, Fiocchi C. Colonic vasoactive intestinal peptide nerves in inflammatory bowel disease. A digitized morphometric immuno-histochemical study. Gastroenterology 1992; 102:1242–1251.

233. Reubi JC, Mazzuchelli L, Laissue JA. Intestinal vessels express a high density of somatostatin receptors in human inflammatory bowel disease. Gastroenterology 1994; 106:951–959.

234. Mazumdar S, Das KM. Immunohistochemical localization of vasoactive intestinal peptide and substance P in the colon from normal subjects and patients with inflammatory bowel disease. Am J Gastroenterol 1992; 87:176–181.

235. Bernstein CN, Robert ME, Eysselein VE. Rectal substance P concentrations are increased in ulcerative colitis but not in Crohn's disease. Am J Gastroenterol 1993; 88:908–913.

236. Grisham MB, Granger DN. Neutrophil-mediated mucosal injury. Role of reactive oxygen metabolites. Dig Dis Sci 1988; 33:6S–15S.

237. Curran FT, Allan RN, Keighley MRB. Superoxide production by Crohn's disease neutrophils. Gut 1991; 32:399–402.

238. Gionchetti P, Campieri M, Guarnieri C, Belluzzi A, Brignola C, Bertinelli E, Ferretti M, Miglioli M, Barbara L. Respiratory burst of circulating polymorphonuclear leukocytes and plasma elastase levels in patients with inflammatory bowel disease in remission. Dig Dis Sci 1994; 39:550–554.

239. Anton PA, Targan SR, Shanahan F. Increased neutrophil receptors for and response to the proinflammatory bacterial peptide formyl-methionyl-leucyl-phenylalanine in Crohn's disease. Gastroenterology 1989; 97:20–28.

240. Simmonds NJ, Allen RE, Stevens TRJ, Niall R, Someren MV, Blake DR, Rampton DS. Chemiluminescence assay of mucosal reactive oxygen metabolites in inflammatory bowel disease. Gastroenterology 1992; 103:186–196.

241. Sandhu IS, Grisham MB. Modulation of neutrophil function as a mode of therapy for gastrointestinal inflammation. In: Academic Press, 1993:51–67.

242. Emerit J, Pelletier S, Tosoni-Verlignue D, Mollet M. Phase II trial of copper zinc super-oxide dismutase (CuZnSOD) in treatment of Crohn's disease. Free Radic Biol Med 1989; 7:145–149.

243. Snook J. Are the inflammatory bowel diseases autoimmune disorders? Gut 1990; 31:961–963.

244. Shorter RG, Huizenga A, Spencer RT. A working hypothesis for the etiology and pathogenesis of inflammatory bowel disease. Am J Dig Dis 1972; 17:1024–1032.

245. Broberger O, Perlmann P. Experimental studies of ulcerative colitis. I. Reactions of serum from patients with human fetal colon cells in tissue culture. J Exp Med 1963; 117:705–715.

246. Lagercrantz R, Hammarström S, Perlmann P, Gustafsson BE. Immunological studies in ulcerative colitis. III. Incidence of antibodies to colon-antigen in ulcerative colitis and other gastrointestinal diseases. Clin Exp Immunol 1966; 1:263–276.

247. Thayer WR, Brown M, Sangree MH, Katz J, Hersh T. *Escherichia coli* O:14 and colon hem-agglutinating antibodies in inflammatory bowel disease. Gastroenterology 1969; 57:311–318.

248. Rabin B, Roger SJ. A cell-mediated immune model of inflammatory bowel disease in the rabbit. Gastroenterology 1978; 75:29–33.

249. Mayer L, Panja A, Lin Y, Siden E, Pizzimenti A, Gerardi F, Chandswang N. Unique features of antigen presentation in the intestine. Ann N Y Acad Sci 1992; 664:39–46.

250. Takahashi F, Das KM. Isolation and characterization of a colonic autoantigen specifically

recognized by colon tissue–bound immunoglobulin G from Idiopathic ulcerative colitis. J Clin Invest 1985; 76:311–318.

251. Das KM, Sakamaki S, Vecehi M, Diamond B. The production and characterization of monoclonal antibodies to a human colonic antigen associated with ulcerative colitis: cellular localization of the antigen by using the monoclonal antibody. J Immunol 1987; 139:77–84.

252. Roche JK, Fiocchi C, Youngman K. Sensitization to epithelial antigens in chronic mucosal inflammatory disease. Characterization of human intestinal mucosa–derived mononuclear cells reactive with purified epithelial cell–associated components in vitro. J Clin Invest 1985; 75:522–530.

253. Fiocchi C, Roche JK, Michener WM. High prevalence of antibodies to intestinal epithelial antigens in patients with inflammatory bowel disease and their relatives. Ann Intern Med 1989; 110:786–794.

254. Perlmann P, Broberger O. In vitro studies of ulcerative colitis. II. Cytotoxic action of white blood cells from patients on human fetal colon cells. J Exp Med 1963; 117:717–733.

255. Kemler BJ, Alpert JE. Inflammatory bowel disease: a study of cell-mediated cytotoxicity for isolated human colonic epithelial cells. Gut 1980: 21:353–359.

256. Shorter RG, McGill DB, Bahn RC. Cytotoxicity of mononuclear cells for autologous colonic epithelial cells in colonic diseases. Gastroenterology 1984; 86:13–22.

257. Shanahan F, Targan SR. Mechanisms of tissue injury in inflammatory bowel disease. In: Targan SR, Shanahan F, eds. Inflammatory Bowel Disease: From Bench to Bedside. Baltimore: Williams and Wilkins, 1994:78–88.

258. Gibson PR, VandePol E, Pullman W, Doe WF. Lysis of colonic epithelial cells by allogeneic mononuclear and lymphokine-activated killer cells derived from peripheral blood and intestinal mucosa: evidence against a pathogenic role in inflammatory bowel disease. Gut 1988; 29:2076–1084.

259. Korsmeyer S, Strickland RG, Wilson ID, Williams RC. Serum lymphocytotoxic and lymphocytophilic antibody activity in inflammatory bowel disease. Gastroenterology 1974; 67:578–583.

260. Strickland RG, Friedler EM, Henderson CA, Wilson ID, Williams RC. Serum lymphocytotoxins in inflammatory bowel disease. Studies of frequency and specificity for lymphocyte subpopulations. Clin Exp Immunol 1975; 21:384–393.

261. Brown DJ, Jewell DP. Cold-reactive lymphocytotoxins in Crohn's disease and ulcerative colitis. I. Incidence and characterization. Clin Exp Immunol 1982; 49:67–74.

262. Korsmeyer SJ, Williams RC, Wilson ID, Strickland RG. Lymphocytotoxic antibody in inflammatory bowel disease: a family study. N Engl J Med 1975; 293:1117–1120.

263. Pelham HRB. Speculations on the function of the major heat shock and glucose regulated proteins. Cell 1986; 46:959–961.

264. Kaufmann SHE. Heat Shock proteins and the immune response. Immunol Today 1990; 11:129–136.

265. Young D, Lathigra R, Hendrix R, Sweetser D, Young RA. Stress proteins are immune targets in leprosy and tuberculosis. Proc Natl Acad Sci U S A 1988; 85:4267–4270.

266. Szewczuk MR, Depew WT. Evidence for T lymphocyte reactivity to the 65 kilodalton heat shock protein of mycobacterium in active Crohn's disease. Clin Invest Med 1992; 15:494–505.

267. Markesich DC, Sawai ET, Butel JS, Graham DY. Investigations on the etiology of Crohn's disease. Humoral immune responses to stress (heat shock) proteins. Dig Dis Sci 1991; 36:454–460.

268. Elsaghier A, Prantera C, Bothamley G, Wilkins E, Jindal S, Ivanyi J. Disease association of antibodies to human and mycobacterial HSP70 and HSP60 stress proteins. Clin Exp Immunol 1992; 89:305–309.

269. Baca-Estrada ME, Gupta RS, Stead RH, Croitoru K. Intestinal expression and cellular immune responses to human heat-shock protein 60 in Crohn's disease. Dig Dis Sci 1994; 39:498–506.

270. Springer TA. Adhesion receptors of the immune system. Nature 1990; 346:425–434.
271. Cronstein BC, Weissmann G. The adhesion molecules of inflammation. Arthritis Rheum 1993; 36:147–157.
272. Greenfield SM, Hamblin A, Punchard NA, Thompson RPH. Expression of adhesion molecules on circulating leucocytes in patients with inflammatory bowel disease. Clin Sci 1992; 83:221–226.
273. Mishra L, Mishra BB, Harris M, Bayless TM, Muchmore AV. In vitro cell aggregation and cell adhesion molecules in Crohn's disease. Gastroenterology 1993; 104:772–779.
274. Pooley N, Ghosh L, Sharon P. Up-regulation of E-selectin and intercellular adhesion molecule-1 differs between Crohn's disease and ulcerative colitis. Dig Dis Sci 1995; 40:219–225.
275. Nielsen OH, Langholz E, Hendel J, Brynskov J. Circulating soluble intercellular adhesion molecule-1 (sICAM-1) in active inflammatory bowel disease. Dig Dis Sci 1994; 39:1918–1923.
276. Malizia G, Calabrese A, Cottone M, Raimondo M, Trejdosiewicz LK, Smart CJ, Oliva L, Pagliaro L. Expression of leukocyte adhesion molecules by mucosal mononuclear phagocytes in inflammatory bowel disease. Gastroenterology 1991; 100:150–159.
277. Schuermann GM, Auer-Bishop AE, Facer P, Lee JC, Rampton DS, Dore CJ, Polak, JM. Altered expression of cell adhesion molecules in uninvolved gut in inflammatory bowel disease. Clin Exp Immunol 1993; 94:341–347.
278. Koizumi M, King N, Lobb R, Benjamin C, Podolsky DK. Expression of vascular adhesion molecules in inflammatory bowel disease. Gastroenterology 1992; 103:840–847.
279. Podolsky DK, Lobb R, King N, Benjamin CD, Pepinsky B, Seghal P, deBeaumont M. Attenuation of colitis in the cotton-top tamarin by anti-alpha4 integrin monoclonal antibody. J Clin Invest 1993; 92:372–380.
280. Halstensen TS, Mollnes TE, Brandtzaeg P. Persistent complement activation in submucosal vessels of active inflammatory bowel disease: immunohistochemical evidence. Gastroenterology 1989; 97:10–19.
281. Halstensen TS, Mollnes TE, Fausa O, Brandtzaeg P. Deposits of terminal complement complex (TCC) in muscularis mucosae and submucosal vessels in ulcerative colitis and Crohn's disease of the colon. Gut 1989; 30:261–366.
282. Halstensen TS, Mollnes TE, Garred P, Fausa O, Brandtzaeg P. Epithelial deposition of immunoglobulin G1 and activated complement (C3b and terminal complement complex) in ulcerative colitis. Gastroenterology 1990; 98:1264–1271.
283. Halstensen TS, Mollens TE, Garred P, Fausa O, Brandtzaeg P. Surface epithelium related activation of complement differs in Crohn's disease and ulcerative colitis. Gut 1992; 33:902–908.
284. Ahrenstedt O, Knutson L, Nilsson B, Nilsson-Ekdahl K, Odlind B, Hallgren R. Enhanced local production of complement components in the small intestines of patients with Crohn's disease. N Engl J Med 1990; 322:1345–1349.
285. Ambrose NS, Johnson M, Burdon DW, Keighley MRB. Incidence of pathogenic bacteria from mesenteric lymph nodes and ileal serosa during Crohn's disease. Br J Surg 1984; 71:623–625.
286. Adenis A, Colombel J-F, Lecouffe P, Wallaert B, Hecquet B, Marchandise X, Cortot A. Increased pulmonary and intestinal permeability in Crohn's disease. Gut 1992; 33:678–682.
287. Bjarnason I, O'Morain C, Levi AJ, Peters TJ. Absorption of 51-chromium-labelled ethylenediaminetetraacetate in inflammatory bowel disease. Gastroenterology 1983; 85:318–322.
288. Hollander D, Vadheim C, Brettholz E, Pettersen GM, Delahunty T, Rotter JI. Increased intestinal permeability in patients with Crohn's disease and their relatives. Ann Intern Med 1986; 105:883–885.
289. Pearson AD, Eastman Ej, Laker MF, Craft AW, Nelson R. Intestinal permeability in children with Crohn's disease and coeliac disease. BMJ 1982; 285:20–21.
290. Hollander D. Crohn's disease—a permeability disorder of the tight junction? Gut 1988; 29:1621–1624.

291. Ainsworth M, Eriksen J, Rasmussen JW, Schaffalitzkydemuckadel OB. 51Cr-labelled ethyl-enediaminetetraacetic acid in patients with Crohn's disease and their healthy relaives. Scand J Gastro 1985; 24:993–998.

292. Katz KD, Hollander D, Vadheim CM, McElree C, Delahunty T, Dadufalza VD, Krugliak P, Rotter JI. Intestinal permeability in patients with Crohn's disease and their healthy relatives. Gastroenterology 1989; 97:927–931.

293. Ruttenberg D, Young GO, Wright JP, Isaacs S. PEG-400 excretion in patients with Crohn's disease, their first-degree relatives, and healthy volunteers. Dig Dis Sci 1992; 37:705–708.

294. Teahon K, Smethurst P, Levi AJ, Menzies IS, Bjarnason I. Intestinal permeability in patients with Crohn's disease and their first degree relatives. Gut 1992; 33:320–323.

295. May GR, Sutherland LR, Meddings JB. Is small intestinal permeability really increased in relatives of patients with Crohn's disease? Gastroenterology 1993; 104:1627–1632.

296. Katz KD, Hollander D, Vadheim CM, McElree C, Delahunty T, Dadufalza VD, Krugliack P, Rotter JI. Intestinal permeability in patients with Crohn's disease and their healthy relatives. Gastroenterology 1989; 97:927–931.

297. Peeters M, Geypens B, Ghoos Y, Nevens H, D'Haens G, Hiele H, Rutgeerts P. The pattern of increased small intestinal permeability abnormalities in families with Crohn's disease: genetic or non-genetic? Gastroenterology 1995; 108:A892.

298. Koenigs KP, McPhedran P, Spiro HM. Thrombosis in inflammatory bowel disease. J Clin Gastroenterol 1987; 9:627–631.

299. Wakefield AJ, Dhillon AP, Rowles PM, Sawyerr AM, Pittilo RM, Lewis AAM, Pounder RE. Pathogenesis of Crohn's disease: multifocal gastrointestinal infarction. Lancet 1989; 2:1057–1062.

300. Wakefield AJ, Sankey EA, Dhillon AP, Sawyerr AM, More L, Sim R, Pittilo RM, Rowles PM, Hudson M, Lewis AAM, Pounder RE. Granulomatous vasculitis in Crohn's disease. Gastroenterology 1991; 100:1279–1287.

301. Hudson M, Piasecki C, Sankey EA, Sim R, Wakefield AJ, More LJ, Sawyerr AF, Dhillon AP, Pounder RE. A ferret model of acute multifocal gastrointestinal infarction. Gastroenterology 1992; 102:1591–1596.

302. Wakefield AJ, Sawyerr AM, Hudson M, Dhillon AP, Pounder RE. Smoking, the oral contraceptive pill, and Crohn's disease. Dig Dis Sci 1991; 36:1147–1150.

303. Wakefield AJ, Pittilo RM, Sim R, Cosby SL, Stephenson JR, Dhillon AP, Pounder RE. Evidence of persistent measles virus infection in Crohn's disease. J Med Virol 1993; 39:345–353.

304. Ekbom A, Helmick C, Zack M, Adami HO. The epidemiology of inflammatory bowel disease: a large, population-based study in Sweden. Gastroenterology 1991; 100:350–358.

305. Ekbom A, Zack M, Adami HO, Helmick HO. Is there clustering of inflammatory bowel disease at birth? Am J Epidemiol 1991; 134:876–886.

306. Ekbom A, Wakefiled A, Zack M, Adami HO. The role of perinatal measles infection in the aetiology of Crohn's disease: a population based epidemiological study. Lancet 1994; 344:508–510.

307. Wurzelmann JI, Lyles CW, Sandler RS. Childhood infection and the risk of inflammatory bowel disease. Gastroenterology 1992; 102:A30.

308. Wakefield AJ, Ekbom A, Dhillon AP, Pittilo RM, Pounder RE. Crohn's disease: pathogenesis and persistent measles virus infection. Gastroenterology 1995; 108:911–916.

309. Rutgeerts P, Goboes K, Peeters M, Hiele M, Penninckx F, Aerts R, Kerremans R, Vantrappen G. Effect of faecal stream diversion on recurrence of Crohn's disease in the neoterminal ileum. Lancet 1991; 2:771–774.

310. Nasmyth DG, Godwin PG, Dixon MF, Williams NS, Johnston D. Ileal ecology after pouch-anal anastomosis or ileostomy. Gastroenterology 1989; 96:817–824.

311. Clausen MR, Tvede M, Mortensen PB. Short-chain fatty acids in pouch contents from patients with and without pouchitis after ileal pouch–anal anastomosis. Gastroeneterology 1992; 103:1144–1153.

312. Ruseler-van-Embden JGH, Schouten WR, vanLieshout LMC. Pouchitis: result of microbial imbalance? Gut 1994; 35:658–664.

313. Workman EM, Jones VA, Wilson AJ, Hunter JO. Diet in the management of Crohn's disease. Hum Nutr Appl Nutr 1984; 38:469–473.

314. Jones VA, Workman EM, Dickenson RJ, Hunter JO. Crohn's disease: maintenance of remission diet. Lancet 1985; 2:77–80.

315. Riordan AM, Hunter JO, Cowan RE, Crampton JR, Davidson AR, Dickenson RJ, Dronfield MW, Fellows IW, Hishon S, Kerrigan HJ, McGouran RC, Neale G, Saunders JH. Treatment of active Crohn's disease by exclusion diet: East Anglian multicentre controlled trial. Lancet 1993; 342:1131–1134.

316. Teahon K, Bjarnason I, Pearson M, Levi AJ. Ten years' experience with an elemental diet in the management of Crohn's disease. Gut 1990; 31:1133–1137.

317. Teahon K, Smethurst P, Pearson M, Levi AJ, Bjarnason I. The effect of elemental diet on intestinal permeability and inflammation in Crohn's disease. Gastroenterology 1991; 101:84–89.

318. Rigaud D, Cosnes J, LeQuintrec Y, Rene E, Gendre JP, Mignon M. Controlled trial comparing two types of enteral nutrition in treatment of active Crohn's disease: elemental vs polymeric diet. Gut 1991; 32:1492–1497.

319. Royall D, Jeejeebhoy KN, Baker JP, Allard JP, Habal FM, Cunnane SC, Greenberg GR. Comparison of amino acid vs peptide based enteral diets in active Crohn's disease: clinical and nutritional outcome. Gut 1994; 35:783–787.

320. Fernandez-Banares F, Cabre E, Gonzalez-Huix F, Gassull MA. Enteral nutrition as primary therapy in Crohn's disease. Gut 1994; (suppl 1):S55–S59.

321. Podolsky DK, Isselbacher KJ. Composition of human colonic mucin. Selective alteration in inflammatory bowel disease. J Clin Invest 1983; 72:142–153.

322. Podolsky DK, Isselbacher KJ. Glycoprotein composition of colonic mucosa. Specific alterations in ulcerative colitis. Gastroenterology 1984; 87:991–998.

323. Raouf A, Parker N, Ryder S, Langdon-Brown B, Milton JD, Walker R, Rhodes JM. Ion exchange chromatography of purified colonic glycoproteins in inflammatory bowel disease: absence of a selective subclass defect. Gut 1991; 32:1139–1145.

324. Rhodes JM, Black RR, Savage A. Altered lectin binding by colonic epithelial glycoconjugates in ulcerative colitis and Crohn's disease. Dig Dis Sci 1988; 33:1359–1363.

COMMENTARY

Derek P. Jewell   *Radcliffe Infirmary, Oxford, England*

How does one piece together a variable clinical picture, the conflicting reports of specific infective agents, the association with smoking, an inexorable tendency to relapse, and a genetic tendency that cannot yet be described in terms of specific genes? Added to this confusion are diverse immunological findings, the role of inflammatory mediators, and observations on neuroendocrine involvement. The potential for chronic disease inducing secondary effects, and the modulating effect on pathogenetic mechanisms of therapeutic endeavors, do not make our understanding any easier. Of course, Crohn's disease may reflect a number of individual diseases with similar phenotypes but with different etiologies. However, our present state of understanding is such that even this possibility sheds little light on the matter.

It is perhaps worth beginning with the clinical course, namely the tendency for disease to recur. The cumulative recurrence rate following resection with anastomosis is well documented, and it is not influenced to any consistent degree by the extent of resection (i.e., whether macroscopic disease is resected with wide margins or by limited resection).

Furthermore, colonoscopy has shown that recurrence occurs within months of resection (1) but may be delayed by corticosteroids (2), 5-aminosalicylic acid (3), or metronidazole (4), although these therapeutic observations are by no means firmly established. It has often been argued that the whole of the intestinal mucosa is abnormal in Crohn's disease and that overt disease breaks out at certain sites, possibly as a result of local stasis. However, as we now know that there is increased trafficking of mucosal lymphocytes in situations of inflammation, it is possible that an increase in mucosal cell populations in areas remote from overt inflammation is merely secondary to this trafficking. The mild increase in colonic mucosal lymphocytes in patients with untreated celiac disease may be a very good example of this phenomenon.

Evidence implicating the fecal stream in the pathogenesis of the disease has become increasingly strong. The importance of intestinal continuity has been emphasized by the observation that Crohn's disease of the colon often goes into remission following fecal diversion (5), in contrast to ulcerative colitis, which shows no such response. More recently this finding has been confirmed (6) in patients having an ileal or ileocecal resection with an ileostomy proximal to the anastomosis. Serial colonoscopic observations showed that there was no endoscopic recurrence in the neoterminal ileum in the subsequent months, but lesions rapidly occurred following closure of the ileostomy. Furthermore, two studies have shown that the instillation of ileostomy contents into the isolated colon initiated a variety of immunological and biochemical changes, and one of the studies suggested that particles greater than 20 nm in size were responsible as ultrafiltrates of ileostomy effluent had no effect (7,8). It is therefore hard to ignore the conclusion that luminal contents play a major role in the pathogenesis of Crohn's disease. Bacteria are clearly one possible factor, and the beneficial effects of metronidazole suggests a role for anaerobes: metronidazole has been shown to be more effective than placebo in treating active disease (9), is equivalent to sulfasalazine (10), and delays endoscopic recurrence following ileocecal resection (4). However, metronidazole has effects other than antibacterial effects, including immunological effects, so it is simplistic to conclude with any certainty that reducing the anaerobe population is the cause of the therapeutic benefit.

Can one fit into this hypothesis the other pathogenetic observations? *Mycobacterium paratuberculosis* is perhaps the easiest, assuming that it genuinely occurs in at least some patients with the disease. We know that not all patients with Crohn's disease have granulomas, although, admittedly, the frequency of granulomas is very dependent on the intensity of the histological search, and that *M. paratuberculosis* can occasionally be detected in water or milk supplies (11). Therefore, it is possible that the organism may be a secondary invader into mucosa that is already inflamed and could then be expected to set up a granulomatous inflammation. This hypothesis predicts that the number of invading organisms from contaminated milk would be minute and might therefore explain the difficulty we have in detecting them. Against this hypothesis is the fact that if an *M. paratuberculosis* organism invaded the colonic mucosa of a patient with ulcerative colitis, then all cases of granulomatous colitis should have an anatomical distribution similar to that of the original colitis. Nevertheless, the hypothesis remains to be disproven.

The evidence for measles virus as an etiological agent is currently so weak that it hardly merits discussion. The virus is known to be ubiquitous, but it is possible to postulate that if inflammation occurred in areas of intestinal mucosa in which measles virus was present as a "slow virus," then it might modulate the nature of the inflammatory response. It would neatly explain the presence of granulomas in the walls of blood vessels (12) and lymphatics (13).

These hypotheses still beg the question as to why a factor (or factors) in the intestinal lumen initiates an inflammatory response in the first place. That is not easily answered but would conceivably be due to permeability abnormalities in the epithelium—induced by genetic factors, drugs, or smoking—or by an immunoregulatory abnormality, which might also be under genetic control. However, if one or the other (or even both) of these mechanisms were operating, then inflammation might be initiated and would then be influenced by luminal contents, bacterial and antigenic absorption, and finally by ischemia secondary to vascular damage induced by cytokines and inflammatory mediators. Even absorption of silicates from toothpaste might occur through an inflamed epithelium and influence the nature of the inflammatory response!

Whether it is helpful to spin hypotheses that attempt to bring together a number of apparently disparate strands of evidence is debatable. In the meantime, better understanding of the many pathogenetic mechanisms so well reviewed by Drs. Katz and Fiocchi is essential. Identification of susceptibility genes in linkage studies using either the candidate gene approach or a systematic search of the genome with microsatellite markers should provide an enormous step forward in our understanding of the disease process.

REFERENCES

1. Rutgeerts P, Geboes K, Vantrappen G, Kerremans R, Coenegrachts JL, Coremans G. Natural history of recurrent Crohn's disease at the ileo-colonic anastomosis after curative surgery. Gut 1984; 25:665–672.
2. Budesonide Study Group. Unpublished observations.
3. McLeod RS, Wolff BG, Steinhart AH, et al. Prophylactic mesalamine treatment decreases post-operative recurrence in Crohn's disease. Gastroenterology 1995; 109: 404–413.
4. Rutgeerts P, Hiele M, Geboes K, et al. Controlled trial of metronidazole treatment for prevention of Crohn's disease recurrence after ileal resection. Gastroenterology 1995; 108:1617–1621.
5. Harper PH, Truelove SC, Lee ECG, Kettlewell MGW, Jewell DP. Split ileostomy and ileocolostomy for Crohn's disease of the colon and ulcerative colitis: a 20 year survey. Gut 1983; 24:106–113.
6. Rutgeerts P, Geboes K, Peeters M. Effect of faecal stream diversion on recurrence of Crohn's disease in the neoterminal ileum. Lancet 1991; 338:771–774.
7. Harper PH, Lee ECG, Kettlewell MGW, Bennett BK, Jewell DP. Role of the faecal stream in the maintenance of Crohn's disease. Gut 1985; 26:279–284.
8. Winslett MC, Andrews H, Allan RN, Keighley MR. Faecal diversion in the management of Crohn's disease of the colon. Dis Colon Rectum 1993; 36:757–762.
9. Sutherland LR, Singleton J, Sessions J, Hanauer SB. Double-blind placebo controlled trial of metronidazole in Crohn's disease. Gut 1991; 32:1071–1075.
10. Ursing B, Alm T, Barany F, Bergelin I, Ganrot-Norlin K. A comparative study of metronidazole and sulphasalazine for active Crohn's disease: the Cooperative Crohn's Disease Study in Sweden II Result. Gastroenterology 1982; 83:550–562.
11. Sanderson JD. Environmental factors—bacterial infection: Crohn's disease and *Mycobacterium paratuberculosis*. In: Monteiro E, Tavarela Velosa F, eds. Inflammatory Bowel Disease. Dordrecht/Boston/London: Kluwer Academic Publishers, 1995:86–90.
12. Wakefield AJ, Sankey EA, Dhillon AP, et al. Granulomatous vasculitis in Crohn's disease. Gastroenterology 1991; 100:1279–1287.
13. Talbot IC, Kamm MA, Leaker BR. Crohn's disease—granulomatous lymphangitis rather than vasculitis. Gut 1992; 33:W32.

3
Epidemiology of Crohn's Disease

Anders Ekbom   *Uppsala University, Uppsala, Sweden*

Crohn's disease is not a new clinical entity, although it was not until 1932 that Dr. Burrill B. Crohn and collaborators introduced the term regional ileitis for the disease to which Crohn's name was later given (1). There were, however, earlier reports. In 1913, a Scottish surgeon, Kenneth Dalziel, reported nine patients with a new entity described as "chronic intestinal enteritis and not tuberculosis" (2). In a retrospective study from Ireland, 29 cases of Crohn's disease were identified in the latter half of the 19th century (3). Crohn's disease also existed outside the British Isles at the beginning of the 20th century. In a retrospective study, we identified the earliest bona fide diagnosis of Crohn's disease in a 13-year-old patient who was operated on in 1918. A bypass procedure was performed because there was stenosis in the terminal ileum and the surgeon dismissed the diagnosis of tuberculosis as highly unlikely. The patient was operated on again in 1969 with a resection, and the histopathological examination revealed changes typical for Crohn's disease.

I. OCCURRENCE

A. Temporal Trends

Until the 1930s, there were only scattered case reports or case series published, and no assessments had been made of the annual incidence of Crohn's disease. Two retrospective incidence studies of Crohn's disease were performed starting from 1935. In one from Olmsted County, Minnesota (4), for the period 1935 to 1975, the authors estimated the annual incidence rate to be 1.9 per 100,000 which was considerably higher than an indicence rate of 0.2 for the period 1935 to 1945 in Cardiff, United Kingdon (5). Since these early studies, there has been an increasing number of incidence studies of Crohn's disease published every year, but they have generally dealt with small populations and the time periods studied have, in most cases, spanned less than ten years. This approach has led to an abundance of publications with little information except unreliable point estimates in which detection bias is a concern. Moreover, in most instances, the point estimates of the annual incidence are not comparable between different populations and time periods because the incidence rates have not been age-standardized and different case finding methods have been used. Some studies were population based (4–41) and others were based mainly or exclusively on hospitalized patients (42–56). It is, therefore, questionable whether more retrospective incidence studies done in a traditional way; that is, by counting "heads" for short periods in areas or populations without a prior assessment of the incidence will yield any additional information. Perhaps the manpower utilized in such studies could be directed in a better way in order to broaden our understanding of Crohn's disease.

There are remarkable similarities in the temporal trends for Crohn's disease in different populations during shifts from low-to high-incidence areas. In Fig. 1, six areas with an assessment of the annual incidence of Crohn's disease for 20 years or more have been summarized (4,5,7–10,13,16,22–24,28,30,31,34). Those figures should not be used to compare the annual incidence but they are a good illustration of the similarities in the temporal trends; the main difference among them is the point in time at which the incidence starts to increase. Although there is a continuous increase in the incidence in two populations in the United Kingdom (5,24), most incidence studies indicate that the annual incidence levels off between 4 and 7 per 100,000 inhabitants per year and, in some instances, a slight decrease ensues (13,16). This finding was confirmed in a study in which Crohn's disease mortality rates in Anglo-Saxon countries were studied. In that study, there was an increase in mortality until the beginning of the 1970s, followed by a decrease (57).

Because of the high incidence of Crohn's disease in the Scandinavian countries (except Finland) during the 1960s and later when compared with that of southern Europe, it has been hypothesized that a north–south gradient exists (24). This hypothesis is further substantiated by results from two studies from the United States. In one (58), Medicare discharge data was analyzed, thus confining the study to hospitalized patients older than

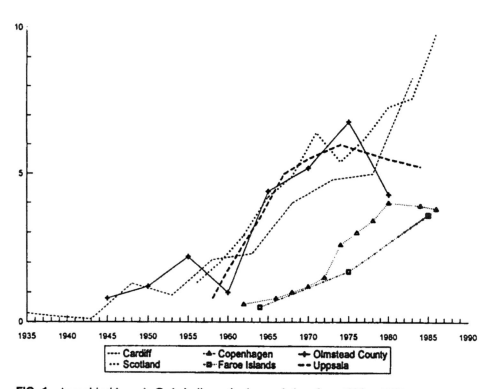

FIG. 1 Annual incidence in Crohn's disease in six populations from 1935 to 1987.

age 65 years. In other (59), data from the Department of Veteran Affairs was used. The results from both studies were in accordance with a north–south gradient in Crohn's disease in the United States. However, recently published data from southern countries of Europe, such as Italy (38,43), France (17), and the urban population in Spain (27), indicate that the north–south gradient has diminished during the last 10 years and has even, in some instances, disappeared. Countries with low GNP such as Portugal (55) and Greece (39) still have a very low incidence of Crohn's disease. One explanation is that this is an effect not from the climate but associated with the GNP or other dynamic exposures in the assessed populations. Moreover, recent data from eastern Europe (40) indicate that there is a very low incidence of Crohn's disease and that, in a European setting, a west–east gradient is perhaps of greater magnitude and interest than a north–south gradient.

There is a strong correlation in incidence between ulcerative colitis and Crohn's disease. Areas or populations with a high incidence or mortality rate attributable to ulcerative colitis also have a high incidence or mortality rate attributable to Crohn's disease and vice versa (60). Although misclassification exists, that is, some cases of Crohn's disease are misclassified as ulcerative colitis and vice versa, it is unlikely to be the only explanation for the correlation. Furthermore, there is a genetic association. Relatives of patients with ulcerative colitis are at higher risk both for ulcerative colitis and, to a lesser extent, for Crohn's disease (61–63). However, in populations or areas where information exists about the temporal trends for the two diseases, it is obvious that an increase in the incidence in ulcerative colitis precedes an increase in Crohn's disease. In Fig. 2, the annual incidence of ulcerative colitis and Crohn's disease is plotted from 1945 until 1983

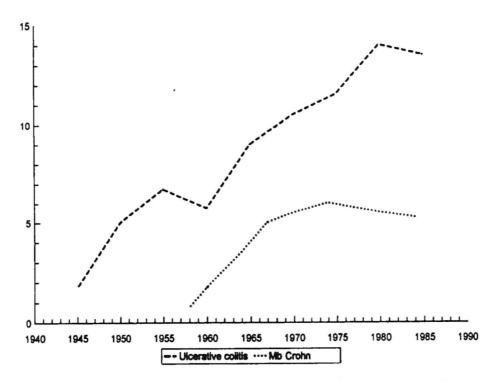

FIG. 2 Annual incidence in Crohn's disease and ulcerative colitis form 1945 to 1983 in Uppsala County, Sweden.

utilizing four different studies from Uppsala County, Sweden (7,13,31,64). This figure shows a time lag of about 15 to 20 years between an increase in incidence of ulcerative colitis and an increase in incidence of Crohn's disease. The same time lag is apparent in studies from Iceland (10,24), Copenhagen (9,30), and the Faroe Islands (8,34). The strong correlation between the two diseases and the genetic link indicates, at least partly, a common etiology. However, the time lag implies that some differences quantitatively and qualitatively in the exposure of interest also have to exist or that "the window of opportunity" differs in the two diseases.

The prevalence of Crohn's disease is often used to compare different populations and areas. However, Fig. 1 shows that prevalence figures in different populations are, to some extent, correlated to when there was a change in incidence because long-term survival among patients with Crohn's disease does not substantially differ from that of the normal population (65). Thus, populations with the same annual incidence can have great differences in the prevalence figures, and the prevalence of Crohn's disease in populations should not be used to compare the incidence.

B. Ethnicity

In areas with a high incidence of Crohn's disease, certain ethnic minorities, especially those with lower socioeconomic status, often have a lower annual incidence. This has been shown among blacks in Baltimore (50), Indian migrants in the United Kingdom (20), blacks in South Africa (41), and Bedouin Arabs in Israel (66). However, those differences do not always persist over time and there are examples in some populations of diminished differences (20,42,67).

In Crohn's original description (1), all 14 patients were Jewish (68). Although Crohn himself refuted the hypothesis of a special susceptibility for Crohn's disease among Jews (68), an association between Jewish ethnicity and an increased risk of Crohn's disease is still widely accepted. Jewish ethnicity has been implicated as a risk factor in at least five analytical epidemiological studies (11,19,41,68,69). There is, however, reason to raise concerns about the validity of the results in at least three of those studies. In the two Swedish studies (11,19), the nominator, that is, the number of subjects with Jewish ethnicity, was assessed mainly through the family name and the denominator was ascertained in a different manner, which could be the reason that excess risk was reported. The analysis done in South Africa (41) had similar drawbacks in that the denominator was ascertained through old census data. Moreover, incidence data from Israel (32,35) indicate that both the annual incidence and prevalence do not exceed the numbers reported from other high incidence areas such as Scandinavia. Moreover, Jews born either in North America or western Europe (32) seemed to be at higher risk compared with other subgroups. One likely explanation for the reports of a higher risk associated with Jewish ethnicity is, therefore, that the increase in annual incidence among Jews occurred earlier than in other populations. This hypothesis is, to some extent, refuted by the findings of a Los Angeles report (70) in which the authors found that Jews originating from middle Europe had an excess risk for Crohn's disease compared with those originating from Poland or Russia. The authors concluded that there is a subset of individuals of Jewish origin with an especially high genetic predisposition for Crohn's disease.

There have also been some concerns that Scandinavian descent should be associated with an increased risk of Crohn's disease (19). Scotland, Scandinavia, and Minnesota, all with large populations of Scandinavian descent, are areas with high annual incidence. The health care system in these areas has, however, many similarities, thus making it easier to conduct descriptive epidemiological studies with an optimal case ascertainment compared with other populations. This is probably, at least partly, one reason for the high incidence in those populations. Scattered reports exist of cases of Crohn's disease in South Korea (71), Japan (72), Kuwait (73), the West Indies (74), and South America (75). Time will tell if there will be an increase in incidence in those populations within the next 10 to 20 years, especially because there seem to be some indications of an increase in incidence in ulcerative colitis in some of those areas.

C. Age-Specific Incidence and Gender

A consistent finding in high incidence areas is a peak in the age-specific incidence of Crohn's disease in the age group of 20 to 30 year old (13,16,24). In Table 1, the age-specific incidence has been estimated in three centers in high-incidence areas (5,13,17), and the similarities in magnitude in Sweden and France are striking. It is also interesting that in low-incidence areas, the peak in the 20- to 30-year age group is missing and that, during periods of an increase of the annual incidence, the increase, in relative terms, is highest in this age group (5,27,31). Some studies have also reported a second, smaller peak in the older age groups (5,46), although other studies have failed to show such a peak (13,17,24). The presence of such a second peak has been questioned and it has been argued that the second peak represents a delayed diagnosis made when the disease once more manifests itself. The existence of undiagnosed cases of Crohn's disease has been shown to be present even in high-incidence areas (76). On the other hand, the increased incidence in Cardiff in the United Kingdon (5), which has one of the highest incidence rates reported, is entirely attributable to an increase in the older age groups (Table 1). It is unlikely that there would be so many overlooked cases in a population, and the existence of a second peak cannot be ruled out.

There is a female predominance in most incidence studies published so far (13,17,24). However, in this respect, there also seem to be differences in high-incidence areas compared with low-incidence areas. In low-incidence areas and during time periods with low incidence in most studies with a duration long enough to follow a shift from low to high incidence, there also seems to be a shift from an even sex distribution or from a male predominance toward a female predominance (31,38,40). Mortality data for Crohn's disease show the same pattern, a male predominance in countries with a low mortality rate for Crohn's disease and a female predominance in countries with a high mortality rate (60). There are also differences in the age-specific incidence rates for males and females in which the peak age in high-incidence areas is the age group with the highest female predominance.

TABLE 1   Age-Specific Incidence Rates in Crohn's Disease in Uppsala Health Care Region, Sweden, 1965–1983 (13), Northern France 1988–1990 (17), and Cardiff, UK, 1981–1985 (5)

Area	Age (years)							
	0–9	10–19	20–29	30–39	40–49	50–59	60–69	70–79
Uppsala	1.2	8.1	16.5	8.0	4.7	2.5	3.0	2.5
Northern France	0.5	6.0	12.5	5.5	4.0	3.0	2.0	2.5
Cardiff	—	6.0	14.5	8.2	5.2	6.2	12.5	10.5

D. Cohort Effects

In a major incidence study of Crohn's disease in Stockholm County by Hellers (19), the author noted a clear tendency that persons born after World War II were at higher risk for Crohn's disease compared with those born during or before World War II. This finding was confirmed in another retrospective incidence study in an adjacent region in Sweden; the authors found a similar cohort phenomena both for Crohn's disease and ulcerative colitis affecting persons born in 1945 and thereafter (13). Although two smaller studies, one from Sweden (26) and one from Denmark (30), failed to show any cohort effect, due to the small number of patients analyzed, these studies do not refute the existence of such an effect. The presence of a birth cohort effect would have important implications for the disease etiology because this would imply that exposures early in life were factors in an important "time window."

II. RISK FACTORS

In Table 2, those risk factors that have been associated with an increased risk of Crohn's disease in different analytical and ecological studies are listed. Several exposures have been implicated. However, the majority of those studies have been criticized based on the methodology used, such as the use of prevalent cases, use of control groups that are not representative of the background population, use of small samples, disregard of potential confounders, and overinterpretation of the results. Moreover, for most exposures, there is a lack of consistency in the results from different studies. A fair statement is, unfortunately, that there are still few established risk factors for Crohn's disease.

A. Familial Aggregation

Familial aggregation for Crohn's disease is, so far, the most established risk factor. A family history of Crohn's disease, especially, and of ulcerative colitis is associated with an increased risk of Crohn's disease (61–63). Familial aggregation of inflammatory bowel disease, especially Crohn's, has been extensively documented and a positive history of inflammatory bowel disease has been found in up to 23% of Ashkenazi Jews in

TABLE 2 Proposed Risk Factors Associated with Crohn's Disease

Familial aggregation	Stressful events
Nicotine	Early life exposures
Smoking	Weaning
Oral moist snuff	Hygiene
Oral contraceptives	Infections
Diet	Dairy products
Refined sugar	Passive smoking
Cereals (cornflakes)	"Sheltered child"
"Fast food"	Infections
Margarine	Mycobacteria
Baker's yeast	Measles
Physical activity	Nonspecific virus
Socioeconomic status	infections

California (77). In a twin study from Sweden (78), there was a high concordance rate for monozygotic twins, that is, 58.3% for Crohn's disease. The concordance rate for Crohn's disease is at the same level as found in diabetes and bronchial asthma (79). For dizygotic twins, the concordance rate was substantially lower (3.9%), indicating that the high concordance rate in monozygotic twins is mainly due to genetic factors and not environmental ones. Most of the concordant twin siblings developed Crohn's disease within a period of two years of each other, and the extent of the disease at presentation was similar in the twin pairs.

B. Smoking

A history of smoking is the most established environmental risk factor for Crohn's disease. The results of an abundance of analytical epidemiological studies have been consistent, showing an elevated risk between 2 and 5 times. Although there are reasons to criticize the methodology used in many of these studies (flaws in the control selection, small number of cases, and disregard of potential confounders in the analysis), the consistency in the results still indicates a causal relationship. In Table 3, the results of 10 studies are presented (80–89). Although the results are consistent for current smokers, the risk estimates for former smokers vary substantially. There is also a tendency toward a dose–response gradient that further strengthens the hypothesis of a causal relationship. However, the lack of a consistent increased risk among former smokers indicates that smoking is not an initiator of the disease but rather a promoting factor. Furthermore, individuals with Crohn's disease who continue to smoke have significantly more relapses, hospital admissions, surgery, pain, diarrhea, and changes in disease activity index compared with nonsmokers or former smokers (90,91). Moreover, the most established association in the epidemiological literature is that smoking causes lung cancer. A strong causal association between smoking and Crohn's disease would, therefore, lead to an increased risk of respiratory malignancies among patients with Crohn's disease. However, in most follow-up studies of Crohn's disease with regard to cancer morbidity and mortality, no such association has been found (92–94), which raises further doubts as to a strong etiological attributable fraction of smoking in Crohn's disease. Changes in smoking habits, especially in females, are therefore unlikely to be the underlying reason for the temporal trends and differences in the male to female ratio over time in Crohn's disease.

The interpretation of an association between Crohn's disease and smoking is further complicated because smoking seemingly decreases the risk of ulcerative colitis, yet former smokers seem to be especially at higher risk (95). These opposite findings for the two diseases have led some authors to speculate that smoking may determine the type of inflammatory bowel disease that develops in a previously exposed individual (87). This speculation, however, assumes that there is an otherwise common etiology of ulcerative colitis and Crohn's disease, which the differences in the temporal trends at least partly contradict.

In the case of ulcerative colitis, a good biological model to explain the protective effect of smoking is still lacking (95). In the case of Crohn's disease, however, an increased risk among smokers could be due to multifocal gastrointestinal infarction potentiated by cigarette smoke (96). Cigarette smoking is a risk factor for arteriosclerosis, and it has been shown to induce morphological injury to endothelial cells. This injury is associated with formation of microthrombi. If part of the pathogenic mechanism for Crohn's disease is due to multifocal gastrointestinal infarction and increased risk with Crohn's disease among

TABLE 3 Risk Estimates for Crohn's Disease for Smokers and Former Smokers Compared with Nonsmokers at Time of Diagnosis

Study (Reference)	Number of Subjects with Crohn's Disease	Risk Estimate for Current Smokers (95% CI)	Risk Estimate for Former Smokers (95% CI)	Dose Response	Type of Study	Case	Control
Benoni et al. 1987 (80)	155	2.18 (p < 0.001)	0.69	—	Case-control	Incident and prevalent	Population-based controls
Franceschi et al. 1987 (81)	109	4.2 (2.3–7.7)	3.5 (1.5–8.0)	Yes, amount and duration	Case-control	Incident and prevalent	Hospital-based controls
Katschinski et al. 1993 (82)	90	3.0 (1.3–6.8)	0.69 (0.1–4.4)	—	Case-control	Incident and prevalent	Population-based controls
Lindberg et al. 1988 (83)	144	2.2 (1.3–3.5)	1.9 (0.8–4.3)	No	Case-control	Prevalent	Population-based controls
Logan and Kay 1989 (84)	42	1.8 (0.9–3.3)	—	—	Cohort	—	—
Persson et al. 1990 (85)	260	Male 1.3 (0.7–2.6) Female 5.0 (2.7–9.2)	Male 1.2 (0.5–3.1) Female 1.0 (0.3–4.0)	Males, yes, duration and amount; Females, no	Case-control	Incident and prevalent	Population-based controls
Sandler et al. 1992 (86)	186	2.64 (1.22–5.75)	0.65 (0.14–2.94)	—	Case-control	Prevalent	Neighborhood controls
Somerville et al. 1984 (87)	81	4.8 (2.4–97)	—	—	Case-control	Prevalent	General Practitioner controls
Tobin et al. 1987 (88)	137	2.9 (1.8–4.9)	—	—	Case-control	Prevalent	General Practitioner controls
Vessey et al. 1986 (89)	18	Increased (p < 0.05)	Not increased	—	Cohort	—	—

smokers, at least partly, can be due to the increased risk for thrombotic vascular disease in smokers, then smoking should be regarded as a promoter and not an etiological agent.

Further credence for an independent association of nicotine and Crohn's disease was given in a Swedish study in which the use of oral moist snuff was analysed as a risk factor in a case-control setting (97). A significantly increased risk for Crohn's disease (relative risk [RR] = 2.1, 95% confidence interval [CI] 1.0–4.6) among users of moist snuff was found and the increased risk persisted even after adjusting for cigarette smoking. Furthermore, the results indicated a synergistic effect between use of moist snuff and smoking. The risk was not increased for snuff use alone but a marked potentiation was found among snuff dippers who were also cigarette smokers.

Exposure to passive smoking during childhood has also been implicated as a risk factor for both Crohn's disease and ulcerative colitis (98), but this result is not in accordance with another case-control study (85), and, in the case of ulcerative colitis, the result is contradicted in two other studies (85,99). Thus, the biological mechanism behind this association remains elusive, and, possibly, the result is likely to be confounded by other exposures during early life that might be associated with an increased risk for Crohn's disease.

C. Oral Contraceptives

At the end of the 1970s, case-reports began to emerge describing an association between the use of oral contraceptives and the occurrence of Crohn's disease (100). As in the smoking studies, those reports were followed by a number of analytical studies (82,84,86,89,101–105), but, in contrast to the smoking data, the results have not been consistent (103) and the point estimates were generally lower than those for smoking. There is also reason to believe that there is an interaction between oral contraceptive use and smoking; an elevated risk has, in some studies, only been found in subgroups of patients based on smoking. In one, the increased risk was only confined to women who were current smokers (86), whereas the opposite finding was reported in another study in which the risk was only present among nonsmokers (82). In a recently published case-control study (101), the authors further strengthen the hypothesis of an association by showing that oral contraceptive use for more than 6 years entailed a relative risk of 5.1 (95% CI 1.8–14.3), which persisted even after adjusting for race, smoking, income, and pregnancy history. However, there was no gradient in the risk when taking into account the estrogen potency. The attributable fraction of the impact of oral contraceptive use and Crohn's disease was also calculated in this study. The authors concluded that almost 16% of Crohn's disease in the American population was due to exposure of oral contraceptives. However, the authors used the highest point estimate ever reported for oral contraceptive use, not taking into account the inconsistencies in the results published so far. A potential mechanism for the role of oral contraceptive use and Crohn's disease could be similar to the one proposed for smoking, that is, multifocal gastrointestinal infarction mediated by chronic mesenteric vasculitis further aggravated by oral contraceptive use (96). In this respect, oral contraceptives should also be regarded as promoters and not as initiators of Crohn's disease.

Differential misclassification cannot be ruled out and the fact that two prospective cohort studies both entailed a less pronounced increased risk for oral contraceptive use indicates that such a bias may be operating. Furthermore, use of oral contraceptives does not seem to affect the recurrence rate or severity of the disease after diagnosis (106). Thus, the hypothesis that the emerging female predominance in Crohn's disease should be caused by the introduction of oral contraceptives (102) seems unlikely, especially because this pattern was evident before the introduction of oral contraceptives.

D. Diet

Because Crohn's disease mainly affects the gastrointestinal channel, it follows that different dietary exposures have been proposed as the major cause for the increase in incidence. However, no dietary ingredients have been consistently implicated as being associated with Crohn's disease. To assess the impact of dietary compounds and disease outcome, researchers are faced with methodologic difficulties because the exposure is most often assessed after diagnosis of disease and the information, therefore, has to be assembled retrospectively. In a Swedish review (107) of all dietary studies conducted up to the mid-1980s, taking into account especially the methodology, the authors were highly critical of the studies and they concluded, in essence, that the methodology used both in study design and in the data analysis made it impossible to infer anything from the results presented.

It is not unlikely that the symptoms in Crohn's disease prompt the patient to change dietary patterns toward a more easily digested diet. Therefore, consumption of refined sugar before or after the diagnosis of Crohn's disease has repeatedly been implicated as a risk factor (108–116). The increased sugar consumption could, however, be a secondary phenomena (108), a hypothesis that is further substantiated by the lack of any association in, at least, one study (117). Moreover, smoking is positively associated with sugar consumption and any analytic study should take that into account. There are two studies in which sugar intake and smoking were independent risk factors for Crohn's disease (110,116), but a combined exposure did not result in a further increase in the risk in one of the studies (110), either because of residual confounding or because those factors may operate through a common mechanism. Cornflakes (118) and fast food (119) have also been implicated as risk factors, results that so far have not been confirmed in other analytical studies.

Margarine has been proposed as a major risk factor, mainly because the introduction of margarine to the westernized world paralleled the beginning of the increase in the annual incidence of Crohn's disease. However, in an ecological study (119) comparing geographic and temporal variations of sugar and margarine consumption in relation to the mortality and incidence in Crohn's disease and sugar and margarine consumption. Finally, exposure to dietary yeast has also been implicated as being associated with an increased risk of Crohn's disease. Antibodies to bakers' yeast have been reported among patients with Crohn's disease but not with ulcerative colitis or other gastrointestinal disorders (120), and one report states that exposure to bakers' yeast affects the activity of Crohn's disease (121). This could, at least partly, be a secondary phenomenon and does not necessarily have any etiological implications.

E. Physical Activity

In an ecological study on mortality and inflammatory bowel disease in England and Wales during eight consecutive years (122), the author analysed occupational exposures in persons who had died from Crohn's disease. A low occurrence of Crohn's disease in men was found in occupations associated with physical work as well as lower social status and farming. A high mortality rate was associated with physically less demanding work, sedentary occupations, and types of work that are performed indoors. Similar results were found in two studies from Germany that studied disability from inflammatory bowel disease (123) and the occupational distribution among patients with Crohn's disease (124). These results were further substantiated in a Swedish analytical study in which the author analysed physical activity through the years preceding the diagnosis. The authors found a protective effect of 0.5 (95% CI 0.3–0.8) for regular daily physical activity compared with that of exercise performed less than weekly (105). Although the authors, by comparing current physical activity with reported physical activity, concluded that their finding was not due to differential underreporting, one has to question the reason for the lower physical activity among the cases before any inference of a casual relationship can be drawn, especially when an underlying biological mechanism has yet to be found.

F. Socioeconomic Status

In the first report of Crohn's disease (1) and the first analytical study (68), there was a finding of higher socioeconomic status as a risk factor for Crohn's disease. The existence of such an association was further strengthened by the lower incidence found among minority groups with lower socioeconomic status (50,67) and in that blue collar workers seem to be protected against Crohn's disease (122–124). However, at least two studies have reported a reverse finding, that is, an increased risk of Crohn's disease associated with low socioeconomic status (125,126). It is not unlikely that socioeconomic status, as such, is of no interest, but differences in socioeconomic status represent different exposures during different time periods or in different populations. That such confounding exists could be inferred from the results of a recently published study from the United Kingdom (127) in which access to a hot water tap during childhood was associated with a substantial increase of Crohn's disease (5.0, 95% CI 1.4–17.3), even after adjusting for socioeconomic status. Therefore, socioeconomic status should probably not be included as a risk factor for Crohn's disease, although it is evident from temporal trends that there are differences in occurrence between time periods and in different populations. These differences are most prominent during periods of increase in the annual incidence, which then can result in the spurious finding of socioeconomic status as a strong risk factor.

Residents of rural communities seem to be at lesser risk for development of Crohn's disease than residents of urban communities (13,24,27). However, urban communities often have better access to health care, and reports of such difference may, therefore, be due to ascertainment bias. However, in a case-control study for residency at time of birth using prospectively assembled data, no association between rural residence and the risk of Crohn's disease was found (126). Moreover, farmers had a significantly lower incidence of Crohn's disease in a study from the United Kingdom (122) but no difference was found in a Swedish study (105). This finding is of special interest because early contact with dairy products has been implicated as an excess risk to exposure to *Mycobacteria paratuberculosis* (128).

G. Stressful Events

An association between psychiatric factors and ulcerative colitis has sometimes been accepted as a causal association, and a similar model has been proposed for Crohn's disease. However, in an extensive review of 138 studies of psychiatric factors and their relation to ulcerative colitis (129), which, to a great extent also includes patients with Crohn's disease, the authors showed, convincingly, that there were serious methodological flaws in most of the studies. The methodological flaws were significantly related to findings of positive associations, and those studies that represented solid systematic investigations all failed to find any association. Although it is probably premature to disregard such an association, especially as a factor aggravating the disease as proposed in two recent studies (130,131), so far no follow-up study of patients with Crohn's disease has found an excess risk for suicide or other psychiatric disorder. On the contrary, patients with Crohn's disease do not seem to differ from the normal population with regard to social adjustment (132).

H. Early Life Exposures and Viral Infections

The notion that early exposures during childhood, perinatally, or even in utero have a causal association with the risk of Crohn's disease was introduced in the 1970s by Whorwell et al. (133). In a case-control study, the authors found that patients with Crohn's disease had a significantly increased incidence of gastroenteritis within the first six months of life independent of bottle-feeding. The authors speculated that the underlying mechanism included an introduction of a persistent pathogenic infection, which manifests later in life. Subacute sclerosing panencephalitis and chronic hepatitis were used as examples of similar mechanisms. A similar finding was reported 10 years later from Canada (134); the authors found an increased risk for Crohn's disease among subjects with a history of childhood diarrhea. Although recall bias is a concern, the fact that a third independent study from the United States found a similar association (135) lends further credence to the hypothesis that early events are of importance. Early weaning has also been proposed as an independent risk factor. Koletzko et al. (134) showed that not being breast fed was an independent risk factor, even after adjusting for childhood diarrhea, and this finding was confirmed in another case-control study in a Swedish setting (136). However, these results have not been consistent; at least five studies (105,125,126,133,135), among them one utilizing prospectively assembled data (126), have failed to show any such association.

The findings of an independent birth cohort effect instead of a period effect in two independent Swedish studies (13,19) also indicates that events early in life influence the risk of Crohn's disease. Furthermore, in one of those studies, the authors claimed that this cohort effect was entirely due to an increased number of future Crohn's disease patients born during the first half of the year (13). Further analysis of this patient cohort revealed significant clustering both by birth date and maternal residence at birth for 845 patients with Crohn's disease born in four counties in central Sweden (137). A similar analysis for ulcerative colitis showed a much weaker tendency toward clustering, indicating, at least partly, that there are different etiologies for the two diseases. The authors speculate that a maternal or a neonatal infection should be the underlying cause for this clustering phenomenon. The existence of an intrauterine or a perinatal exposure to infections was further substantiated by the same group in a case-control study using maternal charts to retrieve information of exposures during the pregnancy and the perinatal period (126). There was an eightfold risk of development of Crohn's disease after exposure to any health event. Viral infections in particular seemed to entail a strong association because those events were only recorded among cases. Influenza, varicella/herpes zoster, and measles were the pathogens specifically mentioned in the charts. There were two cases of measles in the mothers during the last trimester, which is of special interest because even during the prevaccination era, measles was a rare event in adults. It has been estimated that approximately 1 of 20,000 to 30,000 pregnancies during this time was complicated by measles, and two cases among less than 100 patients with Crohn's disease is therefore noteworthy.

The presence of viremia in pregnant women previously immunized either by vaccination or overt measles, was shown by an increased perinatal mortality rate among the offspring of asymptomatic pregnant women in Guinea Bissau who were exposed to measles (138). Therefore, to test whether a measles epidemic in the background population during women's last trimester of pregnancy was associated with an increased incidence in Crohn's disease among their offspring, further analyses were performed in central Sweden (139). Five epidemics of measles were identified during a 10-year period and, by using a time window of 3 months after the peak of the epidemic, the authors showed a 46% increased risk for Crohn's disease in the offspring, but no association was found for ulcerative colitis. Although it can be argued that a risk estimate of 1.5 does not indicate a causal relationship (140), probably only a minority of the expectant mothers in the population was exposed to measles, this the exposures could represent a major contribution to the attributable risk.

The long-term effects of early exposure to measles or inadequate response to measles leading to a persistent infection were shown in a Danish follow-up study among patients with a serologically proven measles infection but without a history of rash (141). Such a disease history indicates an altered immune response either due to early exposure or an incompetence in the immune system. In 252 patients who were followed up, there was one case of Crohn's disease combined with a sarcoidosis; three patients had anal fistula and one had a perianal abscess. The results from the analytical epidemiological studies mentioned previously (126,133–135) indicate that the infectious events associated with an increased risk for Crohn's disease are nonspecific. However, a detailed examination of specimens from 24 cases of Crohn's disease and 22 inflammatory and noninflammatory intestinal control subjects identified measles virus in the endothelium, lymphocytes, and macrophages of the inflammatory foci in Crohn's disease specimens but not in the control specimens (142). This finding implies that measles is specifically associated with Crohn's disease, although an early exposure to a nonspecific pathogen might be needed for a later persistent measles infection.

The proposed underlying biological mechanism is a vasculitis secondary to persistent measles infection in the endothelium. The finding of an association of smoking and oral contraceptive use with Crohn's disease, therefore, fits well into such a model. It is also the case with the finding of the relapse of the disease following restoration of the fecal stream after an ileostomy (143). The blood flow of the intestinal mucosa increases greatly from basal levels after restoration in response to local luminal contents, thus resulting in ischemia and infarction when the demand for blood exceeds the supply. This phenomenon may also explain the transient beneficial effects of an elementary or polymeric diet in patients with Crohn's disease.

There has been a dramatic increase in the incidence of Crohn's disease in children in Scotland in the last two decades (144). Because measles vaccination was introduced in the late 1960s in Scotland, this seemingly contradicts an association between measles infection and Crohn's disease. However, live attenuated measles virus was used in the vaccination process, and the increased incidence in children with Crohn's disease could, therefore, be an effect of the vaccination program. Further credence to this hypothesis is lent by the fact that children who first were subjected to the measles vaccination program in the United Kingdom seem to be a greater risk for Crohn's disease compared with nonvaccinated children (145). This seems to be specifically pronounced if the time of vaccination was before the age of one year.

A report of a strong association between a more hygenic environment in early childhood, with access to a hot water tap as a proxy variable, and an excess risk of Crohn's disease later on (127) seemingly contradicts the hypothesis of early exposures to infectious agents as a risk factor. Similar concerns could be raised about the association found between being a single child or a first child and the increased risk for Crohn's disease (105), that is, both exposures could lead to a delayed infection in life (a "sheltered child"), a hypothesis also proposed for increased risk of multiple sclerosis (146). However, in this century there has been a dramatic decrease in perinatal mortality. Good hygiene, better nutrition, and improved maternal and pediatric care could, therefore, at least partly, be the underlying reasons for the temporal trends in inflammatory bowel disease (both ulcerative colitis and Crohn's disease). In underdeveloped countries or in other populations with high perinatal mortality, potential patients with inflammatory bowel disease would be the first to die of early exposure to infections, and there would be a low incidence of inflammatory bowel disease 20 to 40 years later. Such a model makes the assumption that the exposure for ulcerative colitis, to some extent, differs from Crohn's disease in severity or its time window. Thus, the time lag between the increase in incidence in the two diseases could be explained in that better hygiene and health care for mother and child are needed to create a population of patients with Crohn's disease. This would also explain the tendency to shift from high socioeconomic status as a risk factor in early studies to the recent reports that those with lower socioeconomic status are at higher risk.

I. Mycobacteria

A chronic mycobacterial infection was proposed by Dalziel as early as 1913 (2) to be the underlying cause for Crohn's disease. The similarities between Johne's disease in cattle, sheep, and goats (147) and Crohn's disease, the former due to an early infection by *M. paratuberculosis*, has lent further credence to a causal association. Clusters of patients with Crohn's disease have been reported from both England (148) and Wales (149). It has been proposed (128) that the underlying mechanisms for those clusters are *M. paratuberculosis* spread by clinically or subclinically infected animals in the waters around the implicated areas. According to the author, the increase in incidence in urban areas should be due to the fact that *M. paratuberculosis* can survive pasteurization. Studies performed on milk samples in southern England suggest that this may occur (128). However, this hypothesis has not been unchallenged and the failure to culture mycobacteria from tissues affected by Crohn's disease has been pointed out. The use of DNA fingerprinting has also been inconclusive in that *M. paratuberculosis* is present not only in Crohn's disease but also in ulcerative colitis and other noninflammatory bowel disorders (150). Antituberculosis treatment has been attempted for Crohn's disease but the results have, so far, not been convincing (151,152). Although *M. paratuberculosis* seems to be present in some patients with Crohn's disease (153), it cannot be ruled out that this is a secondary phenomenon.

In conclusion, the hypothesis that *M. paratuberculosis* is a major etiologic agent for Crohn's disease is seductive, but the epidemiological evidence presented so far is mostly indirect, sometimes inconsistent, and, even if it is premature to rule out such an association, a casual relationship remains unproven.

J. Other Infectious Agents

Clusters of Crohn's disease have been reported among neighbors and friends in at least three studies (148,154,155), thus indicating a transmittable agent for Crohn's disease. However, if there is long-term exposure to infectious and environmental factors, there should be an overrepresentation of the disease in married couples in which one spouse or both develop the disease after marriage. There have been such reports, especially from the United Kingdom (156,157), and the findings have been interpreted as supporting a casual role of environmental factors with a long latent period for Crohn's disease. However, because of the increasing prevalence of Crohn's disease and the long time span between the reports, it is possible that the expected number of Crohn's disease in married couples in the United Kingdom is close to that reported. There has been a renewed interest for the hypothesis of a transmittable agent in Crohn's disease after a report of an epidemic of Crohn's disease in which multiple siblings in two French families developed Crohn's disease during a short time period (158). However, an extensive search for a common transmittable agent has so far not yielded any result. Further studies of these two families might, however, provide new clues for such an agent.

Seasonal variations in the clinical presentation of Crohn's disease have been reported in one study (159), indicating the presence of an infectious agent, at least as a trigger factor. A prospective study of 64 patients with Crohn's disease followed for 20 months (160) gives further credence to such a mechanism; the authors reported 54 infections, of which, 23 were associated with exacerbations corresponding to 24% of all recorded exacerbations. Respiratory pathogens were most common. The presence of rubella was implicated as was the presence of Epstein-Barr virus and adenovirus as the infectious agents. Reactivation of latent herpesvirus was also reported. These findings indicate that the infectious agents associated with exacerbations of the disease are nonspecific and that one specific pathogen should, therefore, not yet be nominated as a necessary cause.

III. CONCLUSION

Crohn's disease has shown an increasing trend in incidence during the last 50 years in the westernized world. Except for smoking, no environmental factor has consistently been shown to be associated with the disease. However, recent findings indicate that early life events, especially infections, could be crucial for the risk of a later development of Crohn's disease.

REFERENCES

1. Crohn BB, Ginzburg L, Oppenheimer GD. Regional ioleitis. A pathological and clinical entity. JAMA 1932; 99:1323–1329.
2. Dalziel TK. Chronic interstitial enteritis. BMJ 1913; 2:1068–1070.
3. Walker JF, Fielding JF. Crohn's disease in Dublin in the latter half of the nineteenth century. Ir J Med Sci 1988; 157:235–237.
4. Sedlack RE, Whisnant J, Elveback LR, Kurland LT. Incidence of Crohn's disease in Olmsted County, Minnesota, 1935–1975. Am J Epidemiol 1980; 112:759–763.
5. Rose JDR, Roberts GM, William G, Mayberry JF, Rhodes J. Cardiff Crohn's disease jubilee: the incidence over 50 years. Gut 1988; 29:346–351.
6. Amanta E, Barbara L, Biasco C. Incidence and prevalence of inflammatory bowel disease in Bologna-risk factors. Scand J Gastroenterol 1989; 17(suppl 78):349.
7. Bergman L, Krause U. The incidence of Crohn's disease in central Sweden. Scan J Gastroenterol 1975; 10:725–729.
8. Berner J, Kiaer T. Ulcerative colitis and Crohn's disease on the Faroe Islands 1964–1983. Scand J Gastroeneterol 1986; 21:188–192.
9. Binder V, Both H, Hansen PK, Hendriksen C, Kreiner S, Torp-Pedersen K. Incidence and

prevalence of ulcerative colitis and Crohn's disease in the County of Copenhagen 1962–1978. Gastroenterology 1982; 83:563–568.

10. Björnsson S. Inflammatory bowel disease in Iceland during a 30-year period, 1950–1979. Scand J Gasroeneterol 1989; 24(suppl 170):47–49.

11. Brahme F, Lindström C, Wenckert A. Crohn's disease in a defined population. An epidemiological study of incidence, prevalence, mortality, and secular trends in the city of Malmö. Gastroenterology 1975; 69:342–351.

12. Devlin HB, Datta D, Dellipiani AW. The incidence and prevalence of inflammatory bowel disease in North Tees health district. World J Surg 1980; 4:183–193.

13. Ekbom A, Helmick C, Zack M, Adami HO. The epidemiology of inflammatory bowel disease: a large, population-based study in Sweden. Gastroeneterology 1991; 100:350–358.

14. Fellows IW, Freeman JG, Holmes GK. Crohn's disease in the city of Derby 1951–1985. Gut 1990; 31:1261–1265.

15. Fireman Z, Grosman A, Lilos P, et al. Epidemiology of Crohn's disease in the Jewish population of central Israel 1970–1980. Am J Gastroeneterol 1989; 84:255–258.

16. Gollop JH, Phillips SF, Melton III LJ, Zinsmeister AR. Epidemiologic aspects of Crohn's disease: a population-based study in Olmsted Couny, Minnesota, 1943–1982. Gut 1988; 29:49–56.

17. Gower-Rousseau C, Salomez JL, Dupas JL, et al. Incidence of inflammatory bowel disease in northern France (1988–1990). Gut 1994; 35:1433–1438.

18. Haug K, Schrumpf E, Halvorsen JF, et al. Epidemiology of Crohn's disease in western Norway. Study group of inflammatory bowel disease in western Norway. Scand J Gastroeneterol 1989; 24:1271–1275.

19. Hellers G. Crohn's disease in Stockholm County, 1955–1974. Acta Chir Scand 1979; 490 (suppl 1):1–84.

20. Jayanthi V, Probert CSJ, Pinder D, Wicks ACB, Mayberry JF. Epidemiology of Crohn's disease in Indian migrants and the indigenous population in Leicestershire. Q J Med 1992; 298;125–138.

21. Kildebo R, Breckan K, Nordgaard PG, et al. The incidence of Crohn's disease in northern Norway from 1983 to 1986. Scand J Gastroeneterol 1989; 24:1265–1270.

22. Kyle J. An epidemiological study of Crohn's disease in northeast Scotland. Gastroenterology 1971; 61:826–833.

23. Kyle J, Stark G. Fall in the incidence of Crohn's disease. Gut 1980; 21:340–343.

24. Kyle J. Crohn's disease in the northeastern and northern Isles of Scotland: an epidemiological review. Gastroenterology 1992; 103:392–399.

25. Lee FI, Costello FT. Crohns' disease in Blackpool—incidence and prevalence 1968–80. Gut 1985; 26:274–278.

26. Lindberg E, Järnerot G. The incidence of Crohn's disease is not decreasing in Sweden. Scand J Gastroenterol 1991; 26:495–500.

27. Maté-Jimenez J, Muñoz S, Vicent D, Pajares JM. Incidence and prevalence of ulcerative colitis and Crohn's disease in urban and rural areas of Spain from 1981 to 1988. J Clin Gastroenterol 1994; 18:27–31.

28. Mayberry J, Rhodes J, Hughes LE. Incidence of Crohn's disease in Cardiff between 1934 and 1977. Gut 1979; 20:602–608.

29. Mayberry JF, Dew MJ, Morris JS, Powell DB. An audit of Crohn's disease in a defined population. J R Coll Physicians Lond 1983; 17:196–198.

30. Munkholm P, Langholtz E, Haagen Nielsen O, Kreiner S, Binder V. Incidence and prevalence of Crohn's disease in the County of Copenhagen, 1962–87: a sixfold increase in incidence. Scand J Gastroenterol 1992; 27:609–614.

31. Norlén BJ, Krause U, Bergman L. An epidemiologic study of Crohn's disease. Scand J Gastroenterol 1970; 5:385–390.

32. Odes HS, Locker C, Neumann L, et al. Epidemiology of Crohn's disease in southern Israel. Am J Gastroenterol 1994; 89:1859–1862.

33. Pinchbeck BR, Kirdeikis J. Inflammatory bowel disease in northern Alberta. An epidemiologic study. J Clin Gastroenterol 1988; 10:505–515.

34. Róin F, Róin J. Inflammatory bowel disease of the Faroe Islands, 1981–1988. Scand J Gastroenterol 1989; 24(suppl 170):44–46.

35. Rozen P, Zonis J, Yekutiel P, Gilat T. Crohn's disease in the Jewish population of Tel-Aviv-Yafo. Gastroenterology 1979; 76:25–30.

36. Shivananda S, Pena AS, Nap M, et al. Epidemiology of Crohn's disease in Regios Leiden, The Netherlands, Gastroenterology 1987; 93:966–974.

37. Smith IS, Young S, Gillespie G, O'Connor J, Bell JR. Epidemiological aspects of Crohn's disease in Clydesdale 1961–1970. Gut 1975; 16:62–67.

38. Trallori G, d'Albasio G, Palli D, et al. Epidemiology of inflammatory bowel disease over a 10-year period in Florence (1978–1987). Ital J Gastroenterol 1991; 23:559–463.

39. Tsianos EV, Masalas CN, Merkouropoulos M, Dalekos GN, Logan RFA. Incidence of inflammatory bowel disease in north west Greece: rarity of Crohn's disease in an area where ulcerative colitis is common. Gut 1994; 35:369–372.

40. Vucelic B, Korac B, Sentic M, et al. Epidemiology of Crohn's disease in Zagreb, Yugoslavia: a ten-year prospective study. Int J Epidemiol 1991; 20:216–220.

41. Wright JP, Froggatt J, O'Keefe EA, et al. The epidemiology of inflammatory bowel disease in Cape Town 1980–1984. S Afr Med J 1986; 70:10–15.

42. Calkins BM, Lilienfeld AM, Garland CF, Mendeloff AI. Trends in incidence rates of ulcerative colitis and Crohn's disease. Dig Dis Sci 1984; 29:10:913–920.

43. Cottone M, Cipolla C, Orlando A, Olivia L, Salerno G, Pagliaro L. Hospital incidence of Crohn's disease in the province of Palermo. Scand J Gastroenterol 1989; 24(suppl 170):27–28.

44. Evans JF, Acheson ED. An epidemiological study of ulcerative colitis and regional enteritis in the Oxford area. Gut 1965; 6:311–324.

45. Fahrlander H, Baerlocher CH. Clinical features and epidemiological data on Crohn's disease in the Basle area. Scand J Gastroenterol 1971; 6:657–662.

46. Garland CF, Lilienfeld AM, Mendeloff AI, et al. Incidence rates of ulcerative colitis and Crohn's disease in 15 areas of the United States. Gastroenterology 1981; 81:1115–1124.

47. Gjone E, Orning OM, Myren J. Crohn's disease in Norway 1956–63. Gut 1966; 7:372–374.

48. Halme I, von Smitten K, Husa A. The incidence of Crohn's disease in the Helsinki metropolitan area during 1975–1985. Ann Chir Gynaecol 1989; 78:115–119.

49. Humphreys WG, Brown JS, Parks TG. Crohn's disease in Northern Ireland. Ulster Med J 1990; 59:30–35.

50. Monk M, Mendeloff AI, Siegel CI, Lilienfeld A. An epidemiological study of ulcerative colitis and regional enteritis among adults in Baltimore. Gastroenterology 1967; 53:198–210.

51. Myren J, Gjone E, Hertzberg JN, Rygvold O, Semb LS, Fretheim B. Epidemiology of ulcerative colitis and regional enterocolitis (Crohn's disease) in Norway. Scand J Gastroenterol 1971; 6:511–514.

52. Nunes GC, Ahlquist RE. Increasing incidence of Crohn's disease. Am J Surg 1983; 145:578–581.

53. Nyhlin H, Danielsson Å. Incidence of Crohn's disease in a defined population in northern Sweden. Scand J Gastroenterol 1986; 21:1185–1192.

54. Stowe SP, Redmond SR, Stormont JM, et al. An epidemiologic study of inflammatory bowel disease in Rochester, New York. Gastroenterology 1990; 98:104–110.

55. Veloso FT, Fraga J, Carvalho J. Inflammatory bowel disease in Oporto. A prospective hospital study. Scand J Gastroenterol 1989; 24(suppl 170):32–35.

56. von Brandes JW, Lorenz-Myer H. Epidemiologische Aspecte zur Enterocolitis regionalis Crohn und Colitis ulceroca in Marburg Lahn zwischen 1962 und 1975. Z Gastroenterol 1983; 21:69–78.

57. Sonnenberg A. Mortality from Crohn's disease and ulcerative colitis in England–Wales and the U. S. from 1950 to 1983. Dis Colon Rectum 1986; 29:624–629.

58. Sonnenberg A, McCarty DJ, Jacobsen SJ. Geographic variation in inflammatory bowel disease within the United States. Gastroenterology 1991; 100:143–149.

59. Sonnenberg A, Wasserman IH. Epidemiology of inflammatory bowel disease among U.S. military veterans. Gastroenterology 1991; 101:122–130.

60. Sonnenberg A. Geographic variation in the incidence of and mortality from inflammatory bowel disease. Dis Colon Rectum 1986; 29:854–861.

61. Fielding JF. The relative risk of inflammatory bowel disease among parents and siblings of Crohn's disease patients. J Clin Gastroenterol 1986; 8:655–657.

62. Monsén U, Broström O, Nordenvall B, Sörstad J, Hellers G. Prevalence of inflammatory bowel disease among relatives of patients with ulcerative colitis. Scand J Gastroenterol 1987; 22:214–218.

63. Orholm M, Munkholm P, Langholz E, Haagen Nielsen O, Sörensen TIA, Binder V. Familial occurrence of inflammatory bowel disease. N Engl J Med 1991; 324:84–88.

64. Samuelsson SM. Ulcerös colit och proctit. Uppsala: Department of Social Medicine. Uppsala, Sweden: University of Uppsala, 1976. Thesis.

65. Ekbom A, Helmick CG, Zack M, Holmberg L, Adami HO. Survival and causes of death in patients with inflammatory bowel disease. A population-based study. Gastroenterology 1992; 103:954–960.

66. Odes HS, Fraser D, Krugliak P, Fenuves D, Fraser GM, Sperber AD. Inflammatory bowel disease in the Bedouin Arabs of southern Israel: rarity of diagnosis and clinical features. Gut 1991; 32:1024–1026.

67. Kurata JH, Kantor-Fish S, Frankl H, Godby P, Vadheim CM. Crohn's disease among ethnic groups in a large health maintenance organization. Gastroenterology 1992; 102:1940–1948.

68. Acheson ED. The distribution of ulcerative colitis and regional enteritis in United States veterans with particular reference to the Jewish religion. Gut 1960; 1:291–293.

69. Mayberry JF, Judd D, Smart H, Rhodes J, Calcraft B, Morris JS. Crohn's disease in Jewish people—an epidemiological study in south-east Wales. Digestion 1986; 35:237–240.

70. Roth MP, Petersen GM, McElree C, Feldman E, Rotter JI. Geographic origins of Jewish patients with inflammatory bowel disease. Gastroenterology 1989; 97:900–904.

71. Yoon CH, Kim SB, Park IJ, et al. Clinical features of Crohn's disease in Korea. Gastroenterol Jpn 1988; 23:576–581.

72. Higashi A, Watanabe Y, Ozasa K, Hayashi K, Aoike A, Kawai K. Prevalence and mortality of ulcerative colitis and Crohn's disease in Japan. Gastroenterol Jpn 1988; 23:521–526.

73. Al-Nakib B, Radhakrishnan S, Jacob GS, Al-Liddawi H, Al-Ruwaih A. Inflammatory bowel disease in Kuwait. Am J Gastroenterol 1984; 79:191–194.

74. Bartholomew C, Butler A. Inflammatory bowel disease in the West Indies. BMJ 1979; 2:824–825.

75. D'Oliveira R, Mayberry JF, Newcombe RG, Rhodes J. International comparison of mortality from inflammatory bowel disease in the Latin-speaking countries Venezuela, Italy, and France. Digestion 1984; 29:3239–241.

76. Mayberry JF, Ballantyne KC, Hardcastle JD, Mangham C, Pye C. Epidemiological study of asymptomatic and inflammatory bowel disease: the indentification of cases during a screening programme for colorectal cancer. Gut 1989; 30:481–483.

77. Roth MP, Petersen GM, McElree C, Vadheim CM, Panish JF, Rotter JI. Familial empiric risk estimates of inflammatory bowel disease in Ashkenazi Hews. Gastroenterology 1989; 96:1016–1020.

78. Tysk C, Lindberg E, Järnerot G, Flodérus-Myhred B. Ulcerative colitis and Crohn's disease in an unselected population of monozygotic and dizygotic twins. A study heritability and the influence of smoking. Gut 1988; 29:990–996.

79. Küster W, Pascoe L, Purmann J, Funk S, Majewski F. The genetics of Crohn's disease.

Complex segregation analysis of a family study with 265 patients with Crohn's disease and 5,378 relatives. Am J Genet 1989; 32:105–108.

80. Benoni C, Nilsson Å. Smoking habits in patients with inflammatory bowel disease. Scand J Gastroentrol 1987; 22:1130–1136.

81. Franceschi S, Panza E, La Vecchia C, Parazzini F, Decarli A, Bianchi Porro G. Nonspecific inflammatory bowel disease and smoking. Am J Epidemiol 1987; 125:445–452.

82. Katschinski B, Fingerle D, Scherbaum B, Goebell H. Oral contraceptive use and cigarette smoking in Crohn's disease. Dig Dis Sci 1993; 38:1596–1600.

83. Lindberg E, Tysk C, Andersson K, Järnerot G. Smoking and inflammatory bowel disease. A case-control study. Gut 1988; 29:352–357.

84. Logan RFA, Kay CR. Oral contraception, smoking and inflammatory bowel disease— findings in the Royal College of General Practitioners oral contraception study. Gut 1990; 31:1377–1381.

86. Sandler RS, Wurzelmann JI, Lyles CM. Oral contraceptive use and the risk of inflammatory bowel disease. Epidemiology 1992; 3:374–378.

87. Somerville KW, Logan RFA, Edmond M, Langman MJS. Smoking and Crohn's disease. BMJ 1984; 289:954–956.

88. Tobin MV, Logan RFA, Langman MJS, McConnell RB, Gilmore IT. Cigarette smoking and inflammatory bowel disease. Gastroenterology 1987; 93:316–321.

89. Vessey M, Jewell D, Smith A, Yeates D, McPherson K. Chronic inflammatory bowel disease, cigarette smoking, and use of oral contraceptives: findings in a large cohort study of women of childbearing age. BMJ 1986; 292:1101–1103.

90. Cottone M, Rosselli M, Orlando A, et al. Smoking habits and recurrence in Crohn's disease. Gastroenterology 1994; 106:643–648.

91. Sutherland LR, Ramcharan S, Bryant H, Fick G. Effect of cigarette smoking on recurrence of Crohn's disease. Gastroenterology 1990; 98:1123–1128.

92. Ekbom A, Helmick C, Zack M, Adami HO. Extracolonic malignancies in inflammatory bowel disease. Cancer 1991; 67:2015–2019.

93. Greenstein J, Gennuso R, Sachar DB, et al. Extraintestinal cancers in inflammatory bowel disease. Cancer 1985; 56:2914–2921.

94. Gyde SN, Prior P, Macartney JC, Thompson H, Waterhouse JAH, Allan RN. Malignancy in Crohn's disease. Gut 1980; 21:1024–1029.

95. Calkins BM. A meta-analysis of the role of smoking in inflammatory bowel disease. Dig Dis Sci 1989; 34:1841–1854.

96. Wakefield AD, Sawyerr AM, Hudson M, Dhillon AP, Pounder RE. Smoking, the oral contraceptive pill, and Crohn's disease. Dig Dis Sci 1991; 36:1147–1150.

97. Persson PG, Hellers G, Ahlbom A. Use of oral moist snuff and inflammatory bowel disease. Int J Epidemiol 1993; 22:1101–1103.

98. Lashner BA, Shaheen NJ, Hanauer SB, Kirshner BS. Passive smoking is associated with an increased risk of developing inflammatory bowel disease in children. Am J Gastroenterol 1993; 88: 356–359.

99. Sandler RS, Sandler DP, McDonnell CM, Wurzelman JI. Childhood exposure to environmental tobacco smoke and the risk of ulcerative colitis. Am J Epidemiol 1992; 135:603–608.

100. Rhodes JM, Cockel R, Allan RN, Hawker PC, Dawson J, Elias E. Colonic Crohn's disease and use of oral contraception. BMJ 1984; 1:595–596.

101. Boyko EJ, Theis MK, Vaughan TL, Nicol-Blades B. Increased risk of inflammatory bowel disease associated with oral contraceptive use. Am J Epidemiol 1994; 140:268–278.

102. Calkins BM, Mendeloff AI, Garland CF. Inflammatory bowel disease in oral contraceptive users. Gastroenterology 1986; 91:523–524.

103. Lashner BA, kane SV, Hanauer SB. Lack of association between oral contraceptive use and Crohn's disease colitis. Gastroenterology 1989; 97:1442–1447.

104. Lesko SM, Kaufman DW, Rosenberg L, et al. Evidence for an increased risk of Crohn's disease in oral contraceptive users. Gastroenterology 1985; 89:1046–1049.

105. Persson PG, Leijonmarck CE, Bernell O, Hellers G, Ahlbom A. Risk Indicators for inflammatory bowel disease. Int J Epidemiol 1993; 22:268–272.

106. Sutherland LR, Ramcharan S, Bryant H, Fick G. Effect of oral contraceptive use on reoperation following surgery for Crohns' disease. Dig Dis Sci 1992; 37:1377–1382.

107. Persson PG, Ahlbom A, Heller G. Crohn's disease and ulcerative colitis. A review of dietary studies with emphasis on methodologic aspects. Scand J Gastroenterol 1987; 22:385–889.

108. Jämerot G, Järnemark I, Nilsson K. Consumption of refined sugar by patients with Crohn's disease, ulcerative colitis, or irritable bowel syndrome. Scand J Gastroenterol 1983; 18:999–1002.

109. Kasper H, Sommer H. Dietary fiber and nutrient intake in Crohn's disease. Am J Clin Nutr 1979; 32:1898–1901.

110. Katschinski B, Logan RFA, Edmond M, Langman MJS. Smoking and sugar intake are separate but interactive risk factors in Crohn's disease. Gut 1988; 29:1202–1206.

111. Martini GA, Brandes JW. Increased consumption of refined carbohydrates in patients with Crohn's disease. Klin Wochenschr 1976; 54:367–371.

112. Mayberry JF, Rhodes J, Newcombe RG. Increased sugar consumption in Crohn's disease. Digestion 1980; 20: 323–326.

113. Mayberry JF, Rhodes J, Allan R, et al. Diet in Crohn's disease: two studies of curent and previous habits in newly diagnosed patients. Dig Dis Sci 1981; 26:444–448.

114. Persson PG, Ahlbom A, Hellers G. Diet and inflammatory bowel disease: a case-control study. Epidemiology 1992; 3:47–57.

115. Silkoff K, Hallak A, Yengena L, et al. Consumption of refined carbohydrate by patients with Crohn's disease in Tel-Aviv-Yafo. Postgrad Med J 1980; 56:842–846.

116. Thornton JR, Emmet PM, Heaton KW. Smoking, sugar, and inflammatory bowel disease. BMJ 1985; 290:1786–1787.

117. Brauer PM, Gee MI, Grace M, Thomson AB. Diet of women with Crohn's and other gastrointestinal diseases. J Am Diet Assoc 1983; 82:659–664.

118. James AH. Breakfast and Crohn's disease. BMJ 1977; 1:943–945.

119. Sonnenberg A. Geographic and temporal variations of sugar and margarine consumption in relation to Crohn's disease. Digestion 1988; 41:161–171.

120. Main J, McKenzie H, Yeaman GR, et al. Antibody to *Saccharomyces cerevisiae* (bakers' yeast) in Crohn's disease. BMJ 1988; 297:1105–1106.

121. Barclay GR, McKenzie H, Pennington J, Parratt D, Pennington CR. The effect of dietary yeast on the activity of stable chronic Crohn's disease. Scand J Gastroenterol 1992; 27:196–200.

122. Sonnenberg A. Occupational mortality of inflammatory bowel disease. Digestion 1990; 46:10–18.

123. Sonnenberg A. Disability from inflammatory bowel disease among employees in West Germany. Gut 1989; 30:367–370.

124. Sonnenberg A. Occupational distribution of inflammatory bowel disease among German employees. Gut 1990; 31:1037–1040.

125. Gilat T, Hacohen D, Lilos P, Langman MJS. Childhood factors in ulcerative colitis and Crohn's disease. Scand J Gastroenterol 1987; 22:1009–1024.

126. Ekbom A, Adami HO, Helmick CG, Jonzon A, Zack MM. Perinatal risk factors for inflammatory bowel disease: a case-control study. Am J Epidemiol 1990; 132:1111–1119.

127. Gent AE, Heller MD, Grace RH, Swarbrick ET, Coggon D. Inflammatory bowel disease and domestic hygiene in infancy. Lancet 1994; 343:766–767.

128. Hermon-Taylor J. Causation of Crohn's disease: the impact of clusters. (editorial). Gastroenterology 1993; 104:643–646.

129. North CS, Clouse RE, Spitznagel EL, Alpers DH. The relation of ulcerative colitis to psychiatric factors: a review of findings and methods. Am J Psychiatry 1990; 147:974–981.

130. Duffy LC, Zielezny MA, Marshall JR, et al. Lag time between stress events and risk of recurrent episodes of inflammatory bowel disease. Epidemiology 1991; 2:141–145.
131. Engström I, Lindquist BL. Inflammatory bowel disease in children and adolescents: a somatic and psychiatric investigation. Acta Paediatr Scand 1991; 80:640–647.
132. Binder V, Hendriksen C, Kreiner S. Prognosis in Crohn's disease—based on results from a regional patient group from the County of Copenhagen. Gut 1985; 26:146–150.
133. Whorwell PJ, Holdstock G, Whorwell GM, Wright R. Bottle feeding, early gastroenteritis and inflammatory bowel disease. BMJ 1979; 1:382.
134. Koletzko S, Sherman P, Corey M, Griffiths A, Smith C. Role of infant feeding practices in development of Crohn's disease in childhood. BMJ 1989; 298:1617–1618.
135. Wurzelmann JI, Lyles CM, Sandler RS. Childhood infections and the risk of inflammatory bowel disease. Dig Dis Sci 1994; 39: 555–560.
136. Bergstrand O, Hellers G. Breast-feeding during infancy in patients who later develop Crohn's disease. Scand J Gastroenterol 1983; 18:903–906.
137. Ekbom A, Zack M, Adami HO, Helmick C. Is there clustering of inflammatory bowel disease at birth? Am J Epidemiol 1991; 134:876–886.
138. Aaby P, Bukh J, Lisse IM, et al. Increased perinatal mortality among children of mothers exposed to measles during pregnancy. Lancet 1988; 1:516–519.
139. Ekbom A, Wakefield AJ, Zack M, Adami HO. Perinatal measles infection and subsequent Crohn's disease. Lancet 1994; 344:508–510.
140. Rothwell PM. Interpretation of temporal variation in patterns of birth. Lancet 1994; 344:1161–1162.
141. Rönne T. Measles virus infection without rash in childhood is related to disease in adult life. Lancet 1985; i:1–5.
142. Wakefield AJ, Pittilo RM, Sim R, et al. Evidence of persistent measles virus infection in Crohn's disease. J Med Virol 1993; 39:345–353.
143. Rutgeerts P, Geboes K, Peters M, et al. Effect of faecal stream diversion on recurrence of Crohn's disease in the neoterminal ileum. Lancet 1991; 338:771–774.
144. Barton JR, Gillon S, Ferguson A. Incidence of inflammatory bowel disease in Scottish children between 1968 and 1983; marginal fall in ulcerative colitis, three-fold rise in Crohn's disease. Gut 1989; 30:618–622.
145. Wakefield A. Personal commuication 1995.
146. Alter M, Zsehn-xin Z, Davanipour Z, et al. Multiple sclerosis and childhood infections. Neurology 1986; 36:1386–1389.
147. Morgan KL. Johne's and Crohn's. Chronic inflammatory bowel disease of infectious aetiology? Lancet 1987; i:1017–1019.
148. Allan R, Pease P, Ibbotson JP. Clustering of Crohn's disease in a Cotswold village. Q J Med 1986; 229:473–478.
149. Mayberry JF, Hitchens RAN. Distribution of Crohn's disease in Cardiff. Soc Sci Med 1978; 12:137–138.
150. Ciclith PJ. Does Crohn's disease have a mycobacterial basis? BMJ 1993; 306:733–734.
151. Järnerot G, Rolny P, Wickbom A, Alemayehu G. Antimycobacterial therapy ineffective in Crohn's disease after a year. Lancet 1989; i:164–165.
152. Rutgeerts P, Geboes K, Vantrappen, et al. Rifabutin and ethanbutol do not help recurrent Crohn's disease in the neoterminal ileum. J Clin Gastroenterol 1992; 15:24–28.
153. Fidler HM, Thurrell W, Johnson NMcI, Rook GAW, McFadden JJ. Specific detection of *Mycobacterium paratuberculosis* DNA associated with granulomatous tissue in Crohn's disease. Gut 1994; 35:506–510.
154. Reilly RP, Robinson TJ. Crohn's disease—is there a long latent period? Postgrad Med J 1986; 62:353–354.
155. Aisenberg J, Janowitz HD. Cluster of inflammatory bowel disease in three close college friends? J Clin Gastroenterol 1993; 17:18–20.

156. Lobo AJ, Foster PN, Sobala GM, Axon ATR. Crohn's disease in married couples. Lancet 1988; i:704–705.

157. Rhodes JM, Marshall T, Hamer JD, Allan RN. Crohn's disease in two married couples. Gut 1985; 26:1086–1087.

158. van Kruiningen HJ, Colombel JF, Cartun RW, et al. An in-depth study of Crohn's disease in two French families. Gastroenterology 1993; 104:351–360.

159. Cave DR, Freedman LS. Seasonal variations in the clinical presentation of Crohn's disease and ulcerative colitis. Int J Epidemiol 1975; 4:317–320.

160. Kangro HO, Chong SKF, Hardiman A, Heath RB, Walker-Smith JA. A prospective study of viral and mycoplasma infections in chronic inflammatory bowel disease. Gastroenterology 1990; 98: 549–553.

COMMENTARY

Robert S. Sandler   *University of North Carolina, Chapel Hill, North Carolina*

The excellent critical review of the epidemiology of Crohn's disease by Dr. Ekbom makes one point clear—our understanding of risk factors for this disease is limited. Despite there being more than 100 studies, we still know relatively little about the epidemiology of Crohn's disease.

The chapter by Ekbom nicely summarizes some of the reasons for our difficulties. Perhaps the most important reason is the rarity of the disease. Although Crohn's disease may seem common to the busy gastroenterologist, the incidence is actually quite low. That makes it difficult to assemble a sufficient number of patients to conduct an adequate epidemiologic study. The onset may be insidious, the intestinal and extraintestinal manifestations may be protean, and the disease may be mistaken for other conditions, most often ulcerative colitis. What we view as Crohn's disease may actually represent several different diseases with similar manifestations but different causes. As pointed out by Ekbom, the methodology of many of the previous epidemiologic studies has been flawed in numerous ways, including there being unrepresentative disease populations, inappropriate control groups, misclassification, inadequate control for potential confounding factors, and small sample size. In addition, many of the potential risk factors that have been identified in past studies suffer from lack of a good biological model to explain them.

There are few facts about the epidemiology of Crohn's disease that are clear and potentially helpful in understanding the cause. As pointed out by Ekbom, the disease is not a new one (such as acquired immunodeficiency syndrome), yet it is still primarily a disease of the 20th century. To find the cause, therefore, we might look to other diseases that have become more common in the 20th century, such as cardiovascular disease and cancer. The increased incidence of these diseases is partly due to longer life expectancy, but that is only a partial explanation. There are a number of environmental and lifestyle factors that increase risk for heart disease and cancer. Similar types of factors may help to explain the increased incidence of Crohn's disease. The increase in Crohn's disease incidence in countries such as Japan that have recently adopted a western lifestyle may provide clues.

The explosion in knowledge of molecular biology techniques and the mapping of the human genome have engendered hope that this new knowledge could explain Crohn's disease. Even though there is evidence that Crohn's disease clusters in families, the rapid increase in incidence in many countries over time cannot be entirely accounted for by genes. Such rapid changes in incidence can only be the consequence of environmental factors. Cigarette smoking is a good example of an environmental exposure that is relevant for Crohn's disease. The studies of smoking and Crohn's disease are striking in their consistency. They have been done by different investigators in different countries using different study designs, yet virtually all have reached similar conclusions. Crohn's disease is more likely to develop in smokers, although the precise mechanism is obscure. Genes may still be important, of course. It is reasonable to expect that interactions between genes and the environment will prove to be significant.

Some of the most tantalizing clues to the etiology of Crohn's disease are the data on temporal and seasonal trends and possible perinatal infection. The information suggesting an association with measles infection and measles vaccination is particularly intriguing especially in view of recent proof that peptic ulcer disease is caused by the infectious agent *Helicobacter pylori*. Specific infections could either render an individual more susceptible to development of Crohn's disease, or else the genetic predisposition to Crohn's disease might increase susceptibility to certain infections. In either case, epidemiologic studies of infection and immunity may be profitable areas of inquiry.

The chapter by Ekbom helps to chart the course for future research. Studies that have been done in referral populations suffer from various types of bias that cast doubt on their findings. We will learn the most from large, population-based studies such as the ones conducted in Sweden. The growth of computerized databases and database linkages may also be useful, but only if these databases represent a defined population. Consolidation of health care in large health maintenance organizations may facilitate this type of research. The field would also benefit from closer cooperation between basic scientists and epidemiologists. Hypotheses generated by one discipline can be scrutinized and tested by others. Past epidemiological studies have suffered, to some extent, from poor biological rationale.

Although we don't know as much as we would like about the epidemiology of Crohn's disease, epidemiologists can play an important role in our eventual understanding. When new risk factors are suggested, they must be consistent with the epidemiological characteristics of the disease. It is important that we continue to study the distribution and determinants of Crohn's disease to provide new clues and to test new hypotheses.

4
Consideration of Smoking in Patients with Crohn's Disease

Bret A. Lashner   *Cleveland Clinic Foundation, Cleveland, Ohio*

I. HISTORICAL PERSPECTIVE

The prevailing theory for the pathogenesis of Crohn's disease involves the trigger of an unchecked immune response by one or more environmental toxins in a genetically predisposed individual. The search for the implicated toxin has been unceasing in recent years and has led to many interesting observations, the most important of which has been the relationship of cigarette smoking to inflammatory bowel disease (1).

The first observations linking cigarette smoking to inflammatory bowel disease were described in ulcerative colitis patients. Compared with a smoking rate of 44% among control subjects in a fracture clinic, the rate was 8% of ulcerative colitis patients and 42% of Crohn's disease patients (2). This effect was apparent at any age. Mormons, lifelong nonsmokers, had a high risk of developing ulcerative colitis and a low risk of developing atherosclerotic heart disease (3). The consistent observation that ulcerative colitis developed soon after quitting smoking led to a flurry of epidemiological studies, mostly case-control studies published since 1982, identifying nonsmoking and former smoking as features of ulcerative colitis (2,4–16). Each study, using distinct and disparate control populations from widely diverse geographical regions, showed similar results. A meta-analysis of these studies demonstrated that the risk to smokers for development of ulcerative colitis was 59% less than the risk in nonsmokers (odds ratio 0.41, 95% confidence interval [CI] 0.34–0.48) (17). There was no difference in disease extent or disease activity as measured by colectomy requirement between smokers and nonsmokers (18,19). The risk of ulcerative colitis developing in former smokers also was consistently elevated over that of nonsmokers (20). A meta-analysis quantified a 64% increased risk in former smokers over nonsmokers (odds ratio 1.64, 95% CI 1.36–1.98) (17). Furthermore, passive smoking exposure in childhood may protect against the development of ulcerative colitis as an adult (21). The protection from ulcerative colitis from cigarette smoking is real, yet unexplained.

In earlier years, men smoked more frequently than women; consequently, women developed ulcerative colitis in greater numbers (22). In recent years as cigarette smoking patterns have changed, women are smoking more often and men are quitting more often.

Such changes have equalized the rates of ulcerative colitis incidence in men and women (22). Other epidemiloigical studies have demonstrated that coffee consumption has no effect on ulcerative colitis incidence but increased alcohol consumption attentuates the risk of ulcerative oclitis in nonsmokers only (11).

The harmful effects of cigarette smoking on many organ systems of the body are legion. Hence, smoking cannot be recommended to protect against ulcerative colitis. However, nicotine gum and nicotine patches do benefit some individuals, usually former smokers, as therapy for active disease (23,24). Many other components of cigarette smoke have not been tested nor has the mechanism of action of nicotine been adequately explained.

Once the effects of smoking on ulcerative colitis patients were elucidated, investigators turned to studying smoking in Crohn's disease patients. From consistent cohort and case-control studies, cigarette smoking has been shown to exert a harmful effect in these patients. Smokers, as well as former smokers, are at increased risk of developing Crohn's disease and of recurrence of disease after medically or surgically induced remission. In Scotland, a decreasing smoking rate did not parallel a rising incidence rate for Crohn's disease and the rising incidence remains unexplained (25).

These discrepant effects of cigarette smoking on the development of ulcerative colitis or Crohn's disease may be more than a curiosity. There is excessive concordance for both type of inflammatory bowel disease and cigarette smoking habit among relatives and twins with inflammatory bowel disease (26,27). It has been postulated that the individual genetically predisposed to inflammatory bowel disease may develop disease according to cigarette smoking habit; smokers develop Crohn's disease and nonsmokers develop ulcerative colitis when an unfortunate combination of genetic and environmental factors coincide (1,28). These effects may be especially interesting in monozygotic twins who could develop disease manifestations depending on smoking habit (27). These effects also suggest that physicians redouble efforts to encourage patients with inflammatory bowel disease, especially Crohn's disease, to quit smoking even if cessation requires replacement of nicotine source with nicotine gum or nicotine patches.

II. ETIOLOGICAL ASSOCIATIONS

A. Current Smoking

Current smokers are more likely to develop Crohn's disease than nonsmokers. Cohort studies of large populations suggest that there is an increased incidence of Crohn's disease among smokers. The Royal College of General Practitioners studied a population of more than 23,000 for more than 25 years (29). The statistically significant incidence rate ratio of smokers to nonsmokers for Crohn's disease was 3.9. A dose-response was demonstrated. The rate of developing Crohn's disease per 100,000 population was 18 in smokers of more than 20 cigarettes per day and 13 in smokers of less than 20 cigarettes per day. Oral contraceptive use did not confound the results. In the Oxford Family Planning Association study of 17,032 women, smokers were 2.5 times as likely (p < 0.05) to develop Crohn's disease as nonsmokers (30). There was no increased risk in former smokers and oral contraceptive use did not confound results. A third cohort study from Italy found that smokers, especially women, were more likely to contract Crohn's disease than a non-smoking population (31).

Many case-control studies, too, have found an association between cigarette smoking and Crohn's disease (15,32). Studies of note include a case-control study comparing 115

Crohn's disease patients with irritable bowel syndrome control subjects (33). The risk of Crohn's disease developing in smokers was nearly four times the risk in nonsmokers (odds ratio 3.71, 95% CI 1.93–7.13). A matched case-control study of 51 women with Crohn's disease found that current smoking was associated with the development of Crohn's disease (odds ratio 2.71, 95% CI 1.33–5.53) and the association persisted for any disease location (ileitis, ileocolitis, or Crohn's colitis) (34). Oral contraceptive use did not confound results. Another case-control study of 137 Crohn's disease patients found an odds ratio among smokers of 2.9 (95% CI 1.8–4.9) that was not appreciably affected by gender, socioeconomic status, number of cigarettes smoked per day, site of disease, or age at onset (8). In another case-control study of 82 patients, Crohn's disease was found to be nearly five times as likely to develop in smokers as in nonsmokers (odds ratio 4.8, 95% CI 2.4–9.7) (28). This effect did not depend on site of disease or coincide with the histological finding of granulomas. Another case-control study found smoking to be associated with Crohn's disease and that this effect was potentiated by high intake of refined sugar (27,35). Finally, another case-control study found a threefold increased risk of Crohn's disease among smokers (odds ratio 3.0, 95% CI 1.3–6.8) that eliminated any oral contraceptive use effects on disease incidence (36).

This strong association is consistent among all acceptable case-control studies that examine this issue. Calkins performed a meta-analysis among seven studies that included a total of 781 patients with Crohn's disease (17). The odds ratios of these studies ranged from 0.86 to 4.67. When the results of these studies were combined and weighted by both sample size and magnitude of the effect, a standard methodology for meta-analysis (Mantel-Haenszel method), the common odds ratio was 2.02 with a 95% CI of 1.65 to 2.47 (Fig. 1). This result implies that current smokers are twice as likely as nonsmokers to develop Crohn's disease.

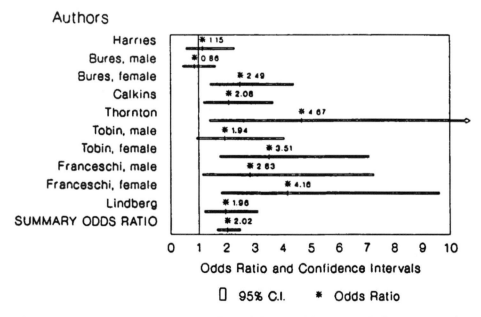

FIG. 1 Individual and summary odds ratios and 95% confidence intervals for current smokers compared with lifetime nonsmokers for Crohn's disease studies included in meta-analysis.

Three of the studies included in the analysis examined the relationship of level of smoking exposure to the risk of development of Crohn's disease (17). The common odds ratio for smokers consuming the most number of cigarettes (actual number varies among studies) was 2.53 and for smokers consuming fewer cigarettes was 2.39. Such a small difference is not clinically significant. In one study, odds ratios were significantly higher among smokers with at least 15 years of exposure (odds ratio 7.5) than among smokers with less duration of smoking (odds ratio 3.2) (9). A strong effect from cigarette smoking on the development of Crohn's disease coupled with a lack of clear dose-response has interesting pathogenetic implications. Dose-response is considered a criterion for epidemiologic causation (37). However, an effect that is apparent when a threshold is reached does not exhibit dose-response. Perhaps, such a threshold effect is present in Crohn's disease patients.

Several other criteria for epidemiologic causation are fulfilled with cigarette smoking and Crohn's disease. Besides dose-response, defining a causal relationship requires (a) a strong association, (b) specificity of risk to disease groups, (c) specificity of risk to exposure categories (lack of interaction effects), (d) a correct temporal relationship between exposure and disease, and (e) biologic plausibility (37). The associations described are quite strong, demonstrate specificity for disease and exposure, and are of the correct temporal relationship. Biologically plausible theories have been proposed but not proved.

B. Former Smoking

Former smokers, too, are more susceptible than nonsmokers to development of Crohn's disease. Six case-control studies looking at this association were evaluated by Calkins in a meta-analysis (17). A total of 750 patients comprised these studies, and the odds ratios ranged from 0.66 to 4.44. When the results were weighted by sample size and magnitude of the effect, the common odds ratio was 1.83 with a 95% CI of 1.33 to 2.51 (Fig. 2). Such an association implies that former smokers are 80% more susceptible than persons who have never smoked to development of Crohn's disease.

Only two of the studies in the analysis examined dose-response (17). Meta-analysis demonstrated that, when compared with persons who never smoked, heavier former smokers had an odds ratio of 2.15 and lighter former smokers had an odds ratio of 2.13. Therefore, no clinically significant dose-response has been demonstrated. In one study, the effect of former cigarette smoking for Crohn's disease disappeared after 5 years had elapsed since the person quit smoking (9). The reason given by quitters was mostly personal choice (53% of Crohn's disease patients compared with 61% in control subjects who quit), but abdominal disturbance was cited as a reason for quitting by 12% of Crohn's disease patients and by none of the control subjects (9).

C. Passive Smoking

Because Crohn's disease develops in children who are rarely smokers or former smokers, recent interest has centered on the association of passive smoking exposure on the development of Crohn's disease. In a matched case-control study of 33 newly diagnosed children with Crohn's disease and peer-nominated control subjects, passive smoking exposure at birth was significantly associated with the development of Crohn's disease (odds ratio 5.32, 95% CI 1.09–25.9) (38). Maternal passive smoking exposure at birth alone had an odds ratio of 2.76. Because the odds ratio from maternal passive smoking exposure was not higher than the odds ratio from exposure by either parent, it is thought

Authors

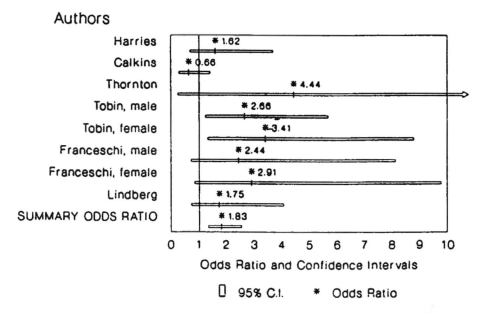

FIG. 2 Individual and summary odds ratios and 95% confidence intervals for former smokers compared with lifetime nonsmokers for Crohn's disease studies included in meta-analysis.

that the toxic exposure is inhaled by the child rather than passed through the placenta or in breast milk. Passive smoking exposure also exhibited dose-response by showing a significantly elevated odds ratio for each pack of cigarettes smoked per day (odds ratio 1.53, 95% CI 1.01–2.30).

Another case-control study of 149 nonsmoking incident cases of Crohn's disease and randomly selected community controls demonstrated an increased risk of Crohn's disease developing in patients exposed to passive smoke during childhood (odds ratio 1.50, 95% CI 1.0–2.3) (39). This effect was slightly greater in women (odds ratio 1.59) than in men (odds ratio 1.37) and adds consistency to the observation that passive smoking exposure during childhood is associated with the development of Crohn's disease in childhood or as an adult.

III. NATURAL HISTORY OF DISEASE

Cigarette smoking tends to induce more severe Crohn's disease symptoms, more difficult complications, and more frequent relapses after surgically induced remission.

A. Severity of Symptoms

Cigarette smoking may influence the natural history of Crohn's disease by affecting the severity of symptoms, type of complications, and rate of recurrence after a surgically induced remission. A cohort study of 74 patients determined that smokers had a 60% increased risk of relapse within 6 months of a medically induced remission than non-smokers (relative risk 1.6, p < 0.01) (40). In this study, 42% of the Crohn's disease population were smokers, of whom 89% relapsed, compared with a 53% relapse rate among nonsmokers. Another study of a 2 million–member health maintenance organization found that active cigarette smokers with Crohn's disease were symptomatic 15.4 days per month compared with 5.0 days per month in nonsmokers (p < 0.001) (41). Smokers with Crohn's colitis tend to have more relapses per year than nonsmokers (3.8 versus 2.5), and they have more pain during relapse (27). Smokers with small bowel Crohn's disease have more frequent bowel movements during relapse, more hospitalizations, more surgery, and higher white blood cell counts than nonsmokers (12).

B. Type of Complication

In a cohort study of South African Crohn's disease patients, cigarette smoking was associated with the development of ileocolitis rather than ileitis or colitis (p < 0.03) (42). Also, smokers had a higher relapse rate and more inflammatory attacks as opposed to obstructive or hemorrhagic attacks or recurrence with perianal abscess (42). In contrast, smokers of more than 10 cigarettes per day developed fistulas and abscesses more often than nonsmokers and were more likely to have small bowel disease than nonsmokers or lighter smokers (43).

Women with Crohn's disease experience menopause at an earlier age than the general population (47.6 years versus 49.6 years) (44). This effect, though, is not influenced by cigarette smoking in that little difference was seen between smokers and nonsmokers.

C. Postsurgical Recurrence

Crohn's disease patients who were smokers of more than 10 cigarettes per day had a risk of first surgery of 14% at 5 years and 24% at 10 years, which was more than that of nonsmokers (45). Defining postsurgical recurrence as the need for repeat surgery, 174 patients who where followed for a mean of 10.8 years had significantly different recurrence rates between smokers (36% at 5 years, 70% at 10 years) and nonsmokers (20% at 5 years, 41% at 10 years) (45). These values correspond to a relative risk of 2.1 (95% CI 1.1–4.1) with even higher relative risks in women (Fig. 3) (45).

In a historical cohort study of 182 patients who underwent surgery for Crohn's

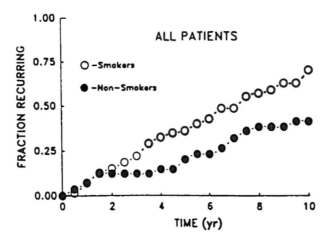

FIG. 3 Five- and 10-year cumulative recurrence rates for smokers (36%, 70%) compared with nonsmokers (29%, 41%) (p = 0.007). Difference between the two groups at 5 years was 16% (CI$_{95\%}$ 2.4–29.6%); at 10 years, the difference was 39% (CI$_{95\%}$ 14–54%).

disease, smokers had twice the risk of needing further surgery (relative risk 2.0, 95% CI 1.2–2.3) and endoscopy (relative risk 2.2, 95% CI 1.2–3.8) as nonsmokers (46). Among Crohn's disease patients requiring a second surgery, the interval between operations was not significantly different between smokers (mean 4.6 years) and nonsmokers (mean 4.0 years) (47).

IV. INDETERMINATE DISEASE

Fully 10% of patients with inflammatory bowel disease and colitis have indeterminate disease. Using clinical, endoscopic, and histologic criteria, it may still be impossible to distinguish between ulcerative colitis and Crohn's disease. In indeterminate patients in whom there is a 50% probability of the patient having either ulcerative colitis or Crohn's disease, an accurate determination of cigarette smoking status at the time of development of symptoms may help to distinguish between the two diseases. If only 10% of ulcerative colitis patients smoke at the time of symptom development and 50% of Crohn's disease patients are expected to smoke at the time of symptom development, then Bayes' theorem can be applied to obtain the "posterior" probabilities of disease occurrence. In an indeterminate population, smokers at the time of symptom onset have an 83% probability of having Crohn's disease and nonsmokers have only a 36% probability of having Crohn's disease. Therefore, a careful cigarette smoking history can help with the diagnosis of indeterminate disease.

V. PATHOGENETIC MECHANISMS

Many theories have been tested to explain pathogenetic mechanisms of Crohn's disease, but none has provided satisfactory explanations. A clear understanding of the mechanism of the relationship between cigarette smoking and Crohn's disease may offer insights into management alternatives.

Polyethylene glycol absorption, a measure of gut permeability, is impaired in Crohn's disease patients (48). This less permeable epithelium is apparent in both smokers and nonsmokers with Crohn's disease, but smokers have greater permeability than nonsmokers. Permeability among smokers with Crohn's disease is especially increased in patients with small bowel disease (49). In theory, greater permeability allows more toxins to cross the epithelial barrier and potentially initiate disease.

Another possible explanation for the effect of cigarette smoking on Crohn's disease involves perturbations of the immune system itself. If present, the modification of the immune system must be specific because the autoimmune disease systemic lupus erythematosus is not associated with current smoking or former smoking (50). Cigarette smoking is a nonspecific immunosuppressant leading to a decrease in IgG, IgM, and IgA, an increase in IgE, and a decrease in the helper/suppresser T-cell ratio (51,52). Furthermore, smoking decreases tissue levels of prostaglandin E, prostaglandin $F_{1\alpha}$, leukotriene B_4, and leukotriene $C_5/D_4/E_4$ (53). With an alteration in the balance of these cytoprotectors and inflammatory mediators, the mucosa may be ripe for unchecked inflammation from a specific toxin and the development of clinically apparent Crohn's disease.

Another theory of pathogenesis involves colonic mucus formation. Cigarette smoking potentiates the quantity of colonic mucus, which, in turn, increases the epithelial barrier to environmental toxins (54). Such a mechanism has been evoked as the mechanism for protection of the colon from smoking in ulcerative colitis patients and may be why small bowel disease and not colonic disease is more likely to develop in smokers with Crohn's disese. However, because colonic mucus in Crohn's disease patients usually is normal and not greatly affected by cigarette smoking, this possible mechanism is less likely to be important (51,52).

Cigarette smoking is associated with a significant decrease in local blood flow in the rectum as measured by laser Doppler flowmetry (55). Delayed healing and higher recurrence rates may be related to the diminished delivery of medical therapy to the affected bowel segments among cigarette smokers.

Smoking contributes to a hypercoagulable state by causing endothelial cell damage, inhibiting vascular prostacycline (PGI_2, an important inhibitor of platelet aggregation), increasing fibrinogen levels, and decreasing plasminogen levels (51). Interestingly, microthrombosis from a hypercoagulable state often results in focal vascular injury of intramural vessels with fibrin deposition, interleukin-1 release, and decreased tissue plasminogen-activator activity, changes indistinguishable from Crohn's disease (1,56). The remarkable similarity of the aphthoid-appearing lesions of ischemia and Crohn's disease and of the changes in the inflammatory response makes microthrombosis a prime candidate for study in the pathogenesis of Crohn's disease among cigarette smokers.

Hypercoagulability from cigarette smoking is potentiated by oral contraceptive use in women. A case-control study of nearly 1000 patients responding to a questionnaire demonstrated that oral contraceptive users were more susceptible than nonusers to development of Crohn's disease (odds ratio 1.49, 95% CI 0.99–2.26) and that there was interaction with cigarette smoking (57). Smokers using oral contraceptives had an odds ratio for development of Crohn's disease of 2.64 (95% CI 1.22–5.75). Even though other studies have failed to show an association between oral contraceptive use and Crohn's disease, perhaps the interaction with cigarette smoking is necessary to demonstrate clinically important effects.

Still, cigarette smoking may not cause a direct toxic effect. Smoking exposure may exert an indirect toxic effect by inducing susceptibility to unique pulmonary infections that may cause disease or may lead to medical therapy (e.g., antibiotics) that contributes to disease initiation. The International Inflammatory Bowel Disease Study Group examined the risk of a number of childhood factors for the development of inflammatory bowel disease in 499 children with inflammatory bowel disease from North America, Europe, and Israel (58). Passive and current smoking were not studied directly, but Crohn's disease patients were significantly more likely to have recurrent respiratory infections and be hospitalized for respiratory diseases than control subjects in all three geographic regions. Furthermore, Crohn's disease patients were significantly more likely to use antibiotics.

VI. TREATMENT OPTIONS

There are many components of cigarette smoke that may be toxic to the gastrointestinal epithelium, including nicotine, tar and nitric oxide. Cigarette smoking cessation is of paramount importance for treating Crohn's disease patients. Nicotine gum or nicotine patches are therapeutic in some patients, especially former smokers, as primary therapy for ulcerative colitis (23,24). Although it has not been proven, it is likely that smoking cessation will lead to lower incidence rates for Crohn's disease, lower rates of recurrence, and less severe complications. A nicotine source to aid smoking cessation can be considered as therapy to treat Crohn's disease and even to prevent disease in predisposed populations. It is extremely difficult to induce a Crohn's disease patient to quit smoking.

After the diagnosis of Crohn's disease is made, patients are 65% less likely to quit than unaffected control subjects (odds ratio 0.35, 95% CI 0.18–0.69) (33).

REFERENCES

1. Sandler RS. Epidemiology of inflammatory bowel disease. In Targan SR, Shanahan F, eds. Inflammatory Bowel Disease: From Bench to Bedside. Baltimore, Williams & Wilkins, 1994.
2. Harries AD, Baird A, Rhodes J. Non-smoking: a feature of ulcerative colitis. BMJ 1982; 284:706.
3. Penny WJ, Penny Em Mayberry JF, Rhodes J. Prevalence of inflammatory bowel disease amongst Mormons in Britain and Ireland. Soc Sci Med 1985; 21:287–290.
4. Jick H, Walker AM. Cigarette smoking and ulcerative colitis. N Engl J Med 1983; 308:261–263.
5. Boyko EJ, Koepsell TD, Perera DR, Inui TS. Risk of ulcerative colitis among former and current cigarette smokers. N Engl J Med 1987; 316:707–710.
6. Logan RFA, Edmond M, Somerville KW, Langman MJS. Smoking and ulcerative colitis. BMJ 1984; 288:751–753.
7. Benoni C, Nilsson Å. Smoking habits in patients with inflammatory bowel disease. Scand J Gastroenterol 1984; 19:824–830.
8. Tobin MV, Logan RFA, Langman MJS, et al. Cigarette smoking and inflammatory bowel disease. Gastroenterology 1987; 93:316–321.
9. Franceschi S, Panza E, LaVecchia C, Parazzinin F, DeCarli A, Bianch-Porro, G. Nonspecific inflammatory bowel disease and smoking. Am J Epidemiol 1987; 125:445–452.
10. Cope GF, Heatley RV, Kelleher J, et al. Cigarette smoking and inflammatory bowel disease. Hum Toxicol 1987; 6:189–193.
11. Boyko EJ, Perera DR, Koepsell TD, Keane EM, Inui TS. Coffee and alcohol use and the risk of ulcerative colitis. Am J Gastroenterol 1989; 84:530–534.
12. Holdstock G, Savage D, Harman M, Wright R. Should patients with inflammatory bowel disease smoke? BMJ 1984; 288:362.
13. Samuelsson S-M, Ekbom A, Zack M, Helmick CG, Adami H-O. Risk factors for extensive ulcerative colitis and ulcerative proctitis: a population based case-control study. Gut 1991; 32:1526–1530.
14. Lorusso D, Leo S, Misciagna G, Guerra V. Cigarette smoking and ulcerative colitis: a case-control study. Hepatogastroenterology 1989; 36:202–204.
15. Lindberg E, Tysk C, Andersson K, Järnerot G. Smoking and inflammatory bowel disease: a case-control study. Gut 1988; 29:352–357.
16. Cope GF, Heatley RV, Kelleher J, Lee PN. Cigarette smoking and inflammatory bowel disease: a review. Hum Toxicol 1987; 6:189–193.
17. Calkins BM. A meta-analysis of the role of smoking in inflammatory bowel disease. Dig Dis Sci 1989; 34:1841–1854.
18. Srivasta ED, Newcombe RG, Rhodes J, Avramidis P, Mayberry JF. Smoking and ulcerative colitis: a community study. Int J Colorectal Dis 1993; 8:71–74.
19. Lashner BA, Kane SV, Hanauer SB. Lack of association between oral contraceptive use and ulcerative colitis. Gastroenterology 1990; 99:1032–1036.
20. Motley RJ, Rhodes J, Form GA, Wilkinson SP, Chesner IM, Asquith P, Hellier MD, Mayberry JF. Time relationships between cessation of smoking and onset of ulcerative colitis. Digestion 1987; 37:125–127.
21. Sandler RS, Sandler DP, McDonnell CW, Wurzelman JI. Childhood exposure to environmental tobacco smoke and risk of ulcerative colitis (abstr). Gastroenterology 1991; 100:A17. 1992; 135:603–609.
22. Tysk C, Järnerot G. Has smoking changed the epidemiology of ulcerative colitis? Scand J Gastroenterol 1992; 27:508–512.

23. Lashner BA, Hanauer SB, Silverstein MD. Testing nicotine gum for ulcerative colitis patients: experience with single-patient trials. Dig Dis Sci 1990; 35:827–832.

24. Pullan RD, Rhodes J, Ganesh S, et al. Transdermal nicotine for active ulcerative colitis. N Engl J Med 1994; 330:811–815.

25. Kyle J. Crohn's disease in the northeastern and northern Isles of Scotland: an epidemiological study. Gastroenterology 1992; 103:392–399.

26. Smith MB, Lashner BA, Hanauer SB. Smoking and inflammatory bowel disease in families. Am J Gastroenterol 1988; 83:407–409.

27. Katchinski B, Logan RFA, Edmond M, Langman MJS. Smoking and sugar intake are separate but interactive risk factors in Crohn's disease. Gut 1988; 29:1202–1206.

28. Somerville KW, Logan RFA, Edmond M, Langman MJS. Smoking and Crohn's disease. BMJ 1984; 289:954–956.

29. Logan RFA, Kay CR. Oral contraception, smoking and inflammatory bowel disease—findings in the Royal College of General Practitioners Oral Contraception Study. Int J Epidemiol 1989; 18:105–107.

30. Vessey M, Jewell D, Smith A, Yeates D, McPherson K. Chronic inflammatory bowel disease, cigarette smoking, and use of oral contraceptives: findings in a large cohort study of women of childbearing age. BMJ 1986; 292:1101–1103.

31. Tragnone A, Hanau C, Bazzocchi G, Lanfranchi GA. Epidemiological characteristics of inflammatory bowel disease in Bologna, Italy—incidence and risk factors. Digestion 1993; 54:183–188.

32. Benoni C, Nilsson Å. Smoking habits in patients with inflammatory bowel disease: a case-control study. Scand J Gastroenterol 1987; 22:1130–1136.

33. Silverstein MD, Lashner BA, Hanauer SB, Evans AA, Kirsner JB. Cigarette smoking in Crohn's disease. Am J Gastroenterol 1989; 84:31–33.

34. Lashner BA, Kane SV, Hanauer SB. Lack of association between oral contraceptive use and Crohn's disease: a community-based matched case-control study. Gastroenterology 1989; 97:1442–1447

35. Thornton R, Emmett PM, Heaton KW. Smoking, sugar, and inflammatory bowel disease. BMJ 1985; 290:1786–1787.

36. Katschinski B, Fingerle D, Scherbaum B, Goebell H. Oral contraceptive use and cigarette smoking in Crohn's disease. Dig Dis Sci 1993; 38:1596–1600.

37. Breslow NE, Day NE. Statistical methods in cancer research. Volume I—The analysis of case-control studies. IARC Scientific Publication No. 32, International Agency for Research on Cancer, Lyon, France, 1980.

38. Lashner BA, Shaheen NJ, Hanauer SB, Kirschner BS. Passive smoking is associated with an increased risk of developing inflammatory bowel disease in children. Am J Gastroenterol 1993; 88:356–359.

39. Persson PG, Ahlbom A, Hellers G. Inflammatory bowel disease and tobacco smoke—a case-control study. Gut 1990; 31:1377–1381.

40. Duffy LC, Zielezny MA, Marshall JR, Weiser MW, Byers TE, Phillips JF, Ogra PL, Graham S. Cigarette smoking and risk of clinical relapse in patients with Crohn's disease. Am J Prev Med 1990; 6:161–166.

41. Kurata JH, Kantor-Fish S, Frankl H, Godby P, Vadheim CM. Crohn's disease among ethnic groups in a large health maintenance organization. Gastroenterology 1992; 102:1940–1948

42. Wright JP. Factors influencing first relapse in patients with Crohn's disease. J Clin Gastroenterol 1992; 15:12–16.

43. Lindberg E, Järnerot G, Huitfeldt B. Smoking in Crohn's disease: effect on localization and clinical course. Gut 1992; 33:779–782.

44. Lichtarowicz A, Norman C, Calcraft B, Morris JS, Rhodes J, Mayberry J. A study of the menopause, smoking, and contraception in women with Crohn's disease. Q J Med 1989; 72:623–631.

45. Sutherland LR, Ramcharan S, Bryant H, Fick F. Effect of cigarette smoking on recurrence of Crohn's disease. Gastroenterology 1990; 98:1123–1128.
46. Cottone M, Rosselli M, Orlando A, Oliva L, Puleo A, Cappello M, Traina M, Tonelli F, Pagliaro L. Smoking habits and recurrence in Crohn's disease. Gastroenterology 1994; 106:643–648.
47. Goldberg PA, Wright JP, Gerber M, Claassen R. Incidence of surgical resection for Crohn's disease. Dis Colon Rectum 1993; 36:736–739.
48. Söderholm J, Olaison G, Sjödahl R, Tagesson C. Smoking and intestinal absorption of oral polyethylene glycols in Crohn's disease. Scand J Gastroenterol 1993; 28:163–167.
49. Bjarnson I, O'Morain C, Levi AJ, Peters TJ. Absorption of chromium-labeled 51-ethylene-diaminetetraacetate in inflammatory bowel disease. Gastroenterology 1983; 85:318–322.
50. Benoni C, Nilsson Å, Nived O. Smoking and inflammatory bowel disease: comparison with systemic lupus erythematosus: a case-control study. Scand J Gastroenterol 1990; 25:751–755.
51. Osborne MJ, Stansby GP. Cigarette smoking and its relationship to inflammatory bowel disease: a review. J R Soc Med 1992; 85:214–216.
52. Cope GF, Heatley RV. Cigarette smoking and intestinal defenses. Gut 1992; 33:721–723.
53. Motley RJ, Rhodes J, Williams G, Tavares IA, Bennett A. Smoking, eicosanoids and ulcerative colitis. J Pharm Pharmacol 1990; 42:288–289.
54. Cope GF, Heatley RV, Kelleher H. Smoking and colonic mucus in ulcerative colitis. BMJ 1986; 293:481.
55. Srivastava ED, Russell MAH, Feyerabend C, Rhodes J. Effect of ulcerative colitis and smoking on rectal blood flow. Gut 1990; 31:1021–1025.
56. Wakefield AJ, Sawyer AM, Hudson M, Dhillon AP, Pounder RE. Smoking, the oral contraceptive pill, and Crohn's disease. Dig Dis Sci 1991; 36:1147–1150.
57. Sandler RS, Wurzelmann JI, Lyles CM. Oral contraceptive use and the risk of inflammatory bowel disease. Epidemiology 1992; 3:374–378.
58. Gilat T, Hacohen D, Lilos P, Langman MJS. Childhood factors in ulcerative colitis and Crohn's disease. Scand J Gastroenterol 1987; 22:1009–1024.

5
Pathology and Pathophysiology of Symptoms

William J. Tremaine *Mayo Foundation, Rochester, Minnesota*

I. INTRODUCTION

Because the etiology of Crohn's disease is unknown, the perception of what constitutes the illness and distinguishes it from others is based on observations of pathology and symptoms that occur together. There is a variety of presentations of the disease; yet, with each presentation, the pathology and symptoms go hand in hand. In this chapter, this relationship of pathology and symptoms is examined.

II. BASIC PATHOLOGY

There is no single pathological feature that is diagnostic of Crohn's disease, but one or more typical histopathological changes are usually present.

A. Aphthous Ulcer

The aphthous ulcer is thought to be the earliest mucosal lesion, and it is characteristic of the disease (1). These pinpoint ulcers are often found in mucosa that overlies enlarged lymphoid follicles, and the ulcers may occur as isolated abnormalitites in mucosa that otherwise appears normal (2). What predisposes the epithelium over a lymph follicle to ulceration is unknown. It may have to do with M cells—specialized epithelial cells that differ in structure and function from the typical gut epithelium. These cells take up foreign particles by pinocytosis and shunt them through the cell into vesicles that are released to migrating lymphocytes. Other epithelial cells also take up particles by pinocytosis, but they package the particles in phagolysosomes where they are destroyed or broken down rather than released. Perhaps it is a dysfunciton of these M cells that allows the entry of agents that cause Crohn's disease, with the subsequent destruction of the surrounding epithelium and the development of an aphthous ulcer (3).

B. Larger Ulcers

The coalescence of aphthous ulcers probably leads to the formation of tiny serpiginous ulcers, which, in turn, connect to form larger ulcers. Both the stellate ulcers and longitudinal ulcers that are found in Crohn's disease may be the result of the merging of smaller ulcers (1).

C. Granulomas

The granuloma is the hallmark of the microscopic findings in Crohn's disease. It may occur as just a loose collection of macrophages or it may be more cellular and contain multinucleated giant cells, neutrophils, eosinophils, and a small area of central necrosis (4). Granulomas are found in up to two-thirds of resected tissue specimens and, in general, the more sections taken, the higher the yield (5). Endoscopic mucosal biopsies from the rectum in a patient with endoscopically visible disease in the rectum yields granulomas in 28% of specimens when two or more biopsies are obtained and the biopsies are meticulously examined with serial sections (6). Granulomas may be found in up to 14% of rectal biopsies in patients with Crohn's disease even when the mucosa looks normal endoscopically (7). Granulomas are more commonly found in Crohn's colitis than in Crohn's ileitis (8). Granulomas are twice as prevalent, are found in higher numbers per cubic millimeter, and are smaller in children than in adults (9). The number of granulomas diminish with increasing duration of disease, with 10% fewer granulomas occurring after 3 years (10). Granulomas may also be found in ulcerative colitis: they were present in 17% of patients in one series (11). Therefore, the presence or absence of granulomas does not confirm or exclude the diagnosis of Crohn's disease.

D. Transmural Inflammation

Transmural inflammation, the presence of lymphoid aggregrates in all layers of the intestine including the serosa, is a characteristic but not invariable finding in Crohn's disease. Typically, the inflammation is most dense in the submucosa, which may be edematous and markedly thickened, with variable involvement in the lamina propria and the muscularis mucosa. Transmural inflammation is found more commonly in patients with chronic and long-standing disease than in patients with acute fulminant disease (12). In areas that are not ulcerated, the inflammation may consist of only isolated chronic inflammatory cells scattered through the layers of the intestine.

E. Disproportionate Submucosal Inflammation

Disproportionate submucosal inflammation refers to the presence of a dense submucosal infiltrate with a relatively normal and noninflamed overlying mucosa. This inflammation in the submucosa distinguishes Crohn's colitis from ulcerative colitis, but endoscopic biopsies are not deep enough to demonstrate the finding. The lymphocytic infiltrates in the submucosa and serosa sometimes develop into follicles that appear to be nodules along the serosal surface (13).

F. Fissures and Fistulas

Fissures arise from aphthous ulcers. They are lined by neutrophils with a surrounding infiltrate of mononuclear cells (12). Fissures may extend perpendicularly to the long axis of the gut and penetrate the muscularis mucosa. In one series, 30% of cases of Crohn's disease had demonstrable fissures (14). Fissures may be branched and complex, and complete penetration of the bowel wall by a fissure is often seen in association with an abscess in the serosal fat (4). Fistulas are presumed to be extensions of fissures, although this progression is unproven. With transmural involvement of the bowel, inflammation of the serosal surface incites an inflammatory exudate that is adherent and attaches the bowel to adjacent structures such as other loops of bowel, muscle, or another structure such as the bladder or vagina. Once the bowel is attached, the fissure advances into the other structure, creating a fistula.

G. Fibrosis and Strictures

Stricture formation is a common complication of the chronic intestinal inflammation in Crohn's disease and, in some patients, it occurs early in the course of the disease (15). The histological features include edema and fibrosis in the submucosa and thickening of the muscularis. In addition, histological examination of the strictures demonstrates a striking proliferation of smooth muscle cells in the muscularis mucosa and an accumulation of submucosal collagen (16). Type V collagen, a subset produced in large quantities in smooth muscle cells, is increased in the submucosal layer of strictures (16). The excesses of type V collagen could lead to the development of structural disturbances in the gut and the formation of strictures (Fig. 1). Type III collagen is synthesized by fibroblasts. It is present in all layers of the intestine, and it is abundant in the strictures of Crohn's disease (17). The fibroblasts are stimulated to make type III collagen by cytokines, such as TGF-β_1 and fibroblasts in strictures are more responsive to stimulation than fibroblasts in inflamed areas that are not strictured (17). An excess of either type III collagen or type V collagen could lead to stricture formation.

H. Vascular Abnormalities

Vascular abnormalities have been reported in 10%-20% of resected tissue from patients with Crohn's disease (18,19). The most common vascular lesion is periarteritis, which may

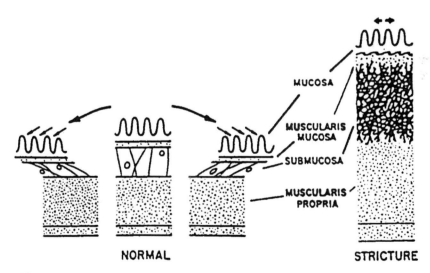

FIG. 1 Postulated role of submucosal collagen in normal and strictured bowel. In the physiological setting, submucosal collagen provides a compliant attachment of mucosa to muscularis propria. *Large arrows* denote mobility of mucosa on muscularis propria. After chronic inflammation, smooth muscle cell proliferation and collagen production within the submucosa lead to thickening of the bowel wall, adhesion of muscularis mucosae to muscularis propria, and a loss of compliance (*short arrows*), which together comprise a stricture. (From Graham et al. Ref 16.)

be granulomatous ro nongranulomatous. True vasculitis with fibroid necrosis may occur and, in long-standing cases, endoarteritis obliterans is common (4). Because of these abnormalities, it has been proposed that Crohn's disease is due to multifocal chronic mesenteric vasculitis in the areas of inflammation in the gut, although this theory has not been widely accepted (20,21).

I. Other Findings

Other histopathological abnormalities that may be found in Crohn's disease include neuronal hyperplasia, lymphangiectasia, and pyloric gland metaplasia. None of these features is specific for inflammatory bowel disease and may be seen with other inflammatory conditions.

III.   DIFFERENTIAL DIAGNOSIS OF BIOPSY FINDINGS

A.   Distinguishing Crohn's Disease from Ulcerative Colitis

Features that favor a diagnosis of Crohn's disease include patchy inflammation, preservation of goblet cells, transmural inflammation, disproportionate submucosal inflammation, and the presence of granulomas, whereas the diagnosis of ulcerative colitis is more likely if there is epithelial destruction, diffuse inflammation, goblet cell depletion, and glandular atrophy (19). The presence of epithelioid granulomas is highly specific for Crohn's disease (6), but not entirely diagnostic. Crypt abscesses in the mucosa are common in Crohn's disease, but they are much less abundant than in patients with ulcerative colitis. When ileal disease is limited to the distal 12 to 15 cm, Crohn's disease must be distinguished from backwash ileitis—the ileal disease that may be seen in approximately 10% of colectomy specimens—from patients with ulcerative colitis with pancolonic involvement (22). Backwash ileitis is probably an inappropriate name because there is no evidence for backwash as the mechanism. The histological changes in backwash ileitis are the same as those found in ulcerative colitis, and the ileocecal valve is dilated—features that are not typical of terminal ileal Crohn's disease.

As noted, the preservation of goblet cells is an important feature to differentiate Crohn's disease from ulcerative colitis. Laxatives and purgative bowel preparations can deplete goblet cells, which can cause misinterpretation of Crohn's colitis as ulcerative colitis.

Despite all efforts, including examination of the resected colon, Crohn's colitis cannot be distinguished from ulcerative colitis by current methods in at least 10% of cases (23).

B.   Diverticular Disease of the Colon

In western countries, colonic diverticular disease occurs in 10% of individuals older than age 40 years and in about one-third of those older than age 60 years, so it is not unexpected that a patient may have both diverticular disease and Crohn's disease (24). The presence of rectal inflammation can differentiate the two conditions. Histologically, it may not be possible to distinguish between an abscess attributable to diverticular disease from an abscess attributable to Crohn's disease.

C.   Ischemic Bowel

Ulcers and strictures in the colon and in the small intestine that are due to ischemia may have radiological or endoscopic appearances similar to those of Crohn's disease, but the histologic distinction is usually straightforward.

D. Lymphoma

Lymphoma of the small intestine may have clinical features that are identical with those of Crohn's disease, including abdominal pain, diarrhea, weight loss, fever, malaise, and a palpable abdominal mass. Symptoms are usually more constant and progressive with lymphoma. In contrast to Crohn's disease, the mass is usually hard and nontender rather than firm and tender. Stenotic lesions are less common in lymphoma than in Crohn's disease, and the total length of small intestinal involvement is usually greater in primary intestinal lymphoma than in Crohn's disease (25). Endoscopic biopsies may not be diagnostic of lymphoma, but confusion in the histological interpretation is more likely to be in distinguishing lymphoma from celiac sprue, not from Crohn's disease.

E. Infection

1. Tuberculosis

It is not possible to differentiate Crohn's disease from tuberculosis based on macroscopic features alone, but the distinction can be made histologically (26). Noncaseating granulomas may be present in both intestinal tuberculosis and Crohn's disease, but, in tuberculosis, the granulomas are bigger and confluent, with a surrounding rim of lymphocytes (19).

2. Yersinia Entercolitica

Terminal ileitis due to *Yersinia enterocolitica* causes disease in the ileocecal region that includes ulceration, granulomatous inflammation, microabscesses, and lymph node enlargement in a picture that can resemble Crohn's disease. The symptoms may be identical to those of Crohn's disease, most commonly with diarrhea, fever, and cramping abdominal pain (27). However, unlike in Crohn's disease, the granulomas in *Yersinia* infections are necrotizing. This gram-negative organism is best identified by stool culture. Serological diagnosis is not sufficiently specific for clinical use (28).

3. Cytomegalovirus

Cytomegalovirus (CMV) infections in the gastrointestinal tract occur in immunosuppressed patients and disease may occur in any part of the gut. The symptoms may be identical to those of Crohn's disease, with abdominal pain, watery or bloody diarrhea, fever, and weight loss. In patients with Crohn's disease who are on treatment with immunosuppresive drugs, CMV infection should be considered as a cause for worsening of symptoms, and patients who are receiving immunosuppressive therapy for other disorders and who develop symptoms compatible with Crohn's disease should be evaluated for possible CMV infection. Endoscopic and radiographical studies usually show nondiagnostic focal inflammatory changes, sometimes with deep ulcers. Biopsies can show typical intranuclear inclusions and, in contrast to Crohn's disease, there is no crypt distortion (29). Viral cultures of tissue biopsy specimens, urine, or blood can be obtained.

4. Other Infections

A number of other bacterial, viral, and fungal infections as well as parasitic infestations may be seen with clinical features similar to those of Crohn's disease (30). The histological changes in some colonic infections can be confused with Crohn's disease, but, in most cases, the histological findings point to an infectious cause (31). A high index of suspicion for an infectious cause and appropriate cultures usually differentiate infectious diseases form Crohn's disease.

F. Behçet's Syndrome

In addition to oral, ocular, and genital lesions, patients with Behçet's syndrome may have ulcers throughtout the gastrointestinal tract. Colonic involvement with ulcers occurs most commonly in Western countries, and this presentation may be difficult to distinguish from Crohn's colitis (32). Microscopically, ulcers are surrounded by an inflammatory infiltrate that may be transmural. As with Crohn's disease, there may be vasculitis in the intestinal vessels and granulomas may be seen. In contrast to Crohn's disease, aggregated lympho-cytic inflammation, strictures, and stenosis are not seen with Behçet's syndrome.

G. Solitary Ulcer Syndrome

The solitary anterior rectal ulcer that occurs, often associated with rectal prolapse, can be misinterpreted as rectal Crohn's disease. However, a biopsy easily distinguishes the condition because of the presence of mucosal fibrosis, crypt hyperplasia, and buried glands beneath the muscularis mucosa known as "colitis cystica profunda." Goblet cell depletion is usually present (33).

H. Medication-Induced Inflammatory Disease

Nonsteroidal anti-inflammatory drugs (NSAIDs) may cause ulceration throughout the gastrointestinal tract, including the small intestine and colon (34). When ulcers occur primarily in the terminal ileum and colon, Crohn's disease may be a major diagnostic consideration. In addition, patients with Crohn's disease and arthralgias may take NSAIDs and develop superimposed ulceration that may be interpreted as an exacerbation of the Crohn's disease. Although some patients who have taken NSAIDs develop characteristic mucosal diaphragms, in many cases, there is nonspecific chronic inflammation without prominent fibrosis. Clinical correlation is necessary to make the correct diagnosis.

IV. PATHOLOGY AND SYMPTOMS: SUBGROUPS

The various clinical presentations of Crohn's disease may be divided into a number of homogeneous subgroups based on anatomical location of the disease, extent of disease, behavior of the disease (primarily inflammatory, fistulizing or fibrostenotic), and operative history (primary or recurrent disease) as delineated by Sachar et al. (Table 1) (35).

Although this classification system has not been tested for its reliability in distinguish-ing clinical responses to treatment, risks for complications, and long-term prognosis, it is useful in providing a framework for characterization of the many manifestations of this disease. In particular, the correlation of pathology and clinical manifestations is more accessible in this schema.

A. Disease Location

Crohn's disease can involve the gastrointestinal tract in any location, from the mouth to the anus, and it is much more common in the ileum and colon than in more proximal locations in the digestive tract.

1. Oral Lesions

Ulcers on the gums, buccal mucosa, lips, and tongue occur in 11% of patients with Crohn's colitis as single or multiple lesions (36). They may be the first manifestation of disease and often herald the onset of an exacerbation of established distal disease. Because

TABLE 1 Subgroups of Crohn's Disease

Modifier	Variables
A. Location[a]	1. Stomach/duodenum
	2. Jejunum
	3. Ileum
	4. Colon
	5. Rectum
	6. Anal, perianal
B. Extent	1. Localized
	2. Diffuse
C. Behavior	1. Primarily inflammatory
	2. Primarily fistulizing
	3. Primarily fibrostenotic
D. Operative history	1. Primary
	2. Recurrent

[a]Sites primarily involved, not those that might be "innocent" recipients of fistulas from elsewhere. In case of multiple locations, indicate all sites (e.g., ileocolon = 3-4) as well as the sites predominantly involved (e.g., ileocolon, predominantly ileum).
Source: Ref. 35.

oral ulcers are common and can occur without other disease associations, there must be more distal disease present to be certain that oral lesions are associated with Crohn's disease. The ulcers may be asymptomatic or painful. Rarely, there are larger and deeper mouth ulcers that cause severe pain and impede oral nutrition.

2. Pharyngeal and Esophageal Disease

Erythema, edema, and strictures may occur in the pharynx and esophagus, usually in conjunction with small intestinal or colonic disease (37,38). Dysphagia is the most common symptom, and patients may have pain and bleeding. Involvement in these locations is rare; fewer than 50 cases of esophageal Crohn's disease have been reported (39). The features vary from mild to severe changes with patchy ulcers, focal deep ulcers, or strictures that can appear malignant. The pathology is similar to that of disease in other sites. Other causes such as peptic reflux, medication-induced lesions, infections, neoplasms, and Behçet's syndrome should be excluded (40).

3. Gastric and Duodenal Crohn's Disease

Older studies using radiographical techniques identified involvement of the stomach and duodenum in up to 4% of patients (41,42). In a more recent prospective study, 13 of 31 (42%) of adolescents with Crohn's disease of the distal intestine who underwent gastroscopy had upper tract involvement, although only 5 (16%) had symptoms and only one (3%) had radiographical findings (43). In the stomach, antral involvement is the most common, but there may be diffuse disease resembling linitis plastica with mural thickening and the stomach may be poorly distensible (44). Symptoms may be similar to those of peptic ulcer disease with epigastric pain, which, in come cases, radiates to the interscapular area of the back, but the pain is rarely relieved by eating or using antacids as may occur in peptic ulcer disease. Fistulas between the colon and the stomach or duodenum are common and usually arise from the colon. Fistulas may also originate in the stomach and extend to the spleen (45). Gastric, pyloric, or duodenal strictures may cause obstruction with nausea, vomiting, abdominal pain, and weight loss. There may be superficial ulcers, deep irregular ulcers and thickened nodular folds, and the mucosa may have a cobblestone appearance; diffuse ulceration of the gastroduodenum is not a feature (19). Granulomas are found in up to 68% of biopsy studies (46). In addition, granulomas are sometimes found in duodenal biopsy studies of normal-appearing mucosa when there is proven Crohn's disease elsewhere in the gut.

The differential diagnosis includes peptic ulcer disease, NSAIDs-induced injury, neoplasm, and other causes of granulomatous disease of the stomach (tuberculosis, syphilis, herpes simplex, sarcoidosis, and isolated granulomatous gastritis) (47). Most of the possibilities in the differential diagnosis can be eliminated by historical data, the histology of gastric or duodenal biopsies, and, for patients at risk, cultures of mucosal biopsies. Differentiating peptic ulcer disease from Crohn's disease may be difficult, particularly when there is no distal bowel involvement and when granulomas are absent. Failure of the patient to improve with standard therapy with H_2-blocker therapy, the absence of *Helicobacter pylori* in the gastric mucosa, and a normal serum gastrin are all clues to the diagnosis.

4. Jejunal Crohn's Disease

In the Cleveland Clinic series of 615 consecutive patients with Crohn's disease, 37 (6%) had involvement of the duodenum or jejunum. Most of the patients also had ileitis, with only 8 patients (1.3%) with only jejunal disease (48). Patients with diffuse inflammation of both the jejunum and ileum may have abdominal pain, diarrhea, fever, malabsorption, and malnutrition. Patients with obstruction due to inflammatory or fibrostenotic changes may have pain, nausea, vomiting, distention, and diarrhea. Because jejunal disease usually occurs in conjunction with ileal disease, the symptoms depend on the total extent and severity of the bowel disease.

5. Ileal Crohn's Disease

In the Cleveland Clinic series of 615 consecutive patients, 391 (63.5%) had ileal involvement, with associated colitis in 252 (41%) and without colitis in 139 (22.5%) (48). Abdominal pain, a feature in two-thirds of the patients, is usually located in the right lower quadrant. On physical examination, there may be a palpable inflammatory mass that has a spectrum of characteristics: it may be diffuse and ill defined or more circumscribed; it may be tender and soft, or hard and irregular, resembling a neoplasm. In patients with involvement that is limited to a relatively short segment of the terminal ileum, less than 50 cm, diarrhea is usually mild with less that 6 stools passed per day. With more extensive small intestinal disease, there may be severe diarrhea. A persistent low-grade fever is common with active disease, this was the sole presenting symptom in 11 of 542 cases reviewed by Crohn and Yarnis (49).

Some patients present suddenly with symptoms indistinguishable from acute appendicitis. At laparotomy, the diagnosis of acute ileitis is made when an inflamed, edematous terminal ileum is found. Some of these presentations are probably due to infection with *Yersinia* or other agent because only the minority eventually develop Crohn's disease. In one series, 15 of 54 patients presenting as acute ileitis developed chronic Crohn's disease after a follow-up period of 25 years (50).

6. Crohn's Disease of the Appendix

Isolated Crohn's disease of the appendix may occur with less than a 10% risk of development of recurrent disease following appendectomy (51). Appendiceal involvement may occur at the same time as disease that is not in continuity, such as the rectum. For patients who have undergone right hemicolectomy for Crohn's colitis, approximately 25% of the specimens have appendiceal disease (52). Typical appendicitis that is not due to Crohn's disease may develop in the setting of Crohn's disease involving the ileum or colon (53).

7. Crohn's Colitis

In the Cleveland Clinic series, isolated colonic disease occurred in 27% of patients and ileocolonic disease was present in another 41% of 615 patients, with a total of 68% of patients with disease in the colon (48). Diffuse colonic disease occurred about twice as commonly as segmental disease. There is rectal sparing in about half of cases of Crohn's colitis (54).

Symptoms depend on the location, extent, and severity of colonic disease. Abdominal pain is the most common symptom, occurring in 55% to 65% of patients, and rectal bleeding occurs in less than half of patients (48). Patients with rectosigmoid disease may have tenesmus and constipation or diarrhea. With more proximal colonic involvement, diarrhea is a common feature, although the frequency and severity of the diarrhea varies so widely that is difficult to quantitate the frequency of occurrence. The role of colonic involvement in nutrition is limited, but up to 22% of patients with colonic involvement may be malnourished, perhaps reflecting a decrease in caloric intake as well as gut loss of protein due to exudation from a diseased mucosa (48). Symptoms due to obstruction and fistulas are reviewed in subsequent paragraphs.

8. Anal Crohn's Disease

Approximately 25% of patients with small bowel disease and 75% of patients with colonic disease have anal lesions during the course of the disease, and approximately 5% of patients with anorectal disease do not have more proximal disease (55). The abnormalities are fissures, fistulas, strictures, and edematous anal tags. Symptoms include local pain, tenderness, fever, drainage of mucus, pus, or stool, and bleeding. Biopsies often show granulomas that differentiate these lesions from other causes of anal disease.

The anal disease may occur and resolve or be surgically treated many years before the onset of Crohn's disease more proximally in bowel. In contrast, anal disease may not improve with removal of proximal areas of bowel involvement with Crohn's disease (56).

V. EXTENT OF DISEASE: IMPLICATIONS FOR SYMPTOMS

In the classification system proposed by Sachar et al. the distribution of disease, whether diffuse or localized, is one of the modifiers used for categorization (35). This distinction also has implications in terms of symptoms.

A. Diffuse Disease

1. Small Intestine

The spectrum of symptoms with extensive involvement of the small bowel, such as more than 1 m of disease, is often different from the symptoms with less extensive involvement. Uncommonly, a patient may have widespread jejunoileal disease that is asymptomatic, or nearly so, and present with only laboratory abnormalities such as anemia or hypoproteinemia. More typically, the patient with extensive disease has generalized abdominal pain that is constant or cramping, weight loss, fever, diarrhea, steatorrhea, and malaise. The weight loss is usually due to damage or destruction of intestinal villi by disease that extends over a large surface area with malabsorption of fat, protein, and specific nutrients. Iron deficiency can be due to iron malabsorption because of duodenal disease or to iron loss from intestinal bleeding. Extensive disease of the distal ileum may result in bile salt and vitamin B_{12} malabsorption.

2. *Diffuse Colonic Disease*

Patients with diffuse colonic involvement may present with symptoms that are indistinguishable from ulcerative colitis with bloody diarrhea, abdominal pain, tenesmus, weight loss, fever, and malaise. When the disease is severely active, dilation with the onset of toxic megacolon is a potential risk, and it is more likely to occur with diffuse than with segmental involvement (57).

B. Localized Disease

Crohn's disease occurs most typically in a segmental pattern with skip areas of normal mucosa, both in the small intestine and in the colon. The length of involved segments varies from a focal stricture of less than 1 cm in length to segments several meters long. The presence of skip lesions in the colon is a distinguishing feature from ulcerative colitis.

VI.   DISEASE BEHAVIOR

Crohn's disease may be classified as primarily inflammatory, or fibrostenotic. In many patients, there may be overlapping features of these categories, but, at any point in time, one of the features dominate the clinical presentation (35). With each pattern, there are characteristic symptoms.

A. Inflammatory Disease

Crohn's disease with exclusive inflammatory features is synonymous with uncomplicated disease, that is, without fistulas, abscesses, or obstructive features. Some patients continue to have only inflammatory changes throughout the course of their illness, without an inevitable progression to complications. In others, inflammatory features represent an early stage of disease that progresses to a more complicated illness. Symptoms of inflammatory-predominant disease include those directly related to the intestinal disease, such as abdominal pain, diarrhea, fever, and rectal bleeding, as well as the extraintestinal symptoms, including peripheral arthritis, erythema nodosum, iritis and uveitis, anemia, and perhaps pyoderma gangrenosum (58). Inflammatory disease is particularly amenable to medical therapy and is potentially completely reversible.

B. Fistulas

Fistulas may occur anywhere from the stomach to the perianal area. Most commonly, fistulas are multiple and arise from the ileum, colon, and anus. Excluding perianal fistulas, enteric fistulas occur in 20% to 40% of cases, equally divided between internal and external fistulas (59). Internal fistulas vary with the site of Crohn's disease; in one series, they occurred in 34% of patients with ileocolic disease, 16% with small intestinal and 17% with colonic disease (19). Internal fistulas develop between loops of bowel and between bowel and bladder, vagina, or uterus. Less commonly, a fistula may develop between the ileum and the sigmoid colon, the ileum and duodenum, or the colon and the stomach or duodenum (60).

1. Enteroenteric and Enterocolic Fistulas

Fistulous connections between adjacent loops of bowel are not uncommon and may be asymptomatic. Bypasses of short segments of intestine due to fistulas are often asymptomatic and do not require treatment. Symptoms may even improve when an internal fistula decompresses a partial bowel obstruction caused by stenosis. Bypasses of long segments of intestine by fistulas are more likely to cause symptoms, though, with diarrhea and the consequences of malabsorption. The fistulas may be side to side between two loops of bowel, or there may be transmural tunneling along the length of a segment of intestine. Fistulas from the colon to the stomach or duodenum usually originate in the colon (61) and fistulas between the ileum and colon usually originate in the ileum (61). More common causes of coloduodenal fistulas are duodenal ulcer, duodenal diverticulitis, appendiceal abscess, foreign body with perforation, and posttraumatic circumstances (62,63).

2. Enterovesical Fistulas

In a series of 65 patients with enterovesical fistulas reported from the Cleveland Clinic, 57% of the fistulas arose from both the ileum and colon, 35% originated in just the ileum, and 8% originated from the colon alone (64). The symptoms are dysuria, pneumaturia, and fecaluria; most patients have all three symptoms.

3. Rectovaginal Fistulas

Fistulas to the vagina in Crohn's disease usually arise from the rectum, and these fistulas occur in up to 23% of women with Crohn's disease (65). The classic symptoms are the passage of gas or stool from the vagina, but some women may have recurrent vaginitis as the only symptom, and 20% of patients are asymptomatic. The fistulas are usually associated with active rectal disease and, in most cases, the presenting symptoms are due to the bowel complaints rather than the rectovaginal fistula (66).

4. Enterocutaneous Fistulas

External fistulas usually occur after surgery for Crohn's disease, probably because the serosa of the inflamed gut adheres more easily to the incised parietal peritoneum; as a result, the fistula develops through the scar. In a study of 47 fistulas occurring after surgery for Crohn's disease, 5% occurred after intestinal resection, 13% occurred after an intestinal bypass procedure, 11% occurred after diagnostic laparatomy, and 24% developed after appendectomy (67). External fistulas to the abdominal wall may arise spontaneously but are much less common than fistulas that develop after laparotomy. Symptoms associated with external fistulas depend on the severity of the fluid loss, either high output (> 500 ml/day) with local skin breakdown, fluid depletion, and nutritional and electrolyte losses or low output (< 500 ml/day), with which the main risk is the potential for local infections.

5. Anal and Perianal Fissures and Fistulas

In most patients with Crohn's disease, anal and perianal fistulas develop after disease has occurred at other locations, but, in 10%, the anal disease may be the first manifestation.

In contrast to other causes of perianal fissures in which the lesions are midline, in Crohn's disease, the fissures are usually located laterally in the anal canal (67). The bases of the fissures are often deep and have undermined edges. The fissures and fistulas of Crohn's disease are usually less painful than those due to other causes. The paths that anal fistulas take are variable and they may open onto the perineum, the buttocks, or into the vagina.

6. Other Fistulas

Fistulas to unusual sites may develop, such as from the stomach to the spleen and from the colon to the bronchial tree, among other (45,68).

C.   Intra-Abdominal and Pelvic Abscess

An abscess develops from a slowly penetrating ulcer of the bowel wall. An abscess may resolve by discharging into the lumen of the bowel or into another organ, resulting in a fistula. Psoas abscess has also been reported as a complication of Crohn's disease (69). When an abscess points to the skin and then opens either spontaneously or surgically, a persistent external fistula usually results. In one series, abscesses were identified pre-operatively in 10% of consecutive patients who underwent surgery for Crohn's disease (70). Most were solitary and developed in patients with small bowel disease. Usually the abscess is small and is not detected by investigations such as computed tomography (CT), gallium scan, leukocyte imaging, or ultrasonography. The white cell count is typically normal. Some patients have a high serum alkaline phosphatase level. In most cases, the abscess is unsuspected. In the same series of patients, postoperative abscess occurred in 14% of the patients and they developed either soon after the operation or within a few months (70). The early abscesses were usually due to anastomotic dehiscence, fecal fistula, or an infected hematoma. Late abscesses were often recurrent in patients who had previously undergone surgical drainage of an abscess. The organisms usually isolated are *Escherichia coli, Bacteroides fragilis,* enterococci, and *Streptococcus viridans.* Treatment is resection of the diseased bowel in continuity with the abscess. Liver abscess is a rare complication of Crohn's disease (71).

The symptoms of an ileal abscess are abdominal pain that can radiate to the right leg if there is psoas involvement and a tender mass in the right lower abdomen. Patients who are already taking anti-inflammatory medications may not have the classic spiking fever, chills, and increased white blood cell count typically found with an abscess.

D.   Fibrosis and Stenosis

As Prantera et al. have pointed out, stenosis and obstruction are not the inevitable consequences of long-standing bowel inflammation; instead they represent a subgroup of Crohn's patients in whom stenosis may develop at any time in the disease course (72). Intestinal obstruction occurs in approximately one-third of patients with Crohn's disease. When examined according to the site of the disease, 44% of patients with obstruction have ileocolonic involvement, 35% have small intestinal involvement, and 17% have disease limited to the colon (48). The symptoms of fibrosis and stenosis depend on the degree of narrowing of the bowel lumen. Nevertheless, patients with marked narrowing of the lumen, as demonstrated by barium x-rays, film, may be asymptomatic because they have restricted their dietary intake of fiber and bulk, sometimes unintentionally. These patients have obstructive symptoms only after eating large or high fiber meals. With tight stenosis, there may be constant pain made worse by drinking or eating, with subsequent abdominal distention, nausea, and vomiting.

VII. OPERATIVE HISTORY

The natural history and responsiveness to medical therapy in Crohn's disease are altered by bowel resections (35). For example, recurrent disease usually appears just proximal to the site of the previous resection for terminal ileal disease with ileocolonic anastomosis. Reflux of colonic contents into the small intestine has been suggested as the cause, but the data regarding this hypothesis are conflicting (73). The risk of recurrence is independent of the presence of microscopic inflammation at the surgical margins, so conservative resections are indicated (74).

VIII. SYMPTOMS AND PSYCHOLOGICAL FACTORS

It is now generally accepted that psychological disorders in individuals with Crohn's disease are a result, not a cause of the underlying illness. Earlier studies that proposed a classic psychosomatic etiology were flawed by selection bias and the lack of appropriate control groups. More recently, Helzer et al. studied 50 subjects with Crohn's disease and 50 control subjects with other chronic medical illness (75). A significantly greater number of patients with Crohn's disease had depression and other psychiatric disorders, but the psychiatric symptoms occur concurrently with exacerbations of the disease and do not appear to be precipitating factors. Patients with inflammatory bowel disease readily discuss symptoms that concern bowel function, pain, and energy level, but the minority volunteer information about emotional problems or social stresses unless prompted (76). Patients with Crohn's disease who also have depression or anxiety may have a more prolonged illness than patients without these coexistent symptoms (77).

IX. NEUROHORMONAL DISTURBANCES AND SYMPTOMS

Marked changes in neuropeptide levels in the bowel and in peptidergic gut innervation patterns have been observed in patients with inflammatory bowel disease (78). Neuropeptides that may play a role include substance P (SP), vasoactive intestinal peptide (VIP), calcitonin gene-related peptide (CGRP), and somatostatin. These peptides have been proposed as possible mediators of neurogenic inflammation, a reaction that includes vasodilation, extravasation of plasma, and contraction of smooth muscles (79). The amounts of SP and immunoreactive VIP are increased in inflammatory bowel disease, and the amount of immunoreactive somatostatin is decreased (80,81). It is possible that alterations in the tissue levels of these peptides may mediate not only the inflammatory response in Crohn's disease but also the immunological alterations and some of the symptoms such as abdominal pain, fever, and diarrhea.

X. DYSMOTILITY AND SYMPTOMS

A. Motility Disorders

Delayed gastric emptying may occur in Crohn's disease and contribute to nausea, but it is not clear if the abnormal emptying is due to direct injury of the gastroduodenum by the disease or an indirect result of weight loss (82). In patients with Crohn's disease who do not have mechanical obstruction, no clinically important abnormalities of small intestinal motility have been identified (83). Approximately 3% of patients with Crohn's disease have fecal incontinence, usually following anorectal surgery (84). Although there are a number of reports about alterations in colonic motility in ulcerative colitis, similar studies of the colonic motility in patients with Crohn's colitis are lacking.

B.   Irritable Bowel Syndrome and Crohn's Disease

Because irritable bowel syndrome (IBS) is so common, with a prevalence of up to 20% in otherwise healthy individuals, it is not uncommon for patients with Crohn's disease to have IBS as well (85). Up to one-third of patients with quiescent ulcerative colitis have symptoms of IBS and presumably the same situation could occur in Crohn's disease (86). The distinction between IBS and inflammatory bowel disease has obvious implications in terms of treatment.

REFERENCES

1.   Price AB, Morson BC. Inflammatory bowel disease: the surgical pathology of Crohn's disease and ulcerative colitis. Hum Pathol 1975; 6:7–29.
2.   O'Leary AD, Sweeney EC. Lymphoglandular complexes of the colon: structure and distribution. Histopathology 1983; 10:267.
3.   Owen RL. And now pathophysiology of M-cells—good news and bad news from Peyer's patches. Gastroenterology 1983; 85:468.
4.   Domizio P. Patholgoy of chronic inflammatory bowel disease in children. Baillieres Clin Gastroenterol 1994; 8(1):35–63.
5.   Chambers TJ, Morson BC. The histopathological evolution of Crohn's disease. In: Pena AS, Weterman IT, Booth CC, Strober W, eds. Recent Advances in Crohn's Disease. The Hague: Martinus Nijhoff, 1981.
6.   Surawicz CM, Meisel JL, Yivisaker T, Saunders DR, Rubin CE. Rectal biopsy in the diagnosis of Crohn's disease: value of multiple biopsies and serial sectioning. Gastroenterology 1981; 81:66–71.
7.   Rotterdam H, Korelitz B 1, Sommers SC. Microgranulomas in grossly normal rectal mucosa in Crohn's disease. Am J Clin Pathol 1977; 67:550.
8.   Chambers TJ, Morson BC. Role of the granuloma in recurrent Crohn's disease. Gut 1979; 20:269–274.
9.   Schmitz-Moorman P, Schag M. Histology of the lower intestinal tract in Crohn's disease of children and adolescents. Multicentric paediatric Crohn's disease study. Pathol Res Prac 1990; 186(4);479–484.
10.   Kelly JK, Sutherland LR. The chronological sequence in the pathology of Crohn's disease. J Clin Gastroenterol 1988; 10:28–33.
11.   Glotzer DJ, Gardner RC, Goldman J, Hinricks HR, Rose H, Zetzel L. Comparative features and course of ulcerative colitis and granulomatous colitis. N Engl J Med 1970; 282:582.
12.   Riddell RH. Pathology of idiopathic inflammatory bowel disease. In: Inflammatory Bowel Disease. 3rd ed. Philadelphia: Lea & Febiger 20. 338–344.
13.   Otani S. Pathology of regional enteritis and regional enterocolitis. J Mt Sinai Hosp 1955; 22:147–158.
14.   Nyhlin H, Stenling R. The small-intestinal mucosa in patients with Crohn's disease assessed by scanning electron and light microscopy. Scand Gastroenterol 1984; 19:433.
15.   Kirsner JB, Shorter RG. Inflammatory Bowel Disease. 2nd ed. Philadelphia: Lea & Febiger, 1980:215, 510.
16.   Graham MF, Diegelmann RF, Elson CO, Lindblad WJ, Gotschalk N, Gay S, Gary R. Collagen content and types in the intestinal strictures of Crohn's disease. Gastroenterology 1988; 94:257–65.
17.   Stallmach A, Schuppan D, Riese HH, Matthes H, Riecken EO. Increased collagen type III

synthesis by fibroblasts isolated from strictures of patients with Crohn's disease. Gastroenterology 1992; 102:1920–1929.

18. Geller SA, Cohen A. Inflammatory arterial involvement in Crohn's disease. Arch Pathol Lab Med 1983; 107:475.

19. Morson BC, Dawson IMP, Day DW. Crohn's disease. In: Morson and Dawson's Gastrointestinal Pathology. 3rd ed. Oxford: Blackwell Scientific 1990:258–276.

20. Wakefield AJ, Dhillon AP, Rowles PM, et al. Pathogenesis of Crohn's disease: multifocal gastrointestinal infarction. Lancet 1989; 2:1057–1062.

21. Talbot IC, Kamm MA, Leaker BR. Pathogenesis of Crohn's disease. Lancet 1992; 340:315–316.

22. Hawk WA, Turnbull RB. Primary ulcerative disease of the colon. Gastroenterolgy 1966; 51:802–805.

23. Marin ML, Geller SA, Greenstein AJ, Marin RH, Gordon RE, Aufses AH Jr. Ultrastructural pathology of Crohn's disease: correlated transmission electron microscopy, scanning microscopy, and freeze fracture studies. A J Gastroenterol 1983; 78:355–365.

24. Manousos ON, Truelove SC, Lumsden K. Prevalence of colonic diverticulosis in the general population of the Oxford area. BMJ 1967; 3:762.

25. Trier JS. Lymphoma. In: Sleisenger MH, Fortran JS, eds. Gastrointestinal Disease. Philadelphia: WB Saunders, 1978:1121–1122.

26. Tandon HD, Prakash A. Pathology of intestinal turberculosis and its distinction from Crohn's disease. Gut 1972; 13:260.

27. Vantrappen G, Agg HO, Geboes K, Ponette E. Yersinia enteritis. Med Clin North Am 1982; 66:639–653.

28. Cover TL, Aber RC. Yersinia entercolitica. N Engl J Med 1989; 321:16–24.

29. Surawicz CM, Belic L. Rectal biopsy helps to distinguish acute self-limited colitis from idiopathic inflammatory bowel disease. Gastreonterology 1984; 86:104–113.

30. Tedesco F. Differential diagnosis of ulcerative colitis and Crohn's ileo-colitis and other specific inflammatory disease of the bowel. Med Clin North Am 1980; 64:1173–1183.

31. Rutgeerts P, Geboes K, Ponette E, Coremans G, Vantrappen G. Acute infective colitis caused by endemic pathogens in western Europe: endoscopic features. Endoscopy 1982; 14:212–219.

32. Lee RG. The colitis of Behçet's syndrome. Am J Surg Pathol 1986; 101:888–893.

33. Levine DS, Surawicz CM, Ajer TN, et al. Diffuse excess mucosal collagen in rectal biopsies facilitates differential diagnosis of solitary rectal ulcer syndrome from other inflammatory bowel diseases. Dig Dis Sci 1988; 33:1345–1352.

34. Allison MC, Howatson AG, Torrance CJ, Lee FC, Russell RI. Gastrointestinal damage associated with the use of nonsteroidal antiinflammatory drugs. N Engl J Med 1992; 327(11):749–754.

35. Sachar DB, Andrews HA, Farmer RG, Pallone F, Pena AS, Prantera C, Rutgeerts P. Proposed classification of patient subgroups in Crohn's disease. Gastroenterology Int 1992; 5(3):141–154.

36. Greenstein AJ, Janowitz HD, Sachar DB. The extra-intestinal complications of Crohn's disease and ulcerative colitis: a study of 700 patients. Medicine 1976; 55:401–412.

37. Rowe PH, Taylor PR, Sladen GE, Owen WJ. Cricopharyngeal Crohn's disease. Post Grad Med J 1987; 63:1101–1102.

38. Miller LJ, Thistle JL, Payne WS, Gaffey TA, O'Duffy JD. Crohn's disease involving the esophagus and colon. May Clin Proc 1977; 52:35–38.

39. Freedman PG, Dieterich DT, Balthazar EJ. Crohn's disease of the esophagus: case report and review of the literature. Am J Gastroenterol 1984; 79:835.

40. Lockhart JM, McIntyre W, Caperton EM. Esophageal ulceration in Behçet's syndrome. Ann Intern Med 1976; 84:572–573.

41. Fielding JF, Cooke WT. Peptic ulceration in Crohn's disease (regional enteritis). Gut 1970; 11:998.

42. Nugent FW, Richmond M, Park SK. Crohn's disease of the duodenum. Gut 1977; 18:115.

43. Mashako M, Cezard JP, Navarro J, et al. Crohn's disease lesions in the upper gastrointestinal tract: correlation between clinical, radiological, endoscopic and histological features in adolescents and children. J Pediatr Gastroenterol Nutr 1989; 8:442–446.

44. Johnson OA, Hoskins DW, Thorbjarnason B. Crohn's disease of the stomach. Gastroenterology 1966; 50:571.

45. Carey ER, Tremaine WJ, Banks PM, Nogorney DM. Isolated Crohn's disease of the stomach. Mayo Clin Proc 1989; 64:776–779.

46. Rutgeerts P, Onette E, Vantrappen G, Geboes K, Broeckaert C, Talloen L. Crohn's diseae of the stomach and duodenum: a clinical study with the emphasis on the value of endoscopy and endoscopic biopsies. Endoscopy 1980; 12:288.

47. Raffin SB. Granulomatous and infectious disease of the stomach. In: Sleisenger MH, Fordtran JS, eds. Gastrointestinal Disease. Philadelphia: WB Saunders 1978:744.

48. Farmer RG, Hawk WA, Turnbull RB. Clinical patterns in Crohn's disease: a statistical study of 615 cases. Gastroenterology 1975; 68:627.

49. Crohn BB, Yarnis H. Regional Ileitis. 2nd ed. New York: Grune & Stratton, 1958.

50. deDombal FT, Burton IL, Clamp SE, Goligher JC. Short term course and prognosis of Crohn's disease. Gut 1974; 15:435.

51. Allen DC, Biggart JD. Granulomatous disease in the vermiform appendix. J Clin Pathol 1983; 36:632.

52. Ariel I, Vinograd I, Hershlag A, et al. Crohn's disease isolated to the appendix. Truths and fallacies. Hum Pathol 1986; 17:1116.

53. Jess P. Acute appendicitis: epidemiology, diagnostic accuracy and complications. Scand J Gastroenterology 1983; 18:161–163.

54. Lockhart-Mummery HE, Morson BC. Crohn's disease (regional enteritis) of the large intestine and its distinction from ulcerative colitis. Gut 1960; 1:87.

55. Lockhart-Mummery HE. Crohn's disease: anal lesions. Dis Colon Rectum 1975; 18:200.

56. Wolff BG, Culp CE, Beart RW, Ilstrup DM, Ready RL. Anorectal Crohn's disease: a long term perspective. Dis Colon Rectum 1985; 28:709.

57. Linssen A, Tytgat GN. Fulminant onset of Crohn's disease of the colon (CDC). Dig Dis Sci 1982; 27:731–736

58. Greenstein AJ, Janowitz HD, Sachar DB. The extra-intestinal complications of Crohn's disease and ulcerative colitis: a study of 700 patients. Medicine 1976; 55:401–412.

59. Williams JA. Surgery and the management of Crohn's Disease. Clinics in Gastroenterology 1972; 1:469.

60. Jacobson IM, Schapiro RH, Warshaw AL. Gastric and duodenal fistulas in Crohn's diseae. Gastroenterology 1985; 89:1347.

61. Annibal R, Pietri P. Fistulous complications of Crohn's disease. Int Surg 1992; 77:19–24.

62. Korelitz B. Colonic-duodenal fistula in Crohn's disease. Am Dig Dis 1977; 22:1040.

63. Ferguson CM, Moncure AC. Benign duodenocolic fistula. Dis Colon Rectum 1985; 28:852.

64. McNamara MJ, Fazio VW, Lavery IC, Weakley FL, Farmer RG. Surgical treatment of enterovesical fistulas in Crohn's disease. Dis Colon Rectum 1990; 33:271–276.

65. Heyen F, Winslet MC, Andrews H, Alexander-Williams J, Deighley MRB. Vaginal fistulas in Crohn's disease. Dis Colon Rectum 1989; 32:379–383.

66. Radcliffe AG, Ritchie JK, Hawley MS, Lennard-Jones JE, Northover JMA. Anovaginal and rectovaginal fistulas in Crohn's disease. Dis Colon Rectum 1988; 31:94–99.

67. Steinberg DM, Cooke WT, Williams JA. Abscess and Fistulae in Crohn's disease. Gut 1973; 14:865.

68. Flueckiger F, Kullnig P, Melzer G, Posch E. Colobronchial and gastrocolic fistulas: rare complication of Crohn's disease. Gastrointest Radiol 1990; 15:288–290.

69. Burul CJ, Ritchie JK, Hawley PR, Todd IP. Psoas abscess: a complication of Crohn's disease. B J Surgery 1980; 67:355.

70. Keighley MRB, Eastwood D, Ambrose NS, Allan RN, Burdon DW. Incidence and micro-biology of abdominal and pelvic abscess in Crohn's disease. Gastroenterology 1982; 83:1271.

71. Mir-Madjlessi SH, McHenry MC, Farmer RG. Liver abscess in Crohn's disease. Report of four cases and review of the literature. Gastroenterology 1986; 91:987.

72. Prantera C, Levenstein S, Capocaccia R, Mariotti S, Luzi C, Cosintino R, Simi M. Prediction of surgery for obstruction in Crohn's ileitis. Dig Dis Sci 1987; 32:1363–1369.

73. Cameron JL, Hanilton SR, Coleman J, Sitzmann JV, Bayless TM. Patterns of ileal recurrence in Crohn's disease: a prospective randomized study. Ann Surg 1992; 215(5):546–552.

74. Speranza V, Simi M, Leardi S, Del Papa M. Recurrence of Crohn's disease after resection: are there any risk factors? J Clin Gastroenterol 1986; 8:640–646.

75. Helzer JE, Chammas S, Norland CC, Stillings WA, Alpers DH. A study of the association between Crohn's disease and psychiatric illness. Gastroenterology 1984; 86:324.

76. Mitchell A, Guyatt G, Singer J, Irvine EJ, Goodacre R, Tomkins C, et al. Quality of life in patients with inflammatory bowel disease. J Clin Gastroenterol 1988; 10:306.

77. Andrews H, Barczak P, Allan RN. Psychiatric illness in patients with inflammatory bowel disease. Gut 1987; 28:1600–1604.

78. Koch TR, Carney JA, Go VLW. Distribution and quantitation of gut neuropeptides in normal intestine and inflammatory bowel disease. Dig Dis Sci 1987; 32:367–376.

79. Reubi JC, Mazzucchelli L, Laissure JA. Intestinal vessels express a high density of somatostatin receptors in human inflammatory bowel disease. Gastroenterology 106(4):951–959.

80. Koch TR, Carney JA, Morris VA, Go VLW. Somatostatin in the idiopathic inflammatory bowel diseases. Dis Colon Rectum 1988; 31:198–203.

81. Lewin MJ. The somatostatin receptor in the GI tract. Ann Rev Physiol 1992; 54:455–468.

82. Grill BB, Lange R, Markowitz R, Hillemeier AC, McCallum RW, Gryboski JD. Delayed gastric emptying in children with Crohn's disease. J Clin Gastroenterol 1985; 7:216–226.

83. Miller LR, Vitti R, Mauer A, et al. Small intestinal transit in symptomatic Crohn's disease (abstr). Gastroenterology 1989; 96:A344.

84. Wilton PB, Goldberg SM. Perianal disease. In: Bayless TM, ed. Current Management of Inflammatory Bowel Disease. Philadelphia: BC Decker. 1989; 298–304.

85. Thompson WG, Heaton KW. Functional bowel disorders in apparently healthy people. Gastroenterology 1980; 79:283–288.

86. Isgar B, Harman M, Kaye MD, Whorwell PJ. Symptoms of irritable bowel syndrome in ulcerative colitis in remission. Gut 1983; 24:190–192.

COMMENTARY

Sidney F. Phillips   *Mayo Clinic and Mayo Medical School, Rochester, Minnesota*

CROHN'S DISEASE IS CROHN'S DISEASE IS CROHN'S DISEASE!

Opportunities for formal, but unrestricted, commentaries are rare in medical writing. This generous offer from the editors, therefore, is taken up with thanks, enthusiasm, and a caveat that these unashamed opinions and speculations are intended only to provoke, by highlighting some of the things we know and some that we do not know.

What's in a Name?

The paraphrasing of Gertrude Stein in my title, although simplistic, offers a reasonable beginning for commentary on the pathology of Crohn's disease. Gross and histological descriptions of circumscribed diseases, what used to be called Special Pathology, are observations founded implicitly on the concept of a single etiology. Thus, we assume that

Crohn's disease, ulcerative colitis, Behçet's syndrome, known and uncertain infections, drug reactions, and perhaps other forms of enterocolitis are discrete entities, and therefore definable by their etiologies. However, fact is, we know this to be almost certainly untrue. Perhaps they are entities, and perhaps they are not! Indeed, it behooves us always to consider the potential dangers of classifications that become too definitive, especially when no etiologies have been established.

These dangers were well summarized by Sir Thomas Lewis (1) who cautioned that designation by a name (e.g., Crohn's disease) should not reassure physicians that they understand the disease. Lewis wrote tellingly that "diagnosis is a system of more or less accurate guessing, in which the endpoint achieved is a name. These names, applied to diseases, come to assume the importance of specific entities, whereas they are for the most part no more than insecure and temporary conceptions." The message is clear and simple. Although we need to make diagnoses for ordered management, we must not delude ourselves, or even worse, obscure progress, by believing that we know precisely what is meant by Crohn's disease or that it can be defined currently by gross pathology or histopathology. Thus, transmural inflammation is a feature of Crohn's disease, at least for the distinction from ulcerative colitis. Moreover, the granuloma was once dominant but, as pointed out by Dr. Tremaine, this feature is now not as distinctive as was once thought. And how might the histopathological features of the infectious colitides, Behçet's syndrome, or certain vasculitides relate to Crohn's disease, if equal scrutiny were applied as has been brought to bear on Crohn's versus ulcerative colitis?

Dr. Tremaine's chapter also points out the multiple pathological faces of Crohn's disease. How should we interpret these subgroups? Do the unusual examples of extensive, and often exclusive, jejunoileitis differ from the far more common presentation as ileocolitis, or from exclusive colitis, or from localized perianal disease? Are the differences related to etiology, genetic expression of an individual's immunology, secondary infection, or other unknown factors? David Sachar's working team developed a set of practical subdivisions by anatomical location and the gross pathology (inflammatory, fibrotic, fistulous); this was a useful, practical beginning (2). Do these distinctive subgroups represent separate etiologies, separate and specific host reactions to tissue injury, or both? The two extraordinary families described from northern France highlight these questions (3). Almost identical clinicopathological features were found in 6 and 7 first degree relatives in these families, with a stunningly high prevalence of the disease overall.

These comments are not meant to denigrate the careful and systematic pathological descriptions upon which this chapter is based. To the reverse, open-minded observations with suitable controls, using other known and unknown chronic enteritides, are needed badly. Detailed histopathology has indeed led to several important hypotheses involving the still unsettled etiological issues of mycobacteria, latent viral infections, and microvascular thrombosis. Perhaps Crohn's disease reflects multiple individual expressions of a common etiology; perhaps multiple etiologies. Before the use of microbiological techniques who would have unified the multiple faces of syphilis, the chancre, secondary disease, tabes dorsalis, and aortic insufficiency? On the other hand, perhaps there are multiple etiologies to explain the broad pathological spectrum summarized so well in this chapter.

Nevertheless, as diagnosticians and therapists, physicians must compute a practical bottom line. An exact name may mean little if the diagnostic and therapeutic approaches are not altered by it; on the other hand, the degree to which an individual patient conforms to the "typical features" determines the confidence with which we approach "standard therapy." Whilst dispensing practical advice, physicians must, at the same time, maintain open minds and not be seduced by blind allegance to a nomenclature that is defined incompletely, and to an etiology that is not defined at all.

CROHN'S DISEASE, GUT DYSFUNCTION, AND SYMPTOMS

Dr. Tremaine is challenging, but I believe correct, in raising the ill-defined duet of Crohn's disease and functional disorders. The challenge resides in the disinclination that many colleagues will have in assigning symptoms of a functional disorder to a patient with a known structural disease. Yet, he is correct in identifying a common but complex circumstance that can be a major cause of inappropriate evaluation and therapy.

What Is the Background?

Crohn's disease is a disease of the terminal ileum. This is the gut segment most often involved and it is the segment most often removed when resective surgery is needed. What is the special role of the ileum in gastrointestinal function and what are the potential relationships between inflammation and dysfunction (4)? The interdigestive complex, the periodic cycle of fasting motor activity in the small bowel, does not pass through the ileum regularly in most humans. However, it is recordable more often from the ileum in patients with irritable bowel syndrome and diarrhea. If the interdigestive complex regularly involves (and presumably empties) the ileum in only a minority of humans, might regular ileal MMCs be relevant to the pathophysiology of symptoms in some patients with Crohn's disease? The ileum is also more likely than the proximal small bowel to develop high-pressure, peristaltic contractions that propel contents distally; these propulsive contractions are also more common in patients with irritable bowel syndrome (4). Might a subset of patients with ileal Crohn's disease exhibit excessive numbers of propulsive contractile events in the ileum, that is, motor phenomena that exacerbate ileal dysfunction and symptoms? Furthermore, the ileum is a selective site for the reabsorption of bile acids, and resection of this locus exposes the colon to the diarrheogenic potential of secretory bile acids. These mechanisms are well known to play a role in the pathogenesis of symptoms after ileocolonic resection; what about before?

Dr. Tremaine correctly points out that up to 20% of otherwise healthy individuals experience symptoms of irritable bowel syndrome (5). We must therefore anticipate that 20% of patients with Crohn's disease will also have the associated pathophysiology of a functional disorder. These interactions bedevil the management of patients with mild Crohn's disease and are even more perplexing when symptoms persist or recur after ileocolonic resection. What is due to Crohn's disease, how much diarrhea is due to irritable bowel syndrome, how vigorous should the anti-inflammatory treatment program be? Prospective endoscopic surveillance after ileocolonic resection for Crohn's disease led to the conclusion that recurrent disease and new or persisting symptoms are poorly related at best (6).

The bottom line is a practical, therapeutic one. Experience dictates that lesser symptoms, such as minor abdominal discomfort, bloating, lethargy, and diarrhea, in the face of little structural disease (new or postoperative), should probably not be treated with potent or potentially dangerous drugs. Unfortunately, referral practice too often includes examples of minimal Crohn's disease being treated with potentially toxic doses of corticosteroids and other drugs. Dr. Tremaine's point, therefore, is well taken. Indeed, these comments are intended to reinforce attempts to curtail the inappropriate practice of treating mild inflammation with steroids, when counseling and the prudent use of anti-diarrheals would be safer and more effective.

REFERENCES

1. Lewis T. Reflections upon reform in medical education. Lancet 1994; 1:619–621.
2. Sachar DB, Andrews HA, Farmer RG, Pallone T, Pena AS, Prantera C, Rutgeert P. Proposed classification of patient subgroups in Crohn's disease. Gastroenterol Int 1992; 5:141–154
3. Van Kruiningen HJ, Colombel JF, Cartun RW, Whitlock RH, Koopmans M, Kangro HO, Hoogkamp-Korstanje JAA, Lecomte-Houcke M, Deired M, Paris JC, Cortot A. An in-depth study of Crohn's disease in five French families. Gastroenterology 1993; 104:351–360.
4. Phillips SF, Quigley EMM, Kumar D, Kamath PS. Motility of the ileocolonic function. Gut 1980; 29:390–406.
5. Drossman DA, ed. The Functional Gastrointestinal Disorders: Diagnoses, Pathophysiology and Treatment. Boston: Little, Brown, 1994.
6. Rutgeerts P, Geboos G, Vantrappen G, Beyls J, Keiremans R, Hiele M. Predictability of the postoperative course of Crohn's disease. Gastroenterology 1990; 99:956–963.

6
Endoscopic Evaluation

Geert D'Haens and Paul Rutgeerts   *University of Leuven, Leuven, Belgium*

I. INTRODUCTION

The management of inflammatory bowel diseases has been greatly refined in the last decades since endoscopic procedures have become routinely available to the treating physician. The direct visual appreciation of lesions, so much more accurate than radiological studies, and the ability to collect biopsy samples have rendered the endoscopic examinations first-line procedures in the initial evaluation of unexplained diarrhea and inflammatory bowel disease.

Nonetheless, the need for an unpleasant bowel preparation, the high cost, and the discomfort caused by the procedure should force the clinician to limit the indications as strictly and correctly as possible.

In this review, we describe the most characteristic lesions of Crohn's disease and their value in the differential diagnosis with other conditions, followed by the proper indications and contraindications for endoscopic procedures and therapeutic interventions in Crohn's disease patients.

II. CHARACTERISTIC ENDOSCOPIC FINDINGS IN CROHN'S DISEASE

The aphthous ulcer is one of the earliest and most characteristic endoscopic findings in Crohn's disease (1). In the "pre-aphthoid phase" focal edema and scattered small red spots appear (2). The inflammatory infiltration then forms a microabscess, originating in the submucosal lymphoid follicles, and penetrates through the superficial layers, which results in a tiny aphthous ulcer (usually smaller than 1 to 3 mm) (3). This ulcer is generally surrounded by a small rim of erythema, and further by entirely normal mucosa with a normal vascular pattern (4,5). Aphthous ulcers can often be seen in groups, tend to enlarge concentrically, and give rise to larger and deeper ulcerations that can become irregular, tortuous, and serpiginous. While aphthous ulcers occur in approximately 30 to 40% of patients with colonic Crohn's disease, some authors find larger ulcers in up to 75%, again surrounded by surprisingly little reactive change, emphasizing the focal nature of the inflammatory reaction (6). This "discontinuity" of lesions is one of the most typical endoscopic features of Crohn's disease.

Ulcerations tend to meet longitudinally. Between interconnecting ulcerations, submucosal edema can create uniform nodulations with a cobblestone appearance, another pathognomonic feature of Crohn's disease (5). The mucosa of cobblestones is intact, although some erythema can be noticed in the center. Cobblestones usually contain few inflammatory cells, but sometimes their appearance hardly differs from inflammatory polyps or pseudopolyps, which also frequently occur in colonic Crohn's disease (7,8). Undermining of inflamed mucosa by adjacent ulcers leads to mucosal bridging when healing and reepithelialization occurs.

Structural changes of the gastrointestinal tract result from either severe inflammatory activity or fibrotic changes accompanying healing. Double-contrast barium enema has been found to be superior to colonoscopy to appreciate them (9). The loss of colonic haustral pattern due to submucosal edema and fibrosis is an abnormality reported in three-fourths of the cases examined in one study (5). Strictures always arise in areas of severe ulceration. Both their length and width vary considerably, ranging from less than 3 to more than 10 cm in length and to less than 5 mm in width. Sites of predilection for stricture development include the pyloric channel, the ileocolonic valve, and the rectosigmoid junction (10,11).

Fistula formation has been reported in up to 8% of patients with Crohn's colitis and is most often seen proximally to strictures, surrounded by extensive inflammatory changes (1).

A. Esophageal Crohn's Disease

Involvement of the esophagus by Crohn's disease is rare (12). There are mainly isolated case reports in which complications such as perforation and stenosis are described (13–17). The earliest lesions, however, consist of aphthous ulcers, similar to the earliest lesions in the ileum and colon. Almost all patients with esophageal Crohn's disease have involvement of other intestinal segments by Crohn's disease and are seriously ill at the time their esophageal disease is diagnosed (18).

In our own series of 14 patients with esophageal Crohn's disease, aphthous ulcers were found in 8 patients, "punched out" ulcers in 4 and isolated or linear erosions in 2 (19). Most lesions disappeared quickly with glucocorticosteroid therapy.

B. Gastroduodenal Crohn's Disease

It is unclear what the true incidence of gross gastroduodenal involvement by Crohn's disease is. Reported frequencies range from 2% to 49% of patients with Crohn's ileocolitis (20–23). The earliest changes include antral aphthae and linear ulcerations, thickening of folds, and eventually antral narrowing. Duodenal strictures can occur. Many patients do not have endoscopically detectable lesions, but examination of biopsy specimens reveals histopathological changes suggestive of Crohn's disease (21–26). These patients' symptoms can often be relieved with conventional anti-inflammatory and antacid therapy, especially omeprazol, but the lesions rarely are seen to disappear when endoscopic follow-up is carried out.

C. Small Bowel Crohn's Disease

The terminal ileum is involved in approximately 75% of Crohn's disease patients. Therefore, ileoscopy should complete every colonoscopy performed in patients with inflammatory bowel disease (IBD). This can be accomplished in 80% to 95% of cases by skilled endoscopists. It can be impossible to intubate the terminal ileum due to narrowing and stricturing of the ileocecal valve, but even then, direct inspection and the collection of biopsy material are of utmost importance. In a prospective study of ileoscopic findings in 110 patients with a radiological diagnosis of ileitis, suspicion of inflammation was rejected in 28 patients (27). In a number of young patients, Peyer's patches (lymphoid tissue covered by normal mucosa) may be pronounced and mislead the radiologist. Nonetheless, for the small bowel as a whole, radiological follow-through studies remain the method of choice to determine the nature and extent of inflammation.

If the terminal ileum can be intubated with the endoscope, a typical sequence of abnormalities can be seen. The area proximal to the ileocecal valve contains large, confluent ulcerations with luminal narrowing, preceded by a second segment with a single long ulceration along the antimesenteric border, and a third most proximal segment with only tiny aphthoid erosions or focal erythema. In many patients without this full-blown picture, only scattered aphthous, irregular or serpiginous ulcers are noted (28).

A number of investigators have examined the small bowel endoscopically at the time of surgical intervention. In 60% of 20 patients undergoing ileocecal resection, mucosal lesions were found proximal to the section margin, that most frequently consisted of aphthous ulcerations. Surprisingly, preoperative x-ray films of this segment of the small bowel had been normal in approximately half of these cases (29).

D. Colonic Crohn's Disease

"Rectal sparing" although considered to be typical for colonic Crohn's disease, is noted in fewer than half of the cases. If the rectum is involved, the disease either begins at the rectosigmoid junction or it accompanies anorectal inflammation. If the whole rectum is involved (5% to 10% of colonic Crohn's disease cases), the inflammatory activity in this area is not indicative of the severity of the disease at a higher level (10). The most common site of involvement is the ileocecal area, affecting approximately 70% of cases. Of these, 20% to 30% have colon involvement exclusively and 40% to 55% have ileocolonic disease (1,11).

The progression of lesions from aphthous to large, serpiginous ulcers takes place in a discontinuous and asymmetric fashion (one side of the colon can be severely inflamed, while the opposite wall is entirely normal), with typical "segmental" inflammation (diseased areas alternating with normal, healthy segments or "skip areas") (4,7). Skip areas tend to be somewhat longer in the left colon, which is less commonly involved than the right colon.

Pseudopolyps occur in both ulcerative colitis and Crohn's disease. They represent regenerative epithelium, but may contain granulation tissue as well. Although visual differentiation from adenomas and carcinomas can be difficult, pseudopolyps have no malignant potential. Endoscopic features suggesting the presence of malignancy include rigidity of the edge, an eccentric lumen, or abrupt shelflike margins (30). Pseudopolyps are often glistening and multiple. Their friable surface is frequently covered by mucopus and bleeds easily when biopsy specimens are taken. Occasionally, polyps become large

TABLE 1 Indications for Colonoscopy in Crohn's Disease

Indications for Ileocolonoscopy in Crohn's Disease
Establishing the correct diagnosis of inflammatory bowel disease
Differential diagnosis Crohn's colitis versus ulcerative colitis or infective/acute self-limited colitis
Assessment of extent and grading of severity
Preoperative delineation of the diseased areas
Postoperative evaluation of recurrent Crohn's disease
Postoperative evaluation of diverted bowel segments
Endoscopic balloon dilatation of ileocolonic strictures
Investigation of radiographic abnormalities (strictures, mass lesions)
Contraindications for Colonoscopy in Crohn's Disease
Severely active disease
Routine monitoring of therapeutic efficacy

and lead to obstruction or intussusception (31,32). If polypectomy seems required in case of possible malignancy, care should be taken to ensure sufficient hemostasis. The same polypectomy technique used for the normal bowel may be applied. Adenomas may be present in approximately 5% of patients with colitis, and their appearance is indistinguishable from pseudopolyps. Only biopsy will identify them to be adenomas.

Colonoscopy also permits direct inspection of colonic strictures. Fibrotic strictures are short and weblike, whereas inflammatory strictures are longer and contain ulcerations (33). If possible, the colonoscope should be advanced through the stricture, so that careful inspection becomes possible. Rather than using the colonoscope as a dilating probe, it may be necessary to use a smaller (pediatric or upper intestinal) scope. Features that suggest possible malignancy within a stricture include rigidity, nodularity at the margins, and an eccentric lumen (30).

III. ROLE OF ENDOSCOPY IN THE DIFFERENTIAL DIAGNOSIS

A. Differentiation Between Chronic Inflammatory Bowel Disease and Other Enterocolitides

A large number of bowel diseases can mimic Crohn's disease. The patient's history, stool cultures, and rectosigmoidoscopy often suffice to establish a correct diagnosis in cases of infective colitis (enterocolitis). On the other hand, the endoscopic and histological features of infective colitis can be similar to those found in IBDs (34). Nevertheless, examination of stool samples does not immediately lead to the correct diagnosis in cases of cytomegalovirus (CMV) colitis, colonic tuberculosis, and amebiasis. In immunosuppressed patients and in those from endemic areas, full colonoscopy with biopsy of all segments is recommended.

Bacterial colitides due to infection with *Salmonella, Shigella,* or *Campylobacter,* common pathogens, can all endoscopically mimic Crohn's disease (34). Hemorrhagic colitis by *Escherichia coli 0157:H7* is characterized by patchy ulceration in the right colon and cecum. *Yersinia* enterocolitis occurs with aphthous, uniform, small ulcers adjacent to normal mucosa. The rectum remains free of disease in 40% of patients (35).

The typical endoscopic picture of subacute colonic amebiasis consists of small ulcers with undermined edges and a reddened rim, amidst almost normal surrounding mucosa. Inflammatory polyps can occur, and the cecum is involved in 80% to 90% of cases (36).

In pseudomembranous, antibiotic-associated colitis caused by *Clostridium difficile*, diagnosis by endoscopy is easy. Small and large confluent yellowish plaques cover a moderately inflamed mucosal wall. In up to 20% to 30% of cases, the rectum is spared to a variable degree (37).

Cytomegalovirus colitis is characterized by shallow "punched-out" ulcers, mimicking Crohn's disease. The lesions can be limited to the cecum. In biopsy samples taken from the edge of the ulcers, CMV inclusions can often easily by recognized (38).

Proctitis in homosexual males can be caused by *Neisseria gonorrheae*, *Chlamydia*, and herpes simplex virus, which can all be indistinguishable from Crohn's disease.

Probably gastrointestinal tuberculosis presents the most difficult visual differential diagnosis. Most often, the ileocecal area is affected by ulcerations of varying size and nodules in the surrounding tissue. The valve, unlike in Crohn's disease, has a "gaping" appearance (39,40).

Acute self-limited colitis is the exclusion diagnosis when the clinical picture and the epidemiological context suggest an infective colitis but stool cultures are negative (in up to 50% of cases). The diagnosis is made by the spontaneous evolution of the disease and sometimes by meticulous examination of colonic biopsy specimens but there is no evidence that standard colonoscopy can readily lead to differentiation from genuine IBD (41,42).

In selected patients, a number of rare conditions must be considered. In chronic ischemic colitis, patchy ulcers, stenosis and pseudopolyps can occur. The solitary rectal ulcer syndrome is characterized by a pathognomonic histological picture of fibromuscular hyperplasia. Also to be considered are graft-versus-host disease in hematologic patients and radiation colitis and drug-induced colitis if the medical history is suggestive.

B. Differentiation Between Crohn's Disease and Ulcerative Colitis

Only approximately 20% of patients with Crohn's disease have involvement of the colon only. In addition, up to one-third suffer from typical anal inflammation, which never occurs in ulcerative colitis. According to a prospective study of 357 patients by Pera et al., complete colonoscopy allows a correct differentiation between Crohn's disease, ulcerative colitis, and "indeterminate colitis" in 89% of cases (43). The most characteristic lesions of Crohn's disease included discontinuous involvement, anal lesions, and cobblestoning (Table 2). A classical pitfall with regard to the patchiness of rectosigmoidal lesions is

TABLE 2 Differentiation of Crohn's Disease and Ulcerative Colitis

Crohn's Disease	Ulcerative Colitis
Discontinuous involvement	Continuous involvement
Cobblestoning	Erosions/microulcers
Aphthous ulcers	Loss of vascular pattern
Deep, longitudinal, serpiginous ulcers	
Rectal sparing or segmental inflammation	Rectal involvement
Anal lesions	
Ileocecal valve stenotic and ulcerated	Ileocecal valve patulous and free of ulceration

former treatment with topical agents, which can convert continuous inflammation into a patchy pattern (44). In Pera's prospective study, errors in diagnosis were more frequent in the presence of severe colonic inflammation. Because the treatment modalities for an acute attack of Crohn's disease or ulcerative colitis do not really differ, endoscopic assessment can best be deferred until the disease activity is under control.

Since long, two criteria have been considered as "absolute" in the differentiation between Crohn's disease and ulcerative colitis: (a) cobblestoning never occurs in ulcerative colitis and (b) the ulcerations in ulcerative colitis never appear in an area of otherwise normal-appearing mucosa (45). The background mucosa in which the ulcers are set hence influences the correct diagnosis more than the ulcers themselves. Even cobblestones carry a normal, though pinkish but not friable mucosa. Furthermore, continuous inflammatory involvement has been observed in approximately 45% of patients with Crohn's disease, which makes the predictive value of this pattern very low. The rectum is free of disease in at least 30% of patients with colonic Crohn's disease. The presence of an ulcerated, stenotic ileocecal valve is another strong indication in favor of Crohn's disease.

IV. ASSESSMENT OF EXTENT AND SEVERITY OF DISEASE

Disease extent tends to be underestimated in both ulcerative colitis and Crohn's disease (43). No uniformly validated system to assess the endoscopic severity of Crohn's disease has been developed. The knowledge of the extent of the colonic inflammation affects management decisions in cases of left-sided disease, in which topical therapy with corticosteroids or aminosalicylates offers an alternative to systemic therapy, and in the preoperative setting. The French GETAID (Groupe d'Etudes Therapeutiques sur les Affections Inflammatoires Digestives) proposed a Crohn's Disease Endoscopic Index of Severity (CDEIS), but was unable to establish any correlation between Crohn's Disease Activity Index (CDAI), biochemical markers, and CDEIS (46,47). The endoscopic index was based on the size and depth of ulcerations, combined with the number of colonic segments involved. Because the localization of the diseased bowel segments appears to change little over time, colonoscopy is only warranted when surgical intervention is considered, when certain therapeutic interventions are to be performed, or to assess the effects of new drugs in therapeutic trials.

V. ENDOSCOPIC MONITORING OF THERAPEUTIC EFFICACY AND ITS VALUE IN CLINICAL TRIALS

Gastroenterologists have long observed that unlike in ulcerative colitis, there is a poor correlation between endoscopic severity and clinical activity in Crohn's disease. The GETAID, in a prospective trial, demonstrated that only approximately one-fourth of patients in clinical remission under corticosteroid treatment also had endoscopic healing of their lesions. Persistence of lesions did not appear to be predictive of early relapse; adjustment of steroid treatment duration based on endoscopic findings proved to be of no benefit. It was concluded that endoscopic monitoring of "healing" is a waste of time and money (6,48).

The pattern of healing of endoscopic lesions under glucocorticoid therapy depends on the location of lesions: esophageal lesions almost completely disappear; gastric lesions hardly show any change under therapy, even with symptomatic relief; ileal lesions have the same tendency to persist and colonic lesions heal slowly after tapering of the steroids (49,50). In a small pilot study with monoclonal tumor necrosis factor (TNF)α antibodies, complete healing of colonic lesions was demonstrated only a few weeks after intravenous administration of a single dose (51). Further studies with this drug are being performed.

VI. INDICATIONS FOR PREOPERATIVE ENDOSCOPY IN CROHN'S DISEASE PATIENTS

When performing ileocolonic resection for Crohn's disease, the surgeon removes grossly involved areas and anastomoses healthy segments of bowel. By means of preoperative colonoscopy, the exact extent of active disease can be assessed. Segments of burnt-out disease should be defined so that the length of surgical resection can be limited. Surgery is often carried out for strictures or fistulas and endoscopy allows better evaluation of the presence of intrinsic bowel disease near fistula orifices.

VII. POSTOPERATIVE INDICATIONS FOR ENDOSCOPY IN CROHN'S DISEASE

Approximately 80% of patients develop endoscopic recurrence of Crohn's disease at the ileal side of the anastomosis within the first two years after "curative" ileocecal resection. We developed an endoscopic score to describe the severity of lesions at the ileal side: grade i0 = no lesions, grade i1 = fewer than 5 aphthous ulcers, grade i2 = more than 5 aphthous lesions with normal mucosa in between or lesions confined to the anastomosis, grade i3 = diffuse aphthous ileitis, grade i4 = diffuse ulcerations with large ulcers and/or stenosis. This scoring system is not only a valuable tool for clinical studies, but it also allows the prediction of the clinical course of the disease in the years ahead. Patients with grade 3 or 4 recurrence after 1 year often suffer from an aggressive course of their recurrent disease (52). However, as is true for Crohn's disease in general, the correlation between symptoms and endoscopic lesions remains poor, so that the endoscopic findings hardly contribute to therapeutic decisions.

In recurrent Crohn's disease of the neoterminal ileum, as in "primary" Crohn's disease, the "aphthous ulcer" is one of the earliest lesions. It seems that the natural evolution of the lesions in the recurrence setting mimics the course of the disease at onset. This makes the recurrence model a valuable tool to study the pathogenesis of the disease.

Treatment modalities to "prevent" or defer clinical and/or endoscopic recurrence are limited. A number of studies have demonstrated benefit from 5-aminosalicylates started shortly after surgery (53). Metronidazole appears to diminish the severity of recurrent lesions, but not the incidence (54). As long as there is no more effective therapy available, routine endoscopy after surgery does not seem to be of any benefit.

Patients with an ileostomy can also develop recurrent inflammation in the most distal ileal segments, but the risk is much lower than after an ileocolonic reanastomosis. Endoscopic examination of the bowel proximal to the stoma allows easy and precise evaluation of the abnormalities. Whenever reanastomosis is considered, endoscopic evaluation of the segments to be anastomosed is useful.

VIII.   THERAPEUTIC ENDOSCOPIC INTERVENTIONS IN CROHN'S DISEASE

Stricture formation is a common phenomenon in the healing phase of the inflammatory lesions. It often occurs at the ileocecal junction and at the ileocolonic anastomosis, but it can affect any part of the gastrointestinal tract. Selected cases can be treated endoscopically with "through the scope" (TTS) balloon dilatation (55). The procedure is performed under direct endoscopic visualization, usually with general anesthesia. The size and length of the semirigid balloon to be used depends on the length and diameter of the stenosis. The balloon is inflated twice for about 2 minutes or until the scope can be advanced through the stenosis. We published one of the first series of 18 patients who underwent balloon dilatation of the ileocolonic anastomosis. An 18-mm balloon was used and the treatment was successful in 16 patients, with immediate symptom relief in 14. No complications occurred. Long-term benefit was greater in patients with inactive disease at the time of dilatation (56). A few isolated reports have suggested potential benefit from injection of corticosteroids into the stricture following dilatation (57).

Patients with anal strictures should not be treated with balloon dilatation, for fear of laceration of the sphincter. Instead, gradual dilatation with Savary dilators can be applied.

IX.   ENDOSCOPIC ULTRASONOGRAPHY

Anal fissures, fistulas, abscesses, and stenoses are common in Crohn's disease. Transrectal ultrasonography provides useful information about the extent and depth of the lesions, and it can demonstrate the presence of lesions missed by routine examination, such as pararectal or para-anal abscesses and fistulas (58). The technique is also useful in the evaluation of the anal sphincter, certainly if surgical interventions are considered.

X.   CONCLUSIONS

The endoscopic evaluation of patients with Crohn's disease is extremely valuable and has greatly changed the management of the disease. Ileocolonoscopy has replaced contrast enemas in the first evaluation of patients with suspected IBD. Nonetheless, these procedures are only justified when they are likely to influence therapeutic management. Ileocolonoscopy can be necessary to establish an exact ("tissue") diagnosis, to determine the extent of inflammatory activity, in the preoperative setting to "guide" the surgeon, and to examine the bowel proximal to stomas. Early endoscopic examination of the ileocolonic anastomosis after resection of the terminal ileum and part of the colon enables evaluation of the severity of recurrence of Crohn's disease, predicting clinical outcome. Routine postoperative colonoscopy is, however, not warranted, because we do not have an effective medical treatment influencing evolution of the disease. Colonoscopy is also useful in the management of dilatable strictures.

Endoscopic examination of the upper gastrointestinal tract should be performed whenever upper gastrointestinal symptoms develop. It is important for the treatment to differentiate between intrinsic Crohn's lesions, peptic disease, gastrointestinal or drug-associated lesions in the esophagus, stomach, or duodenum. Upper gastrointestinal lesions are present in a high number of Crohn's disease patients.

On the other hand, endoscopic procedures are not helpful in guiding medical therapy, and there appears to be little correlation between clinical and endoscopic disease activity.

Therefore, the number of endoscopies in a single Crohn's disease patient should be restricted to the moments of important management decisions.

REFERENCES

1. Mekhjian HS, Switz DM, Melnyk CS, Rankin GB, Brooks RK. Clinical features and natural history of Crohn's disease. Gastroenterology 1979; 77:898–906.
2. Watier A, Devroede G, Perey B, Haddad H, Madarnas P, Grand-Maison P. Small erythematous mucosal plaques: an endoscopic sign of Crohn's disease. Gut 1980; 21:835–839.
3. Rutgeerts P, Geboes K. Crohn's disease and pre-aphthoid lesions (editorial). Lancet 1993; 341:1443–1444.
4. Hogan WJ, Hensley GT, Geenen JE. Endoscopic evaluation of inflammatory bowel disease. Med Clin North Am 1980: 64:1083–1102.
5. Meuwissen SGM, Pape KSSB, Agenant D, Oushoorn HH, Tytgat GNJ. Crohn's disease of the colon: analysis of the diagnostic value of radiology, endoscopy and histology. Am J Dig Dis 1976; 21:81–88.
6. Modigliani R, Mary JY, Simon JF, et al. Clinical, biological and endoscopic picture of attacks of Crohn's disease. Evolution on prednisolone. Gastroenterology 1990; 98:811–818.
7. Waye JD. The role of colonoscopy in the differential diagnosis of inflammatory bowel disease. Gastrointest Endosc 1977; 23:150–154.
8. Fishman RS, Fleming CR, Stephens DH. Roentgenographic simulation of colonic cancer by benign masses in Crohn's disease. Mayo Clin Proc 1978; 54:447–449.
9. Geboes K, Vantrappen G. The value of colonoscopy in the diagnosis of Crohn's disease. Gastrointest Endosc 1975; 22:18–23.
10. Blackstone MO. Inflammatory bowel disease. In: Blackstone MO, ed. Endoscopic Interpretation. New York: Raven Press, 1984;464–494.
11. Farmer RG, Hawk WA, Turnbull RB. Clinical patterns in Crohn's disease: a statistical study of 615 cases. Gastroenterology 1975; 68:627–635.
12. Fruhmorgen P, Rosch W. Endoskopischer Aspekt des Morbus Crohn in Osophagus, Magen, Duodenum, Jejunum, Ileum und Kolon. Z. Gastroenterol 1974; 12:592.
13. Miller LJ, Thistle JL, Payne WS, Gaffey TA, O'Duffy JD. Crohn's disease involving the esophagus and colon. Mayo Clin Proc 1977; 52:35–38.
14. Ghahremani GG, Gore RM, Breuer RI, Larson RH. Esophageal manifestations of Crohn's disease. Gastrointest Radiol 1982; 7:199–203.
15. Kuboi H, Yashiro K, Shindou H, Hayashi N, Nagasako K. Crohn's disease in the esophagus— report of a case. Endoscopy 1988; 20:118–121.
16. Cynn WS, Chon H, Gureghian PA, Levin BL. Crohn's disease of the esophagus. AJR Am J Roentgenol 1975; 125:359–364.
17. Peix, JL, Moulin G, Evreux M, Berger N, Magis M. Localisations buccooesophagienne de la maladie de Crohn. Gastroenterol Clin Biol 1987; 11:604–606.
18. Bagby RJ, Rogers JV, Hobbs C. Crohn's disease of the esophagus, stomach and duodenum: a review with emphasis on the radiographic findings. South Med J 1972; 65:515–523.
19. D'Haens G, Rutgeerts P, Geboes K. Esophageal Crohn's disease: three patterns of evolution. Gastrointest Endosc 1994; 40:296–300.
20. Danzi JT, Farmer RG, Sullivan BH, et al. Endoscopic features of gastroduodenal Crohn's disease. Gastroenterology 1976; 70:9–13.
21. Harary AM, Rogers AI. Gastroduodenal Crohn's disease. Differential diagnosis and treatment. Postgrad Med 1983; 74: 129–137.
22. Danesh BJZ, Park RHR, Upadhyay R, Howatson A, Lee F, Russell RI. Diagnostic yield of upper gastrointestinal endoscopic biopsies in patients with Crohn's disease. Gastroenterology 1989; 96:A108.

23. Schmitz-Moorman P, Malchow H, Pittner PM. Endoscopic and bioptic study of the upper gastrointestinal tract in Crohn's disease patients. Pathol Res Pract 1985; 179:377–387.
24. Haggitt RC, Meissner WA. Crohn's disease of the upper gastrointestinal tract. Am J Clin Pathol 1993; 59:613–622.
25. Nugent FW, Richmond M, Park SV. Crohn's disease of the duodenum. Gut 1977; 18:115–120.
26. Rutgeerts P, Ponette E, Vantrappen G, et al. Crohn's disease of the stomach and duodenum: a clinical study with emphasis on the value of endoscopy and endoscopic biopsies. Endoscopy 1980; 12:288–294.
27. Coremans G, Rutgeerts P, Geboes K, Vanden Oord J, Ponette E, Vantrappen G. The value of ileoscopy with biopsy in the diagnosis of intestinal Crohn's disease. Gastrointest Endosc 1984; 30: 173–178.
28. Tytgat GNJ, Van Olffen GH. Role of ileocolonoscopy in diagnosis and follow-up in inflammatory bowel disease. Acta Endoscopica 1983; 13: 245–259.
29. Lescut D, Vanco D, Bonniere P, et al. Perioperative endoscopy of the whole small bowel in Crohn's disease. Gut 1993; 34: 647–649.
30. Waye J. Colitis, cancer and colonoscopy. Med Clin North Am 1978; 62:211.
31. Jones B, Abbruzzese A. Obstructing giant pseudopolyps in granulomatous colitis. Gastrointest Radiol 1978; 3:437.
32. Forde K, et al. Giant pseudopolyposis with colonic intussusception. Gastroenterology 1978; 75:1142.
33. Waye J. Endoscopy in inflammatory bowel disease: indications and differential diagnosis. Med Clin North Am 1990; 74:51–65.
34. Rutgeerts P, Geboes K, Ponnette E, Coremans G, Vantrappen G. Acute infective colitis caused by endemic pathogens in western-Europe: endoscopic features. Endoscopy 1980; 6:212–219.
35. Vantrappen G, Geboes K, Ponette F. Yersinia enteritis. Med Clin North Am 1982; 66: 639–653.
36. Kaplan LR, Pries JM. A case of endemic amebic colitis: diagnosis with colonoscopic biopsy. Dis Colon Rectum 1979; 573–574.
37. Seppala K, Hjelt L, Sipponen P. Colonoscopy in the diagnosis of antibiotic-associated colitis. Scand J Gastroenterol 1981; 16:465–468.
38. Meiselman MS, Cello JP, Margaretten W. Cytomegalovirus colitis: report of the clinical, endoscopic and pathologic finding in two patients with the acquired immune deficiency syndrome. Gastroenterology 1985; 88:171–175.
39. Franklin GO, Mohapatra M, Perrillo RP. Colonic tuberculosis diagnosed by colonoscopic biopsy. Gastroenterology 1979; 76:362–364.
40. Shah S, Thomas V, Mathan M, et al. Colonoscopic study of 50 patients with colonic tuberculosis. Gut 1992; 33:437–351.
41. Nostrant T, Kumar N, Appelman H. Histopathology differentiates acute self-limited colitis from ulcerative colitis. Gastroenterology 1987; 92:318–328.
42. Surawicz CM, Belic L. Rectal biopsy helps to distinguish acute self-limited colitis from idiopathic inflammatory bowel disease. Gastroenterology 1984; 86:104–113.
43. Pera A, Bellando P, Caldera D. Colonoscopy in inflammatory bowel disease. Diagnostic accuracy and proposal of an endoscopic index. Gastroenterology 1987; 92:181–185.
44. Tytgat GNJ, Reijers MHE, Van Dullemen HM. Pitfalls in the diagnosis of Crohn's disease. In: Rachmilewitz D, ed. Inflammatory bowel disease 1994. Dordrecht: Kluwer Academic Press, 1994:165–173.
45. Teague RH, Waye JD. Endoscopy in inflammatory bowel disease. In: Hunt RH, Waye JD, eds. Colonoscopy: Techniques, Clinical Practice and Colour Atlas. London: Chapman and Hall, 1981:343–362.
46. Mary JY, Modigliani R. Development and validation of an endoscopic index of the severity of Crohn's disease: a prospective multicenter study. Gut 1989; 30:983–989.
47. Cellier C, Sahmoud T, Froguel E, et al. Correlations between clinical activity, endoscopic

severity, and biological parameters in colonic or ileocolonic Crohn's disease. A multicenter prospective study of 121 cases. Gut 1994; 35:231–235.

48. Landi B, Anh TN, Cortot A, et al. Endoscopic monitoring of Crohn's disease treatment: a prospective, randomized clinical trial. Gastroenterology 1992; 102:1647–1653.

49. Modigliani R, et al. Acute attacks of colonic and ileocolonic Crohn's disease: is colonoscopic follow-up useful to adjust steroid treatment duration? Gastroenterology 1990; 98:A193.

50. Olaison B, Sjodahl R, Tagesson C. Glucocorticoid treatment in ileal Crohn's disease: relief of symptoms but not of endoscopically viewed inflammation. Gut 1990; 31:325–328.

51. Van Dullemen HM, Van Deventer SJH, Hommes DW, Bijl HA, Jensen J, Tytgat GNJ, Woody J. Treatment of Crohn's Disease with Anti-Tumor Necrosis Factor Chimeric Monoclonal Antibody (cA2). Gastroenterology 1995; 109: 129–135.

52. Rutgeerts P, Geboes K, Vantrappen G, Beyls J, Kerremans R, Hiele M. Predictability of the postoperative course of Crohn's disease. Gastroenterology 1990; 99:956–962.

53. Caprilli R, Andreoli A, Capurso L, D'Albasio G, Gioieni A, et al. Oral mesalazine (Asacol) for the prevention of postoperative recurrence of Crohn's disease. Aliment Pharmacol Ther 1994; 8:35–43.

54. Rutgeerts P, Peeters M, Hiele M, Kerremans R, Penninckx F, Aerts R, et al. A placebo controlled trial of metronidazole for recurrence prevention of Crohn's disease after resection of the terminal ileum. Gastroenterology 1992; 102:A688.

55. Blomberg B, Rolny P, Jarnerot G. Endoscopic treatment of anastomotic strictures in Crohn's disease. Endoscopy 1991; 23:195–198.

56. Breysem Y, Janssens JF, Coremans G, Vantrappen G, Hendrickx G, Rutgeerts P. Endoscopic balloon dilation of colonic and ileocolonic Crohn's strictures: long-term results. Gastrointest Endosc 1992; 38:142–147.

57. Lavy A. Steroid injection improves outcome in Crohn's disease strictures (letter). Endoscopy 1994; 26:366.

58. Van Outryve MJ, Pelckmans PA, Michielsen PP, Van Maercke YM. Value of transrectal ultrasonography in Crohn's disease. Gastroenterology 1991; 101:1171–1177.

7

The Role of Contrast Barium X-Rays vs. Endoscopy

Burton I. Korelitz   *Lenox Hill Hospital and New York University School of Medicine, New York, New York*

In the 1970s, when the potential benefits of colonoscopy in inflammatory bowel disease (IBD) became apparent, radiologists vigorously debated that the barium enema in expert hands maintained an advantage without risk. Subsequently, years and experience have served to eliminate the advantages of contrast x-rays of the colon, with exceptions. Surprisingly, it is the expert endoscopist whose writings and lectures have served to lessen the role of colonoscopy in management of IBD. It is my own conviction, based on my experience with diagnosis and management of Crohn's disease (and ulcerative colitis) and my experience in the performance of both barium enema and colonoscopy in these diseases, that the role of the x-ray has been progressively reduced but still maintains advantages over endoscopy in these diseases, that the role of the x-ray has been progressively reduced but still maintains advantages over endoscopy of the rectum and colon in a few instance. In evaluation of small bowel Crohn's disease, the barium contrast x-ray study remains supreme.

I. DIAGNOSIS OF CROHN'S DISEASE OF THE COLON BY BARIUM ENEMA

A. Pro

If the disease is sufficiently advanced to reveal loss of normal mucosal pattern, deep ulcerations, linear ulcerations, cobblestoning, pseudopolyposis, pseudodiverticula, discontinuous involvement, asymmetry, strictures, and skip lesions, then introducing barium by rectum can reveal many characteristic features of Crohn's disease as well as extent of involvement (Fig. 1) (1,2). If barium is refluxed into the terminal ileum and reveals characteristic features of ileitis, there is a great advantage, but if the disease is advanced, the terminal ileum is likely to be strictured and this advantage is lost. Air contrast serves no advantage when the barium enema is used for this purpose and should probably be contraindicated.

B. Con

Hopefully, Crohn's disease is recognized soon after onset of clinical symptoms. Under these circumstances, the barium enema can appear completely normal, whereas colon-

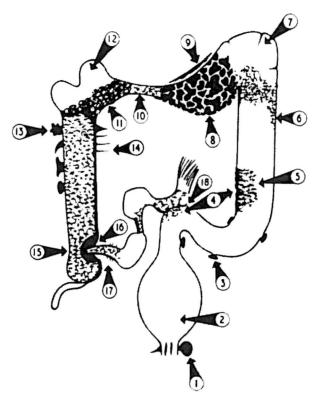

FIG. 1 The barium enema in Crohn's ileocolitis. (From Simpkins KC, Ref. 2.)

oscopy may reveal many of the characteristic features of the Crohn's disease listed above, in addition to rectal sparing or relative sparing, exudate, friability, and aphthous ulcers. Furthermore, colonoscopic biopsies can secure the diagnosis of Crohn's disease. The most productive areas have been from the normal or relatively normal appearing rectal mucosa (3) and from the edges of aphthous ulcers (4). The yield of diagnostic granulomas and microgranulomas (5) from these areas is the highest. Other histological lesions can be suggestive but not diagnostic (6).

II. DIFFERENTIAL DIAGNOSIS OF CROHN'S DISEASE OF THE COLON BY BARIUM ENEMA

A. Pro

If the characteristic features of Crohn's disease are found, all other types of colitis are excluded. This is unlikely to be the case, however, unless the involvement in the colon is advanced. Early in the course of the disease, x-ray features are probably lacking to separate Crohn's colitis from ulcerative colitis, infectious colitis, amebic colitis, pseudo-membranous colitis, ischemic colitis, radiation colitis, cytomegalovirus (CMV) colitis, and diversion colitis.

B. Con

The barium enema can appear normal in all of the above conditions, or, if abnormal, probably present features that are noncharacteristic. On the other hand, the colonoscopic appearance may include features that are typical of ulcerative, amebic, and pseudomembranous colitis. Biopsies can lead to a diagnosis of amebic, pseudomembranous, ischemic, radiation, and CMV colitis; if performed early, biopsies can help to separate infectious colitis from ulcerative and Crohn's colitis (7), and biopsies from normal or relatively normal appearing rectal mucosa can separate Crohn's disease from ulcerative colitis (8–9).

III. USE OF BARIUM ENEMA IN MANAGEMENT OF CROHN'S DISEASE

A. Pro

Most endoscopists state that colonoscopy is not necessary in managing Crohn's disease of the colon and imply that the barium enema is not necessary either, once the diagnosis is established. However, the barium enema can be used once the colon has narrowed or formed a specific stricture that cannot usually be suspected by clinical symptoms and cannot be passed by colonoscope. The barium contrast x-rays can then serve to determine progression of the narrowing and its extent and features regarding benignancy versus malignancy. Furthermore, if surgery is being considered, information might be provided concerning the state of the colon proximal to a stricture and its extent would influence the decision of whether to perform colectomy or segmental resection.

B. Con

Modigliani et al. in France have provided an endoscopic index of Crohn's disease activity, based on the following (10):

1. Superficial ulcerations
2. Deep ulceration
3. Mucosal edema
4. Erythema
5. Pseudopolypi
6. Aphthoid ulcers
7. Ulcerated stenosis
8. Nonulcerated stenosis

Using this index, the authors conclude that there is no correlation between clinical activity and the endoscopic findings, in that only 38 of 131 patients in clinical remission were also in endoscopic remission after 7 weeks of prednisolone therapy. This conviction is further accentuated by the additional correlation between clinical activity, endoscopic severity, and biological parameters, with the conclusion that Crohn's disease clinical activity seems to be virtually independent of the severity of the mucosal lesions and biological activity (11,12).

Nevertheless, the fact that clinical response to steroid therapy preceded the objective endoscopic response was recognized even before the advent of modern day colonoscopy and should not be considered a surprise. Active colitis could be seen via the sigmoidoscope after the patient responded to steroids and was in clinical remission. The same group of endoscopic observers submitted their correlation between the clinical and colonoscopic results to a randomized trial as to whether prolonged therapy with prednisolone would improve the endoscopic index of response—and it does (13). I believe that an important point is omitted here. Because steroids have not proven to be of value as maintenance drugs, both the clinical and the endoscopic remission should be accomplished as quickly as possible to "buy time" for a therapeutic/maintenance program to be established. Therefore, intravenous steroid preparations should be favored over oral prednisone to effect a more rapid and perhaps a more enduring clinical remission to buy this time for slower acting maintenance drugs to be effective. The question arises whether full endoscopic remission provides more time than merely the clinical remission to accomplish successful maintenance. It is my impression that this is so. The major value of clinical trials of drugs to prevent relapse should therefore continue to include the endoscopic appearance and start from a baseline of colonoscopic remission. The colonoscope will then continue to have a role in management of Crohn's disease, if only for this purpose. Moreover, it is better to seek and recognize recurrent Crohn's disease activity by colonoscopy or flexible sigmoidoscopy before symptoms recur so that drug management can be altered.

There is little advantage to endoscopic biopsies over examination of gross appearance except in the realm of surveillance for cancer and for recognition of recurrence after surgery.

IV. RECOGNITION OF ILEITIS AND JEJUNITIS BY GASTROINTESTINAL X-RAYS

A. Pro

The small bowel x-ray series remains the most effective facility for demonstrating Crohn's disease involving the terminal ileum and other segments of small bowel. The findings of edematous folds, superficial and deep ulcerations, linear ulcerations, nodularity, cobblestoning, skip lesions, transverse fissures, fistulas, strictures, and masses are almost always diagnostic. Demonstration by small bowel x-rays of fistulous communications to the urinary bladder (Fig. 2), the mesenteries, the sigmoid (Fig. 3) and other segments of the colon, and the rectum (Fig. 4) still provide visual images of the most outstanding features of Crohn's disease (14,15). The barium enema also maintains a role in the demonstration of small bowel Crohn's disease. When the barium can be refluxed into the terminal ileum, this modality occasionally shows the ileitis even better than a small bowel x-ray study. When a fistula between colon and small bowel (Fig. 5), stomach, or duodenum (Fig. 6) has its origin in the colon, the barium introduced under pressure by the barium enema is more likely to demonstrate the fistula than when barium is given from above (16,17). Air contrast is almost never an advantage in the barium enema study of a Crohn's disease patient.

B. Con

Small bowel endoscopy rarely reveals Crohn's disease that is missed by barium x-rays, but, rarely, biopsies of small bowel lesions performed by endoscopy provide histological

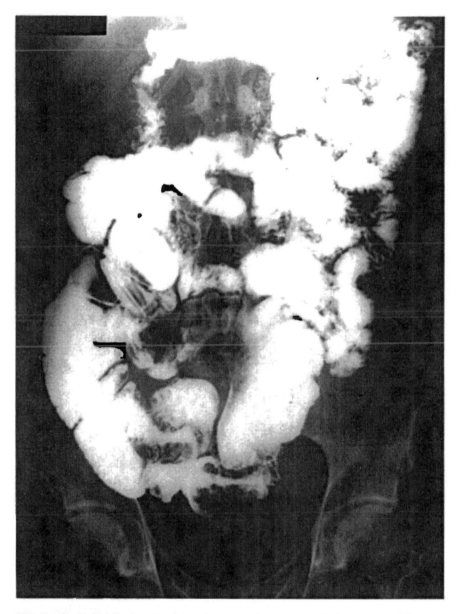

FIG. 2 Ileovesical fistulas. Small bowel x-ray series showing distal segments of ileum involved with Crohn's disease wrapped around the superior surface of the urinary bladder with fistulas penetrating its wall.

evidence confirming the diagnosis. Nevertheless, small bowel enteroscopy may show severe disease not obvious by x-rays and also clarify the severity of strictures (Fig. 7). Perhaps dilatations are feasible through this route. Recognition of ileitis involving the terminal ileum can sometimes be accomplished by endoscopic introduction at colonoscopy when the ileitis is not appreciated by barium x-rays (18).

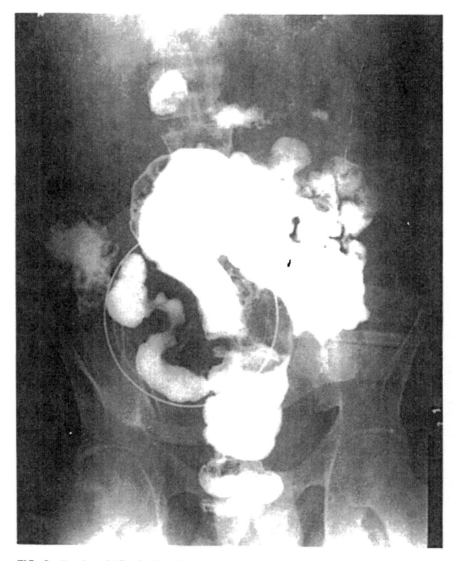

FIG. 3 Ileosigmoid fistula. Small bowel x-ray series showing Crohn's disease of the distal ileum with skip areas approximating the sigmoid colon with filling of the sigmoid and rectum with barium before filling of the transverse and descending colons.

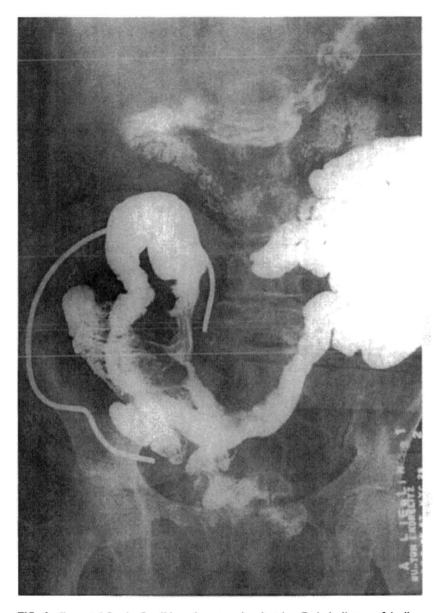

FIG. 4 Ileorectal fistula. Small bowel x-ray series showing Crohn's disease of the ileum and filling of the rectum with barium before filling of the colon.

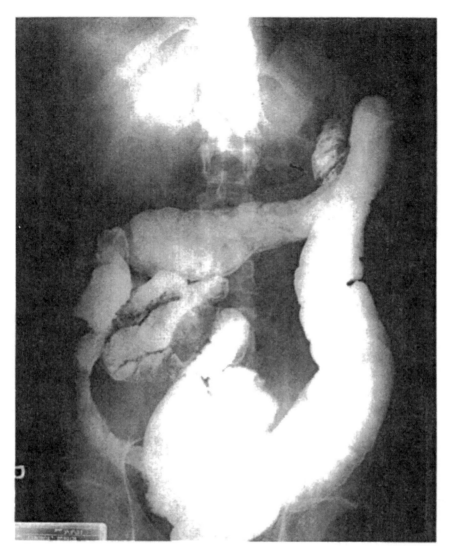

FIG. 5 Colonic jejunal fistula. Barium enema x-ray examination showing Crohn's disease of the transverse colon, ascending colon (shortened), cecum (contracted), and terminal ileum with reflux of barium from the distal transvere to a loop of jejunum.

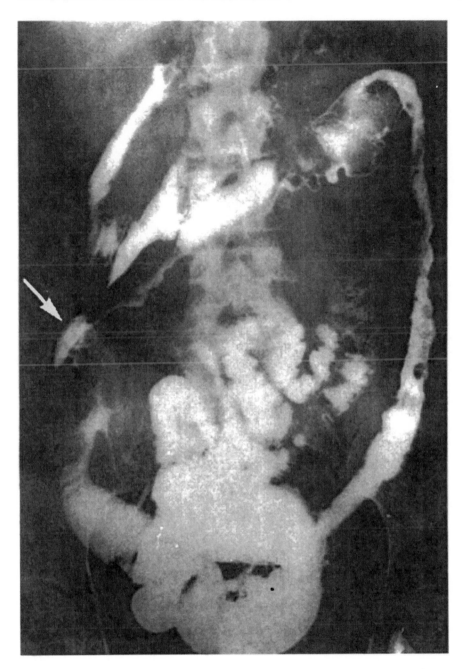

FIG. 6 Colonic–duodenal fistula. A barium enema x-ray series showing extensive Crohn's disease of the colon with reflux of barium from the hepatic flexure into the descending duodenum.

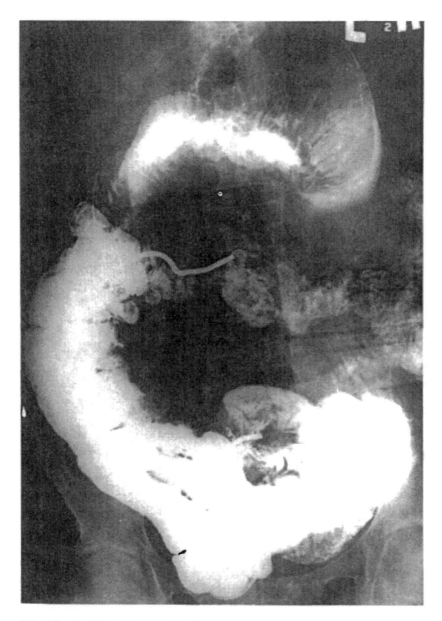

FIG. 7A Small bowel x-ray series showing extensive jejunoileitis with dilated jejunum proximal to a Crohn's disease stricture.

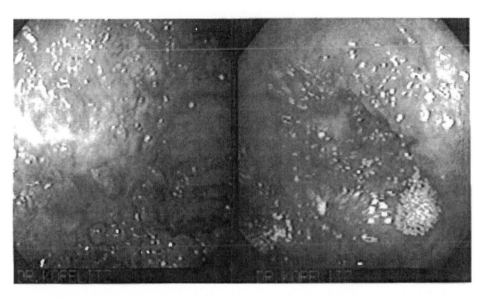

FIG. 7B The same jejunal stricture seen on enteroscopy with cobblestoning adjacent to the stricture and retained ethyl-cellulose beads of Pentasa.

V. UPPER GASTROINTESTINAL TRACT

A. Pro

Clinical symptoms that suggest upper gastrointestinal (GI) disease before the diagnosis of Crohn's disease is made often lead directly to esophagogastroscopy, which then reveals ulceration or diffuse inflammation in the esophagus, stomach, or duodenum. The upper GI x-ray series, usually performed in conjunction with a small bowel series, is more likely to demonstrate the full extent and degree of the inflammatory process. Esophageal Crohn's disease is rare and, when seen, does not show a consistent pattern (19). Crohn's disease of the stomach is more often a diffuse process in the distal stomach but discrete irregular ulcers are seen with or without the adjoining extensive inflammation. Crohn's disease of the duodenum is also a diffuse process with thickening of folds, granularity, and perhaps friability. There may be compromise of the sphincter of Oddi with reflux of barium into the common duct or pancreatic duct (20). Usually, involvement of the stomach and duodenum occur together. Almost always there is more distal involvement with terminal ileitis, even if it is less severe than in the proximal GI tract.

B. Con

In this particular distribution of Crohn's disease, one modality is not better than another because they complement each other, and management ideally includes both esophagogastroscopy and upper GI x-ray series, not necessarily during the same period of time.

VI. RECURRENT ILEITIS
AFTER RESECTION WITH ANASTOMOSIS

A. Pro

The recurrence of ileitis occurs in almost all patients after transection of the bowel, and it occurs earlier after anastomosis than after ileostomy. By the time the recurrence can be demonstrated by small bowel x-ray series (or by barium enema), the patient is usually symptomatic with diarrhea, abdominal pain, or both. With progressive narrowing, the course of the recurrent ileitis or jejunitis can be best monitored by the small bowel x-ray to determine the degree of stricturing, the extent of involvement, skip lesions, fistula formation, and the presence of a mass (Fig. 8). Endoscopy of the neoterminal ileum cannot achieve these goals.

B. Con

Soon after the ileocolic anastomosis (or ileostomy), colonoscopy (or ileoscopy) can serve to recognize early recurrences that would not yet be clinically manifest or be seen by small bowel x-ray. Rutgeerts et al. have proposed an index of recurrent ileitis at the anastomosis based on inflammation, aphthous ulcers, and histological findings that can be recognized in advance of any meaningful narrowing of the bowel lumen (21). This index is the basis of a randomized controlled trial of 6-mercaptopurine versus Pentasa versus placebo in the prevention of recurrence of Crohn's disease at the anastomosis site. It also offers the opportunity to substitute alternate therapy before onset of symptoms. The combination of colonoscopy and small bowel x-rays annually after resection with anastomosis is the best guide for ongoing drug management. This is the case after ileostomy as well. The ileoscopy is better for finding early changes in the neoterminal ileum and the small bowel x-rays are better for following lesions recognized but not resected at the time of surgery or not recognized but progressing in severity.

VII. STRICTURES OF THE COLON
OR ILEOCOLIC ANASTOMOSIS

A. Pro

The GI series or barium enema can demonstrate the extent of stricture, degree of narrowing, associated fistulas, and masses, all of which are important to clinical management of strictures of the colon. Furthermore, the x-ray might show features of malignancy in the stricture such as an apple core defect.

B. Con

Colonoscopy can reach the stricture. A pediatric colonoscope or gastroscope might even be passed through the stricture. Biopsy specimens should be taken at the proximal and distal edges of the stricture as well as from representative areas within the stricture, when feasible. If biopsies through the stricture are not possible, then a brush should be passed to collect cells for cytology.

When a stricture appears to be caused by the primary Crohn's disease inflammation and is responsible for the current symptoms, dilation of the stricture can be attempted.

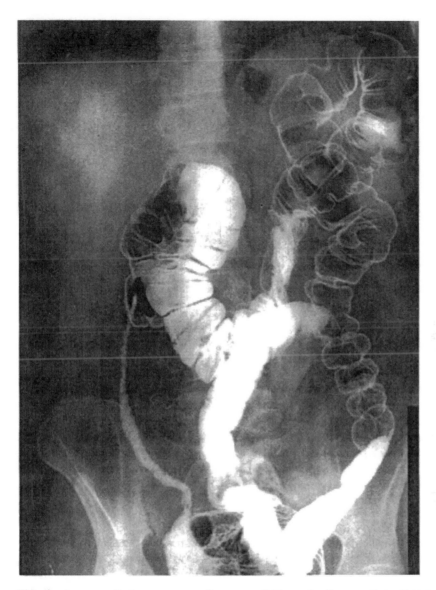

FIG. 8 An unusually long segment of recurrent ileitis at the ileoascending anastamosis after resection for Crohn's disease. Transverse fissures (rose thorn lesions) as in Fig. 1 are noted.

Whereas some endoscopists use a balloon for dilation, others successfully use the endoscope itself. The scope should be advanced through the stricture cautiously because the risk of perforation is high. Furthermore, the successful dilation will be in vain and the strictures will soon revert to their previously narrowed state unless the instrumentation is combined with new drug therapy chosen to counteract the inflammatory process and maintain the integrity of the lumen.

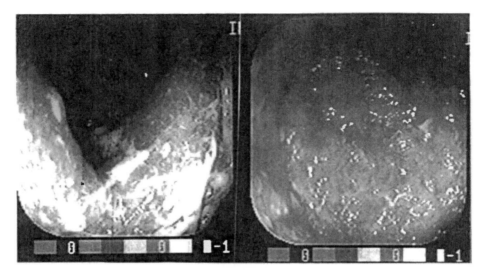

FIG. 9A Severe pouchitis after ileopouch–anal anastomosis for ulcerative colitis.

VIII. EVALUATION OF THE ILEOPOUCH–ANAL ANASTOMOSIS

A. Pro

Although the pouch is the choice surgical procedure for some patients with ulcerative colitis, postoperative pouchitis is common and, in a few cases, provides the diagnosis in retrospect of Crohn's colitis and not ulcerative colitis (22). Differential features within the pouch itself are not usually satisfactorily seen on barium x-rays. If the inflow tract is narrowed or strictured, however, or fistulas have originated from the pouch or the inflow or outflow tract, the barium studies might demonstrate these, in which case, the diagnosis of Crohn's disease would be recognized (Fig. 9A).

B. Con

Gross features of the inflammatory process can usually be better identified by endoscopic examination of the pouch and both the inflow and outflow tracts (Fig. 9B). Furthermore, biopsies can reveal granulomas or microgranulomas, which makes the diagnosis of Crohn's disease conclusive.

IX. FULMINANT COLITIS AND TOXIC MEGACOLON

A. Pro

A barium enema, whether for diagnosis, differential diagnosis, or management, is contra-indicated in the presence of a truly fulminating Crohn's colitis. This is not absolutely true for GI/small bowel x-ray series when involvement of the small bowel with Crohn's disease would alter management and there is no obstruction or impending perforation in the colon to contraindicate it. Neither barium enema nor GI x-rays series should be performed in the presence of toxic megacolon. Plain x-rays of the abdomen would serve the same purpose.

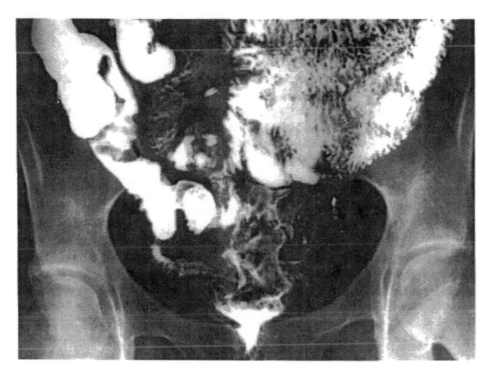

FIG. 9B Small bowel x-ray series showing recurrent ileitis of the inflow tract proximal to the pouch supporting the diagnosis of Crohns' disease. There are transverse fissures in the segment of ileum immediately proximal to the pouch.

B. Con

Flexible sigmoidoscopy or limited cautious colonoscopy is not contraindicated for a fulminating colitis when it would identify the nature of the colitis or lead to a change in management (23,24). This is also true of a toxic megacolon when the findings would clarify response to therapy and help to determine whether further nonoperative therapy would be futile or promising.

X. SURVEILLANCE FOR CANCER IN CROHN'S DISEASE OF THE COLON

A. Pro

When a stricture of the colon prevents advancement of the colonoscope, barium studies might reveal features of the stricture that would favor benign versus malignant disease as well as define the status of the bowel proximal to the stricture.

B. Con

Just as in ulcerative colitis, the risk of cancer of the colon increase with extent and duration of Crohn's disease (25). Furthermore, the colon involved with Crohn's disease is subject to the same premalignant dysplasia as that found in ulcerative colitis (26). Therefore, colonoscopic surveillance is warranted using the same criteria as that for ulcerative colitis.

XI. DIVERSION COLITIS VERSUS CROHN'S COLITIS AFTER ILEOSTOMY OR COLOSTOMY

The barium enema is of no value in distinguishing diversion colitis and its differential diagnosis from active Crohn's disease in the diverted rectum or colon. Colonoscopy or flexible sigmoidoscopy can be used to identify the gross features of the colitis, which are nonspecific for diversion colitis and might be nonspecific for Crohn's disease as well (27). Biopsies might reveal granulomas, microgranulomos, or merely nonspecific inflammation, leading to the decision as to whether to proceed with a reanastamosis.

XII. BARIUM X-RAYS VERSUS ENDOSCOPY AND BIOPSY

There is no diagnostic modality better than a small bowel x-ray series to make the diagnosis of Crohn's disease of the small bowel and demonstrate its many clinical features. Perhaps with time and experience, computerized axial tomography will be the preferred technique for total small bowel evaluation as it is now for identification of intramural abscesses and fistulas and for abdominal masses. Although barium enema x-rays serve the same purpose for Crohn's disease involving the colon for subsequent management and sometimes even as the primary procedure, colonoscopy can be used to identify most of the same lesions and allow biopsies and dilatations as well (28). The two procedures should supplement each other, and that which is preferred at one time may not be preferred later in the course of the disease. Only as a generality, the combination of colonoscopy and small bowel x-rays series is best to follow and manage the course of most cases of Crohn's disease.

REFERENCES

1. Wolf BS, Marshak RH. Granulomatous colitis (Crohn's disease of the colon.) Roentgen features. AJR Am J Roentgenol 1962; 88:662–670.
2. Simpkins KC. The barium enema in Crohn's colitis. In: Weterman IT, Pena AS, Booth CC, eds. The Management of Crohn's Disease. Proceedings of Workshop on Crohn's Disease. Leyden, 1976. Amsterdam: Exerpta Media, 1976:62–67.
3. Korelitz BI, Sommers SC. Rectal biopsy in Patients with Crohn's disease. JAMA 1977; 237:2742–2744.
4. Waye JD. X-ray or endoscopic examination for initial evaluation and follow-up in patients with colonic inflammatory bowel disease. In: Korelitz BI, Sohn N, eds. Management of Inflammatory Bowel Disease. St Louis: Mosby-Year Book, 1992:105–117.
5. Rotterdam HZ, Korelitz BI, Sommers SC. Micro-granulomas in grossly normal rectal muscosa in Crohn's disease. Am J Clin Pathol 1977; 67:550–555.
6. Korelitz BI. Appropriate use of biopsies in inflammatory bowel disease. In: Korelitz BI, Sohn N, eds. management of inflammatory bowel disease. St Louis: Mosby-Year Book, 1992:118–125.
7. Surawicz CM, Belic L. Rectal biopsy helps to distinguish acute self-limited colitis from idiopathic inflammatory bowel disease. Gastroenterology 1984; 86:104–113.
8. Korelitz BI, Sommers SC. Differential diagnosis of ulcerative and granulomatous colitis by sigmoidoscopy, rectal biopsy, and cell counts of rectal mucosa. Am J Gastroenterol 1974; 61:410–419.
9. Yardley JH. Pathology of idiopathic inflammatory bowel disease and relevance of specific findings. In: Bayless TM, ed. Current Management of Inflammatory Bowel Disease. Philadelphia: BC Decker 1989:16–21.

10. Groupe D'Etudes Therapeutiques des Affections Inflammatoires Du Tube Digestif. Development and validation of an endoscopic severity index for Crohn's disease. Gut 1989; 30:983–989.

11. Modigliani R, Mary J-Y, Simon J-F, et al. Clinical, biological and endoscopic picture of attacks of Crohn's disease. Evolution on prednisolone. Gastroenterology. 1990; 98:811–818.

12. Cellier C, Sahmoud T, Froguel E, et al. Correlations between clinical activity, endoscopic severity and biological parameters in colonic or ileocolonic Crohn's disease. A prospective multicentre study of 121 cases. Gut 1994; 35:231–235.

13. Landi B, N'Guyen ANH T, Cortot A, et al. Endoscopic monitoring of Crohn's disease treatment: a prospective randomized clinical trial. Gastroenterology 1992; 102:1647–1653.

14. Margolin ML, Korelitz BI. Management of bladder fistulas in Crohn's disease. J Clin Gastroenterol 1989; 11:399–402.

15. Korelitz BI. The Ileorectal and ileosigmoidal fistula in Crohn's disease. Clinical–radiological correlation. Mt Sinai J Med 1984; 51:341–346.

16. Leichtling JJ, Garlock JH. Granulomatous colitis complicated by gastrocolic, duodenocolic and colo-pulmonic fistulas. Gastroenterology 1962; 43:151–165.

17. Korelitz BI. Colonic–duodenal fistulas in Crohn's disease. Am J Dig Dis 1977; 22:1040–1048.

18. Zwas ER, Bonheim NA, Berken CA, Gray S. Ileoscopy as an important tool for the diagnosis of Crohn's disease; a report of seven cases. Gastrointest Endosc 1993; 40:89–91.

19. D'Haens G, Rutgeerts P, Geoboes K, Vantrappen G. The natural history of esophageal Crohn's disease: three patterns of evolution. Gastrointest endosc 1994; 40:296–300.

20. Meltzer SJ, Korelitz BI. Pancreatitis and duodenopancreatic reflux in Crohn's disease. Case report and review of the literature. J Clin Gastroenterol 1988; 10:555–558.

21. Rutgeerts P, Geboes K, Van Trappen G, et al. Predictability of the postoperative course of Crohn's disease. Gastroeneterol 1990; 99:956–963.

22. Cohen Z. Results of ileo pouch anal anastomosis. In: Korelitz BI, Sohn N, eds. Management of Inflammatory Bowel Disease. St Louis: Mosby-Year Book, 1992:164–172.

23. Ale Mayehu G, Jarnerot G. Colonoscopy during an attack of severe ulcerative colitis in a safe procedure, and of great value in clinical decision making. Am J Gastroenterol 1991; 86:187–190.

24. Carbonnel F, LaVergne A, Le'mann M, et al. Colonoscopy of acute colitis. A safe and reliable tool for assessment of severity. Dig Dis Sci 1994; 39:1554–1557.

25. Choi PM, Zelig MP. Similarity of colorectal cancer complicating Crohn's disease and ulcerative colitis. Gastroenterology 1993; 104:A682.

26. Cooper DJ, Weinstein MA, Korelitz BI. Complications of Crohn's disease predisposing to dysplasia and cancer of the intestinal tract: considerations of a surveillance program. J Clin Gastroenterol 1984; 6:217–224.

27. Korelitz BI, Cheskin LJ, Sohn N, Sommers SC. The fate of the rectal segment after diversion of the fecal stream in Crohn's disease; its implication for surgical management. J Clin Gastroenterol 1985; 7:32–43.

28. Holdstock G, DuBoulay CE, Smith CL. Survey of the use of colonoscopy in inflammatory bowel disease. Dig Dis Sci 1984; 29:731–734.

COMMENTARY: ENDOSCOPIC AND RADIOLOGIC EVALUATION

Robert Modigliani *Saint-Louis Hospital, Paris, France*

Morphological assessment of the gut in patients with Crohn's disease raises several practical questions:

1. What are the respective roles of endoscopy and radiology for the diagnosis of Crohn's disease?

When Crohn's disease is suspected, ileocolonoscopy with biopsy should be performed first, followed by small bowel barium x-rays, and, when needed, upper digestive fibroscopy. In inflammatory bowel disease, as in most other fields of gut pathology, direct inspection and biopsy sampling of a lesion is more informative than indirect x-ray imaging. That endoscopy is superior to radiology for the diagnosis of Crohn's disease has been repeatedly proven. It may be argued that ileocolonoscopy needs an unpleasant preparation, may be painful, carries a small but definite risk of perforation, and is costly. These disadvantages must be balanced against the discomfort, health hazard, pain, and cost of a delayed or erroneous diagnosis. Endoscopy should be performed by an endoscopist with experience in inflammatory bowel disease. Rectosigmoidoscopy is of limited help in Crohn's disease although it may be diagnostic in distal disease. Inspection of the anal margin and anoscopy may also lead to diagnosis.

Small bowel x-rays must be obtained also, regardless of whether ileocolonoscopy is normal, to search for more proximal disease, or, if it is diagnostic, to evaluate the extent of the disease. Total enteroscopy may prove to be better than small bowel radiology in the future, but its role in the diagnosis of Crohn's disease remains to be evaluated.

If there is diagnostic doubt between Crohn's disease and ulcerative colitis, upper digestive endoscopy may show lesions typical of the former, with a good yield of tuberculoid granulomas shown on biopsy samples.

There are a few indications left for barium (or double contrast) x-rays of the colon: (a) patients who refuse colonoscopy or those in whom it fails; (b) presence of a stenosis precluding the progression of the endoscope; and (c) search for a fistula, better evidenced by radiology.

2. *What are the indications for morphological investigations in Crohn's disease once the diagnosis is made and before resection?*

They are few:

1. There is no need for repeating endoscopy at each attack of the disease, unless the clinical picture changes.

2. There is no need to check the mucosal pattern when, after a flare of the disease, a clinical remission is obtained on prednisone. We now know that: (a) active mucosal lesions will be found in about 70% of cases of patients in clinical remission; (b) persistance of those lesions has not any prognostic implications; (c) prolonging prednisone therapy will induce more endoscopic remissions but no change of the subsequent evolution in terms of corticodependance or timing of relapse after steroid weaning (1,2).

3. It is probably useful to have a morphological workup before surgery for Crohn's disease.

3. *Indications for endoscopic monitoring after intestinal resection?*

We know that 1 year after ileocolonic resection, about 75% of patients have endoscopic recurrence in the perianastomotic area (3). The risk of clinical relapse is strongly correlated with the severity of endoscopic lesions, reaching 100% within 4 years in those subjects with most severe mucosal recurrences (3). Several attempts have been made to prevent endoscopic recurrences by prescribing the tested drug immediately after surgery and for 1–2 years. No definite result has yet been published, but data suggest a positive effect of 5-aminosalicylic acid (5-ASA) on the rate of endoscopic recurrence.

For the time being, several possibilities are open to manage a patient who has just undergone a "curative" intestinal resection:

1. Follow-up without endoscopy or any recurrence-preventing treatment.
2. To start oral 5-ASA (2–3 g/day) immediately after the postoperative period.
3. Endoscopy 1 year after surgery and 5-ASA prescribed to those with severe mucosal lesions.
4. Include the patient in a controlled trial on postoperative recurrence prevention.

Attitude (4) and, if impossible, (3) are the most appealing.

4. Is it licit to perform a colonoscopy in patients with severe acute colitis?

The answer to this question is usually negative, because of the risk of perforation. We routinely endoscope this type of patient without complications. We obtain thereby precious information on the severity of mucosal lesion (which bears no relationship with the intensity of the clinical picture), which may be useful for the choice of treatment.

5. Is endoscopic cancer surveillance necessary in Crohn's disease?

There is increasing evidence that extensive Crohn's colitis carries a risk of colorectal adenocarcinoma similar to that of ulcerative colitis (4). Dysplasia has been associated with cancer in Crohn's disease (5). In the absence of any large-scale prospective evaluation of the yield of endoscopic surveillance in extensive Crohn's colitis in terms of dysplasia, cancer, and survival, it seems reasonable to opt for the same policy as in ulcerative colitis.

6. Therapeutic intervention in Crohn's disease may be useful in intestinal strictures, as discussed?

REFERENCES

1. Modigliani R, Mary JY, Simon JF, Cortot A, Soule JC, Gendre JP, Rene E, the Groupe d'Etudes Thérapeutiques des Affections Inflammatories Digestives: Clinical, biological and endoscopic pictures of attacks of Crohn's disease. Evolution on prednisolone. Gastroenterology 1990; 98:811–818.
2. Landi B, N'Gyuen anh T, Cortot A, Soulé JC, Rene E, Gendre JP, Bories P, See A, Metman EH, Florent C, Lerebours E, Mary JY, Modigliani R, and GETAID. Endoscopic monitoring of Crohn's disease ? A prospective randomized clinical trial. Gastroenterology 1992; 102:1647–1653.
3. Rutgeerts P, Geboes K, Vantrappen G, Beyls J, Kerremans R, Hiele M. Predictability of the postoperative course of Crohn's disease. Gastroenterology, 1990; 99:956–962.
4. Gillen CD, Walmsley RS, Prior P, Andrews HA, Allan RN. Ulcerative colitis and Crohn's disease: a comparison of the colorectal cancer risk in extensive colitis. Gut 1994; 35:1590–1592.
5. Cooper DJ, Weinstein MA, Korelitz BI. Complications of Crohn's disease predisposing to dysplasia and cancer of the intestinal tract: considerations of a surveillance program. J Clin Gastroenterol 1984; 6:217–224.

8
Cross-Sectional Imaging in the Evaluation of Crohn's Disease

Richard M. Gore and Gary G. Ghahremani   *Evanston Hospital–McGaw Medical Center of Northwestern University, Evanston, Illinois*

Frank H. Miller   *Northwestern University Medical School and Northwestern Memorial Hospital, Chicago, Illinois*

I. INTRODUCTION

Fiberoptic endoscopy and gastrointestinal barium studies are the principal methods for evaluating patients with known or suspected Crohn's disease. Both techniques provide superb visualization of the bowel mucosa and its abnormal surface patterns. Double-contrast radiography and endoscopy, however, cannot reliably detect the extraluminal complications of Crohn's disease, such as abscess, creeping fat of the mesentery, and associated extraintestinal abnormalities such as sclerosing cholangitis (1). Furthermore, approximately 10% to 15% of patients with inflammatory bowel disease do not present with sufficiently characteristic radiographic or endoscopic findings to permit accurate classification as either ulcerative or granulomatous colitis, so-called indeterminate colitis (2).

Because computed tomography (CT), ultrasonography, and magnetic resonance (MR) imaging can directly image pathological changes in the bowel wall, serosa, surrounding mesentery, and lymph nodes, they can provide crucial information for accurate diagnosis and management of many of the complications of Crohn's disease. These techniques can also be used to guide percutaneous abscess drainage and monitor the therapeutic response (2,3).

This chapter describes the current clinical applications and relative merits of various cross-sectional imaging techniques in evaluating patients with Crohn's disease.

II. TECHNICAL CONSIDERATIONS

A. Ultrasonography

In the early years of sonographic use, the peristaltic activity and gas–fluid content of intestinal loops were considered detriments to sonographic demonstration of intra-abdominal organs. Technical advances in the past decade have led to development of high-resolution gray-scale and real-time scanners, transrectal and endovaginal transducers, and Doppler and color-flow computed sonography. These techniques have greatly expanded the applications of ultrasound in evaluating alimentary tract disorders (4,5).

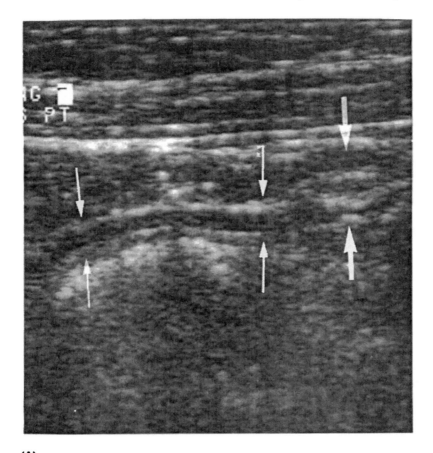

(A)
FIG. 1 Transabdominal sonographic features of normal gut versus Crohn's ileitis. A, Oblique sonogram of the right lower abdomen shows a longitudinally imaged segment of distal ileum (*small arrows*) as it joins the collapsed cecum (*large arrows*). The intestinal wall is approximately 3 mm thick and appears as an echogenic center (mucosa and submucosa) and hypoechoic periphery (muscularis propria). B, Longitudinal image of distal ileum in a patient with Crohn's disease demonstrates marked mural thickening of the intestinal wall (*W*) to about 11 mm. The inflamed loop (*arrows*) appears more hypoechoic and has a narrowed lumen (*L*).

1. Conventional Transabdominal Sonography

Real-time ultrasound of the small bowel and colon should use the highest frequency transducer possible, usually 3.5 or 5.0 MHz. The gut should be imaged axially and longitudinally as the transducer is angulated to visualize each segment. The following elements should be carefully scrutinized: mural thickness with its symmetrical stratification and homogeneity, presence of mucosal folds (haustra and valvulae conniventes), frequency and amplitude of peristalsis, diameter of bowel loops, and distribution of intraluminal gas or fluid content (6–9).

On axial images, the wall of the small bowel or colon appears as an echogenic structure with a "target" appearance (Fig. 1A). Five to seven layers of bowel wall can be appreciated with transrectal ultrasound. However, only two distinct layers representing an echogenic center and hypoechoic periphery can be visualized in nondistended loops on

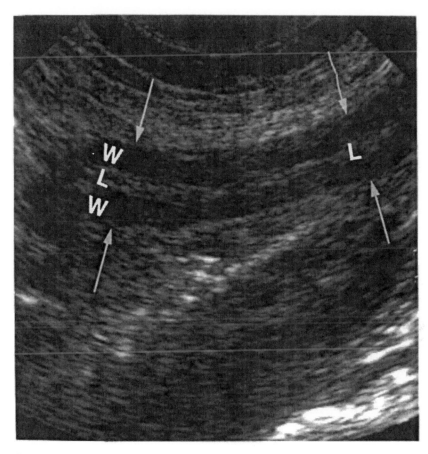

(B)

transabdominal scans. The thickness of the intestinal wall measured from the lumen to the outer edge of the hypoechoic layer should be less than or equal to 5 mm in nondistended segments or less than 3 mm when the gut is well distended. If the bowel wall is thicker than 5 mm, either diffusely or asymmetrically, then a pathological process should be suspected (see Fig. 1B) (10–15).

Normal fluid-filled small bowel loops show segmental contractions and distal propagation of their content during peristalsis when observed by real-time sonography. A functional or organic disorder should be suspected when a segment of bowel fails to change configuration over a 30- to 60-second period. Also, change in the distribution of gas within a loop during peristalsis or with transducer compression should normally be observed. Similarly, when observed over a 1-minute period, fluid- and stool-filled colon should change configuration because of peristalsis. These changes are best appreciated in the ascending colon (16–20).

2. Hydrocolonic Sonography

With hydrocolonic sonography, the large bowel is examined after adequate luminal distention with water instilled by retrograde enema (21,22). This allows improved sonographic visualization of the colonic wall, from the rectosigmoid to the cecum, with clear

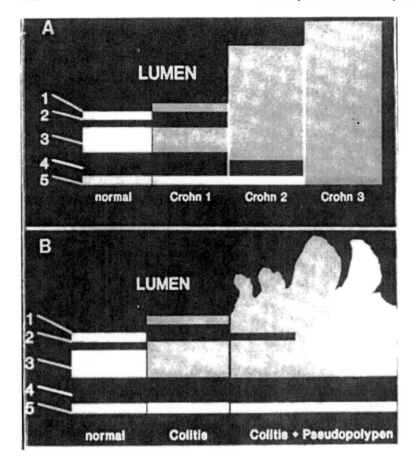

FIG. 2 Sonographic features of inflammatory bowel disease. **A,** Five layers are recognizable within the normal colon wall on endorectal and hydrocolonic sonography: 1 = mucosa; 2 = muscularis mucosae; 3 = submucosa; 4 = muscularis propria; 5 = serosa. In the early phase of Crohn's disease (*Crohn 1*), there is mild mural thickening and the wall is less echogenic, but all five layers are still visible. Progression of inflammatory changes (*Crohn 2*) results in marked mural thickening. The wall becomes hypoechoic and layers 1 through 3 are not distinguishable. In advanced chronic phase (*Crohn 3*), the colon wall is clearly thickened, hypoechoic, and mural stratification can no longer be appreciated. **B,** Comparison of normal versus ulcerative colitis. In acute ulcerative colitis, the wall is only slightly thickened and mural stratification is pronounced. The wall is less echogenic than normal colon wall or the surrounding connective tissue. In patients with more advanced disease, the colon wall is thickened and multiple pseudopolyps are demonstrable. In such cases, mural stratification can be obliterated which can interfere with differentiation from Crohn's colitis. (From Ref. 21.)

depiction of typical mural stratification. In one series, hydrosonography detected active colonic Crohn's disease and ulcerative colitis with a sensitivity of 91% and 89%, respectively (Figs. 2,3) (23).

3. Transrectal Ultrasound

Endorectal sonography was initially developed for the evaluation of carcinoma of the prostate. Because of its ability to define the layers of the rectal wall and perirectal soft tissues, it has recently been adapted for staging rectal carcinoma and evaluating the spectrum of benign and malignant rectal or perirectal disorders. Initial reports indicate usefulness of this technique in evaluating patients with Crohn's disease and associated anorectal conditions such as fissures, ulcers, fistulas, and perirectal or pelvic abscesses. Anatomical changes caused by soft-tissue masses, cysts, calcification, and fluid collections can be readily identified (24–26).

With this technique, a tubular transducer with inflatable balloon attachment is covered by a condom, lubricated with scanning gel, and inserted per anus. A series of axial images are obtained at 1-cm intervals from the anorectal junction to approximately 15 cm above it, which is the usual maximal depth of insertion. A cleansing enema administered before the procedure and the examination itself are generally well tolerated by the patient (24–26).

When a 7-MHz transducer is used, endosonograms show five to seven layers of rectal wall (see Fig. 2). These consist of the following: (a) inner white line representing the interface between the water-filled balloon of the transducer and the rectal mucosa; (b) inner black line representing the mucosa–muscularis mucosae junction; (c) middle black line representing the submucosa; (d) outer black line representing the muscularis propria; (e) outer white border indicating the interface between the muscularis propria and perirectal fat. Occasionally, a seven-layered wall can be seen where the hypoechoic (dark) muscularis propria layer is divided by a thin echogenic (white) line of connective tissue into an inner circular muscle layer and an outer longitudinal muscle layer. The normal wall of distended rectum is 2 to 3 mm thick and perirectal tissue has an inhomogeneous echo pattern consistent with its fibrofatty components (27–31).

Transrectal ultrasound can show the following abnormalities: (a) mural thickening; (b) perianal and perirectal abscesses (Fig. 4) and fistulas; (c) heterogeneity of the anal sphincter. Rectal wall thickening (> 4 mm) is often accompanied by loss of mural stratification in Crohn's disease. Fistula and sinus tracts appear as dotted columns of echo-rich gas bubbles with reverberation. Abscesses are characterized sonographically as predominantly hypoechoic areas that contain echogenic elements corresponding to debris and gas bubbles. The wall of the abscess is usually thick and irregular, and some posterior acoustic enhancement may be seen. The anal sphincter derives from the rectal muscular layer as a sharply delineated ellipsoid that is uniformly hypoechoic. When involved by Crohn's disease, the sphincter becomes heterogeneous with echogenic zones interspersed between the normal hypoechoic regions. Also, in patients with active proctologic disease, the shortening and narrowing of the anal canal during squeezing and the elongation with dilatation during straining are less pronounced. Some authors advocate routine screening with transrectal ultrasound because this technique is capable of defining pararectal and para-anal abscesses and fistula that develop extramurally without mucosal lesions (32).

B. Magnetic Resonance Imaging

Magnetic resonance imaging provides a similar perspective as CT in that images demonstrate the overall topography of the abdomen. This imaging technique has several inherent advantages: lack of ionizing radiation, multiplanar imaging capability, and superb soft-tissue contrast (33–42). Disadvantages that have generally precluded the routine use of MR imaging in the evaluation of inflammatory bowel disease (IBD) include respiratory and bowel motion artifact, lack of a satisfactory oral contrast agent, high signal intensity of intra-abdominal fat, and long imaging times used in conventional spin-echo sequences.

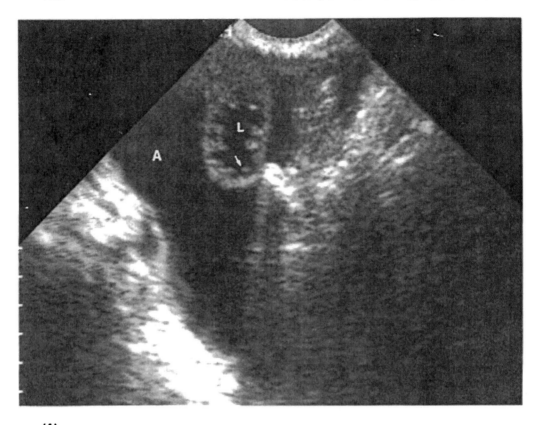

(A)
FIG. 3 Hydrocolonic sonography. A, Normal sigmoid colon is axially imaged and shows intraluminal water (*L*) and the haustra (*arrow*). Ascites (*A*) is also present. B, Crohn's disease. The colon wall
is thickened and has lost its typical haustration on this axially oriented scan. Wall layers 1 through
3 are no longer visible and layers 4 and 5 are only rudimentarily recognizable. (From Ref. 21.)

Many of the limitations of MR imaging have been overcome by using breath-holding
imaging (fast low angle shot [FLASH]) to reduce artifacts, fat suppression techniques
to reduce the signal intensity of fat, and an intravenous contrast agent, gadopentate
dimeglumine (Gd-DTPA). With these new techniques, MR imaging can show the extent
and severity of inflammatory changes (Fig. 5) of the gut that correlate with endoscopic
and histological findings from surgical specimens (34). There are also certain MR features
than can help differentiate Crohn's disease from ulcerative colitis (vide infra). Further
studies, however, are needed to determine the role of this elegant, but expensive examination in the clinical management of patients with IBD.

C. Computed Tomography

Computed tomography provides an important and often unique diagnostic perspective and
therapeutic tool in the evaluation and management of patients with Crohn's disease
(43–46). It has emerged as the single most useful cross-sectional imaging technique in
patients with IBD. Indeed, in the acutely ill patient, CT is usually the only radiological
examination needed. In a recent study of a large number of patients with clinically

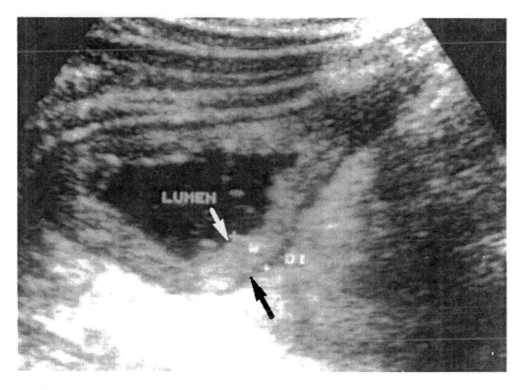

(B)

symptomatic Crohn's disease, CT demonstrated significant, previously unsuspected findings that led to a change of medical and surgical management in 28% of cases (47).
Additionally, CT proved reliable in confirming or excluding complications suggested
clinically or by barium techniques (48,49).

Excellent opacification of the gut is necessary when evaluating the bowel wall and
surrounding mesentery on CT scans of patients with known or suspected inflammatory or
infectious bowel disease. Unopacified bowel may stimulate an abscess, mass, or lymph
node and is a common source of diagnostic error. Additionally, proper distention of the
lumen either by contrast or air is essential in detecting bowel wall thickening, an important
CT sign of IBD. Several techniques have proved successful in achieving adequate bowel
opacification and distention in these patients (50,51).

Intravenous contrast material is helpful in the search for abscess but is not strictly
necessary is assessing bowel wall thickness. With bolus administration of contrast media
and dynamic scanning, bowel wall enhancement can be seen with active inflammation.
Intravenous contrast material is also needed to establish the diagnosis of ischemic gut of
splanchnic venous thrombosis.

On CT, the normal thickness of the wall of the small bowel and colon is 2 to 3 mm
when the lumen is distended. This measurement should be made on scans in which the gut
is fully distended and imaged transaxially or when the scan plane is parallel with the
segment of bowel (e.g., transverse colon, sigmoid, and stomach). Oblique scanning planes
may artificially increase this measurement. Mural thickness greater than 4 mm for the

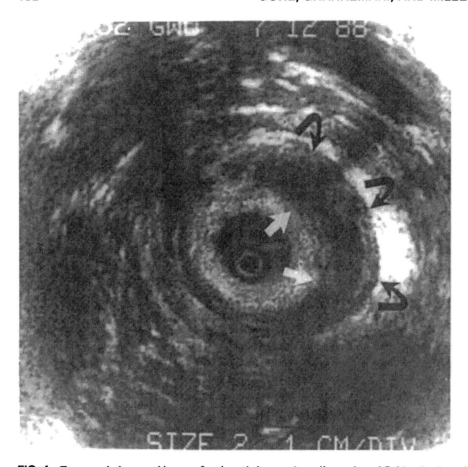

FIG. 4   Transrectal ultrasound image of perirectal abscess. A semilunar-shaped fluid collection with internal echoes (*arrows*) is identified at the level of anal sphincter, just below the supralevator ani muscle in a patient with Crohn's disease. (From Hill MC, Smith LE, Huntington DK, et al. Endorectal sonography in the evaluation of the rectum. Ultrasound 1992; 10:29–56.)

small bowel and colon or 11 mm for the stomach is abnormal. The bowel wall should also have a homogeneous attenuation (43,52).

The mesentery and omentum normally contain blood vessels and small lymph nodes that are less than 3 to 5 mm in size, as well as fat having an attenuation value ranging between –75 and –125 Hounsfield units (HU). A higher CT number may indicate the presence of fluid, cellular infiltrate, hemorrhage, or fibrosis (43).

In patients with inflammatory bowel disease, the following CT features should be carefully considered: (a) bowel wall thickness and homogeneity; (b) mesenteric, perirectal, retroperitoneal, and omental fat attenuation and homogeneity; (c) lymph node size; (d) abscess, fistulas, sinus tracts, and extraluminal contrast collections; (e) mesenteric or perivisceral masses; (f) dimensions of the presacral space; (g) liver abnormalities (e.g., sclerosing cholangitis or steatosis); (h) hydronephrosis and renal or gallbladder stones; (i) sacroiliitis and spinal ligamentous ossification; (j) osteomyelitis; (k) avascular necrosis of the femoral heads (43).

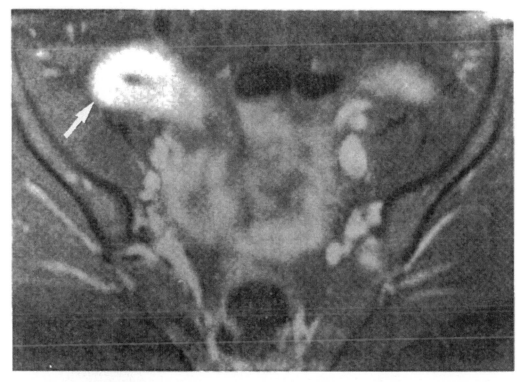

FIG. 5 Crohn's disease of the terminal ileum: contrast-enhanced MR findings. Axial scan of the pelvis obtained after the intravenous administration of Gd-DTPA shows severe inflammation with marked wall thickening and mural enhancement of the distal ileum (*arrow*). The degree of enhancement correlates with the degree of inflammation. (From Ref 34.)

III. MURAL DISEASE

Pathologically, Crohn's disease involves all layers of the gut, producing a bowel wall that is thickened by edema, inflammatory cell infiltration, and lymphangiectasia acutely, and by granulation tissue proliferation and fibrosis chronically. Bowel wall thickening can be impressive, and these mural changes can be appreciated on cross-sectional imaging.

A. Computed Tomography

On CT, mural disease is manifested by bowel wall thickening (Fig. 6) ranging between 1 and 3 cm, occasionally reaching 10 times normal thickness (44–46). These changes, which occur in up to 83% of patients, are most frequently observed in the terminal ileum, but other portions of the small bowel, colon, duodenum, stomach, and esophagus may be similarly affected (43). The mural thickening is often discontinuous and the skip areas correlate with abnormalities seen on barium studies. This does not suggest, however, that all patients with Crohn's disease have mural thickening demonstrable on CT. In early Crohn's disease with superifical ulceration, the CT may appear normal. Conversely, in patients with quiescent disease, the mucosa may be normal while CT shows wall thickening. Rarely, mural changes may antedate mucosal changes seen on barium enema studies (45–50).

Depending on the chronicity and level of disease activity, the presence of sinus tracts,

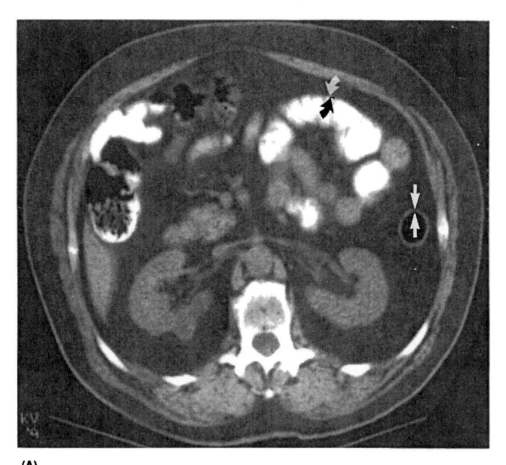

(A)
FIG. 6 Computed tomographic evaluation of the gut wall: normal versus Crohn's disease. A, Computed tomographic section of the abdomen shows normally thin bowel wall (≤ 3 mm) when the lumen is well distended. This is apparent both in the air-filled descending colon (*straight arrows*) and contrast-filled jejunal loops (*curved arrows*). B, In this patient with long-standing Crohn's disease, there is obvious mural thickening of the ileum (*arrows*) associated with narrowing of its lumen. C, In another case of Crohn's disease, there is gradual transition of normal proximal transverse colon (*small arrows*) to enormously thickened walls of splenic flexure with its irregularly narrowed lumen (*large arrows*).

and the corticosteroid intake, the thickened bowel wall typically has a homogeneous appearance with loss of mural stratification. Less frequently, a "double-halo" appearance of the small bowel and colon can be seen in the early active, noncicatrizing phase of Crohn's disease. A soft-tissue density ring (corresponding to mucosa) is surrounded by a low-density ring with an attenuation similar to that of water (corresponding to severe submucosal edema) or fat (corresponding to submucosal fat deposition), which, in turn, is surrounded by a higher density ring of muscularis propria and serosa (51–55).

This "double-halo" appearance is nonspecific and has also been described in ulcerative colitis, radiation enteritis, ischemic colitis, mesenteric venous thrombosis, acute pancreatitis, and pseudomembranous colitis. Inflamed mucosa and bowel wall may show significant contrast enhancement following bolus intravenous contrast administration, and the intensity of enhancement has been reported to correlate with the clinical activity of disease (54).

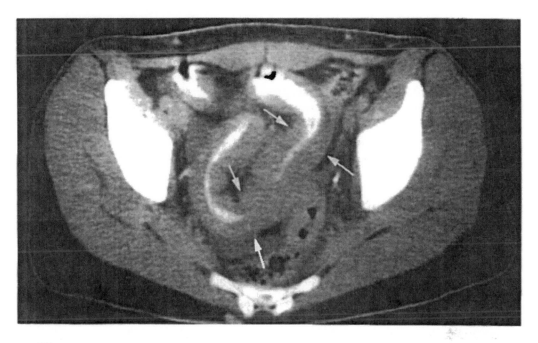

(B)

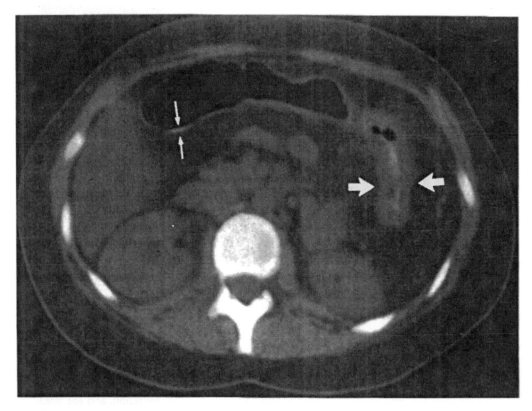

(C)

B. Ultrasound

The thickness of the colonic and small bowel wall can be appreciated sonographically, and the validity of using mural thickening in the diagnosis of inflammatory bowel disease has a reported sensitivity of between 67% and 86% and a specificity of 87% to 100% (4,7,10,15,19,22,23). Some authors suggest using sonography as a screen for Crohn's disease (10). When suspicion of disease is low, normal ultrasonography may be sufficient to avoid barium examination (10). When abnormal gut is seen or clinical suspicion is high, despite a normal ultrasound study, barium examination should be performed (10).

In patients with active Crohn's disease, the colon wall can be up to 1.5 cm thick (see Figs. 1B, 2). Mural stratification is typically lost as well. Using criteria listed in Table 1, the sensitivity of ultrasound in detecting active Crohn's disease was 91% with a specificity of 100% and it was 89% and 97%, respectively, for active ulcerative colitis (22). There are several sonographic caveats. In patients with only aphthoid ulcerations, there is typical wall stratification in Crohn's disease, suggesting the disease is not yet transmural. In patients with ulcerative colitis who have large and extensive pseudopolyps, the thickness of the colon wall may approach 1.5 cm and mural stratification may be lost (21–23).

Several authors, however, have questioned the use of ultrasound in differentiating ulcerative colitis and Crohn's colitis on the basis of bowel wall changes alone (28,29). Documentation of continuous or discontinuous involvement combined with evidence of mesenteric disease, abscess, and/or fistulas can assist in the differentiation.

In a recent study using hydrocolonic sonography, 93% of patients with Crohn's disease showed loss of mural stratification, and the wall appeared hypoechoic and clearly thickened (see Fig. 3B). In contrast, mural stratification was maintained in patients with ulcerative colitis (see Fig. 2). Indeed, hydrocolonic sonography differentiated Crohn's disease form ulcerative colitis in 93% of cases. Colonic Crohn's disease and ulcerative colitis were detectable by this technique with a sensitivity of 96% and 91%, respectively (21).

The thickened bowel wall in Crohn's disease produces a "target," "bulls-eye," or "cockade" appearance that must be differentiated from chronic ulcerative colitis, diverticulitis, lymphoma, ischemic colitis, and pseudomembranous colitis.

Sonography has also been successful in diagnosing recurrent disease in patients who have had surgical resections (20).

TABLE 1 Crohn's Disease Versus Ulcerative
Colitis: Sonographic Features

Active Crohn's Disease
  Loss of mural stratification
  Clearly thickened, hypoechoic bowel wall
  Haustral loss
  Decreased compressibility
  Diminished peristalsis
Acute Ulcerative Colitis
  Mural stratification maintained
  Moderately thickened, hypoechoic bowel wall
  Haustral loss
  Decreased compressibility
  Diminished peristalsis

Source: Ref. 22.

C. Magnetic Resonance Imaging

Mural thickening of the gut (see Fig. 5) can also be appreciated with MR imaging (33–38). When fast imaging sequences are combined with intravenous contrast (Gd-DPTA) administration and fat-suppressed imaging, a good correlation between bowel wall thickness, length of diseased bowel, and severity of inflammation has been reported (34). Indeed, the percent of contrast enhancement compared well with severity of inflammation based on endoscopic and surgical findings (34). Gd-DTPA is a nonspecific extracellular space contrast agent that increases the T1 relaxation of surrounding water protons, which produces relative tissue brightening. This tissue brightening is transmural in Crohn's disease but not present in the submucosa in ulcerative colitis, an important differentiating feature of these two colitides. The actively inflamed wall enhances because of increased delivery of the agent and increased capillary permeability.

IV. MESENTERIC DISEASE

The palpation of an abdominal mass or separation of bowel loops seen on a small bowel series in a patient with Crohn's disease evokes a large differential diagnosis with significantly different prognostic and therapeutic implications: abscess, phlegmon, "creeping fat" or fibrofatty proliferation of the mesentery, thickening of the bowel wall, and enlarged mesenteric lymph nodes. This diagnostic dilemma is further complicated because many of the patients are receiving immunosuppressive therapy that can mask signs and symptoms and there may be a large psychological overlay. These extraluminal complications of Crohn's disease can readily be differentiated on cross-sectional imaging. Computed tomography has emerged as the premier imaging technique in their characterization.

A. Abscess

Approximately 15% to 20% of patients with Crohn's disease develop an intra-abdominal abscess at some time. Abscesses are most frequently associated with small bowel disease of ileocolitis. Once developed, an abscess can burrow through the adjacent tissue or break open and drain spontaneously into another part of the bowel and/or adjacent organ. Abscesses usually result from sinus tracts, fistulas, perforations, or surgical operations for Crohn's disease (56–58).

An intra-abdominal abscess may be difficult to diagnose on clinical grounds in patients with Crohn's disease because symptoms may be inconspicuous, masked by the effects of corticosteroids, or mistaken for an exacerbation of the disease. Barium studies and endoscopy can only suggest the presence of an abscess indirectly by mass effect, spiculation of the mucosa, or demonstration of the presence of a fistula. Also, these studies do not evaluate the ischiorectal fossa, psoas muscle, or other solid organs in which abscesses occur (57). Cross-sectional imaging is required to confirm the diagnosis and reveal the full extent and location of the abscess cavity.

1. Computed Tomography

Computed tomography is the procedure of choice for both the diagnosis and percutaneous management of intra-abdominal abscesses (59–77). On CT scans, abscesses appear as circumscribed round or oval soft-tissue density masses with an attenuation between +10 to +30 HU (Fig. 7). If the abscess has a well-formed capsule, it may show contrast enhancement, whereas the central area of the abscess, which contains necrotic material, does not. Intralesional, extraluminal gas is an important diagnostic feature seen in 30% to

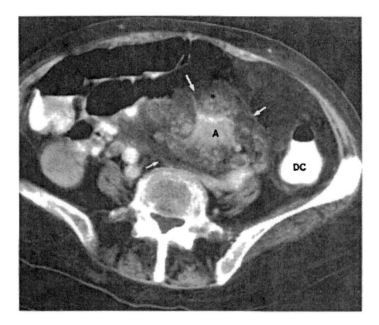

(A)

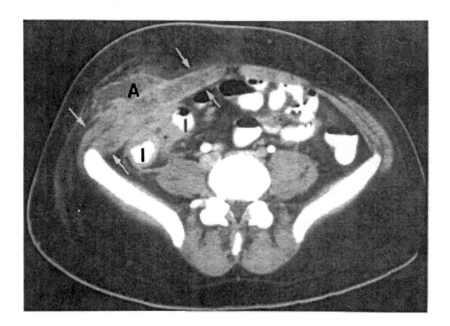

(B)
FIG. 7 Computed tomographic appearance of abscesses complicating Crohn's disease. A, Mesenteric interloop abscess presenting as a central fluid density (*A*) and surrounding inflammatory changes (*arrows*) medial to the contrast-filled descending colon (*DC*). B, Abdominal wall/subcutaneous ab-

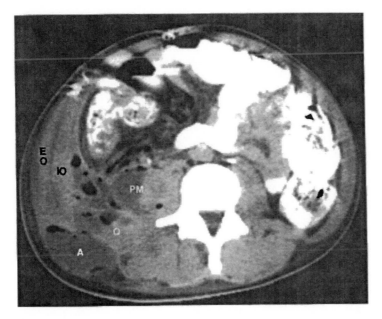

(C)

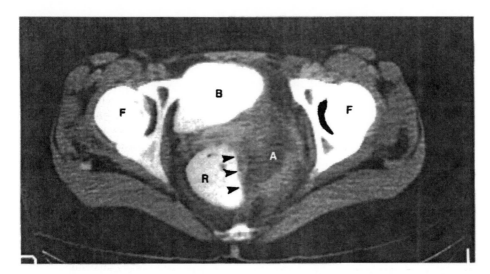

(D)

scess. Direct extension of transmural inflammation from the ileocecal segment (*I*) has involved the adjacent abdominal wall muscles (*arrows*), causing their swelling and associated subcutaneous abscess (*A*). C, Psoas abscess. Note the low attenuation and gas within the right psoas muscle (*PM*). The quadratus lumborum muscle (*Q*), and internal (*IO*) and external (*EO*) oblique muscles are also involved. A right flank subcutaneous fat abscess cavity (*A*) is also present. D, Perirectal abscess. A low attenuation abscess (*A*) is identified along the left lateral aspect of the rectum (*R*), causing deformity of the rectal wall (*arrowheads*). B = bladder; F = femoral heads.

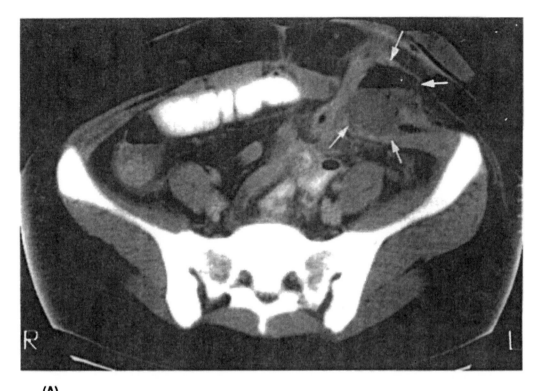

(A)
FIG. 8 Computed tomography directed percutaneous abscess drainage. A, Peristomal abscess presenting as a well-defined air-filled collection adjacent to descending colostomy (*arrows*). B, This abscess was percutaneously drained under CT guidance. Injected contrast delineates the abscess cavity (*arrows*).

50% of cases. The gas may result from gas-forming bacteria but most often results from sinus tracts communicating with the skin surface or the gastrointestinal tract. The gas may be distributed as finely dispersed air bubbles throughout the collection or as an air-fluid level (14,57). Complete bowel opacification is essential to establish the diagnosis of abscess with confidence.

2. Ultrasound

The internal sonographic architecture of an abscess is variable, ranging from anechoic to a complex echogenic mass. Abscesses often have thick echogenic walls. Intracavitary gas appears highly echogenic with or without acoustic shadowing. Although ultrasound has a reported accuracy of 80% to 90% in detecting intra-abdominal abscesses, this technique is operator dependent and is limited by the presence of drains, wounds, obesity, and bowel gas (57).

3. Magnetic Resonance Imaging

Magnetic resonance imaging is too expensive and time consuming to be used as a primary screening tool for abdominal abscesses (57). Abscesses appear as homogenous or heterogeneous areas of low signal intensity on T1-weighted images with an increase in signal intensity on T2-weighted images. On gradient echo images, the abscess wall may show

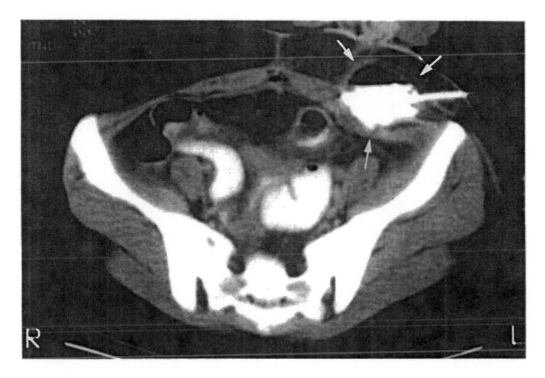

(B)

enhancement after the intravenous administration of Gd-DTPA. Areas of gas within the abscess have no signal.

4. Percutaneous Abscess Drainage

The treatment of abscesses in patients with Crohn's disease is difficult (66,69,70,75,76). If surgically drained, these abscesses reform in 40% to 90% of cases, with a death rate of 2% to 4% (58). Because these abscesses usually have accompanying fistulas and may be multiloculated, in the past there has been a reluctance to drain them percutaneously.

Recent studies, however, have reported success in the percutaneous management of these abscesses. Casola et al. reported success in draining 15 of 15 abscesses in patients with Crohn's disease (74). Fistulas closed in four of seven patients, and the remaining three required surgery for excision of diseased bowel and enteric fistulas (74). Other authors have noted that this procedure may only be palliative in patients with enteric communication and serves as an effective temporizing measure that provides time to improve nutritional and clinical status. Also, two-stage surgical resections that initially bypass the diseased gut can often be simplified into single-stage surgery (76). In the series reported to date, no patients have developed an entercutaneous fistula as a result of catheter drainage.

Computed tomography is the catheter guidance procedure of choice in these patients and may obviate the need for surgery in many cases (Fig. 8). Because 70% to 90% of patients with regional enteritis require surgery at some times, avoidance of an operation is an advantage.

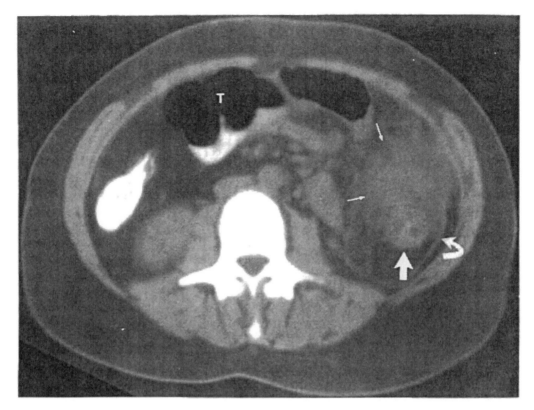

FIG. 9   Phlegmon: CT findings. There is an ill-defined region of increased attenuation (*small arrows*) representing a phlegmon along the anterior aspect of a thickened descending colon (*large arrow*). The transverse colon (*T*) is uninvolved. Curved arrow = thickened lateroconal fascia.

B.   Phlegmon

A phlegmon is an ill-defined, inflammatory mass in the mesentery that may resolve completely with antibiotic therapy or progress to abscess formation (53). It is another common cause of mesenteric mass effect in patients with Crohn's disease (49).

On CT, a phlegmon produces loss of definition of surrounding organs and a "smudgy" or "streaky" appearance of the adjacent mesenteric fat (Fig. 9). Fine needle aspiration may be needed to differentiate this entity from abscess (43,44,49,50). On ultrasound, the mesenteric fat becomes heterogeneous, and it becomes hypoechoic when involved by a phlegmon (54). On MR scans, the involved mesentery has a lower signal intensity on T1-weighted sequences and higher signal intensity on T2-weighted sequences than normal mesenteric fat (54).

C.   Fibrofatty Proliferation

Fibrofatty proliferation, also known as "creeping fat" of the mesentery, is the most common cause of separation of bowel loops seen on small bowel series (43,44,49,50). On CT, the sharp interface between bowel and mesentery is lost and the attenuation value of the fat, usually between −90 and −130 HU, is elevated by 20 to 60 HU because there is an influx of inflammatory cells and fluid (Fig. 10A). Mesenteric adenopathy with lymph nodes ranging in size between 3 and 8 mm may also be present. If these lymph nodes

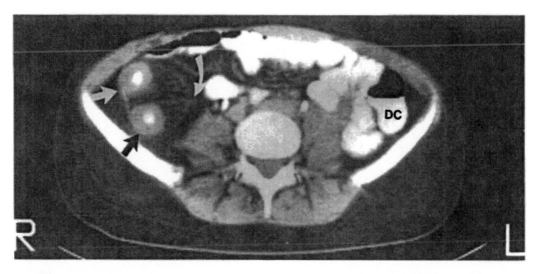

(A)

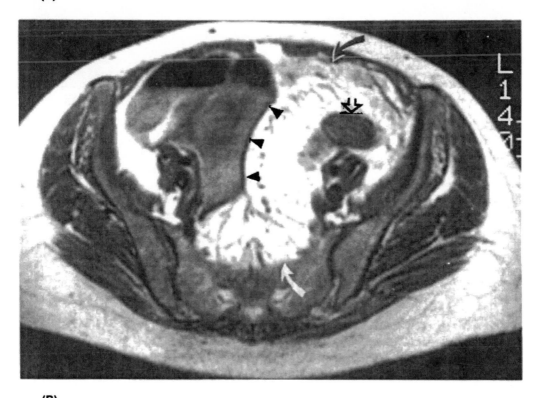

(B)

FIG. 10 Mesenteric disease: creeping fat of the mesentery. A, Computed tomography abnormal mesenteric fat (*curved arrow*) along the medial aspect of disease-thickened loops of distal ileum (*straight arrows*). This abnormal fat has an increased number of strandlike densities and is separating bowel loops. DC = descending colon. B, T1-weighted MR scan of the pelvis shows thickening of the sigmoid colon (*open arrow*) and creeping fat of the sigmoid mesocolon (*curved arrows*). This fat in the mesocolon has an abnormal number of strandlike areas of decreased signal because of the presence of fluid and is producing a mass effect (*arrowheads*) on adjacent small bowel loops.

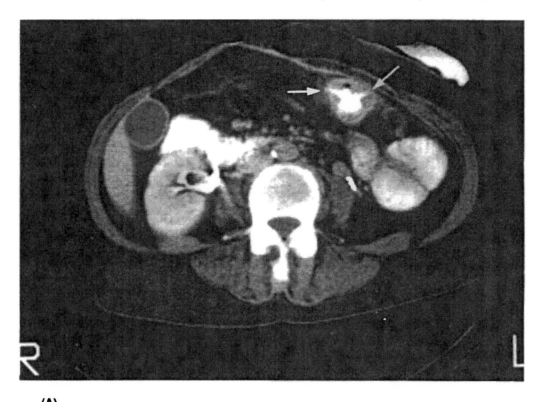

(A)

FIG. 11 The utility of CT in demonstrating fistulas and sinus tracts. A, Recurrent Crohn's disease of the ileum following creation of an ileostomy causing mural thickening of the involved segment and deep sinus tracts (*arrows*) extending through the serosa into the adjacent fat. B, Double-contrast barium enema of a different patient showing recurrent disease with intramural fistulas (*arrows*) following an ascending colon–sigmoid anastomosis. C, Computed tomography scan in the same patient as in view B showing mural thickening of the involved segment, the lumen of the colon (*straight arrows*), and intramural fistulas (*curved arrows*). D, Lateral film of a small bowel series in a different patient shows sinus tracts and fistulas anterior to the L5 vertebral body (*arrows*). E, Computed tomography scan in the same patient as in view D shows the full extent of the disease as well as the presence of an abscess cavity. The presence of contrast within the cavity (*arrows*) confirms communication with the gut.

become larger than 1 cm in size, the presence of lymphoma or carcinoma (both of which occur with greater frequency in Crohn's disease) should be excluded (43,50).

Sonographically, edema causes creeping fat of the mesentery to be hypoechoic compared with normal fat (11,14). On T1-weighted MR sequences (see Fig. 10B), the fat may have low signal intensity streaks and strands. These area may be enhanced after Gd-DTPA administration on gradient echo images (34).

D. Fistulas and Sinus Tracts

Fistulas and sinus tracts (Fig. 11) are a hallmark of Crohn's disease, affecting approximately 20% to 40% of individuals (77–88). A sinus tract is close-ended, usually

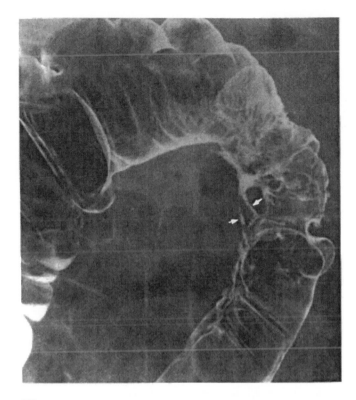

(B)

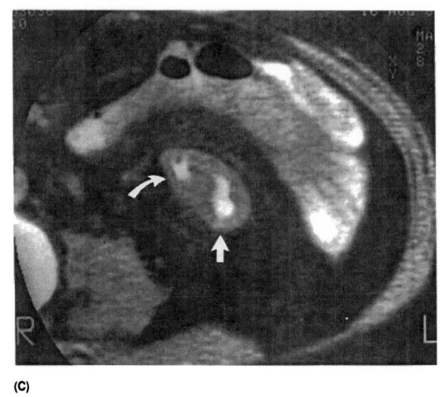

(C)

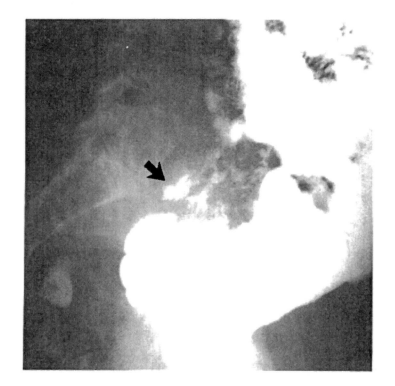

(D)

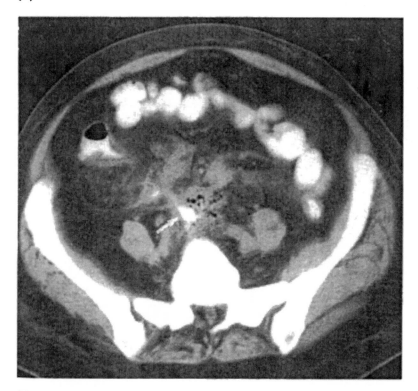

(E)
FIG. 11 (Continued)

extending into the fat of the mesentery, omentum, or ischiorectal fossa, whereas fistulas extend to other viscera or open through the skin. The morphology and anatomical sites of fistulas are protean: enteroenteric, enterocolic, enterovesical, enterovaginal, enterocutaneous, anorectal, duodenopancreatic, gastrocolic, colobronchial, and enterospinal (77–88).

The origin, anatomical course, and sites of communication of sinus tracts and fistulas should first be evaluated by conventional barium studies, excretory urography, cystography, and sinography. These studies may be limited because the origin of the fistula may be edematous and prevent contrast opacification. Additionally, tiny fistulous tracts may not be seen and anorectal fistula and sinus tracts are often painful and difficult to evaluate on barium studies.

If surgical or percutaneous intervention is planned for symptomatic fistulas, then cross-sectional imaging should be obtained to precisely define their anatomical relationships. This is particularly true for anorectal disease (Figs. 12 and 13).

V. EXTRAINTESTINAL COMPLICATIONS

Extraintestinal manifestations develop in one-fourth to one-third of patients with Crohn's disease (89–94). They can be divided into three categories: (a) those intimately related to disease activity or extent of disease and which are responsive to therapy directed at the bowel disease (i.e., arthritis, iritis); (b) those whose course is independent of underlying bowel disease (i.e., sclerosing cholangitis, ankylosing spondylitis); (c) those due to an inadequate or disordered intestinal function (i.e., cholelithiasis, nephrolithiasis).

A. Hepatobiliary Complications

The most frequent serious manifestations of extraintestinal Crohn's disease occur in the liver and the biliary tract. These complications generally do not correlate with disease activity, duration, or severity, except when there is fatty infiltration, which occurs in patients who tend to be more seriously ill, debilitated, and malnourished (95,96).

1. Hepatic Steatosis

Fatty liver is found on liver biopsy in 20% to 25% of patients with Crohn's disease and may be caused by fat malabsorption, hyperalimentation, sepsis, protein-losing enteropathy, malnutrition, or corticosteroids (97,98).

The imaging features of fatty liver depend on the amount of fat deposited, its distribution within the liver, and the presence of associated hepatic disease. Computed tomography is the best noninvasive technique for the detection of hepatic steatosis because there is an excellent correlation between hepatic parenchymal CT attenuation and the amount of hepatic triglyceride found in liver biopsy specimens. Increased hepatic fat decreases mean hepatic CT density which is best appreciated on noncontrast scans. The liver, which is normally more dense than the spleen, becomes less dense (darker) than the spleen. The hepatic and portal venous structures are also more clearly outlined. Fatty deposition is usually diffuse (Fig. 14A), however, involvement can be focal, lobar, segmental, or scattered in a bizarre pattern that rapidly appears and disappears (98).

Sonographically, the fatty liver is usually diffusely echogenic (see Fig. 14B), with the

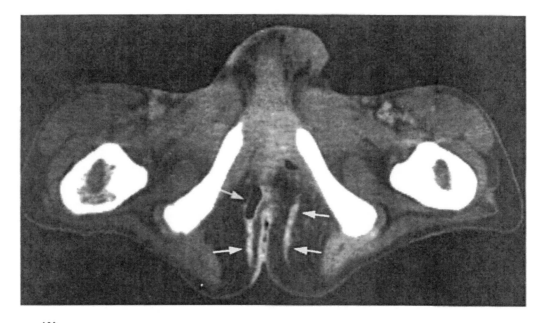

(A)

FIG. 12 Computed tomography evaluation of anorectal fistulas and sinus tracts. A, Bilateral perianal sinus tracts (*arrows*) are extending into the buttocks in this patient with long-standing Crohn's disease. B, C, Contrast was instilled through the skin wound of this different patient with perineal Crohn's disease. The fistula (*large arrow*) can be seen extending between the levator ani muscle (*small arrow*) and the rectum (*R*). IRF = left ischiorectal fossa.

degree of echogenicity being roughly proportional to the level of steatosis. The hepatic and portal venous systems are less well visualized as well. These sonographic changes tend to parallel biochemical and clinical dysfunction.

Despite the exquisite tissue characterization afforded by MR imaging, most of the commonly used imaging pulse sequences do not demonstrate fatty infiltration well.

2. Cholelithiasis

Approximately 30% to 50% of patients with Crohn's disease develop gallstones, especially those with extensive terminal ileal disease or after they have undergone ileal resection (95–99). These patients form lithogenic bile because of bile salt malabsorption or loss of the enterohepatic circulation. Ultrasound is the premier means of evaluating gallbladder disease, and there are three major sonographic criteria for establishing the diagnosis of cholelithiasis. A gallstone appears as an echogenic focus that casts an acoustic shadow and seeks gravitational dependence. Computed tomography demonstrates only 79% of gallstones depicted sonographically, because CT cannot discern stones that have the same radiographic attenuation as bile. Stones denser than bile are well seen as are those with rim or nidus calcification (98). Computed tomography is superior to ultrasound in the detection of choledocholithiasis, with endoscopic retrograde cholangiopancreatography (ERCP) being the "gold standard" for detection.

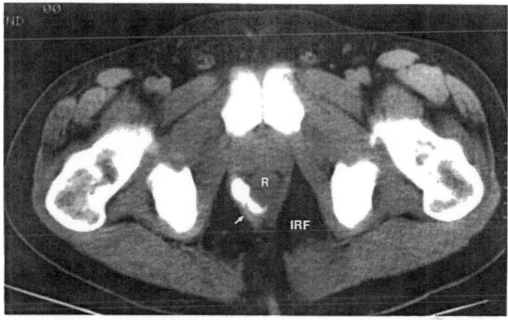

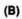

(B)

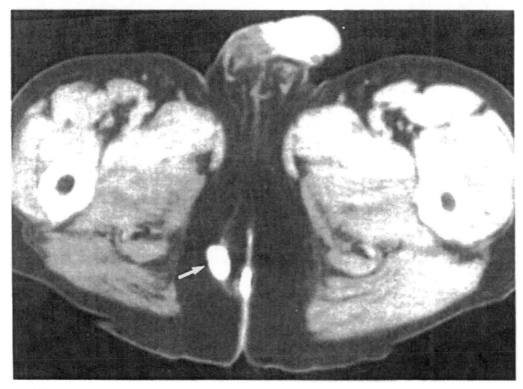

(C)

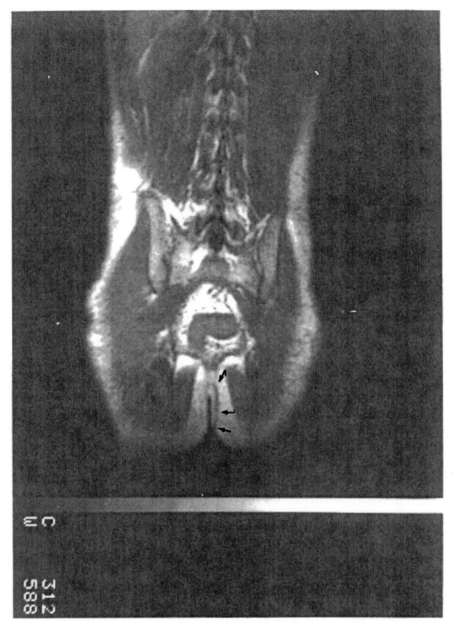

(A)
FIG. 13 Magnetic resonance evaluation of fistulas. A, Coronal T1-weighted image demonstrates intermediate signal intensity of a fistula (*arrows*) reaching the skin surface along the medial aspect of the left buttock. B, Axial T2-weighted image shows an area of increased signal intensity (*arrows*) in the infralevator region consistent with active inflammation of the fistulous tract. (Courtesy of Richard B. Rafal.)

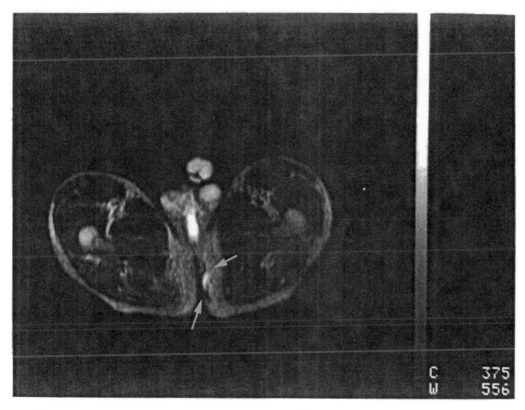

(B)

3. Primary Sclerosing Cholangitis

Primary sclerosing cholangitis occurs in fewer than 2% of patients with Crohn's disease; it is more commonly associated with ulcerative colitis (93,99). Ultrasound (Fig. 15) and CT (Fig. 16) can directly visualize the fibrous mural thickening of the larger bile ducts that characterize this disease. The thickening may be concentric or asymmetric and usually measures 2 to 5 mm. Other signs suggesting the diagnosis include focal duct dilatation, discrepancy between the size of the intrahepatic and extrahepatic bile ducts, focal clustering of intrahepatic ducts, and discontinuous areas of minimal intrahepatic biliary dilatation without associated hepatic, porta hepatis, or pancreatic masses. The cholangiographic signs of beading, pruning, and nodular mural thickening can also be seen on cross-sectional imaging, but usually with less detail and precision.

Ultrasound and CT offer three major advantages in evaluating patients with known or suspected sclerosing cholangitis (98,99). First, they are noninvasive techniques that are quite safe in these patients who often need multiple serial examination. Second, they can visualize the entire biliary tract in cases in which strictures obstruct the flow of contrast medium during cholangiography, occasionally leaving large portions of the intrahepatic ducts unexamined. Third, CT and ultrasound can depict complications of sclerosing

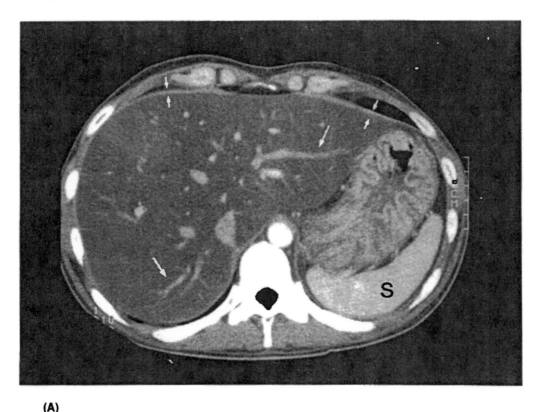

(A)
FIG. 14 Fatty infiltration of the liver. A, Note the low density of the liver in comparison with the spleen (S), permitting clear visualization of the portal branches (*large arrows*) and liver capsule (*small arrows*). Normally, the liver is denser than the spleen. B, Longitudinal sonogram shows a strikingly echogenic liver (*L*). Normally, at least 3 to 4 hepatic and portal venous structures should be visualized. None are seen in this case. The sound is so attenuated by the steatosis that the deep areas of the liver cannot be interrogated. K = right kidney.

cholangitis such as cirrhosis and portal hypertension, as well as soft-tissue masses associated with cholangiocarcinoma.

4. Liver Abscess

More than 30 cases of hepatic abscess (Fig. 17) complicating Crohn's disease have been reported. In one institution, they accounted for 8% of all liver abscesses (100). They most commonly develop in patients with long-standing disease but may occur as the initial manifestation of Crohn's disease. Steroids and other immunosuppressive agents, perforation, intra-abdominal abscess, and anastomic leaks are all predisposing factors to the development of a hepatic abscess in patients with Crohn's disease.

B. Pancreatic Complications

Approximately 1% to 2% of patients with Crohn's disease develop pancreatitis due to a variety of causes: (a) drugs such as steroids, azathioprine, metronidazole; (b) choledo-

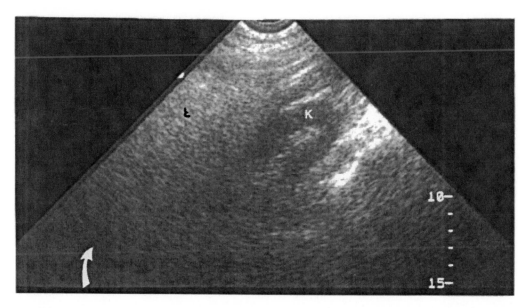

(B)

cholithiasis; (c) fistula from the adjacent gut; (d) sclerosing cholangitis; (e) dysfunction of the sphincter of Oddi or stenosis of the descending duodenum leading to obstruction of the duct or reflux of duodenal contents into the duct; (f) autoantibodies against pancreatic acinar cells (100–104). Regardless of the cause, cross-sectional imaging is needed to help confirm the diagnosis of pancreatitis and, more importantly, its complications.

Computed tomography is the premier imaging test for the diagnosis of pancreatitis (105). In milder forms of the disease, CT may show slight to moderate increase in pancreatic size. Alternatively, mild peripancreatic inflammation may be present around an otherwise normal-appearing gland. The entire gland may become diffusely enlarged with a shaggy irregular contour, and the parenchyma appears slightly heterogeneous in density. In more advanced cases (Fig. 18), fluid collections can be seen in the substance of the gland, anterior pararenal space, lesser sac, small bowel mesentery, and transverse mesocolon. In severe forms of pancreatitis, the gland becomes massively enlarged and heterogeneous. The peripancreatic inflammation, fluid, phlegmon, and abscess that complicate pancreatitis are superbly depicted on CT. Computed tomography can also help stage these lesions, suggest prognosis, and guide percutaneous drainage of fluid collections (105).

C. Urinary Tract Complications

1. Nephrolithiasis

Between 2% and 10% of patients with Crohn's disease develop nephrolithiasis due to water and electrolyte losses in diarrhea, malabsorption, and large ileostomy output (106). Oxalate stones are most common and, because they are not calcified, may not be visible with conventional radiological techniques. Noncontrast CT scans and, to a lesser degree, ultrasound detect these stone more readily.

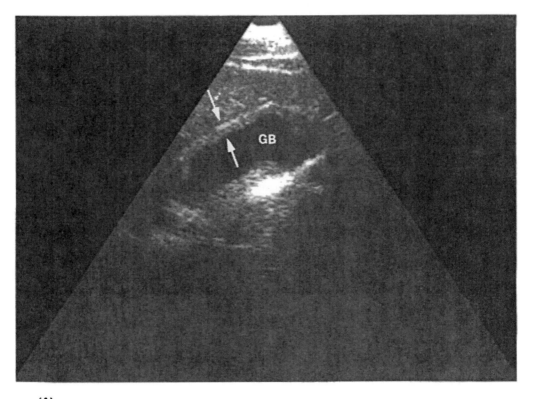

(A)
FIG. 15 Sclerosing cholangitis associated with Crohn's disease: ultrasound findings. A, Mural thickening (*arrows*) of the gallbladder (*GB*) is identified in this patient with Crohn's disease. B, The wall of the common hepatic duct is also thickened (*straight arrows*). Curved arrow = narrowed lumen of common hepatic duct; V = portal vein. C, Endoscopic retrograde cholangiography shows irregularly narrowed intrahepatic branches casued by sclerosing cholangitis.

2. Hydronephrosis

Hydronephrosis may develop in patients with Crohn's disease for a variety of reasons including calculous disease or obstruction caused by the inflammatory effect of an abscess or phlegmon or the mass effect of creeping fat of the mesentery. Computed tomography is useful in detecting both the hydronephrosis and the obstructing mass (106).

3. Fistulas

Fistulas may develop between diseased gut and the kidney in patients with Crohn's disease, leading to a renal or perinephric abscess. More commonly, enterovesical fistulas develop. These fistulas should first be evaluated with conventional barium studies, excretory urography, and cystography, but the origin of the fistula may be edematous, which may prevent contrast opacification, and tiny fistulous tracts may not be seen. Indeed, conventional studies detect fewer than 50% of enterovesical fistulas; CT has a nearly 90% success rate (87). Computed tomography scans are initially obtained with only oral and rectal contrast administration (84). The presence of gas and small amounts of contrast entering through the fistula may be obscured if the bladder is opacified following the intravenous injection of iodinated contrast medium.

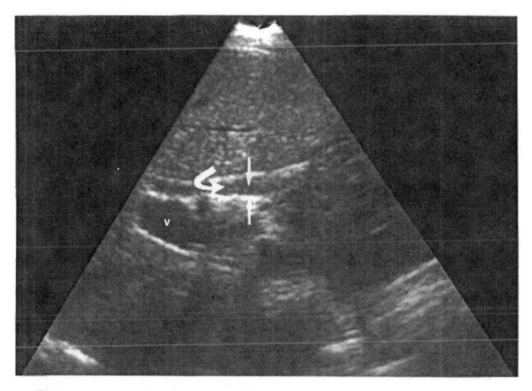

(B)

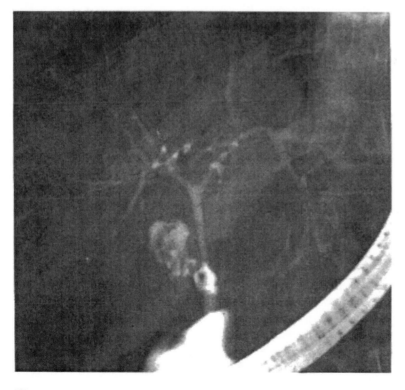

(C)

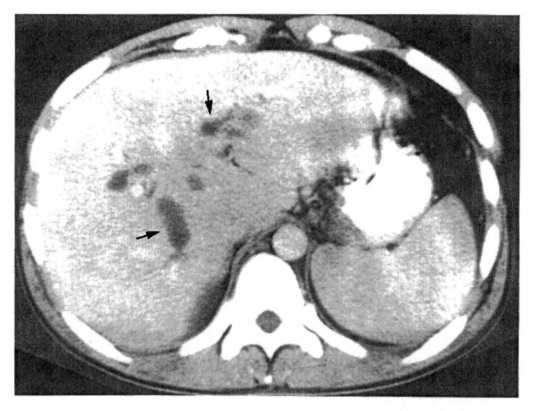

FIG. 16 Sclerosing cholangitis: CT findings. Focally dilated segments (*arrows*) of the intrahepatic biliary system are seen, whereas the narrowed more central ducts are not visible.

D. Musculoskeletal Complications

1. Arthropathy

Arthritis is one of the most common extraintestinal manifestations of Crohn's disease, and it is manifested as a peripheral arthritis and/or sacroiliitis-spondylitis (107–111). The radiological findings of peripheral enteropathic arthritis are usually minimal and are best seen, if at all, with conventional radiographs. The changes in the axial skeleton (affecting 3% to 16% of patients with Crohn's disease) are similar to ankylosing spondylitis (107). Computed tomography and MR imaging can often detect the subtle changes of early sacroiliitis (bilateral, usually symmetrical joint narrowing with osseous erosions followed by sclerosis, more pronounced on the iliac side of the articulation) before they become apparent on plain films. Eventually, bony ankylosis occurs.

2. Avascular Necrosis

Osteonecrosis has been reported as a rare complication in patients with inflammatory bowel disease in the following clinical settings: during or after corticosteroid therapy; during total parenteral nutrition, especially with lipid emulsions; and, most recently, as a direct complication of the disease without other precipitating factors (112,113).

Magnetic resonance imaging is the best imaging technique for establishing this diagnosis, with a reported sensitivity of 97% and a specificity of 98%. On T1-weighted

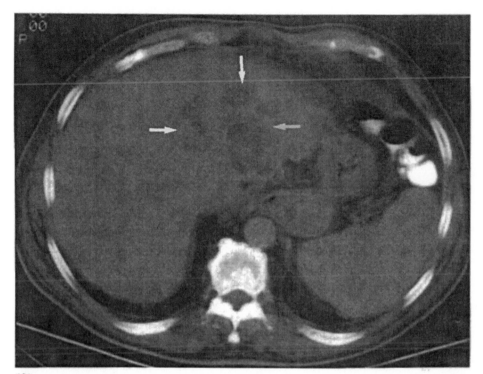

(A)

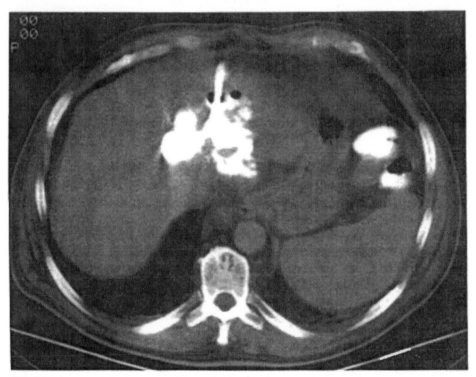

(B)

FIG. 17 Liver abscess associated with Crohn's disease. A, Noncontrast CT scan shows a multi-located, low-density mass in the left lobe of the liver (*arrows*). B, This abscess, in which all the locules communicated, was percutaneously drained.

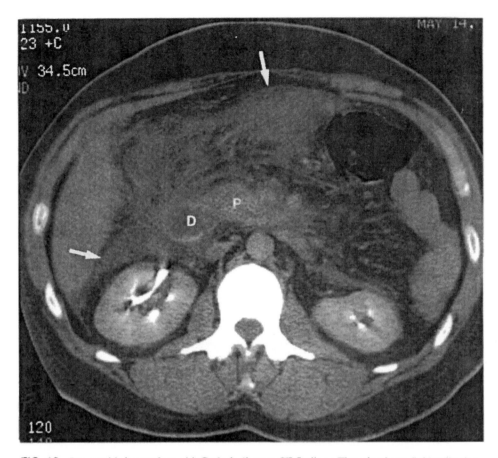

FIG. 18 Pancreatitis in a patient with Crohn's disease: CT findings. There is a large fluid collection with mesenteric changes due to phlegmon in the anterior pararenal space and transverse mesocolon (*arrows*). P = uncinate process of pancreas; D = descending duodenum.

images, areas of low signal intensity may be seen beneath the articular surface. Alternatively, a band or bands of low signal intensity are seen surrounding a central area of higher signal intensity. On T2-weighted images, areas of low signal intensity can become bright, and regions of high signal intensity remain high.

Asymptomatic and radiologically normal hips may have early signs of avascular necrosis on CT studies. These include subtle alterations in trabecular pattern, joint space integrity, femoral head contour, and acetabulum, which may be undetected or poorly defined on plain films.

3. Osteomyelitis-Septic Arthirits

Septic arthritis of the hip can complicate a psoas abscess or a retroperitoneal abscess tracking through the greater sciatic notch. Magnetic resonance imaging and CT may show these changes before they are recognizable on plain films.

The iliac bone and sacrum are the most frequent sites of osteomyelitis in patients with Crohn's disease (114–116). They are almost invariably the result of an adjacent pelvic abscess or enteric fistula (Fig. 19). Accordingly, osteomyelitis is usually diagnosed on

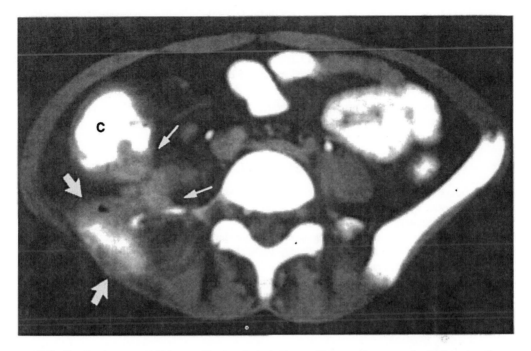

FIG. 19 Pelvic osteomyelitis complicating Crohn's disease. Computed tomography thickened wall of the cecum (*C*) with adjacent soft-tissue swelling (*small arrows*) due to Crohn's disease. An associated fistula penetrates deep into the right iliac fossa, causing osteomyelitis and partial destruction of right iliac bone (*large arrows*).

cross-sectional imaging when the abscess is identified. Computed tomography findings in osteomyelitis include cortical bone destruction, intraosseous gas, increase attenuation of the bone marrow, narrowing of the medullary cavity, serpentine drainage tracts, and the presence of an involucrum or sequestrum. On MR imaging, the marrow space of the involved bone demonstrates decreased signal on T1-weighted images and increased signal on T2-weighted images. Cortical destruction or thickening and edema or abscess formation in the soft tissues can also be demonstrated on MR imaging.

Spinal epidural abscess has been reported from fistulization of a presacral or psoas abscess in patients with Crohn's disease (86). Indeed, prevertebral, intraforaminal, and epidural gas may be seen on CT and MR imaging studies (82,84).

4. Psoas Abscess

Crohn's disease complications account for 73% of all psoas abscesses (65–69). On the right, a psoas abscess may develop secondary to terminal ileal disease (see Fig. 7C); on the left, it can result from sigmoid or jejunal involvement. Most patients with psoas abscess have well-established Crohn's disease but the clinical manifestations may be nonspecific. Occasionally, psoas abscess may be seen at the initial presentation of disease. Computed tomography has emerged as the best means of examination for its diagnosis. Computed tomography can also direct percutaneous abscess drainage in these patients (65–69,71).

Primary rectus sheath abscesses have also been reported as a complication of Crohn's disease and may be visualized on CT, MR imaging, or ultrasound (70).

VI. CONCLUSION

Computed tomography, ultrasound, and MR imaging are useful in evaluating the mural and extraintestinal manifestations of Crohn's disease. Although barium studies have been and remain the primary radiographical means of detecting inflammatory bowel disease, the cross-sectional imaging modalities can play a critical role in detecting abscesses, in differentiating various causes of mesenteric abnormalities, and in discovering extraintestinal complications that commonly afflict patients with inflammatory bowel disease.

REFERENCES

1. Gore RM, Laufer I. Ulcerative and granulomatous colitis: idiopathic inflammatory bowel disease. In: Gore RM, Levine MS, Laufer I, eds. Textbook of Gastrointestinal Radiology. Philadelphia: WB Saunders, 1994:1098–1141.

2. Gore RM. Cross-sectional imaging of the colon. In: Gore RM, Levine MS, Laufer I, eds. Textbook of Gastrointestinal Radiology. Philadelphia: WB Saunders, 1994:1051–1063.

3. Vecchioli A, De Franco A, Maresca G, Gore RM. Cross-sectional imaging of the small bowel. In: Gore RM, Levine MS, Laufer I, eds. Textbook of Gastrointestinal Radiology. Philadelphia: WB Saunders, 1994:789–801.

4. Bozkurt T, Richter F, Lux G. Ultrasonography as a primary diagnostic tool in patients with inflammatory disease and tumors of the small intestine and large bowel. J Clin Ultrasound 1994; 22:85–91.

5. Limberg B. Diagnosis of inflammatory and neoplastic large bowel diseases by conventional abdominal and colonic sonography. Ultrasound Q 1988; 6:151–156.

6. Robbins PA. Ultrasound demonstration of bowel wall thickness in inflammatory bowel disease. Clin Radiol 1984; 35:227–231.

7. Pera A, Cammarota T, Comino E, et al. Ultrasonogrpahy in the detection of Crohn's disease and in the differential diagnosis of inflammatory bowel disease. Digestion 1988; 4:180–189.

8. Limberg B. Diagnosis of inflammatory and neoplastic colonic disease by sonography. J Clin Gastroenterol 1987; 9:607–611.

9. Pedersen BH, Gronvall S, Dorph S, et al. The value of dynamic ultrasound scanning in Crohn's disease. Scan J Gastroeneterol 1986; 21:969–974.

10. Sheridan MB, Nicholson DA, Martin DF. Transabdominal ultrasonography as the primary investigation in patients with suspected Crohn's disease or recurrence: a prospective study. Clin Radiol 1993; 48:402–404.

11. Sonnenberg A, Erckenbrecht J, Peter P, et al. Detection of Crohn's disease by ultrasound. Gastroenterology 1982; 83:430–434.

12. Worlicek H, Lutz H, Heyder N, et al. Ultrasound findings in Crohn's disease and ulcerative colitis: a prospective study. J Clin Ultrasound 1987; 153:153–163.

13. Kimmey MB, Wang KY, Haggitt RC, et al. Diagnosis of inflammatory bowel disease with ultrasound. Invest Radiol 1990; 25:1085–1090.

14. Kaftori JK, Pery M, Kleinhaus U. Ultrasonography in Crohn's disease. Gastrointest Radiol 1984; 9:137–142.

15. Schwerk WB, Beckh K, Raith M, et al. A prospective evaluation of high resolution sonography in the differential diagnosis of inflammatory bowel disease. Eur J Gastroenterol Hepatol 1992; 4:173–182.

16. Dubbins PA. Ultrasound demonstration of bowel wall thickness in inflammatory bowel disease. Clin Radiol 1984; 35:227–331.

17. Holt S, Samuel E. Gray scale ultrasound in Crohn's disease. Gut 1979; 20:590–595.

18. Yeh HC, Rabinowitz JG. Granulomatous enterocolitis: findings by ultrasonography and computed tomography. Radiology 1983; 149:253–259.

19. Wellmann Von W, Gebel M, Freise J, Grote R. Sonographic in der Diagnostik der Ileitis Terminalis Crohn. Forschr Röntgenstr 1980; 133:146–148.

20. DiCandio G, Mosca F, Campatella A, et al. Sonographic detection of postsurgical recurrence of Crohn's disease. AJR Am J Roentgenol 1986; 146:523–526.

21. Limberg B, Osswald B. Diagnosis and differential diagnosis of ulcerative colitis and Crohn's disease by hydrocolonic sonography. Am J Gastroenterol 1994; 89:1051–1057.

22. Limberg B. Diagnosis of acute ulcerative colitis and colonic Crohn's disease by colonic sonography. J Clin Ultrasound 1989; 17:25–31.

23. Limberg B. Sonographic features of colonic Crohn's disease: comparison of in vivo and in vitro studies. J Clin Ultrasound 1990; 18:161–166.

24. St. Ville EW, Jafri SZH, Madrazo BL, et al. Endorectal sonography in the evaluation of rectal and perirectal disease. AJR Am J Roentgenol 1991; 157:503–508.

25. Tio TL, Weijers O, Hulsman F, et al. Endosonography of colorectal disease. Endoscopy 1992; 24:309–314.

26. Tio TL, Mulder CJJ, Wijers OB, et al. Endosonography of peri-anal and peri-colorectal fistula and/or abscess in Crohn's disease. Gastrointest Endosc 1990; 36:331–336.

27. Van Outryve MJ, Pelckmans PA, Michielsen PP, Van Maercke YM. Value of transrectal ultrasonography in Crohn's disease. Gastroenterology 1991; 101:1171–1177.

28. Kimmey MB, Martin RW, Haggitt RC, et al. Histologic correlates of gastrointestinal ultrasound images. Gastroenterology 1989; 96:433–441.

29. Lim JH, Ko YT, Lee DH, et al. Sonography of inflammatory bowel disease: findings and value in differential diagnosis. AJR Am J Roentgenol 1994; 163:343–347.

30. Adams LS, Peltekian KM, Mitchell MJ. Detection of Crohn's ileitis by endovaginal ultrasonography. Abdom Imaging 1994; 19:400–402.

31. Hata J, Haruma K, Yamanaka H, et al. Ultrasonographic evaluation of the bowel wall in inflammatory bowel disease: comparison of in vivo and in vitro studies. Abdom Imaging 1994; 19:395–399.

32. Hata J, Haruma K, Suenaga K, et al. Ultrasonographic assessment of inflammatory bowel disease. Am J Gastroenterol 1992; 87:443–447.

33. Smelka RC, Shoenut JP, Silverman R, et al. Bowel disease: prospective comparison of CT and 1.5T pre- and post-contrast MRI imaging with T1-weighted fat-suppressed and breath-hold FLASH sequences. JMRI 1991; 1:625–632.

34. Shoenut JP, Semelka RC, Silverman R, et al. Magnetic resonance imaging in inflammatory bowel disease. J Clin Gastroenterol 1993; 17:73–78.

35. Shoenut JP, Semelka RC, Silverman R, et al. MRI in the diagnosis of Crohn's disease in pregnant women. J Clin Gastroenterol 1993; 17:244–247.

36. Pels Rijcken TH, Davis MA, Ros PR. Intraluminal contrast agents for MR imaging of the abdomen and pelvis. JMRI 1994; 4:291–300.

37. Anderson CM, Brown JJ, Balfe DM, et al. MR imaging of Crohn disease: use of perflubron as a contrast agent. JMRI 1994; 4:491–496.

38. Giovagnoni A, Misericordia M, Terilli F, et al. MR imaging of ulcerative colitis. Abdom Imaging 1993; 18:371–375.

39. Outwater E, Schiebler ML. Pelvic fistulas: findings on MR images. AJR Am J Roentgenol 1993; 160:327–330.

40. Koelbel G, Schmiedl U, Majer MC, et al. Diagnosis of fistulae and sinus tracts in patients with Crohn disease: value of MR imaging. AJR Am J Roentgenol 1989; 152:999–1003.

41. Van Beers H, Grandin C, Kartheuser A, et al. MRI of complicated anal fistulae: comparison with digital examination. J Comput Assist Tomogr 1994; 18:87–90.

42. Myhr GE, Myrvold HE, Nilsen G, et al. Perianal fistulas: use of MR imaging for diagnosis. Radiology 1994; 191:545–549.

43. Gore RM. CT of inflammatory bowel disease. Radiol Clin North Am 1989; 27:717–730.

44. Goldberg HI, Gore RM, Margulis AR, et al. Computed tomography in the evaluation of Crohn disease. AJR Am J Roentgenol 1983; 140:277–282.

45. Jabra AA, Fishman EK, Taylor GA. CT findings of inflammatory bowel disease in children. AJR Am J Roentgenol 1994; 162:975–979.

46. Klein VHM, Wein B, Adam G, et al. Computed tomography of Crohn's disease and ulcerative colitis. Fortschr Röntgenstr 1995; 163:9–15.

47. Gore RM, Cohen MI, Vogelzang RL, et al. Value of computed tomography in the detection of complication of Crohn's disease. Dig Dis Sci 1985; 30:701–709.

48. Gore RM, Goldberg HI. Computed tomographic evaluation of the gastrointestinal tract in diseases other than primary adenocarcinoma. Radiol Clin North Am 1982; 20:781–798.

49. Gore RM. Cross-sectional imaging of inflammatory bowel disease. Radiol Clin North Am 1987; 25:115–133.

50. Gore RM, Marn CS, Kirby DF, et al. CT findings in ulcerative, granulomatous, and indeterminate colitis. AJR Am J Roentgenol 1983; 143:279–284.

51. Fishman EK, Wolf EJ, Jones B, et al. CT evaluation of Crohn's disease: effect on patient management. AJR Am J Roentgenol 1987; 148:537–540.

52. Philpotts LE, Heiken JP, Westcott MA, Gore RM. Colitis: use of CT findings in differential diagnosis. Radiology 1994; 190:445–449.

53. Geller SA. Pathology of inflammatory bowel disease: a critical appraisal in diagnosis and management. In: Targan SR, Shanahan F, eds. Inflammatory Bowel Disease: From Bench to Bedside. Baltimore: Williams & Wilkins, 1994:336–351.

54. Simpkins KC, Gore RM. Multiorgan involvement in Crohn's disease. In: Gore RM, Levine MS, Laufer I, eds. Textbook of Gastrointestinal Radiology. Philadelphia: WB Saunders, 1994:2660–2681.

55. Jones B, Fishman EK, Hamilton SR, et al. Submucosal accumulation of fat in inflammatory bowel disease: CT/pathologic correlation. J Comput Assist Tomogr 1986; 10:759–763.

56. Keighley MRB, Eastwood D, Ambrose NS, et al. Incidence and microbiology of abdominal and pelvic abscess in Crohn's disease. Gastroenterology 1982; 83:1271–1275.

57. Hyde C, Gerzof SG. Abdominal abscess. In: Gore RM, Levine MS, Laufer I, eds. Textbook of Gastrointestinal Radiology. Philadelphia: WB Saunders, 1994:1553–1569.

58. Rolandelli RH. Surgical Treatment of Crohns' Disease: From Bench to Bedside. Baltimore: Williams & Wilkins, 1994:582–609.

59. Fukuya T, Hawes DR, Lu CC, et al. CT of abdominal abscess with fistulous communication to the gastrointestinal tract. J Comput Assist Tomogr 1991; 15:445–449.

60. Gore RM, Ghahremani GG. Radiologic investigation of acute inflammatory bowel disease. Gastroenterol Clin North Am 1995; 24:353–384.

61. Orel SG, Rubesin SE, Jones B, et al. Computed tomography vs. barium studies in the acutely symptomatic patient with Crohn disease. J Comput Assist Tomogr 1987; 11:1009–1016.

62. Jabra AA, Fishman EK, Taylor GA. Crohn disease in the pediatric patient: CT evaluation. Radiology 1991; 179:495–498.

63. Guillaumin E, Jeffrey RB, Shea WJ, et al. Perirectal inflammatory disease: CT findings. Radiology 1986; 161:153–157.

64. Yousem DM, Fishman EK, Jones B. Crohn's disease: perirectal and perianal findings at CT. Radiology 1988; 167:331–334.

65. Lev S-Y, Leonard MB, Baert RW, Dozois RR. Psoas abscess: changing patterns of diagnosis and etiology. Dis Colon Rectum 1986; 29:694–698.

66. Procaccino JA, Lavery IC, Fazio VW. Psoas abscess: difficulties encountered. Dis Colon Rectum 1991; 34:784–789.

67. Gray RR, St. Louis EL, Grosman H, Newman H. Ilio-psoas abscess in Crohn's disease. J Can Assoc Radiol 1983; 34:36–38.

68. Ricci MA, Meyer KK. Psoas abscess complicating Crohn's disease. Am J Gastroenterol 1985; 80:970–977.
69. Agha FP, Woolsey EJ, Amendola MA. Psoas abscess in IBD. Am J Gastroenterol 1985; 80:924–928.
70. Sung W-C, McKinley MJ, Harvey LP. Rectus sheath abscess in Crohn's disease. Am J Gastroeneterol 1993; 88:793–794.
71. Lamport RD, Cheskin LJ, Moscatello SA, Nikoomanesh P. Sterile epidural and bilateral psoas abscesses in a patient with Crohn's disease. Am J Gastroeneterol 1994; 89:1086–1087.
72. Mir-Madjless SD, McHenry MC, Farmer RG. Liver abscess in Crohn's disease. Gastroenterology 1986; 91:987–993.
73. Vakil N, Hayne G, Sharma A, et al. Liver abscess in Crohn's disease. Am J Gastroenterol 1994; 89:1090–1095.
74. Casola G, vanSonnenberg E, Neff CC, et al. Abscess in Crohn's disease: percutaneous drainage. Radiology 1987; 163:19–22.
75. Safrit HD, Mauro MA, Jaques PF. Percutaneous abscess drainage in Crohn's disease. AJR Am J Roentgenol 1987; 148:859–862.
76. Milward SF, Ramsewak W, Fitzsimons P, et al. Percutaneous drainage of iliopsoas abscess in Crohn's disease. Gastrointest Radiol 1986; 11:289–290.
77. Cohen JL, Stricker JW, Shoetz DJ, et al. Rectovaginal fistula in Crohn's disease. Dis Colon Rectum 30 1989; 32:492–496.
78. Michelassi F, Stella M, Balestracci T, et al. Incidence, diagnosis and treatment of enteric and colorectal fistulae in patients with Crohn's disease. Ann Surg 1993; 218:660–666.
79. Pichney LS, Fantry GT, Graham SM. Gastrocolic and duodenocolic fistulas in Crohn's disease. J Clin Gastroenterol 1992; 15:205–211.
80. Ajzen SA, Gibney RG, Cooperberg PL, et al. Enterovenous fistula: unusual complication of Crohn's disease. Radiology 1988; 106:745–746.
81. Flueckiger F, Kullnig P, Melzer G, Posch E. Colobronchial and gastrocolic fistulas: rare complication of Crohn's disease. Gastrointest Radiol 1990; 15:288–290.
82. West D, Russell TR, Brotman M. Rectal epidural fistula complicating Crohn's entercolitis. Dis Colon Rectum 1983; 26:622–624.
83. Richtermann RL, Caroline DF, Friedman AC, et al. Enterobronchial fistula. Gastrointest Radiol 1987; 12:194–196.
84. Pontari MA, McMillen MA, Garvey RH, Ballantyne GH. Diagnosis and treatment of enterovesical fistulae. Am Surg 1992; 58:258–263.
85. Jakobson IM, Schapiro RH, Warshaw AL. Gastric and duodenal fistulas in Crohn's disease. Gastroenterology 1985; 89:1347–1352.
86. Piontek M, Hengels K-J, Hefter H, et al. Spinal abscess and bacterial meningitis in Crohn's disease. Dig Dis Sci 1992; 37:1131–1135.
87. Merine D, Fishman EK, Kuhlman JE, et al. Bladder involvement in Crohn disease: role of CT in detection and evaluation. J Comput Assist Tomogr 1989; 13:90–93.
88. Koelbel G, Schmiedl V, Major MC, et al. Diagnosis of fistulae and sinus tracts in patients with Crohn's disease: value of MR imaging. AJR Am J Roentgenol 1985; 144:1229–1233.
89. Lichtman SN, Sartor RB. Extraintestinal manifestations of inflammatory bowel disease: clinical aspects and natural history. In: Targan SR, Shanahan F, eds. Inflammatory Bowel Disease: From Bench to Bedside. Baltimore: Williams & Wilkins, 1994:317–335.
90. Levine DS. Clinical features and complications of Crohn's disease. In: Targan SR, Shanahan F, eds. Inflammatory Bowel Disease: From Bench to Bedside. Baltimore: Williams & Wilkins, 1994:296–316.
91. Farmer RG, Hawk W, Turnbull RB. Clinical patterns in Crohn's disease: a statistical study of 615 cases. Gastroenterology 1975; 68:627–635.

92. Danzi JT. Extraintestinal manifestations of idiopathic inflammatory bowel disease. Arch Intern Med 1988; 148:297–302.

93. Greenstein AJ, Janowitz HD, Sachar DV. The extraintestinal complications of Crohn's disease and ulcerative colitis: a study of 700 patients. Medicine 1976; 55:401–412.

94. Rankin GB, Watts HD, Melnyk CS, Kelley ML. National cooperative Crohn's disease study: extraintestinal manifestations and perianal complications. Gastroenterology 1979; 77:914–920.

95. Vierling JM. Hepatobiliary diseases in patients with inflammatory bowel disease. In: Targan SR, Shanahan F, eds. Inflammatory Bowel Disease: From Bench to Bedside. Baltimore: Williams & Wilkins, 1994:654–667.

96. Wewer V, Gluud C, Schlichting P, et al. Prevalence of hepatobiliary dysfunction in a regional group of patients with chronic inflammatory bowel disease. Scand J Gastroenterol 1991; 26:97–102.

97. Schrumpf E, Fausa O, Elgjo K, Kolmannskog F. Hepatobiliary complications of inflammatory bowel disease. Semin Liver Dis 1988; 8:201–209.

98. Williams SM, Harned RK. Hepatobiliary complications of inflammatory bowel disease. Radiol Clin North Am 1987; 25:175–188.

99. MacCarty RL. Noncalculous inflammatory disorders of the biliary tract. In: Gore RM, Levine MS, Laufer I, eds. Textbook of Gastrointestinal Radiology. Philadelphia: WB Saunders, 1994:1727–1745.

100. Vakil N, Hayne G, Sharma A, et al. Liver abscess in Crohn's disease. Am J Gastroenterol 1994; 89:1090–1094.

101. Weber P, Seibold F, Jenss H. Acute pancreatitis in Crohn's disease. J Clin Gastroenterol 1993; 17:286–291.

102. Eisner TD, Goldman IS, McKinley MJ. Crohn's disease and pancreatitis. Am J Gastroenterol 1993; 88:583–586.

103. Spiess SE, Braun M, Vogelzang RL, Craig RM. Crohn's disease of the duodenum complicated by pancreatitis and common bile duct obstruction. Am J Gastroenterol 1992; 87:1033–1036.

104. Matsumoto T, Matsui T, Iida Y, et al. Acute pancreatitis as a complication of Crohn's disease. Am J Gastroenterol 1989; 84:804–807.

105. Balthazar EJ. Pancreatitis. In: Gore RM, Levine MS, Laufer I, eds. Textbook of Gastrointestinal Radiology. Philadelphia: WB Saunders, 1994:2132–2160.

106. Banner MP. Genitourinary complications of inflammatory bowel disease. Radiol Clin North Am 1987; 25:199–204.

107. Levine JB. Arthropathies and ocular complications of inflammatory bowel disease. In: Targan SR, Shanahan F, eds. Inflammatory Bowel Disease: Bench to Bedside. Baltimore: Williams & Wilkins, 1994:668–681.

108. Schorr-Lesnick B, Brandt LJ. Selected rheumatologic and dermatologic manifestations of inflammatory bowel disease. Am J Gastroenterol 1988; 83:216–223.

109. Björkengren AG, Resnick D, Sartoris DJ. Enteropathic arthropathies. Radiol Clin N Am 1987; 25:189–198.

110. Münch H, Purrmann J, Reis HE, et al. Clinical features of inflammatory joint and spine manifestations in Crohn's disease. Hepatogastroenterology 1986; 33:123–127.

111. Gravallese EM, Kantrowitz FG. Arthritic manifestations of inflammatory bowel disease. Am J Gastroenterol 1988; 83:703–709.

112. Vakil N, Sparberg M. Steroid-related osteonecrosis in inflammatory bowel disease. Gastroenterology 1989; 96:62–67.

113. Freeman HJ, Kwan WCP. Brief report: non–corticosteroid-associated osteonecrosis of the femoral heads in two patients with inflammatory bowel disease. N Engl J Med 1993; 1314–1316.

114. Schwartz CM, Demos TC, Wehner JM. Osteomyelitis of the sacrum as the initial manifestation of Crohn's disease. Clin Orthop 1987; 222:181–185.
115. Ghahremani GG. Osteomyelitis of the ilium in patients with Crohn's disease. AJR Am J Roentgenol 1973; 118:364–370.
116. Miller LK, Miller JW. Pelvic osteomyelitis complicating Crohn's disease: diagnosis by computed tomography. Am J Gastroenterol 1987; 82:371–372.

COMMENTARY

Daniel Maklansky *Mount Sinai School of Medicine and Mount Sinai Hospital, New York, New York*

The authors in their excellent text and superb illustrations have detailed the merits and deficiencies of the imaging modalities available for the evaluation of Crohn's disease. The ability of cross-sectional imaging to visualize primary mural disease, mesenteric complications, and, significantly, extraintestinal complications, including hepatobiliary, pancreatic, urinary tract, and musculoskeletal complications, is lucidly presented by the authors.

I agree with the authors that the initial evaluation of patients with known or suspected Crohn's disease should be with gastrointestinal barium studies and/or fiberoptic endoscopy. My colleagues and I have shared the same office as Burrill Crohn, Richard Marshak, and Henry Janowitz and, therefore, have had the opportunity to examine more than 8000 cases of gastrointestinal Crohn's disease. It has been our experience that, in the absence of surgery, there is rarely linear extension of involvement. The apparent discrepancies to this dictum are usually resolved by review of the prior or initial studies that reveal that segments of minimal involvement were initially overlooked. Once the diagnosis is established, subsequent follow-up barium studies demonstrate the progression of the initial inflammatory phase to eventual fibrosis and stricture in some patients, or the sequelae of progressive ulceration, sinus tracts, and fistula formation in others. In the overwhelming majority of cases, the initial diagnosis of small bowel disease is not difficult for the experienced radiologist familiar with the roentgenographic findings of inflammatory bowel disease. Indeed, we have found that, most frequently, there is already extensive involvement of the small intestine at the time of the initial presentation to the radiologist.

In a few patients, the degree of small bowel disease may be extensive enough to cause confusion at differential diagnosis. In these cases, cross-sectional imaging, especially by CT scan, is essential in distinguishing Crohn's disease of the small bowel from carcinoid, retractile mesenteritis, lymphoma, or metastatic disease to the small bowel. In many of these instances, the characteristic presentation of transmural, extraenteric, mesenteric, or lymph node involvement is best demonstrated by CT which may obviate more invasive procedures including laparotomy.

Furthermore, in clinical follow-up and in the evaluation of possible complications, cross-sectional imaging is superior to the gastrointestinal barium study (whether dedicated follow through or enteroclysis) in the accurate depiction of the type and extent of complication. Specifically, the exact nature of mesenteric disease is best evaluated by cross-sectional imaging whereas involvement of the mesentery can only be inferred on the barium study as "separation" of the loops or a "soft-tissue mass." Further analysis of loop separation, including the differentiation of mural thickening from fatty proliferation, phlegmon, or an actual abscess, is best accomplished by CT scan as is shown by the authors. Additionally, the linear extent of mural disease can be further delineated by cross-sectional imaging. Hepatobiliary, pancreatic, urinary tract, and musculoskeletal extraintestinal complications are beyond the scope of the barium study.

However, there is another entity for which barium studies are more effective. The incidence of small bowel cancer in Crohn's disease of long duration is 6 to 7 times more than the expected rate of specific cancer in standard populations. The lesion is mucosal in origin, usually unincentric, and thereby can be more easily diagnosed by a careful barium study, either using enteroclysis or dedicated follow through.

Overall, the authors provide the clinician with a valuable guide to the often perplexing question of the nature and extent of IBD once the mucosa is penetrated, at which juncture the value of the barium study is diminished.

9
Proposed Measures of Disease Activity: How Useful Are They?

Cosimo Prantera and Anna Kohn *Ospedale Nuovo Regina Margherita, Rome, Italy*

I. ACTIVITY INDICES

Assessing health status, evaluating response to treatment, and determining prognosis and timing of surgery are the essence of clinical medicine in the treatment of patients with Crohn's disease—a process whose subjectivity is influenced by the degree of competence of the physician as well as by the patient's state of mind. The consequent need to make clinical judgment more objective has, therefore, raised the interest of many researchers.

The difficulty of clinically assessing Crohn's disease is well known to every gastroenterologist. Unlike ulcerative colitis, Crohn's disease, for the most part, occurs outside direct vision, and there is often a discrepancy between clinical manifestations and pathological abnormalities. During the 1970s, when clinical trials in the field of Crohn's disease were first initiated, researchers were faced with the need to construct a mathematical model (a) that could easily be used by researchers in different clinical centers, (b) whose numerical values would reproduce the clinical assessment of the various researchers, and (c) that would allow for an evaluation of response to ongoing therapy. Because of the complexity of Crohn's disease, treatment has principally been directed toward combatting symptoms, and, because the symptoms are connected with the phases of activity, the mathematical models were initially "indices of clinical activity" (Table 1).

A. Before the Crohn's Disease Activity Index

The earliest scoring systems devised to rate disease as mild, moderate, or severe included subjective complaints, physical signs, and simple laboratory tests. In 1974, using Truelove's three-category scale for ulcerative colitis, De Dombal et al. devised a comparable classification for Crohn's disease (1). The severity of attack was classified as mild, moderate, or severe according to a system that encompassed such factors as bowel habit, rectal bleeding, abdominal pain, pulse rate, temperature, hemoglobin level, and weight. In 1971, a numerical scoring system was used by Willoughby et al. in an early trial of azathioprine in Crohn's disease and, in 1976, by Talstad and Gjone in a study of disease activity in ulcerative colitis and Crohn's disease (2,3). Willoughby et al. graded a number of clinical features from 0 to 3 and considered simple laboratory findings (hemoglobin

TABLE 1 Clinical and Laboratory Variables in Crohn's Activity Indices Validated Against Physicians' Assessment of Crohn's Disease Activity Index

Features	CDAI[a] (4)	Harvey Bradshaw score[b] (8)	van Hees Index[a] (12)	NCDAI[a] (15)	IOIBD Index[a] (10)	Sandler score[b] (9)	LCDAI[b] (16)
Sex			×				
Pain	×	×			×	×	
Bowel habits	×	×	×	×	×	×	
General well-being	×	×				×	
Abdominal mass	×	×	×		×		
Abdominal tenderness					×		
Perianal disease	×				×		
Fistula	×			×	×		
Other complications	×	×	×		×		
Previous resection			×				
Lomotil or opiates	×						
Temperature	×		×	×	×		
Body weight	×		×		×		
Hemoglobin/Hct	×				×		
Erythrocyte sedimentation rate			×				×
Albumin			×				
C-reactive protein				×			×
Alpha-1-glycoprotein				×			×
Serum iron				×			
Alpha-2-globulin				×			
Alpha-1-antitrypsin							×
White blood cell count							×

[a]Validation by physician's assessment.
[b]Validation by CDAI.
CDAI = Crohn's Disease Activity Index; NCDAI = New Crohn's Disease Activity Index; IOIBD = International Organization for the Study of Inflammatory Bowel Disease; LCDAI = Laboratory Crohn's Disease Activity Index.

level, erythrocyte sedimentation rate, serum albumin), each of which received 1 point, up to a theoretical maximum score of 38 (2). The method proposed by Talstad and Gjone was based on symptoms and laboratory tests that measured sedimentation rate (ESR), serum albumin, total iron binding capacity, hemoglobin level, leukocytes, thrombocytes, vitamin B_{12} absorption, and serum folic acid (3). Neither of these scoring systems was validated against other indices or general clinical assessment.

B. Crohn's Disease Activity Index

The Crohn's Disease Activity Index (CDAI), used by the National Cooperative Crohn's Disease Study (NCCDS) and subsequently by many other multicenter trials, is the most used index in the management of Crohn's disease (4). The statistical procedure used for the construction of this mathematical model has been repeated by other authors for the construction of successive indices.

The American gastroenterologists involved in the preparation of the NCCDS listed the usual clinical symptoms and signs (independent-item variables) that they considered important indicators of active Crohn's disease; subsequently, they numerically weighted these independent variables according to the severity and importance of the symptom/sign. The dependent variable with which the independent variables were then compared was the physician's clinical evaluation of severity of disease, subdivided into four categories ranging from "very well" to "very poor." A multiple regression analysis with stepwise deletion was then carried out, thus providing the eight final independent variables that best predicted the physician's overall evaluation (see Table 1).

During the following years, the CDAI was the subject of much criticism. Attempts to improve it have not been as successful as the CDAI itself, which is still widely used in clinical trials.

Several commentators pointed out that the CDAI was not a true measure of disease activity, but a measure of degree of illness (5,6). This criticism was not merely theoretical; the result could have been the application of incorrect therapies. In fact, the variables of the CDAI could not only reflect "activity" but could also reflect the consequences of scarring or of previous intestinal resection. This is particularly true in patients with burnt-out stenotic disease, in whom steroids are as useless as they are to patients crippled by stable deformities from burnt-out rheumatoid arthritis. Use of the variables, "pain" and "well-being," was criticized because, although they were strongly influenced by subjective evaluations, they were heavily rated and could unbalance the CDAI score (7). Furthermore, CDAI was considered cumbersome in practice; a simplified index was therefore proposed by Harvey and Bradshaw and compared with CDAI in a prospective study of 112 patients (8).

The Harvey Bradshaw index was based on five clinical variables (see Table 1) calculated at a single outpatient visit without consideration of weight factors or laboratory tests, and without completion of a 1-week diary card. Because no laboratory tests were included in this index, it was dependent on subjective patient reporting of symptoms and was strongly influenced by the number of liquid stools passed per day. It showed, however, a very good correlation with CDAI ($r = 0.93$).

An even simpler index that does not require direct physician assessment has recently been developed by Sandler et al. for epidemiological studies (9). This index is based exclusively on data about well-being, abdominal pain, and stool frequency and correlates well with CDAI ($r = 0.87$) and with clinical judgment.

A simpler system than CDAI was also proposed in Oxford by the International Organization for the study of Inflammatory Bowel Disease (IOIBD) and reported by Myren et al. in 1984 (10). It proposed a 10-item index, scoring each item as either present or absent, the factors taken into account being those listed in Table 1. The Oxford (or IOIBD) assessment showed good correlation with the CDAI and with the "clinical opinion" measured by linear analog scale.

In 1980, Present et al. used the "goal system" as criterion of efficacy in their trial on 6-mercaptopurine (11). This system overcame another criticism of the CDAI: whether it was acceptable to base clinical assessment on a number that would group together patients with different problems and disease localizations. In the "goal system," the clinical assessment was no longer represented by a number, but the clinical problems of each patient were identified and the goal was the success in resolving them. Achieving a treatment goal is, in essence, how the clinician and the patient judge the efficacy of a drug. However, this excellent method was not widely used because a numerical index such as CDAI was more easily statistically analyzable and comparable.

The methodology by which the CDAI was obtained was the subject of another important criticism: comparison of the independent variables with a dependent variable (physician's clinical evaluation) expressed on the basis of those same independent variables was a circular procedure. This criticism raised the question of whether there was a laboratory or instrumental test that was an objective measure of the quantity of inflammation and whether that measurement could be used as a dependent variable. Unfortunately, no such "gold standard" for measuring disease acitvity existed then, nor does it exist now. Although they cannot represent a complete measure of the activity of Crohn's disease, laboratory tests are often used in clinical practice to aid diagnosis and therapeutic decision-making. They were, therefore, incorporated into the indices to increase the "portion" of objectivity.

C. Inflammatory Indices

An activity index based on more objective variables was developed by van Hees et al. using physical examination and laboratory studies (12). Regression analysis of 19 variables used to rate the activity of inflammation in 85 patients with Crohn's disease yielded nine variables that correlated well (r = 0.95) with the physician's assessment of disease activity (see Table 1). The van Hees or Dutch Index, also called the Activity Index (AI), included some variables of CDAI plus qualifications of serum albumin, ESR, previous resection, and sex. Abdominal pain and general well-being were excluded as variables from this index because of their subjectivity. Serum albumin and body temperature were weighted more heavily than other clinical features so that, to a large extent, they determined the index value. Patients with malabsorption due to extensive resections or with ileostomies and colonostomies could not be evaluated with this index. When the AI is compared with the CDAI, the correlation tends to be low because the indices measure different things; one is a clinical index and the other is an inflammatory index (5,10,12,13).

Subsequently, André et al. found that acute-phase proteins correlated significantly with disease activity as measured by the physician-rated four points of the Likert scale and by the CDAI (14). In view of their strong correlation with clinical disease activity, seromucoids, erythrocyte sedimentation rate (ESR), and C-reactive protein (CRP) were proposed to be measured as the most suitable laboratory tests to add to a clinical index of Crohn's disease activity.

In 1981, Prantera et al. devised another index, the Italian or New Crohn's Disease Activity Index (NCDAI), based on easily quantifiable clinical variables: fever, anal fistula, number of bowel movements, and four laboratory parameters (serum iron, CRP, alpha-2-globulin, and seromucoids) (15). When compared with the CDAI, the NCDAI—because of the acute-phase reactants in the blood—disclosed a higher diagnostic accuracy in the early asymptomatic phase of disease or in postoperative recurrence (13). However, the usefulness of a diagnosis of early recurrence of inflammation in the presymptomatic phase remains to be demonstrated.

In 1986, an activity index based only on laboratory parameters was developed by

Brignola et al. (16). Nine tests were evaluated, each of which historically showed some proof of being an indicator of inflammatory activity. A combination of five variables correlated best with the CDAI. In decreasing order of accuracy, these included alpha-1-glycoprotein, CRP, ESR, alpha-1-antitrypsin, and white cell count. Evaluation of the relationships between this laboratory index and the CDAI showed that, in patients with clinical activity, the laboratory index was constantly altered. This also occurred in 55% of cases in clinical remission (CDAI < 150), which suggested a permanent inflammatory activity, also in the absence of symptoms.

It is evident, from the proliferation of indices and their contrasting correlations, that confusion stems from difficulty in clarifying the purpose that an activity index is to serve; that is, the concept of activity itself, which can be either activity of the inflammatory process or the degree of illness. In using any kind of index, we must consider what to measure and what the index measures. Clinical indices mainly measure the degree of illness, including the impact of the disease on the single patient, whereas laboratory assessments measure the quantity of inflammation independently of the development of clinical symptoms. From the practical point of view, a correct guideline to treatment of Crohn's disease must take more account of the functional consequences in the severity of disease than of its pathological essence. Assessment of the patient's quality of life requires a clinical index, whereas an index using laboratory tests can be useful in therapeutic trials, in prognostic evaluation in Crohn's disease, or in determining whether symptoms are due to inflammation.

A general criticism of any type of index concerns the interobserver variation in the use of these indices. An IOIBD survey showed that, when using the CDAI and the Dutch Index, there was a wide variation in individual assessment by six experienced gastroenterologists who independently interviewed and examined six patients (17).

D. Pediatric Indices

Gastroenterologists caring for pediatric patients found that the previously mentioned indices could not be used for their young patients, in whom other factors such as growth rate had to be considered. Two scoring systems were therefore constructed for children with Crohn's disease (18,19). One index included six levels of disease activity, ranging from asymptomatic with normal laboratory tests to incapacitating disease (18). Growth data were not included in activity assessment but were evaluated separately. A subsequent clinical scoring system was developed by Lloyd-Still and Green for children with either Crohn's disease or ulcerative colitis (19). It included growth data in the calculation of the activity score, but it also required an endoscopic and radiological evaluation, which are not easily obtained.

More recently, a scoring system constructed for use with children and adolescents, the Pediatric Crohn's Disease Activity Index (PCDAI), has been proposed for classification by disease severity (20). This index takes into account disturbances in growth as well as the commonly obtained laboratory measurements of hematocrit, albumin, and ESR, which comprise 20% of the total index score. Good interobserver agreement and a strong correlation between PCDAI and physician's global assessment were reported.

Neither of these indices has been widely used in the assessment of pediatric Crohn's disease activity.

II. LABORATORY TESTS

The need for a "gold standard" other than clinical assessment performed by experienced physicians led investigators to search for a single laboratory marker that would independently measure disease activity. Laboratory tests proposed as markers of disease activity include the acute-phase reactants, measures of intestinal permeability and mucosal injury, and indicators of general state of nutrition; each group reflects different aspects of disease activity that is poorly correlated with the others.

A. Acute Phase Response

Erythrocyte sedimentation rate and nonspecific acute-phase plasma proteins such as CRP, seromucoids (and alpha-1-acid glycoprotein), alpha-2-globulin, serum amyloid-A protein, and cholinesterase are sensitive markers of a general inflammatory process in some part of the body (3,14–16,21–31). The amount of CRP increases within a few hours after tissue damage and decreases shortly after the inflammatory response subsides; it is a good test for evaluating the onset of inflammation and its response to treatment (32). C-reactive protein seromucoid levels are markedly elevated in most patients with active Crohn's disease and the levels correlate well with the clinical assessment (23,25,27). The level of CRP probably reflects the amount of tissue involved in the inflammation. CRP levels respond most rapidly with large incremental changes and correlate with fecal granulocyte excretion, which seems to closely reflect the extent of tissue-damaging inflammatory activity in the lesions (24,33). However, although CRP is well correlated with superficial extent of inflammation in ulcerative colitis, it is not equally well correlated with the superficial extent of active lesions in ileal Crohn's disease (34,35). This difference is probably due to the different pathological process of the two diseases: in Crohn's disease the amount of damaged tissue is determined by the extension of lesion in depth and, in ulcerative colitis, quite often, by the superficial extent.

Because the major function of CRP in humans is the defense against bacteria, some authors have speculated that increased levels of CRP reflect the amount of infected gut rather than the amount of inflamed gut (25,36). The ESR reflects a rise in the plasma concentration of proteins; it increases late after inflammation begins and decreases in terms of days after inflammation subsides. Thus, ESR has little value for monitoring rapid changes in the onset or resolution of acute-phase response (32,37). It is considered to be unreliable as a predictor of an attack (26). In active disease, it is useful as an indicator of colonic inflammation but does not appear to be helpful in assessing ileal Crohn's disease (38). The use of ESR in following the course of the inflammatory process is, nevertheless, limited because many factors such as erythrocyte characteristics, serum protein, and lipid levels influence it in a complex fashion (39).

Serum amyloid A (SAA) is an acute-phase protein synthesized by hepatocytes, and it is thought to be the circulating precursor of tissue amyloid AA. It may be involved in the binding and removal of cholesterol from inflammatory lesions and it increases markedly during acute inflammation (29,40). Serum amyloid A is considered to be the most sensitive acute-phase protein known that correlates well with clinical activity in Crohn's disease (41). Increased concentration of SAA has been observed when other acute-phase proteins remain within the reference range (29). However, clinical usefulness is limited by the lack of specificity, because increased concentration was observed even though no clinical evidence of underlying inflammatory bowel disease was detectable and none subsequently developed (29). The recent development of specific immunoassays with a suitable greater specificity may overcome this limitation (42).

Human leucocyte elastase (HLE) is a proteinase considered to be an important mediator of inflammation; it is normally stored in the polymorphonuclear leucocytes and released during phagocytosis. The serum concentration of HLE in patients with Crohn's disease reflects the intestinal disease activity and correlates with the disease activity index scores (43).

In general, acute-phase response is variably associated with severity and extension of the disease in the bowel, owing to anatomical location, bacterial infection, extraintestinal symptoms, and general state of nutrition (23,35,38,44,45). Acute-phase reactants persistently raised in asymptomatic patients with Crohn's disease are associated with a greater risk of clinical relapse (16,25,26).

B. Iron Stores

Decline of serum iron levels during active inflammation is significantly correlated with the extension of the lesion when located in the small bowel (15,26,35). The mechanism of this decline is probably due to a redistribution of the body iron stores, with a movement of the iron into the liver and reticuloendothelial system, as well as to a loss of iron via microhemorrhage from erosions and ulcerations, which would seem to increase with greater lesion length (46). The measurement of ferritin concentration, which mirrors the amount of iron stores, is helpful in determining whether the low serum iron is caused by inflammation or by blood loss. A value below 15 µg/L confirms iron deficiency by loss, whereas a value of 50 µg/L or more suggests an inflammatory activity (47,48).

In anemia caused by chronic inflammatory activity, the transferrin levels are also low, but ferritin measurement can replace other tests such as those for iron-binding capacity and transferrin saturation (49,50).

C. Gastrointestinal Protein Loss

A different approach to assessing inflammatory activity is based on the fact that proteins are lost in the lumen from diseased mucosa. In fact, low serum albumin levels are not infrequently found in Crohn's disease patients. Serum albumin has been correlated with intestinal protein loss and with lesion extension; it has also been associated with disease activity and has been included in the van Hees Activity Index (12,15,31,35). Serial measurements of serum albumin concentration were considered to provide a useful guide in assessing activity and response to medical treatment. However, low serum albumin level is not only the result of protein loss as measured in gut lavage fluid, but it may also be caused by malnutrition and abnormal turnover (51–53). It is not clear to what extent this decreased level depends on diminished hepatic synthesis or increased catabolism (54). A direct measure of the leakage of circulating blood proteins into the gut lumen is provided by the fecal concentration of radiolabelled proteins and, more recently, of alpha-1-antitrypsin (alpha-1-AT), an alpha-glycoprotein that is a protease inhibitor synthesized by the liver and present in normal serum (55,56). The clearance of alpha-1-AT seems to be a more reliable method of measuring intestinal protein loss; alpha-1-AT fecal concentration alone correlates well with clinical activity expressed by an activity index and with the extent as well as the severity of inflammation (57–59). Estimation of alpha-1-AT loss in the stool is a practical tool for quantifying protein loss because it does not require use of radioisotopes and can be accurately evaluated on a single sample.

TABLE 2 Combination of Variables and Clinical Situation in Crohn's Disease

	Symptoms and Signs	Laboratory Tests	Lesions
Active disease	+	+	+
Disorder of immune response	+	−	+
Function symptoms plus inflammation outside the gut or early postsurgical period	+	+	−
Early recurrence	−	−	+
Recurrence in asymptomatic phase	−	+	+
Scars/obstruction/consequence of operation	+	−	−
Inflammation outside the gut	−	+	−

D. Laboratory Tests in Clinical Practice

Laboratory tests are frequently used in clinical practice to aid in making a diagnosis and in therapeutic decision-making. In clinical practice, laboratory tests of inflammation may be normal or abnormal in the presence or absence of symptoms and in the presence or absence of active lesions as shown by endoscopy/radiology. Knowledge of the pathological process in Crohn's disease can clarify the clinical meaning of these three variables (Table 2). In different situations, symptoms, laboratory tests, and presence or absence of lesions are combined: a clinically and pathologically active disease nearly always shows an abnormality of laboratory tests, whereas the recurrence of disease after an operation is characterized by the appearance of a mild lesion at the site of anastomosis, followed by an early asymptomatic phase of elevated acute-phase reactants (60). This is followed, sometimes years later, by a third phase of frank activity, when humoral signs of inflammation closely parallel the severity of symptoms (25).

III. MEASURE OF HEALTH STATUS IN CROHN'S DISEASE

It is well known that a patient's health status cannot be adequately explained by any kind of indices or by instrumental evaluations such as laboratory tests, histopathology, or endoscopic and x-ray findings. Illness, in fact, can be experienced in different ways according to the patient's perceptions of symptoms, inability to work, and impairment of social and sexual life. The illness experience is influenced by psychological, social, and cultural factors. Because the CDAI is too rough an instrument for accurate measurement of the complex impact of the disease on the sick person, more appropriate methods have been studied for gauging the quality of life of patients suffering from Crohn's disease (61–63). Through the use of questionnaires, patients with inflammatory bowel disease have reported impairment that was worse in psychological and social functioning rather than in physical functioning (61).

Criticisms of indices based on quality of life are mainly directed toward the complexity of the questionnaires and the difficult validation of these scales because a "gold standard" for quality of life does not exist (64). A comparison with the CDAI could validate a quality of life test, but if the CDAI were well correlated with a more complex index, who would adopt it?

However, the physician should be aware of the complexity of Crohn's disease and of the influence that the patient's emotional state and social life can have on the results of therapy.

IV. CONCLUSIONS

No mathematical model has been able to satisfactorily evaluate such a complex illness as Crohn's disease, and it is unlikely that such a model will ever do so. The usefulness of an index is directly linked to the reason for which it is used; monocenter and, especially, multicenter trials will have need of different indices according to the goals that they aim to achieve. The main goal of every trial on the efficacy of drugs in Crohn's disease has been the improvement or disappearance of symptoms, inasmuch as no specific therapy is yet known for Crohn's disease. In the future, indices that take a more global view of the patient's quality of life could fulfill this role better than the CDAI, but since the ultimate aim of every therapy is that of healing pathological lesions, other types of indices that measure phlogosis inside and outside the bowel will always be useful and sometimes necessary. In clinical practice, however, increased knowledge about the significance of alterations in laboratory tests will facilitate understanding of the symptoms and, as a result, the choice of the most suitable therapy.

Except in the case of clinical trials, the usefulness of any index will always be overridden by a good penetrating clinical eye and by a wise interpretation of the alteration in laboratory tests.

REFERENCES

1. De Dombal FT, Burton, IL, Clamp SE, Goligher JC. Short term course and prognosis of Crohn's disease. Gut 1974; 15:435–443.
2. Willoughby JMT, Kumar PJ, Beckett J, Dawson AM. Controlled trial of azathioprine in Crohn's disease. Lancet 1971; ii:944–947.
3. Talstad I, Gjone E. The disease activity of ulcerative colitis and Crohn's disease. Scand J Gastroenterol 1976; 11:403–408.
4. Best WR, Bektel JM, Singleton JW, Kern F. Development of a Crohn's disease activity index: National Cooperative Crohn's Disease Study. Gastroenterology 1976; 70:439–444.
5. Maratka Z. Crohn's disease activity index: needs for distinguishing activity from severity. Hepatogastroenterology 1981; 28:187–188.
6. Singleton JW. Clinical activity assessment. In: Inflammatory Bowel Disease. Dig Dis Sci 1987; 32(suppl):42s–45s.
7. Goldstein F, Thornton JJ, Abramson J. Comments on National Cooperative Crohn's Disease Study (NCCDS). Gastroenterology 1980; 78:1647–1648.
8. Harvey RF, Bradshaw JM. A simple index of Crohn's disease activity. Lancet 1980; i:514.
9. Sandler RS, Jordan MC, Kupper LL. Development of a Crohn's index for survey research. J Clin Epidemiol 1988; 41:451–458.
10. Myren J, Bouchier IAD, Watkinson G, et al. The O.M.G.E. multinational inflammatory bowel disease survey 1976–1982: a further report on 2657 cases. Scand J Gastroenterol 1984; 19(95)(suppl):1–27.
11. Present DH, Korelitz BI, Wisch N, et al. Treatment of Crohn's disease with 6-mercaptopurine. N Engl J Med 1980; 302:981–987.
12. van Hees PAM, van Elteren PH, van Lier HJJ, van Tongeren JHM. An index of inflammatory activity in patients with Crohn's disease. Gut 1980; 21:279–286.
13. Prantera C, Levenstein S, Andreoli A, et al. Assessing disease activity in Crohn's disease: a comparison of two indices (Is Best best?). Ital J Gastroenterol 1982; 14:152–155.

14. André C, Descos L, Landais P, Fermanian J. Assessment of appropriate laboratory measures to supplement the Crohn's Disease Activity Index. Gut 1981; 22:571–574.

15. Prantera C, Baiocchi G, Levenstein S, et al. Clinical and Laboratory parameters in Crohn's disease: relation to disease activity, morphology and extent. Ital J Gastroenterol 1981; 13:24–27.

16. Brignola C, Campieri M, Bazzocchi G, et al. A laboratory index for predicting relapse in asymptomatic patients with Crohn's disease. Gastroenterology 1986; 91:1490–1494.

17. De Dombal FT, Softley A. I.O.I.B.D. Report No.1: observer variation in calculating indices of severity and activity in Crohn's disease. Gut 1987; 28:474–481.

18. Whittington PF, Barnes HV, Bayless TM. Medical management of Crohn's disease in adolescence. Gastroenterology 1977; 72:1338–1344.

19. Lloyd-Still JD, Green OC. Clinical scoring system for chronic inflammatory bowel disease in children. Dig Dis Sci 1979; 24:620–624.

20. Hyams JS, Ferry GD, Mandel FS, et al. Development and validation of a pediatric Crohn's disease activity index. J Pediatr Gastroenterol Nutr 1991; 12:439–447.

21. Beck IT. Laboratory assessment of inflammatory bowel disease. Dig Dis Sci 1987; 32(12) (suppl):26s–41s.

22. Sachar DB, Smith H, Chan S, et al. Erythrocytic sedimentation rate as a measure of clinical activity in inflammatory bowel disease. J Clin Gastroenterol 1986; 8:647–650.

23. Fagan EA, Dyck RP, Maton PN, et al. Serum levels of C-reactive protein in Crohn's disease and ulcerative colitis. Eur J Clin Invest 1982; 12:351–359.

24. Saverymuttu SH, Hodgson HJF, Chadwick VS, Pepys MB. Differing acute phase response in Crohn's disease and ulcerative colitis. Gut 1986; 27:809–813.

25. Boirivant M, Leoni M, Tariciotti D, et al. The clinical significance of serum C-reactive protein levels in Crohn's disease. Results of a prospective longitudinal study. J Clin Gastroenterol 1988; 10:401–405.

26. Wright JP, Alp MN, Young GO, Tigler-Wybrandi N. Predictors of acute relapse of Crohn's disease: a laboratory and clinical study. Dig Dis Sci 1987; 32:164–170.

27. Cook WT, Prior P. Determining disease activity in inflammatory bowel disease. J Clin Gastroenterol 1984; 6:17–25.

28. Weeke B, Jarnum S. Serum concentration of 19 serum proteins in Crohn's disease and ulcerative colitis. Gut 1971; 12:297–302.

29. Chambers RE, Stross P, Barry RE, Whicher JT. Serum amyloid A protein compared with C-reactive protein, alpha 1-antichymotrypsin and alpha 1-acid glycoprotein as a monitor of inflammatory bowel disease. Eur J Clin Invest 1987; 17:460–467.

30. Khalil SN, Dudrick S, Mathieu A, et al. Low levels of pseudocholinesterase in patient with Crohn's disease. Lancet 1980; ii:267–268.

31. Tromm A, Tromm CD, Huppe D, et al. Evaluation of different laboratory tests and activity indices reflecting the inflammatory activity of Crohn's disease. Scand J Gastroenterol 1992; 27:774–778.

32. Stuart J, Lewis SM. Monitoring the acute phase response. BMJ 1988; 297:1143–1144.

33. Camilleri M, Proano M. Advances in the assessment of disease activity in inflammatory bowel disease. Mayo Clin Proc 1989; 64:800–807.

34. Prantera C, Davoli M, Lorenzetti R, et al. Clinical and laboratory indicators of extent of ulcerative colitis. J Clin Gastroenterol 1988; 10(1):41–45.

35. Prantera C, Luzi C, Olivotto P, et al. Relationship between clinical and laboratory parameters and length of lesion in Crohn's disease of the small bowel. Dig Dis Sci 1984; 29:1093–1097.

36. Pepys MB. C-reactive protein fifty years on. Lancet 1981; i:653–657.

37. International Committee for Standardization in Haematology (Expert Panel on Blood Rheology). Guidelines on selection of laboratory tests for monitoring the acute phase response. J. Clin Pathol 1988; 41:1203–1212.

38. Sachar DB, Luppescu NE, Bodian C, et al. Erythrocyte sedimentation as a measure of Crohn's disease activity: opposite trend in ileitis versus colitis. J Clin Gastroenterol 1990; 12:643–646.

39. Crawford J, Eye-Boland MK, Cohen HJ. Clinical utility of erythrocyte sedimentation rate and plasma protein analysis in the elderly. Am J Med 1987; 82:239–246.
40. Benditt EP, Hoffman JS, Eriksen N, et al. SAA, an apoprotein of HDL: its structure and function. Ann N Y Acad Sci 1982; 389:183–189.
41. Maury CPJ. Comparative study of serum amyloid A protein and C-reactive protein in disease. Clin Sci 1985; 68:233–238.
42. Liuzzo G, Biasucci LM, Gallimore JR, et al. The prognostic value of C-reactive protein and serum amyloid A protein in severe unstable angina. N Engl J Med 1994; 331:417–424.
43. Adeyemi EO, Neumann S, Chadwick VS, et al. Circulating human leucocyte elastase in patients with inflammatory bowel disease. Gut 1985; 26:1306–1311.
44. Powell-Tuck J, Day DW, Bucknell NA. Correlation between defined sigmoidoscopic appearances and other measures of disease activity in ulcerative colitis. Dig Dis Sci 1982; 27:533–537.
45. Rose PE, Johnsdon SA, Meakin M, et al. Serial study of C-reactive protein during infection in leukemia. J Clin Pathol 1981; 34:263–266.
46. Beisel WR. Trace elements in infectious processes. Med Clin North Am 1976; 60:831–849.
47. Atkins D. Test for determination of iron-deficiency anemia: a metanalysis. ACP J Club July/August 1992:23.
48. Blake DR, Waterworth RF, Bacon PA. Assessment of iron stores in inflammation by assay of serum ferritin concentrations. BMJ 1981; 283:1147–1148.
49. Lee GR. The anemia of chronic disease. Semin Hematol 1983; 62:61–67.
50. Guyatt GH, Oxman AD, Ali M, et al. Laboratory diagnosis of iron-deficiency anemia: an overview. J Gen Intern Med 1992; 7:145–153.
51. Choudari CP, O'Mahony S, Brydon G, et al. Gut lavage fluid protein concentration: objective measures of disease activity in inflammatory bowel disease. Gastroenterology 1993; 104:1064–1071.
52. André C, Descos L, André F, et al. Biological measurements of Crohn's disease activity—a reassessment. Horm Metab Res 1985; 17:135–137.
53. Meryn S, Lochs H, Bettelheim P, et al. Serum proteinkonzentrationen-Parameter fur die Krank-heits-activitat bei Morbus Crohn? Leber Magen Darm 1985; 15:160–164.
54. Kushner I. The phenomenon of the acute phase response. Ann N Y Acad Sci 1982; 82:40–48.
55. Beeken WL, Busch HJ, Sylvester D. Intestinal protein loss in Crohn's disease. Gastroenterology 1972; 62:207–215.
56. Crossley JR, Elliot RB. A simple method for diagnosing protein losing enteropathies. BMJ 1977; 1:428–429.
57. Bernier JJ, Florent CH, Desmazures CH. Diagnosis of protein losing enteropathy by gastrointestinal clearance of alpha 1-antitrypsin. Lancet 1978; ii:763–764.
58. Meyers S, Wolke A, Field SP, et al. Fecal alpha-1 antitrypsin measurement: an indicator of Crohn's disease. Gastroenterology 1985; 89:113–118.
59. Crama-Bohbouth G, Pena AS, Biemond I, et al. Are activity indices helpful in assessing active intestinal inflammation in Crohn's disease? Gut 1989; 30:1236–1240.
60. Rutgeerts P, Geboes K, Vantrappen G, et al. Predictability of the postoperative course of Crohn's disease. Gastroenterology 1990; 99:956–963.
61. Drossman DA, Patrick DL, Mitchell CM, et al. Health related quality of life in inflammatory bowel disease: functional status and patient worries and concerns. Dig Dis Sci 1989; 34:1379–1386.
62. Garrett JW, Drossman DA. The assessment of quality of life in inflammatory bowel disease. In: Spilker B, ed. Quality of Life Assessments in Clinical Studies. New York: Raven Press, 1990:367–379.
63. Garrett JW, Drossman DA. Health status in inflammatory bowel disease. Gastroenterology 1990; 90:90–96.
64. Love JR, Irvine EJ, Fedorak RN. Quality of life in inflammatory bowel disease. J Clin Gastroenterol 1992; 14(1):15–19.

COMMENTARY

John W. Singleton   *University of Colorado School of Medicine, Denver, Colorado*

As so well presented in Drs. Prantera and Kohn's chapter, activity indices in Crohn's disease remain a controversial issue in evaluation of patients with this disease. It may be illuminating to compare the attempts at a Crohn's disease index with what appear to be more successful classification schemes for arthritis or heart disease. The American Heart Association classification system for severity of heart disease, for example, is widely used in practice and clinical research (1). Its simple four-point scale expresses the patient's ability to carry on normal daily activities. Would such a system be useful in Crohn's disease? Probably not, because the effect of Crohn's disease symptoms on daily activities is so complex and so dependent on the individual patient's response to his or her symptoms. A closer parallel may be the American College of Rheumatology core set of disease activity measures, which combines number of joints involved and severity of impairment into a single scale (2). However, in this case, all of the impairment relates to a limited range of symptoms, all affecting a single structure, namely the joints. In Crohn's disease, a wide variety of symptoms occur as a result of disease of a complex organ and its associated structures. Thus, Crohn's disease presents unique problems in formulation of an index of disease activity or illness severity.

In designing controlled clinical trials, clinical investigators found that they needed numerical measures of Crohn's disease activity and patients' severity of illness. For these applications, indices of disease activity have been and continue to be extremely useful. Attempts to incorporate such indices into everyday practice, however, have been largely unsuccessful. Doctors prefer to make their own global assessment fo the patient's degree of illness. This will probably always be true, because no single system of evaluating patients will ever satisfy all clinicians.

The Crohn's Disease Activity Index (CDAI) developed for the American National Cooperative Crohn's Disease Study has been used in the great majority of subsequent clinical trials. Other indices have been less popular. The relatively complex Inflammatory Bowel Disease Quality of Life Questionnaire (IBDQ) has proven very useful in clinical trials, but it may be too cumbersome for daily clinical practice in which expert clinicians gain accurate assessment of a patient's quality of life with a few penetrating questions (3).

One successor to the CDAI that was carefully evolved from the CDAI and tested in a large group of patients is Severity-Activity Index (SI) of Goebell et al. (4). This index overcomes the objections leveled at the CDAI of too much subjectivity while still retaining a close correspondence to the actual clinical situation. It should be given serious consideration as the standard index for future clinical trials.

An index of Crohn's disease activity might be useful when an accurate and objective measure of a patient's response to therapy is needed. Here, a numerical expression for the degree of illness might enable the patient and physician to judge more accurately the effect of a treatment new to the patient.

If it could be shown that an activity index, a biological measurement, or a combination of the two could actually predict incipient clinical deterioration and, further, that therapeutic intervention at that point would prevent the predicted adverse clinical course from occurring, such an index or measurement would immediately become clinically important. Several reasonably successful attempts have been made to develop such an index, but it has never been shown that therapeutic intervention on that basis improved patients' subsequent course (5,6). A carefully designed randomized clinical trial of this proposition is needed.

REFERENCES

1. Criteria Commitee, New York Heart Association, Inc. Diseases of the Heart and Blood Vessels. Nomenclature and Criteria for Diagnosis. 6th ed. Boston: Little, Brown, 1964:114.
2. Felson DT, Anderson JJ, Boers M, et al. The American College of Rheumatology preliminary core set of disease activity measures for rheumatoid arthritis clinical trials. Arthritis Rheum 1993; 36:729–740.
3. Guyatt G, Mitchell A, Irvine EJ, et al. A new measure of health status for clinical trials in inflammatory bowel disease. Gastroenterology 1989; 96:804–810.
4. Goebell H, Malchow H, Wienbeck W, et al. Evaluation of an index for severity and activity of Crohn's disease (Severity-Activity Index). Eur J Gastroenterol Hepatol. In press.
5. Brignola C, Campieri M, Bazzocchi G, et al. A laboratory index for predicting relapse in asymptomatic patients with Crohn's disease. Gastroenterology 1986; 91:1490–1494.
6. Wright JP, Alp MN, Young G, et al. Predictors of acute relapse in Crohn's disease: a laboratory and clinical study. Dig Dis Sci 1987; 32:164–170.

10
Different Patterns of Crohn's Disease

Lloyd R. Sutherland   *Foothills Hospital and University of Calgary, Calgary, Alberta, Canada*

I. OUTLINE

This chapter reviews the evidence that clinical patterns of Crohn's disease can be identified. The possible uses for such patterns and the pitfalls of the current literature are also discussed.

A summary of each of the various attempts to classify Crohn's disease to determine whether there are consistent patterns of disease activity restricted to various subgroups of patients follows. Following the description of each pattern, a brief critique is given. After examining the simplest classification, that based on the anatomical location of disease, other classifications focusing on the type of disease activity or the lesions identified are reviewed. Disease activity is examined from a temporal point of view (aggressive, indolent) as well as from a mechanistic perspective (perforating, nonperforating). The results of the deliberations of a group of experts in the field are summarized. Finally, a brief consideration of other modifiers that might describe patterns of disease including family status, life-style, age, laboratory parameters, or functional status are presented.

II. WHY SEARCH FOR DIFFERENT PATTERNS IN CROHN'S DISEASE?

A. The Need to Provide Information to Patients Regarding Prognosis

From its earliest descriptions, Crohn's disease has been characterized as an unpredictable sequence of flares and remissions punctuated from time to time by the need for a resection. Consider the patients' perspective when given the diagnosis of Crohn's disease. They are ill, medications are prescribed, and it is natural to want to know what the prognosis is. Many physicians prefer not to predict the future. Perhaps they would refer to the Scandinavian publications and offer the reassurance that as a group, Crohn's disease patients have a normal life expectancy. However, as to the prediction of flares, need for resections, or use of potent medications, most physicians would decline to speculate.

From a patient's perspective, this is unsettling. As recently noted by Hodgson, aside from a cure, patients expect the research community to provide objective information by which physicians can answer their questions regarding prognosis (1). Growing literature suggests that providing patients with knowledge about their disease and its management results in improvements in symptoms and health care savings (2,3).

B. The Need to Assist in Identifying the Causes of Crohn's Disease

The refusal by many members of the medical community to attempt to classify the various manifestations or presentations of Crohn's disease may have held back new insights into the etiology of the disease. By being "splitters" rather than "lumpers," we should be able to determine whether there is a sole cause of Crohn's disease or, more likely in my opinion, there are multiple causes that assault the gut, combined with a limited repertoire of responses by the host.

The search for a phenotypical classification of Crohn's disease has begun. Support for this strategy is drawn from classification of other chronic diseases, which should encourage further research. Identification of a phenotype will expedite the search for a corresponding gene. For example, autosomal dominant polycystic kidney disease is a common genetic condition affecting 1 in 1000 people. It has a characteristic phenotype that includes extra renal manifestations (hepatic and pancreatic cysts, cardiac valvular disease, colonic diverticulum). Recently, an abnormal gene on chromosome 16 was described and should identify most patients at risk of disease development. Alterations in clinical management might include careful observations for development of hypertension before development of renal failure in the identified population at risk (4).

C. The Need to Assist in Decision-Making

A recent study in the field of rheumatoid arthritis illustrates the potential for genetic markers to identify phenotypes, in this case, subsets of patients at greater risk of serious disease. As in the therapy of inflammatory bowel disease, rheumatologists have traditionally used a pyramidal or stepped approach to therapy of rheumatoid arthritis, beginning with anti-inflammatories and reserving immunosuppressants or cytotoxic agents for patients who fail treatments that have fewer side effects.

Weyand et al. studied the HLA-DRB1 region in 102 seropositive patients with rheumatoid arthritis and compared each genotype with the presence or absence of major organ involvement and the requirement for surgical procedures. Patients homozygous for the 04 allele (i.e., DRB1*04/04) had more severe disease compared with patients who did not have extra-articular disease (61% versus 11%, $p < 0.0001$) or require joint surgery (61% versus 25%, $p < 0.004$). The investigators speculated that because patients homozygous for DRN1*04 appear to have a greater risk for serious disease, early intervention with second-line agents could be more appropriate and effective (5).

In Crohn's disease, the classification of patterns of disease might also identify particular therapeutic subgroups for which different classes of therapies are warranted. For example, the use of immunosuppressants is often restricted to patients who have already failed therapy with either corticosteroids or 5-aminosalicylates. Identification of patients at high risk for extensive unremitting disease might lead to treatment strategies that initiate early therapy with more potent agents rather than therapy delayed until after the gut has been extensively damaged or scarred. If fibrostenotic disease were predictable, efforts might be made to develop therapies that focus on the prevention of fibrosis rather than on dampening inflammation.

III.   INTERPRETING THE CURRENT LITERATURE

A.   Essentials of Studies of Natural History

Studies of the natural history of disease could provide the data required to determine the clinical patterns, if they exist, of Crohn's disease. There are a variety of criteria, reviewed by Sackett and Whelan, used to evaluate studies of natural history of disease to determine their acceptability (6). They include the identification of an inception cohort (e.g., all consecutive, newly diagnosed patients with Crohn's disease seen during a certain period of time), a description of referral patterns (patients seen within a certain geographic area or referral from elsewhere), and completeness of follow-up. Other features include objective outcome criteria (clear definitions of outcome variables, for example, indications for surgery), blinded assessments (those who assessed the outcome were unaware of the prognostic implications at issue), and adjustment for extraneous prognostic factors (e.g., treatment).

If recurrence is the outcome of interest, a clear definition as to what is meant should be given. Lennard-Jones and Stadler offered three definitions of recurrence: recurrent symptoms, symptomatic relapse with radiological or surgical evidence of recurrence, and need for a second operation (7).

Studies should include a sufficient number of patients on which to base any clinical projections. It is unlikely that patterns of activity are so consistent that they can be appreciated after studying a few patients. Because Crohn's disease is a chronic affliction and certain complications may take several years to manifest, sufficient follow-up should transpire so that definitive conclusions can be drawn.

In general, the best studies include only incident (i.e., newly diagnosed) patients. Prevalent patients have already received treatment including surgery and cannot be considered to be without bias. Basing a study on all patients that attend a clinic (i.e., incident and prevalent cases) may result in an overrepresentation of ill patients because those who are well may not return to the clinic.

If these criteria are strictly applied, it is impossible for most centers to meet all of the standards. Long-term follow-up is often difficult in North America because patients may seek other providers of health care and move easily throughout the continent. Only the Scandinavian studies, because of their relatively low migration patterns and superb patient registries, approach this degree of perfection. However, by reviewing these principles, it should be easier for clinicians to critically interpret the current literature.

B.   Treatment and Investigation Bias

Another potential difficulty in reviewing the literature is related to biases of treatment and investigation. Various classifications have been proposed and findings such as the need for medical therapy, requirements for surgery and so on, have been reported. Unless there are clearly enunciated guidelines related to treatment (i.e., the use of corticosteroids or the indications for surgery), the outcomes reported may be more influenced by the treatment bias of that particular institution rather than the classification itself.

As an example, a center has a tradition of early resection of limited disease occurring in the terminal ileum. If this treatment strategy is not specifically enunciated, a natural history study based on the experience at that center would conclude that patients with limited small bowel disease require early surgical intervention for the management of their disease. The best solution to this problem is repetition, for example, encouraging other centers to use the same classification system to determine whether the outcomes are similar.

Biases in the investigation of patients may also be present and are potentially important in studies of natural history. Many of the reports include patients identified in the 1960s when flexible endoscopy was not available and disease extent was determined using barium techniques. This may have underestimated the contribution of right-sided colonic disease, this could be important if different clinical patterns are claimed for disease confined to the terminal ileum compared with ileocolonic involvement.

Centers may differ as to whether they routinely perform biopsies on endoscopically normal-appearing mucosa at the time of colonoscopy or gastroduodenoscopy to detect microscopic disease. Because there is little evidence to suggest that routine repetition of barium or endoscopic investigations is warranted, the patient phenotype in terms of gut involvement may change and the investigator may not be aware of it.

C. Referral Bias

A further problem in reviewing studies related to the natural history of disease is the identification of a referral bias. A referral bias occurs when the results of a natural history study are contaminated by the introduction of patients referred because of the difficulty of their cases.

The influence of referral bias in Crohn's disease has been documented by Truelove and Pena in their description of the long-term follow-up of patients attending the Radcliffe Infirmary (8). They characterized their patients as to whether or not they came from the Oxfordshire Health District or were specifically referred from outside the district. Significant differences in survival between the two groups could be demonstrated. The local patients had a similar probability of survival as the general United Kingdom population. The referred patients had a significantly reduced survival rate compared with the normal population. In reviewing articles related to prognosis, it is not always possible to determine the mix between local patients and those referred from outside the community.

D. Other Sources of Data

It has been suggested that a potential source of information on natural history might be analyses of disease characteristics of patients participating in large multicenter trials of therapy. Both the National Cooperative Crohn's Disease Study (NCCDS) and the European Cooperative Crohn's Disease Study (ECCDS) reported their data related to the disease milestones for patients who participated (9,10). Although the trials are important guides to the therapy of Crohn's disease, their impact in terms of prognosis or the definition of clinical pattern is limited because they do not reflect incident or newly diagnosed cases. As with most studies of therapy, they represent a select subgroup of patients, many of whom may be refractory to current therapies. For example, in the NCCDS, most patients were diagnosed for at least 3 years before entering the study. Of the 77 patients randomized to placebo in part I, phase 1, only 13 (17%) had never received medication before study entry. Data from such studies can be used, not to generate hypotheses but perhaps to corroborate findings in other studies.

IV. PREVIOUS CLASSIFICATIONS

A. Anatomical Location and the Clinical Pattern

1. The Pattern

As discussed, it is almost impossible in North America to conduct a natural history study, because of the easy migration and the ease of changing physicians. The Cleveland Clinic, however, has provided an important approximation to a natural history study. However, its reputation as an inflammatory bowel disease center leaves it open to the possibility of a referral bias. Their reports are of interest because of the large numbers of consecutive, generally newly diagnosed patients enrolled and the good long-term follow-up. The majority of patients returned to the Cleveland Clinic on a regular basis for evaluation and treatment. For the few patients who did not return, telephone contacts were attempted. Reports of the patient cohort assembled between January 1966 and December 1969 were published in 1975, 1985, and 1987 (11–13). Follow-up has been excellent, with data available on more than 95% of patients who entered the study.

In their initial report, Farmer et al. stressed the importance of disease location as a predictor of the "clinical pattern" that patients might expect (11). They initially divided their patients into four groups: ileocolonic (distal ileum and right colon, 41%), small bowel only (29%, 139 of 176 [78%] with disease confined to the terminal ileum, 8 with duodenal/jejunal disease alone), colonic (27%), and localized anorectal disease (3%). Eventually, all patients with localized anorectal disease developed more extensive colonic disease, and the two groups were later combined into the colonic stratum.

The first report emphasized a series of associations under the overall scheme of a clinical pattern. Patients with ileocolonic disease were more likely to have rectal fistulas at the time of diagnosis than those with small bowel disease alone. During the early years of follow-up, a greater chance of developing internal fistulas was also apparent (34% compared with less than 20% of patients with disease elsewhere). Fistulas, either perianal or internal, were often associated with abscesses. In the first report, patients with ileocolonic disease had a greater risk of surgery (73%) compared with 51% of the remainder of the patients. The primary indications for surgery were internal fistulas (38%), intestinal obstruction (37%), and perianal disease (15%). By the time of the 1985 report, 92% of patients with ileocolonic disease reported having at least one resection.

Patients with disease confined to the small intestine had a different clinical pattern. Intestinal obstruction developed twice as often as in patients with exclusively colonic disease. Conversely, there was less risk of development of perianal fistulas (14% compared with nearly 40% of those with either ileocolonic or colonic disease alone). The primary indications for surgery were obstruction (54%) and internal fistulas (29%). By 1985, the percentage of patients undergoing resection increased to 66%.

Patients with colonic disease had the greatest risk of rectal bleeding. Rectal fistulas were more common at the time of diagnosis in patients with colonic disease compared with patients with small bowel disease alone. Episodes of toxic megacolon were generally confined to this group. Extracolonic manifestations were more common (16% compared with 4% of patients with disease elsewhere). Half of the patients underwent resection during the early years of follow-up. Indications for surgery varied and included internal fistulas (25%), perianal disease (23%), toxic megacolon (19%), obstruction (12%), and refractory disease (21%). By 1985, 58% of patients with colonic disease required surgery.

In concluding their second report, Farmer et al. emphasized their hypothesis that the anatomical location was an important determinant of clinical course. Links were described between small bowel disease and obstruction, ileocolonic disease and fistula/abscess development, and colonic disease and toxic megacolon. Disease morbidity was greatest with ileocolonic disease. As a general rule, patients with malnutrition, abscesses, sepsis, or megacolon had a poorer prognosis. Patients with segmental colonic or isolated ileal disease had the best prognosis. Perianal disease was generally identified at disease onset rather than appearing later in the course of disease.

The most recent report of the Cleveland cohort focused attention on the subgroup of 139 patients who had a minimum of 15 years of follow-up at the Cleveland Clinic (13). The authors noted that, after 15 years of follow-up 72% of patients who originally presented with localized small bowel disease progressed to ileocolonic disease. Conversely, 24 of 39 (61%) patients who presented with colonic disease continued to have disease confined to the large intestine. However, it is possible that the apparent extension in patients with ileal disease reflects a reliance on barium enema to determine colonic disease during the early phases of the study.

Anatomical location still predicted the indication for surgery. Patients with small bowel disease tended to undergo resections for obstruction, whereas, intractability was the most frequently cited complication for ileocolonic and colonic disease. One-third of all patients had proctocolectomy, including 18% of patients who presented initially with only small bowel disease and 30% of those with ileocolonic disease.

2. Critique

It is possible that the Cleveland concept is based on material that suffers from a referral bias, but other researchers have examined the concept of a clinical pattern based on disease location. Holdstock et al. suggested that the anatomical location distinguished the course of Crohn's disease of the small intestine from Crohn's disease of the colon in terms of symptoms, the number of surgeries, and the number of relapses per year (15). Patients with small bowel disease had more problems. Provocatively, the researchers found few differences in the clinical symptoms, complications, disease duration, and number of relapses when patients with Crohn's colitis were compared with patients with ulcerative colitis (15). They argued that distinguishing between Crohn's colitis and ulcerative colitis was unnecessary. Although this may be true in terms of clinical symptoms and medical therapy, distinctions between the two in terms of surgical options are clearly required.

In Copenhagen, one group described the natural history of 185 consecutive patients with Crohn's disease diagnosed between 1960 and 1978 (16). Their patient population is ideal for a natural history studies because the investigators have access to all patients with Crohn's disease in Copenhagen. However, they did not explore relationships between disease location, clinical patterns, and prognosis.

There are numerous case series related to the follow-up of patients who have undergone resection for Crohn's disease. For example, Higgins and Allan reviewed the outcome of 227 patients in Leeds (17). Two-thirds of the subjects had isolated terminal ileal disease; the remainder had cecal or minimal right colonic disease, in addition to involvement of their terminal ileum. Based on the clinical pattern associated with small bowel disease, one would expect obstruction to be a common indication for surgery. In this series, the most likely indication for resection was obstruction, followed by fistula with abscess formation. Specific proportions were not given.

In a report of 87 patients with Crohn's disease assessed in Malmo, Sweden, between 1958 and 1974, symptoms of weight loss, pain, and diarrhea were the most common indications for surgery, with only 10% of patients complaining of intestinal obstruction (18). This report is an excellent example of treatment bias. The treatment plan in Malmo, as reported in the paper, was to offer surgery early to patients before "serious" complications arose. Only 25% of the patients received medical therapy before surgery. This aggressive approach would clearly alter the perception of indications for surgery.

B.   Indolent Versus Aggressive Disease

1.   The Pattern

De Dombal et al. reviewed their experience at Leeds, a tertiary referral center for inflammatory bowel disease (19). The series included 169 patients who had undergone their first resection for Crohn's disease and were available for follow-up (19). Two groups of patients were identified. One presented with recurrent disease within 2 years after surgery ("early"); the other ("late") reported recurrence 5 to 10 years later. When the two groups were compared, differences in the duration of symptoms and disease location were apparent. Patients with early recurrence tended to have disease symptoms for only a short period of time before undergoing resection. Patients with late recurrence had a longer duration of symptoms. Another observation was that patients with colonic resections tended to fall into the early recurrence group. The authors concluded that there might be two forms of Crohn's disease: an aggressive form, which required surgery soon after diagnosis, and a more benign or indolent form, which did not require early surgery and only recurred several years after resection.

2.   Critique

The concept of two forms of Crohn's disease, one aggressive, the other indolent, has received support from other studies. Sachar et al. reviewed the risk factors for postoperative recurrence in 93 patients who underwent their first resection at the Mt. Sinai Hospital between 1964 and 1973. They confirmed the suggestion that recurrence rates were significantly lower in patients with a longer duration of symptoms before surgery. Specifically, the risk of recurrence in patients with symptoms for less than 10 years before surgery was twice that of patients who had symptoms for more than 10 years (20).

In the 110 patients randomized to placebo in the ECCDS, the majority (67%) who entered with inactive disease remained in remission during the next 2 years. Conversely, only one-third of patients who entered with active disease entered a sustained remission during the study period.

There is biological evidence to support the hypothesis of different patterns of recurrence. The phenomenon of early endoscopic recurrence has been described by Rutgeerts et al. and confirmed by Olaison et al. (21,22). Two extremes are encountered: the first is represented by a few scattered aphthous ulcerations in the neoterminal ileum, which is associated with a low risk of early clinical recurrence; the other is characterized by large serpiginous ulcers associated with rapid clinical recurrence. When Rutgeerts et al. attempted to model recurrence, however, duration of disease was not an important factor in predicting rapid recurrence.

Not every group has confirmed this pattern. In Boston, a trend in the opposite direction was noted. Patients with disease symptoms of short duration (< 2 years) appeared to have a lower risk of recurrence compared with those with a longer history of antecedent disease. This finding, however, did not reach statistical significance (23). In a study of 82 children with Crohn's disease who had undergone surgery, a longer duration of symptoms was associated with more recurrences (24).

An early Swedish study of recurrence found no difference in recurrence rates when patients were characterized by duration of symptoms (< 1 year or > 1 year; 39% versus 43%) (25). A Dutch study was unable to identify disease duration as a predictor of repeat resection (26). Hellers also failed to find an association betweeen duration of disease before surgery and recurrence (27).

C. Perforating Versus Nonperforating

1. The Pattern

Stimulated by the work of De Dombal and their own observations, the Mt. Sinai group suggested that aspects of disease behavior could predict the future course of patients with Crohn's disease. In their classification scheme, patients were divided into two groups based on the indication for surgery: perforating or nonperforating (28). The series consisted of 770 patients who had either all surgery done at the Mt. Sinai institution or for whom surgical notes from other institutions were available to clearly state the indication for surgery. Perforating indications included acute free perforation, subacute perforation with abscess formation, and chronic perforation with internal fistulization. Nonperforating indications included obstruction, intractability, hemorrhage, and toxic dilation. If any perforating indication was identified, then the presence of a concurrent nonperforating indication was ignored. Surgical indications for successive surgeries were reviewed independently from the original surgery.

In terms of the primary resection, approximately equal proportions of patients underwent surgery for perforating or nonperforating indications. However, 70% of patients who underwent a second resection remained in the original perforating or nonperforating category. This division of surgical indications remained, even when patients were categorized by disease location. The observation was also consistent when patients undergoing their third resection were analyzed separately. Finally, the authors noted that the time interval between the first and second resection and the second and third resection was approximately double for nonperforating compared with perforating indications. They speculated that perforating indications signified a disease pathogenesis characterized by deep ulceration whereas many of the nonperforating indications could be more likely associated with the development of fibrosis. Whether or not the perforating or nonperforating phenotype indicated different disease etiologies or different host inflammatory or immune responses to a single etiological factor was left open to question.

2. Critique

To date, there have been few attempts to validate this classification. In the Beth Israel (Boston) series, reported before the Mt. Sinai paper, the presence of a fistula as the indication for the first resection did not predict that fistula would be the indication for the second surgery (23).

Italian investigators reviewed the clinical course of 58 patients who underwent resection of the terminal ileum. Recurrence was defined as the need for a second resection or the occurrence of symptoms with either radiological or endoscopic evidence of recurrent disease. Of the 29 patients who presented with obstruction as the indication for the first resection, 19 (67%) developed obstructive symptoms again. In terms of fistulizing disease, however, only 1 of 11 patients with fistula as the primary indication reported a fistula as the indication at the second recurrence (29).

D. Roma 91 Classification

1. The Pattern

A working group, consisting of several experienced experts in the field of inflammatory bowel disease, reviewed potential classification schemes including etiopathogenic, biochemical or immunological, life-style, and pathological or endoscopic and found them all unsatisfactory (30). Their solution was to link the anatomical classification of the Cleveland Clinic with the disease behavior model of the Mt. Sinai group. At the same time, additional descriptors related to extent of disease and the surgical history were added.

They proposed that each patient with Crohn's disease be characterized in four dimensions, specifically disease location, extent, behavior, and operative history. As shown in Table 1, disease location is subdivided into stomach/duodenum, jejunum, ileum, colon, and rectum–perianal. The extent of disease is dichotomized to localized (< 1 m) or diffuse. The primary disease behavior is described as inflammatory, fistulizing, or fibrostenotic. The operative history is categorized as primary (never resected) or recurrent.

2. Critique

The classification represents an important attempt to categorize large groups of patients with Crohn's disease. When and if candidate genes are proposed, it will provide a framework on which to search for a genotypical expression for each phenotype. Hundreds of patients will be required for such a project because the patient population will be divided into many segments. For example, using the four stated modifiers with their variables creates 72 ($6 \times 2 \times 3 \times 2$) subgroups. The analysis becomes more difficult when patients have disease in two sites, for example, ileocecal, possibly creating additional subgroups.

Another problem in implementing the classification could be interobserver differences. Although there should be little disagreement between observers in terms of extent of disease or the operative history, there may be differences of opinion related to the primary disease behavior.

Past experience with the reproducibility of activity indices is not encouraging for future attempts. In a previous report, De Dombal et al. asked experienced clinicians to calculate Crohn's Disease Activity Index on a group of patients. Each clinician was given the same information, but the range of indices calculated was broad (31).

TABLE 1 Proposed Classification of Patient Subgroups in Crohn's Disease

Location	Extent	Primary Behavior	Operative History
Stomach/duodenum	Localized (< 100 cm)	Inflammatory	Primary
Jejunum	Diffuse	Fistulizing	Recurrent
Ileum		Fibrostenotic	
Colon			
Rectum			
Anal–perianal			

Source: Ref. 30.

Ideally such a classification system would be tested in a prospective fashion, but this would entail years of effort. Retrospective studies can be performed more efficiently, assuming that the data were collected in a satisfactory format. Assessments have already begun. Musso et al. reviewed 141 patients with a mean follow-up of 14 years (range 10–34); their study has been reported only as an abstract (32). They did not, perhaps because of the number of cases, explore the complete classification. They collapsed the disease location variable into the traditional small bowel, ileocolon, and colon groupings and did not report either the extent of disease or history of surgery. In terms of disease behavior, only 10 of the 141 were unclassifiable. Differences in corticosteroid use and the need for resection or multiple resections were apparent when the "fibrostenotic," "penetrating," and "inflammatory" groups were compared. Patients with "penetrating" or "fibrostenotic" disease almost invariably required surgery. Patients with "inflammatory" disease rarely required surgery and had longer intervals on corticosteroid treatment.

V. OTHER POSSIBLE CLASSIFICATION SYSTEMS

A. Genetic/Familial

1. The Pattern

Another potential classification would be to categorize patients as having either familial or nonfamilial Crohn's disease. Farmer et al. reported that 35% of patients with inflammatory bowel disease had at least one relative with the disease (33). Others report frequencies as low as 10% (34). From a research perspective, the advantage to implementing this classification would be that studies into the etiology of Crohn's disease might be more efficiently performed if confined to those with a positive family history who are theoretically at higher risk of developing disease. To date, studies that examine the relationship between disease characteristics within families have focused on either twins or attendees at an inflammatory bowel disease center.

Twins, either monozygotic or dizygotic, offer an opportunity to examine genetic and environmental factors. Although it is generally accepted that there is greater concordance (i.e., both twins having the disease) for Crohn's disease compared with ulcerative colitis, it is possible that reporting bias may be operative. In this case, a physician might be more interested in reporting concordant twin pairs rather than discordant twins. Studies based on regional populations would guard against this bias.

Tysk examined the Swedish twin registry, which contains information on most twin pairs identified in Sweden (35). Of the 18 monozygotic twin pairs identified, 8 were concordant for Crohn's disease; only 1 of 26 dizygotic twin pairs were concordant. Of the eight, five had identical distribution of disease. The disease presented within 2 years of the diagnosis in the index case in five patients. The twin pairs did not appear to be similar in terms of intestinal complications, but the most were similar with regard to the presence or absence of extraintestinal complications (35). Unfortunately, a search for the presence or absence of disease in other family members was not performed. Long-term follow-up of this unique patient resource would be of interest.

At Johns Hopkins, one group has carefully analyzed the disease milestones of patients with a positive family history of inflammatory bowel disease. In their review of 490 patients with Crohn's disease, the researchers reported that 54 patients had at least one relative with inflammatory bowel disease. Among the relatives, concordance with the index case could be demonstrated for disease location (88%), pattern of transmural aggressiveness (67%), and age at onset (within 10 years) 68% (36).

B. Life-Style

1. The Pattern

Patients with Crohn's disease generally are interested in life-style modification as potential disease modifiers. Three issues have been identified: diet, use of oral contraceptives, and smoking. To date, there is little evidence, either from trials or case-control studies, that alteration of diet or avoidance of oral contraceptives influences disease activity.

There is abundant evidence that smoking is a risk factor for the development of Crohn's disease (37). A growing amount of literature implicates smoking as a risk factor for continued disease activity (38–41). The evidence that alteration in smoking habits may influence disease activity is limited but suggests that cessation of smoking alters disease activity (40,41). It might be reasonable to suggest that future classifications include stratification related to smoking status. Smoking is discussed in Chapter 4 of this volume.

C. Extremes of Age

1. The Pattern

It is not clear whether there are significant differences in the clinical patterns of patients with Crohn's disease who develop their disease at either extreme of the age range. When studies of disease recurrence in the pediatric population are reviewed, the prognostic factors do not fit as well as they appear to do in the adult literature. This could be used as evidence either for different patterns of disease or that the putative patterns described in adult patients are not valid. Differences in recurrence rates following surgery have been reported using different cutpoints for patient age. Results are conflicting.

Chapters 18 and 19 of this volume, respectively, deal with issues related to the pediatric and geriatric populations with Crohn's disease.

D. Functional Status

1. The Pattern

Although various attempts at clinical classification have focused on disease location, indications for surgery, and recurrence, another potential classification framework could be constructed. Patients could be classified in terms of the impact of disease on their activities of daily living. Attempts have been made to measure the impact of disease on patient quality of life and concerns (42). Within the context of a clinical trial, quality of life measurements are often performed and one has been specifically developed for Crohn's disease (43).

Perhaps these instruments should now be applied to larger populations. Such a functional classification might have merit. It would allow the description of clinical populations to be used for comparative purposes. The classification could be tested to determine whether patients remain within strata, and it might be used to assist in identifying those patients who may require disability support.

E. Other Considerations

It is possible that associations between particular gene types and histological features or inflammatory or immunological processes (for example, cytokine metabolism) will be found. Currently, studies are confusing and a pattern cannot readily be perceived. Studies involving larger number of patients are required.

VI. CONCLUSION

Classification systems are relatively easy to derive. The measure of their validity is dependent on others repeating the study and finding similar outcomes. Their importance lies in providing carefully categorized cohorts of patients on which to base the search for the causes of Crohn's disease.

Until there is definite evidence for the involvement of a particular gene in Crohn's disease, advances in classification may be limited. Using the example of Weyand et al. it may be easier to move from finding the genotype to finding the phenotype (5).

REFERENCES

1. Hodgson HJF. The natural history of treated ulcerative colitis. Gastroenterology 1994; 107:300–308.
2. Lorig K, Lubeck D, Kraines RG, Seleznick M, Holman HR. Outcomes of self-help education for patients with arthritis. Arthritis Rheum 1993; 36:439–485.
3. Lorig K, Mazonson PD, Holman HR. Evidence suggesting that health education for self-management in patients with chronic arthritis has sustained health benefits while reducing health care costs. Arthritis Rheum 1993; 36:439–447.
4. The European Polycystic Kidney Disease Consortium. The polycystic kidney disease 1 gene encodes a 14 kb transcript and lies within a duplicated region on chromosome 16. Cell 1994; 77:881–894.
5. Weyand CM, Hicok KC, Conn DL, Goronzy JJ. The influence of HLA-DRB1 genes on disease severity in rheumatoid arthritis. Ann Intern Med 1992; 117:801–806.
6. Sackett DL, Whelan G. Cancer risk in ulcerative colitis: scientific requirements for the study of prognosis. Gastroenterology 1980; 78:1632–1634.
7. Lennard-Jones JE, Stadler GA. Prognosis after resection of chronic regional ileitis. Gut 1967; 8:332–336.
8. Truelove SC, Pena AS. Course and prognosis of Crohn's disease. Gut 1976; 17:192–201.
9. Mekhjian HS, Switz DM, Melnyk CS, Rankin GB, Brooks RK. Clinical features and natural history of Crohn's disease. Gastroenterology 1979; 77:898–906.
10. Steinhardt HJ, Loeschke K, Kasper H, Holtermuller KH, Schafer H. European Cooperative Crohn's Disease Study (ECCDS): clinical features and natural history. Digestion 1985; 31:97–108.
11. Farmer RG, Hawk WA, Turnbull RB Jr. Clinical patterns in Crohn's disease: a statistical study of 615 cases. Gastroenterology 1975; 68:627–635.
12. Whelan G, Farmer RG, Fazio VW, Goormastic M. Recurrence after surgery in Crohn's disease. Relationship to location of disease (clinical pattern) and surgical indication. Gastroenterology 1985; 88:1826–1833.
13. Harper PH, Fazio VW, Lavery IC, et al. The long-term outcome in Crohn's disease. Dis Colon Rectum 1987; 30:174–179.
14. Farmer RG, Whelan G, Fazio VW. Long-term follow-up of patients with Crohn's disease. Gastroenterology 1985; 88:1818–1825.

15. Holdstock G, Savage D, Harman M, Wright R. An investigation into the validity of the present classification of inflammatory bowel disease. Q J Med 1985; 54:183–190.

16. Binder V, Hendriksen C, Kreiner S. Prognosis in Crohn's disease—based on results from a regional patient group from the County of Copenhagen. Gut 1985; 26:146–150.

17. Higgins CS, Allan RN. Crohn's disease of the terminal ileum. Gut 1980; 21:993–940.

18. Lindhagen T, Ekelund G, Leandoer L, Hildell J, Lindstrom C, Wenckert A. Crohn's disease in a defined population course and results of surgical treatment 1. Small bowel disease. Acta Chir Scandinavia 1983; 149:407–413.

19. De Dombal FT, Burton I, Goligher JC. Recurrence of Crohn's disease after primary excisional surgery. Gut 1971; 12:519–527.

20. Sachar DB, Wolfson DM, Greenstein AJ, Goldberg J, Styczynski R, Janowitz HD. Risk factors for post-operative recurrence of Crohn's disease. Gastroenterology 1983; 85:917–921.

21. Rutgeerts P, Geboes K, Vantrappen G, Beyls J, Kerremans R, Hiele M. Predictability of the postoperative course of Crohn's disease. Gastroenterology 1990; 99:956–963.

22. Olaison G, Smedh K, Sjödahl R. Natural course of Crohn's disease after ileocolic resection: endoscopically visualised ileal ulcers preceding symptoms. Gut 1992; 33:331–335.

23. Trnka YM, Glotzer DJ, Kasdon EJ, Goldman H, Steer ML, Goldman LD. The long-term outcome of restorative operation in Crohn's disease. Ann Surg 1982; 196:345–355.

24. Griffiths AM, Wesson DE, Shandling B, Corey M, Sherman PM. Factors influencing post-operative recurrence of Crohn's disease in childhood. Gut 1991; 32:491–495.

25. Krause A, Bergman L, Norlen BJ. Crohn's disease A clinical study based on 186 patients. Scand J Gastroenterol 1971; 6:97–108.

26. Shivananda S, Hordijk ML, Pena AS, Mayberry JF. Crohn's disease: risk of recurrence and reoperation in a defined population. Gut 1989; 30:990–995.

27. Hellers G. Crohn's disease in Stockholm County. Acta Chir Scandinavia 1979; 490(suppl):1–84.

28. Greenstein AJ, Lachman P, Sachar DB, et al. Perforating and non-perforating indications for repeated operations in Crohn's disease: evidence for two clinical forms. Gut 1988; 29:588–592.

29. Pallone F, Boirivant M, Stazi MA, Cosintino R, Prantera C, Torsoli A. Analysis of clinical course of postoperative recurrence in Crohn's disease of distal ileum. Dig Dis Sci 1992; 37:215–219.

30. Sachar DB, Andrews HA, Farmer RG, et al. Proposed classification of patient subgroups in Crohn's disease. Gastroenterol Int 1992; 5:141–154.

31. De Dombal FT, Softley A. IOBID Report No. 1: observer variation in calculating indices of severity and activity in Crohn's disease. Special Report. Gut 1987; 28:474–481.

32. Musso A, Fiorentini MT, Sostegni R, et al. Subgroups classification in Crohn's disease: treatment and outcome in long-term follow-up (abstr). Gastroenterology 1994; 106:A742.

33. Farmer RG, Michener WM, Mortimer EA. Studies of family history among patients with inflammatory bowel disease. Clin Gastroenterol 1980; 9:271–280.

34. Orholm M, Munkholm P, Langholz E, Haagen Nielsen O, Sorensen TIA, Binder V. Familial occurrence of inflammatory bowel disease. N Eng J Med 1991; 324:84–88.

35. Tysk C, Lindberg E, Jarnerot G, Floderus-Myrhed B. Ulcerative colitis and Crohn's disease in an unselected population of monozygotic and dizygotic twins. A study of heritability and the influence of smoking. Gut 1988; 29:990–996.

36. Tokayer AZ, Ryedel B, Bayless TM. Possible role of heredity in site and transmural aggressive of Crohn's disease (abstr). Gastroenterology 1992; 102:A705.

37. Calkins BM. A meta-analysis of the role of smoking in inflammatory bowel disease. Dig Dis Sci 1989; 34:1841–1854.

38. Sutherland LR, Ramcharan S, Bryant H, Fick G. Effect of cigarette smoking on recurrence of Crohn's disease. Gastroenterology 1990; 98:1123–1128.

39. Persson P-G, Ahlbom A, Hellers G. Inflammatory bowel disease and tobacco smoke—a case-control study. Gut 1990; 31:1377–1381.

40. Cottone M, Rosselli M, Orlando A, et al. Smoking habits and recurrence in Crohn's disease. Gastroenterology 1994; 106:6431–648.
41. Russel MG, Bergers JM, Dorant E, Stockbrugger R, South Limburg IBD Study Group. Smoking worsens quality of life in Crohn's disease but not in ulcerative colitis (abstr). Gastroenterology 1994; 106:A763.
42. Drossman DA, Patrick DL, Mitchell CM, Zagami EA, Appelbaum MI. Health-related quality of life in inflammatory bowel disease: functional status and patient worries and concerns. Dig Dis Sci 1989; 34:1379–1386.
43. Irvine EJ, Feagan B, Rochon J, et al. Quality of life: a valid and reliable measure of therapeutic efficacy in the treatment of inflammatory bowel disease. Gastroenterology 1994; 106:287–296.

COMMENTARY

David B. Sachar   *The Mount Sinai Medical Center, New York, New York*

The Crohn's and Colitis Foundation of America recently convened a task force to propose a "Clinical Research Agenda" for the coming years. This group concluded, among other recommendations, that "inflammatory bowel disease is all too often considered as one disease process, or else is defined simply in terms of Crohn's disease or ulcerative colitis. However, the identification of sub-clinical markers combined with extensive epidemiological characterization supports the hypothesis that there are potentially several subgroups within each disease category." Focusing more specifically on Crohn's disease, an International Working Team (Gastroenterol Int 1994; 5:141–154) wrote "Crohn's disease is not a single homogeneous clinical entity. The various forms in which it appears are so fundamentally diverse in their course, prognosis, and responses to standard therapies that it is virtually meaningless to identify a case as 'Crohn's disease' in the absence of additional, more detailed descriptors."

Since Dr. Lloyd Sutherland is an experienced clinician, talented investigator, and critical observer in this field, it is not surprising that his chapter provides such an insightful review of the nearly 30-year search for "different patterns of Crohn's disease." As a confirmed "splitter" myself, I heartily endorse Dr. Sutherland's strong arguments for seeking to classify different subgroups of patients who present with the widely varied manifestations that we currently "lump" under the time-honored but uninformative name "Crohn's disease."

In my view, this chapter makes at least four important contributions to the ongoing debate over disease classification. First, it solidly outlines several justifications for dividing patients into phenotypical subgroups. To the benefits of providing prognostic information, we might add the opportunity for genetic counseling; to the etiological implications, we might add the alluring hopes for gene therapy; to the facilitating of individual treatment choices, we might add more refined selection of populations for clinical trials.

Second, Dr. Sutherland encourages our efforts by citing the precedents of other chronic diseases in which phenotypical classification has yielded valuable etiological or therapeutic lessons. To his examples of polycystic kidney disease and rheumatoid arthritis, we might add such other obvious models as type I and II diabetes, as well as the closer-to-home analogy of the belated distinction between ulcerative colitis and Crohn's disease of the colon—not to mention the further "splitting off" of various infectious and ischemic colitides.

Third, this chapter focuses welcome attention on the criteria needed for studies of natural history, including clear definitions of diseases and outcomes and corrections for biases and other compounding factors. Unfortunately, not only do we lack an unambiguous definition of Crohn's disease to start with, we do not even have readily available or reliable means of ruling out the diagnosis in presumed "normal" populations or "unaffected" relatives.

In the absence of any subclinical markers, such as insulin antibodies or impaired glucose tolerance for diabetes mellitus, we are in a position akin to being unable to recognize diabetes unless or until it presents with symptomatic hyperosmolarity or ketoacidosis. If, as Dr. Sutherland points out, our studies of "natural history" suffer from problems in distinguishing between reports of local versus referred or treated versus untreated patients, how much greater are our difficulties if we do not know how to date "onset" of disease or even how to tell the difference betweeen people who have the disease and people who don't.

Fourth, Dr. Sutherland has done a splendid job of reviewing and critiquing previous efforts at classifying Crohn's disease. Appropriately, he devotes most attention to the traditional anatomical classification based on small bowel versus colonic location. Not only is this system useful in predicting "clinical patterns" and complications, but as we and others have noted, some standard laboratory indicators may vary in their correlations with disease activity depending on anatomical distribution (J Clin Gastroenterol 1990; 12:643–646).

I will not comment in any detail on Dr. Sutherland's evaluations of these previous classifications because his critiques speak so well for themselves (and also because I have been heavily involved in promoting three of the four schemas he reviews). However, I must commend both his imaginativeness in proposing other possible classification systems and his caution in not jumping prematurely onto any of the current immunogenetic band wagons. The final chapter on this subject has yet to be written.

11
Immunosuppressive Therapy of Crohn's Disease: A Historical Perspective

Burton I. Korelitz   *Lenox Hill Hospital and New York University School of Medicine, New York, New York*

When I arrived at Mt. Sinai Hospital as an intern, many years had passed since the publication on regional ileitis by Crohn, Ginzburg, and Oppenheimer but management remained primarily in the hands of the surgeons (1). Drug therapy in recent years had been limited to a variety of sulfonamides, and gastroenterologists were slow to acknowledge that sulfasalazine should be favored. Even so, it did not work as well for ileitis as it did for ulcerative colitis.

The first edition of Dr. Crohn's book included data on course, complications, and treatment of ileitis, but not on corticosteroids, which became available soon afterward. Never before had such dramatic improvements been seen as those that followed treatment with corticosteroids and adrenocorticotropic hormone (ACTH). The outcome was favorably influenced, surgery could be postponed and performed electively, and the gastroenterologist inherited the primary responsibility for management and for clinical observation (2).

In retrospect, this period was one of relative complacency, particularly in the sense that there was a lack of search for new drugs. The initial euphoria warranted by the obvious elimination of the inflammatory process yielded to the stark realization and disappointment that (a) the effect was transient, (b) the inflammation returned not only with termination of drug therapy but also with its reduction in dose, (c) the inflammation responded less dramatically with subsequent courses of treatment, and (d) corticosteroids were no more effective than placebo in maintaining remission (3,4).

In the 1960s, nine prevalent phenomena merged to rekindle the effort to provide new treatment for inflammatory bowel disease (IBD):

1. The cause remained unknown.
2. The concept of autoimmune diseases had become popular (5,6).
3. The question was frequently raised as to whether Crohn's disease (and ulcerative colitis) could be autoimmune diseases.
4. Studies demonstrating autoantibodies in ulcerative colitis were being reported (7).
5. Elion and Hitchings concluded their experiments with azathioprine, demonstrating its ability to prevent rejection of the donor's transplanted kidney (8).

6. Reports demonstrated not only the success of long-term corticosteroid therapy but also its toxicity (9).

7. Winkelman and Brown reported a favorable experience with nitrogen mustards in the treatment of both ulcerative colitis and regional enteritis (10).

8. Bean had successfully treated an ulcerative colitis patient with 6-mercaptopurine (6-MP), a metabolic product of azathioprine, and was pursuing this early success (11,12).

9. Brooke et al. reported unheard of reversals of advanced Crohn's disease using azathioprine. Patients included those with complex fistulas and patients in whom all surgical efforts had failed.

Although later epidemiological data showed that the incidence of Crohn's disease was on the rise while that of ulcerative colitis was stable, in the 1960s, this was not yet apparent. After extensive exposure to ulcerative colitis with Banks and Zetzel at the Beth Israel Hospital in Boston, I was impressed with the many children with ulcerative colitis at Mt. Sinai who failed corticosteroid therapy, who were physically and emotionally traumatized by the toxicity of these drugs, who required colectomy and ileostomy, and who died (15,16). Accordingly, in January 1967, what was to prove to be a lifetime experience with 6-MP in the treatment of IBD was launched (17). This drug was used for ulcerative colitis patients who were considered failures of therapy with adrenal steroids and sulfaoalazine but who did not have an absolute indication for surgical intervention. My coworker in this study was Nathaniel Wisch, a hematologist, who favored 6-MP over azathioprine only because he had experience with its use in treating childhood leukemia. Furthermore, there was Food and Drug Administration (FDA) approval for that indication. As an outcome of this study, it was clear that 6-MP had no dramatic influence on the course of the disease as did ACTH and corticosteroids and that transient nausea and vomiting occurred frequently. Therefore, it had no role in fulminating disease. This had already been demonstrated for azathioprine by Bowen et al. whose report of toxicity when the drug was used in the sickest patients suggested that future consideration of immunosuppressives for ulcerative colitis be eliminated. The favorable results of our own study impressed us with a choice of candidates being those with prolonged ulcerative colitis, those with imcomplete response to steroids, those with complications of steroids or contraindications to their use, and those in whom sulfasalazine had failed, but not for those with fulminating disease or toxic megacolon.

Perhaps the most important observation was that the value of 6-MP could not be realized without long-term observation (17). Only 1 out of 14 patients remained incapacitated; the remaining 13 either went into remission or improved significantly. Based on this study—and later when the series had been increased to 25 patients—a long-term double-blind controlled study was planned (19).

Coincidentally, in the latter half of the 1960s, a few events occurred:

1. Daniel Present completed his fellowship in gastroenterology at Mt. Sinai. We had become friends, found that we shared common interests for clinical investigation in the field of IBD, and his enthusiasm for conducting a double-blind trial of immunosuppressive therapy was similar to my own.

2. The Ileitis Foundation was launched by Rosenthal, Modell, and Chief of Gastroenterology at Mt. Sinai, Henry D. Janowitz. The primary goal of the foundation was to encourage and support research in IBD, and Present became its first fellow.

My own early participation was encouraged by the founders because of my accumulated experience with ulcerative colitis. Soon thereafter, the name of the organization was changed to the National Foundation for Ileitis and Colitis.

3. Dr. Janowitz, in our discussion with him on our projected protocol, suggested a change of direction toward Crohn's disease rather than ulcerative colitis because it was already known that the letter was predisposed to the development of cancer of the colon but not yet known that this was also true of the former.

In 1969, Present and I launched our 2-year placebo-controlled, double-blind, crossover study of 6-mercaptopurine in the treatment of refractory Crohn's disease (20). The study was conducted primarily through our private offices, and, rather than using an index of Crohn's disease activity so that the response in diverse cases could be interpreted, we established goals of therapy for each case as had been done in the usual management of Crohn's disease until then and subsequently. The most common goals were elimination of corticosteroids, closing of fistulas, and prevention of small bowel obstruction. Elimination of the primary bowel symptoms was not a frequent goal because steroids, usually administered intravenously, temporarily accomplished this. Rather than stopping the steroids when the 6-MP was started, the steroids were reduced and eliminated when clinically feasible, serving as a variable measuring response to therapy.

Coincidentally, the National Cooperative Crohn's Disease Study was being conducted at 14 centers using Crohn's Disease Activity Index as a measure of response and comparing four treatment modalities: prednisone, sulfonamide, azathioprine, and placebo (22). This study led to its conclusion that azathioprine was ineffective (21). Based on their experience with azathioprine, Goldstein et al. provided a critique of the study which was soon followed by our own in which we pointed out the shortcomings of the NCCDS and encouraged clinical researchers to not yet disregard the use of immunosuppressive drugs (23,24). The major shortcoming of the NCCDS had been as follows:

1. The study was terminated at 17 weeks.
2. Azathioprine was eliminated because it caused pancreatitis before there were enough entries in this category to be statistically significant.
3. Steroids were eliminated before the assigned drug or placebo was started.
4. The amount of azathioprine used was relatively small (6-MP = 54% azathioprine by weight).

In 1980, our own study was published, showing conclusively that 6-MP was effective in Crohn's disease (20). The most clear-cut features of the study included:

1. Overall success in two out of three patients. Of the 83 patients, 39 received both placebo and 6-MP for 1 year each; 26 (67%) improved while receiving 6-MP and only 3 (8%) improved with placebo. This difference was highly statistically significant ($p < 0.0001$) (Table 1). Of the 83 patients, 33 received only one drug, either 6-MP or placebo; for the 19 receiving 6-MP, the rate of improvement was 79% compared with 29% in the 14 patients treated with placebo ($p < 0.05$) (see Table 1). To determine whether the outcome of the first year of trial influenced the outcome of the second year, a separate analysis was performed for 36 patients. This showed a significant difference favoring 6-MP: 26 (67%) versus 5 (14%) of 36 patients improved ($p < 0.0001$) (see Table 1).
2. Steroids were eliminated in 55% and the dose was reduced in 20% of patients.

TABLE 1   Results in Crossover and Noncrossover Patients

Treatment	Improved No. of Patients	Not Improved No. of Patients
39 Crossover patients[a]		
6-MP	26/39	13/39
Placebo	3/39	36/39
33 Noncrossover patients[b]		
6-MP	15/19	4/19
Placebo	4/14	10/14
Combined results in first year[c]		
6-MP	26/36	10/36
Placebo	5/36	31/36

[a]Whereas 67% of patients improved with 6-MP, only 8% improved with placebo. The difference is 59% with 95% confidence limits of 32% to 86% (p < 0.0001).
[b]Whereas 79% of patients improved with 6-MP, only 29% improved with placebo. The difference is 50% with 95% confidence limits of 20% to 80% (p < 0.05).
[c]Whereas 72% of patients improved with 6-MP, only 14% improved with placebo. The difference is 58% with 95% confidence limits of 40% to 77% (p < 0.001).

3. Fistulas were able to be closed.
4. It was confirmed that the drug was slow acting (mean response time 3.1 months) and, in most instances, required continuation or reintroduction of steroids to achieve full benefit (Table 2).
5. Toxicity was modest and there was no early mortality.

More specific data on fistulas followed (25). The 6-MP seemed to close fistulas in one-third of patients within 3½ months. The 6-MP (and azathioprine) proved to be the first drug to have this influence on Crohn's disease fistulas, except for metronidazole which had a favorable effect on perirectal fistulas. Abdominal wall fistulas improved or closed in 10 of 12 patients (83%), rectovaginal fistulas in 4 of 6 patients (67%), and enteroenteric

TABLE 2   Time Required for a Response to 6-MP

No. of Months	No. of Patients	Cumulative Percent Responding
< 1	4	10
2	19	56
3	5	68
4	5	81
5	2	85
6	3	93
> 6	3	100

fistulas in 5 of 7 patients (71%). The perirectal abscess and fistulas have sometimes led to diversionary surgery, usually with a colostomy. The results here have been disastrous, with recurrent Crohn's colitis in the stoma, diversionary colitis in the rectum, and persistence of perirectal sepsis. Even perirectal fistulas have closed or improved in 9 of 18 patients (50%). A modified Parks' operation combined with therapy with 6-MP often eradicates perirectal abscesses and fistulas in patients with recurrence following an incision and drainage procedure.

Other early observations regarding 6-MP in the treatment of Crohn's disease included:

1. The drug was more effective when the colon was involved (colitis and ileocolitis) than when the small bowel alone was involved.

2. O'Donoghue et al. showed that remission once established, was maintained by azathioprine in 79% of patients at 1 year but was not maintained with placebo (26) (Fig. 1). Early observations following completion of our controlled trial showed maintenance of remission in 19 of 20 patients (95%) after a mean of 37 months on 6-MP, whereas 26 of 32 (81%) relapsed after a mean of 6 months after their earlier favorable response.

3. When 6-MP was reintroduced in 16 patients after relapse, all patients improved with a mean response time of 1.5 months, considerably more rapidly than the first response (27).

Subsequently, my colleagues at Lenox Hill Hospital and I reported our long-term experience with 6-MP in the treatment of Crohn's disease (28). Again, therapeutic goals were established for each of the 148 patients and an index of Crohn's disease activity

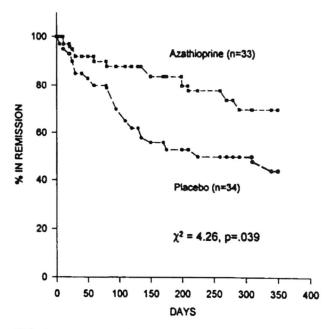

FIG. 1 Maintenance of remission by azathioprine.

created by a joint committee of the Crohn's and Colitis Foundation of America and the International Organization of Inflammatory Bowel Disease (CCFA/IOIBD) was calculated before and after therapy as well. Table 3 lists the goals and the successes observed.

Defined therapeutic goals were achieved in 68% of patients. The major successes included (a) elimination of steroids (66%, p < 0.001), (b) healing of internal fistulas and abscesses or improvement by elimination of discharge and tenderness (64%, p < 0.05), and (c) healing or improvement by elimination of pain, tenderness, and discharge of perirectal fistulas and abscesses (87%, p < 0.05). Other therapeutic goals that achieved 100% success were (a) healing or marked improvement of Crohn's disease of the stomach and duodenum and (b) permitting surgery to be performed electively after 6-MP allowed margins for surgical resection to be delineated. The 6-MP was less effective in achieving the therapeutic goals of preventing recurrent small bowel obstruction (43%) and eliminating abdominal masses (55%).

Other new findings included a 50% success rate in eliminating ileovesical fistulas, success in preventing recurrence of extraintestinal manifestations such as arthritis, erythema nodosum, pyoderma gangrenosum after steroids were eliminated, restoration of normal growth rate after steroids were eliminated, and promise that 6-MP would have prophylactic value after surgical resection. Only 10 patients (5%) who had gone into remission on 6-MP experienced exacerbation.

TABLE 3 Results of Therapeutic Goals

Goals	Patients (No.)	Goals (No.)	Achieved (%)
Eliminate steroids	125	82	65.6
Heal or improve internal fistulas	49	32	64.1
Rectovaginal	7	6	86.7
Ileorectal and ileosigmoidal	15	11	73.0
Other entero-enteric	5	2	40.0
Ileocutaneous	10	6	60.0
Colocutaneous	2	2	100.0
Ileovesical	10	5	50.0
Heal or improve perirectal abscesses/fistulas	34	23	67.6
Prevent recurrent small bowel obstruction	21	9	43.0
Prevent recurrent colonic obstruction due to strictures	7	6	85.7
Eliminate abdominal mass	9	5	55.5
Heal or improve recurrent ileitis in ileostomy	5	4	80.0
Heal or improve stomal abscess	3	2	66.6
Heal or improve Crohn's disease of stomach and duodenum	3	3	100.0
Heal pyoderma gangrenosum	1	1	100.0
Eliminate arthritis	8	7	87.5
Restore normal growth rate when retarded	4	3	75.0
Eliminate narcotics	3	2	66.0
Permit elective resection	5	5	100.0
Prophylaxis after resection (ongoing mean follow-up 41 months)	10	9	90.0
All goals	293	199	68.0

I. TOXICITY OF IMMUNOSUPPRESSIVE AGENTS

A. Historical Aspects

Experience with 6-MP in the treatment of leukemia and with azathioprine in treatment of rheumatoid arthritis and prevention of rejection of organ transplants disclosed that bone marrow suppression was dose related in such treatment. Both leukopenia and thrombocytopenia were reported. Hepatotoxicity was observed in both animals and humans, especially at a dosage of greater than 2.5 mg/kg per day.

Any kind of superinfection was theoretically possible, and induction of immunity to vaccines could have been compromised. The incidence of infection was markedly greater in the transplant cases than in the rheumatoid arthritis cases treated with azathioprine.

6-Mercaptopurine and azathioprine cause chromosomal aberrations in animals and humans, but these are reversible in humans. The drugs are carcinogenic in animals at the dosages used and, therefore, may increase the risk of neoplasia in humans. Because of the higher dosages used, the risk has been greater in transplant cases than in arthritis cases.

Allopurinol used to lower blood uric acid concentration, may delay the catabolism of 6-MP, accentuating its toxicity. When the two drugs are used concurrently, the 6-MP should be reduced by one-half to one-third.

B. Toxicity Clearly Related to 6-MP in the Treatment of Crohn's Disease

Data on the toxicity to 6-MP have been compiled for 396 patients seen by Present and Korelitz in their private practices in New York. Four types of toxicity directly attributable to 6-MP were identified, including pancreatitis, bone marrow depression, idiosyncratic/hypersensitivity reactions, and drug-induced hepatitis.

1. Pancreatitis

In 3% of patients, 12 with Crohn's disease and 1 with ulcerative colitis, pancreatitis was observed. The peak incidence was 21 days after starting the drug, and all but one case occurred within 32 days. Clinically, each case was mild, with symptoms of abdominal pain, nausea, vomiting, and elevation of serum amylase, all resolving quickly upon discontinuation of the drug. No hemorrhagic pancreatitis, hypocalcemia, pancreatic abscess, or pseudocyst formation was observed. Seven patients were later rechallenged with 6-MP or azathioprine, and, in each, the symptoms recurred rapidly (30). Clinically, the pancreatitis behaved like a sensitivity reaction, but attempts at desensitization were unsuccessful. Therefore, a single bout of 6-MP pancreatitis is considered a contraindication for future use, but a trial with a small dose of azathioprine may be clinically warranted.

2. Bone Marrow Depression

In 2% of patients, bone marrow suppression sufficient to necessitate hospitalization occurred, all during the early years before experience was gained in blood count monitoring and individual dosage adjustment (29). In these eight patients, the lowest white blood cell count (WBC) ranged from 300 to 2500, fever was present in seven, and blood cultures were positive in three. Septic complications were major in one patient, but none died. Characteristically, the bone marrow depression was followed by prolonged remission of the Crohn's disease or ulcerative colitis. This important observation has also been noted by others in relation to ulcerative colitis (31).

Leukopenia was noted at some time in most patients. White blood cell counts above

3500 were rarely associated with clinical problems and were managed by temporarily stopping the 6-MP and then resuming it at a lower dosage.

Subsequently, Connell et al. reported the experience from St. Mark's in London in 739 IBD patients treated with azathioprine (32). Only nine (1.2%) developed severe leukopenia (WBC < 2000); five of the nine had complications, which resulted in two deaths. Our experience suggests that use of current methods of monitoring would avoid this complication as would the availability of granulocyte-stimulating agents.

3. Idiosyncratic/Hypersensitivity Reactions

In addition to pancreatitis, other allergic-type reactions occurred within the first 3 weeks of treatment with 6-MP in 2% of patients: drug fever in eight, skin rash in two, arthralgia in one, and abdominal pain with normal serum amylases in one. I have also seen severe muscle pain occurring soon after treatment with 6-MP was initiated. Rechallenging the patient with 6-MP or azathioprine produced similar reactions. Nevertheless, desensitization with gradually increased doses, similar to the successful desensitization for sulfasalazine, has been tolerated and rewarding (33). Whether these reactions are idiosyncratic or represent an allergic phenomenon is unknown because no definitive immunological hypersensitivity mechanism has been defined.

4. Drug-Induced Hepatitis

Eleven patients in this study developed a type of hepatitis, but in only one patient could it clearly be attributed to 6-MP. In this patient, whose severe ulcerative colitis had gone into remission, liver tests normalized after cessation of the drug and again became abnormal after rechallenge. This is the only allergic type form of toxicity that seems to occur late in the course in most cases. It is also unique in that rechallenge is often tolerated. The only instances of immediate toxicity occurred at a later date in a patient whose 6-MP was initiated at 3 mg/kg of body weight.

C. Infections

Almost every type of infection reported in the IBD patinet treated with 6-MP has also been reported in patients not treated with immunosuppressive drugs. This is especially true of the patients with Crohn's disease, in whom infectious complications are frequent.

All of our patients on 6-MP who develop fever are instructed to discontinue the drug regardless of whether we think the fever is related to the underlying bowel disease, the drug, or an incidental illness such as an upper respiratory infection or flu. The most severe septic complication occurred in a young woman with ileocolitis who developed fever but did not stop the 6-MP for many weeks. She developed intra-abdominal abscesses requiring drainage, followed by a pyogenic liver abscess requiring further drainage. Cytomegalovirus and other organisms were cultured from different areas of the peritoneal cavity including a site of perforation. The patient recovered, and like other patients with profound immunosuppression in the course of 6-MP therapy, she had no sign of recurrence of Crohn's disease activity for 10 years, but she did at a later date.

One other patient developed a liver abscess that required drainage; there had been no bone marrow suppression in that case.

Five patients developed pneumonia; all responded to antibiotics and cessation of 6-MP therapy. Subsequently, the patients with pneumonia responded equally well to antibiotics while continuing 6-MP. Some patients reported frequent colds and upper respiratory infections, and some elected to discontinue 6-MP on that basis; it is difficult, however, to document a true increased incidence compared with the general population.

Herpes zoster occurred in eight patients while they were taking 6-MP. In all cases, the "shingles" took its usual course, even though 6-MP was continued at half dosage. Many years later, one patient had a recurrence of herpes zoster on his trunk when he was again taking 6-MP, and he suffered a 3-day syndrome consistent with encephalitis. There was no residual effect during a 9-year follow-up, and the patient's ulcerative colitis remained in remission. Subsequent experience suggests that there is no advantage to stopping the 6-MP during the course of herpes zoster infection.

D. Neoplasms

Like many infections, many neoplasms occur in patients with IBD not receiving immunosuppressives and among people without IBD. In Crohn's disease, an increased risk of extraintestinal neoplasms has been recognized (34). An appraisal of neoplastic risk has been made during or after 6-MP therapy (29). In one instance, the neoplasm was considered probably related to the 6-MP. This was a diffuse cerebral histiocytic lymphoma in a man with Crohn's disease who had taken 6-MP for approximately 9 months. He had stopped the drug 11 months before the onset of headaches, an evaluation of which led to the diagnosis. The tumor did not respond to therapy. Subsequently, 2 more cases of cerebral lymphoma in Crohn's disease patients treated with azathioprine were reported (35).

Other neoplasms occurring in patients who had earlier received 6-MP included an islet cell carcinoma of the pancreas, carcinomas of the lung in heavy cigarette smokers, one carcinoma of the breast, and a basal cell carcinoma. None of these was thought to be due to the immunosuppressive therapy. I have subsequently seen three patients who developed carcinoma of the breast who had previously been on 6-MP.

Cancer of the colon could be a complication of particular concern because Crohn's disease of the colon is a disease prone to the development of cancer, even without immunosuppressive drugs. Present and I looked back to our experience. I could identify seven patients in whom carcinoma of the ileum or colon developed; one had been treated with 6-MP. Present identified 10 patients, with 1 receiving 6-MP. Together, of 17 patients, 2 had received 6-MP therapy and 15 had not. Although these figures are not controlled and do not include a denominator, carcinoma seems to be far more common in Crohn's disease independent of immunosurrpressive therapy than associated with it. Connell et al. have reported that the incidence of colon cancer and death from cancer are not higher in IBD patients treated with azathioprine than IBD patients who are not (36).

Benign tumors disclosed at follow-up of patients previously on 6-MP included one prolactinoma, a papilloma in the bladder, and a follicular adenoma of the thyroid. None of these was thought to be related to the 6-MP.

E. Nausea

Nausea is seen as a fairly common side effect during the first month of 6-MP therapy. Occasionally, the dose of 6-MP has to be temporarily reduced. Rarely does does the drug need to be eliminated on this basis.

F. Mortality

Except in the patient with cerebral lymphoma, no deaths have been attributable to 6-MP. Lymphomas of the brain and other lymphomas have been reported in transplant patients on immunosuppressive therapy (37,38). It must, therefore, be assumed that cerebral lymphomas may in fact caused by 6-MP. There are, however, reports of increasing numbers of lymphomas in patients with Crohn's disease who are not taking immunosuppressives (39,40).

II. CONSIDERATIONS IN PREGNANCY

6-Mercaptopurine and azathioprine cause reversible chromosome damage in humans, but the true teratogenic effect of these drugs has not been studied in a systematic or controlled manner. On theoretical grounds, conception has been contraindicated in all patients on 6-MP therapy, whether male or female. Before initiating the drug, women should be tested for human chorionic gonadotropin (HcG) serum to eliminate the possibility of early pregnancy, and all couples should have a reliable method of birth control with which they are practiced and comfortable.

When pregnancy becomes a priority, we have recommended stopping the drug before eliminating contraceptives. In our toxicity study, we found that 16 pregnancies had occurred (29). In 10, the 6-MP had been terminated before contraception was recommended, but, in 6, the 6-MP had been continued for 3 to 4 weeks before the pregnancy was recognized. In 3 of the 6 as well as the 10 who stopped 6-MP earlier, the patient continued the pregnancy, and all 13 delivered full term. No abnormalities have been found in any of the 13 children. Subsequently, data from Alstead et al. served to conclude that there is no danger to the mother and fetus by taking azathioprine throughout pregnancy (41).

III. METHOTREXATE

Kozarek et al. called attention to the success of methotrexate, a folic acid inhibitor with both immunosuppressive and anti-inflammatory effects, in the treatment of inflammatory bowel disease (42). Their acute-phase trial resulted in improvement of Crohn's disease in 80% of patients using 25 mg intramuscular one time/week for 12 weeks, followed by 15 mg orally one time/week thereafter with tapering of the dose. At the time of intermediate follow-up, two of three patients with Crohn's disease who had responded remained in remission (43).

Subsequently, a group at St. Louis Hospital in Paris treated 39 patients with refractory Crohn's disease with 1 M methotrexate, and 72% were in remission at 3 months, but only 25% maintained the remission at 18 months (44). Side effects were reported in 56%. Methotrexate toxicity includes nausea, stomatitis, leukopenic abnormal liver function tests, pneumonitis, and teratogenesis. A preliminary report of the first placebo-controlled trial has concluded that the drug offers no significant advantage (45). Nevertheless, the drug retains a role in the treatment of Crohn's disease patients who have either failed or have not tolerated 6-MP.

IV. CYCLOSPORINE

The marked difference between cyclosporine and 6-MP/azathioprine in the treatment of inflammatory bowel disease is that when they work, the former works fast and the latter works slowly. Cyclosporine acts on T lymphocytes rather than B lymphocytes and inhibits their proliferation while at the same time activating their primary helper T cells. Ultimately, the rapid onset of action is due to inhibiting the secretion of interleukin 2.

Brynskov et al. conducted the first controlled trial of oral cyclosporine given at 5 to

7 mg/kg per day to chronically ill patients with Crohn's disease (46). It showed a response rate of 59% and a coincident 32% response for placebo (46). As with previous uncontrolled trials, the response was rapid (2 weeks). In short, the trial was successful but the results were not impressive. Hanauer and Smith treated Crohn's disease patients with various fistulas with cyclosporine intravenously at 4 mg/kg per day for 14 days and then orally thereafter at 6 to 8 mg/kg per day. Eighty-eight percent responded in the acute phase to intravenous cyclosporine with closure of fistulas in 44% and improvement in another 44%. Two-thirds of patients maintained improvement in the chronic phase and steroids could be discontinued in 75%. Another trial has shown no value for oral cyclosporine added to conventional treatment (48). A study of oral cyclosporine versus placebo to prevent relapses in Crohn's disease in 305 patients led to the conclusion that cyclosporine is ineffective for this purpose as well (49).

Presumably, malabsorption is the factor in Crohn's disease that accounts for a more favorable response to intravenous rather than oral cyclosporine.

Toxicity is of great concern when considering use of cyclosporine, particularly intravenously. The foremost toxic effect is nephrotoxicity, which can be kept at a minimum by careful monitoring of the blood urea nitrogen and creatinine, by keeping the cyclosporine blood level in a therapeutic range, and by avoiding non-steroidal anti-inflammatory drugs while they may potentiate the effect. Lymphoma and carcinoma are also of concern, but the doses and duration used in the treatment of IBD have not served to dominate consideration in management. Other complications such as tremors, hirsutism, gingival hyperplasia, paresthesias, headaches, and hypertension, although common, are almost always transient.

Although the experience with cyclosporine in Crohn's disease is limited, a preliminary conclusion is that its major role will prove to be in the intravenous treatment of very sick patients with ulcerative colitis and in those who have failed treatment with intravenous steroids. Presumably, malabsorption is the factor in Crohn's disease that accounts for a poorer response to oral medication than in ulcerative colitis.

V. T-LYMPHOCYTE APHERESIS

Remission has been achieved using T-lymphocyte apheresis in sick patients with Crohn's disease but treatment is long, expensive, and not long lasting (50). A recent study has since raised doubt of any further role for this technique (51).

VI. WHEN TO INITIATE IMMUNOSUPPRESSIVE THERAPY

The question arises whether more goals would be achieved if 6-MP were started earlier in the course of Crohn's disease when complications of the disease are less severe. Inflammation and strictures composed of cellular infiltrate and edema are more likely to be reversible than the more advanced fibrotic phase of longer-standing disease. It has been our policy that once the diagnosis of Crohn's disease is made and its manifestations are mild to treat first with sulfasalazine or one of the oral 5-aminosalicylic (5-ASA) products. This is true whether the distribution of disease is colitis, in which the opportunity for success is best; ileocolitis, in which the drug is usually effective; or ileitis, in which the response is least. In each distribution, there are some patients who never require an additional drug. For the sicker patient, we generally use corticosteroids either by the intravenous or the oral route in proportion to severity to bring the disease into remission.

The 5-ASA products may then have a better chance of success. If, however, the steroids cannot be eliminated after repeated attempts with recurrent activity, we recommend using 6-MP either alone or coincident with the reintroduction of steroids at a high dosage to allow time for the 6-MP to be effective.

There are exceptions to the above policy. If the dominating symptoms are those of perirectal fistula and/or abscess, we favor a trial of metronidazole rather than 6-MP. If this drug fails, 6-MP would be appropriate treatment, or, in some cases, drainage of the abscess or a modified Parks' procedure would be indicated followed by introduction of the 6-MP.

Only generalizations can be made about indications for 6-MP other than failure of sulfasalazine, corticosteroids, and, in some cases, metronidazole. It is certainly indicated more often when the Crohn's disease is totally colonic, but, even with small bowel disease already complicated by obstruction, 6-MP has been successful (28). The most severely ill patients that we have treated have been those with extensive refractory Crohn's disease with complication of high-dosage steroid therapy imposed on the primary bowel disease. 6-Mercaptopurine has been effective in all kinds of fistulas, extensive disease, recurrent disease, retarded growth and development, Crohn's disease of the stomach and duodenum, narcotic-dependence, and resistant extraintestinal manifestions. A trial of 6-MP should be favored in any patinet who depends on any dosage of corticosteroids for long periods to control the disease. The absolute indications for surgery in Crohn's disease have been reduced to free perforation, massive hemorrhage, possible appendicitis, and carcinoma. All other indications are relative.

VII. THE CURRENT AND THE FUTURE

Of all the drugs available with immunosuppression as the primary mechanism, 6-MP and azathioprine have had the most enduring role and continue to show the most promise for the future. Despite the disadvantage of its longer period in becoming effective, 6-MP, once introduced, has been consistently effective in two-thirds of patients with otherwise refractory Crohn's disease and in half of those with ulcerative colitis. Azathioprine has also been effective for the same groups of patients. Because 6-MP is a metabolic by-product of azathioprine, presumably, weight for weight, its favorable effect is not as great as the purer compound, 6-MP. Nevertheless, this has never been studied by controlled trial.

More importantly, why are favorable results of treatment consistently approximately 66% in Crohn's disease rather than 100%? What accounts for the other one-third? Perhaps the answer lies in the pathology of Crohn's disease, particularly in the small bowel where repeated attacks of inflammation result in fibrosis, which, to date, has been irreversible. After all, success with 6-MP in preventing small bowel obstruction has been consistently less than for other indications such as elimination of steroids and closure of fistulas.

Perhaps the answer lies in the role of inducing leukopenia with 6-MP/azathioprine. In retrospect, those patients who did develop leukopenia had greater success than those who did not (Fig. 2 and Table 4) (52). Furthermore, the success came earlier and was longer lasting, and those who did develop leukopenia had no clinical bone marrow depression. This can be attributed, in part, to what has been learned about careful monitoring of blood counts. My own approach is to have the patient undergo a complete blood count weekly for the first 3 weeks. Then, if the white blood cell count does not decrease and there is no clinical indication for increasing the dose of 6-MP, the time between blood counts may be extended. If, at any time the symptoms recur, however, and the white blood cell count permits, the dose of 6-MP should be increased. At this point, monitoring should return to

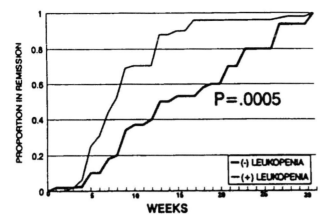

FIG. 2 Remission rate by presence or absence of leukopenia.

being weekly for 3 weeks. Another time to monitor the blood count particularly carefully is when the steroids are reduced or are to be eliminated. Because the steroids raise the white blood cell count, this counteraction is lost, and the patient may be vulnerable. In all cases, the patient must contact the physician's office after each blood count measurement to receive new directions as to dose and when the next count should be done. Platelets should be included in the count because infrequently thrombocytopenia also is caused by 6-MP therapy.

Another consideration is why leukopenia develops so easily in one patient but not in another. While some patients tolerate as much as 200 mg/day without apparent effect on white blood count, others tolerate only tiny doses such as 12.5 mg/week, or even less. When leukopenia is first recognized in these patients, they are almost always doing better than those without leukopenia, but when the dose of 6-MP is further and further reduced, the value of leukopenia is replaced by loss of overall drug efficacy.

Hematologists/oncologists have accumulated a large experience with 6-MP in the treatment of childhood leukemias (53). They have made us aware of the enzyme thiopurine methyltransferase, which hastens the metabolism of 6-MP. In those patients with a high enzyme level, we would expect rapid degradation of 6-MP, no leukopenia, and less therapeutic effect, whereas those with little or no enzyme may develop leukopenia, bone marrow depression, and an early response. These possibilities must be submitted to close scrutiny. Perhaps we should aim for higher doses of 6-MP in treating Crohn's disease (54).

When should 6-MP therapy be stopped? There are, as yet, no rules, and toxicity does not seem to be in proportion to duration of therapy. There is preliminary evidence that the longer the duration of therapy, the longer the remission ending after the drug is stopped

TABLE 4 Recurrence Rate and Time to Recurrence in 77 Patients Achieving Remission According to Leukopenia

	Leukopenia (No., %)	No Leukopenia (No., %)
Recurrence	5, 10.6%	4, 13.3%
Time to recurrence (mo)	21	12

(55). The most influential factor in stopping 6-MP therapy is its failure. This usually takes a full year to determine. In those whose treatment has been successful, the most common priority in stopping the drug is the desire for pregnancy. The next greatest indication is fear. At the end of 2 years of remission on 6-MP, I usually stop the drug for this indication. For those with less fear, no fear at all, or the need to be well far outweighing any fear, I usually reduce the dose of the drug rather than stop it, and then repeat this exercise at a later date. The reward for this approach is the mildness of the recurrence compared with that which occurs when the drug is stopped and the greater likelihood of response when the dose is increased once again.

A fairly dramatic response of resistant Crohn's Disease to an anti-Tumor Necrosis Factor (TNF) monoclonal antibody has been reported by Van Dullimen [56] and colleagues in Amsterdam and Centocor Inc. of Malvern, Pennsylvania. TNF has been considered a major mediator of inflammation in Crohn's Disease.

Impressive results were obtained in at least 8 out of 10 patients and the drug seemed to be quite safe. Perhaps this opens a door to still more focused immunosuppressive therapy than so far offered by 6-MP, azathioprine, methotrexate, and cyclosporine.

REFERENCES

1. Crohn BB, Ginzburg L, Oppenheimer GD, Regional ileitis: a pathological and clinical entity. JAMA 1932; 99:1323–1329.
2. Korelitz BI, Lindner AE. The influence of corticotrophin and adrenal steroids in the course of ulcerative colitis. Gastroenterology 1964; 46:671–679.
3. Spencer SA, Kirsner JB, Mlynaryk P, Reed PI, Palmer WL. Immediate and prolonged therapeutic effects of corticotrophin and adrenal steroids in ulcerative colitis: observations in 340 cases of period up to ten years. Gastroenterology 1962; 42:113–129.
4. Jones JH, Lennard-Jones JE. Corticosteroids and corticotrophin in the treatment of Crohn's disease. Gut 1966; 7:181–187.
5. Mackay IR, Burnet FM. Autoimmune disease: pathogenesis, chemistry, and therapy. Springfield, IL: Charles C Thomas, 1963:237–239.
6. Skinner MD, Schwartz RS. Medical progress: immunosuppressive therapy. N Engl J Med 1972; 287:221–227.
7. Broberger O. Immunologic studies in ulcerative colitis. Gastroenterology 1964; 47:229–240.
8. Elion GB, Hitchings GH. Azathioprine. Handbook of Experimental Pharmacology. New York: Springer-Verlag, 1975:404–425.
9. Sparberg M, Kirsner JB. Long term corticosteroid therapy for regional enteritis. Am J Dig Dis 1966; 11:865–880.
10. Winkelman EJ, Brown GH. Nitrogen mustard in the treatment of chronic ulcerative colitis and regional enteritis. Cleveland Clin Q 1965; 32:165.
11. Bean RHD. The treatment of chronic ulcerative colitis with 6-Mercaptopurine. Med J Aust 1962; 2:592–593.
12. Bean RHD. Treatment of ulcerative colitis with antimetabolites. BMJ 1966; 1:1081–1084.
13. Brooke BN, Hoffmann DC, Swarbrick ET. Azathioprine for Crohn's disease. Lancet 1969; 12:612–614.
14. Brooke BH, Javett SL, Davison OW. Further experience with azathioprine for Crohn's disease. Lancet 1970; 2:1050–1053.
15. Banks BM, Korelitz BI, Zetzel L. The course of nonspecific ulcerative colitis. Reviewing twenty years experience and late results. Gastroenterology 1957; 32:983–1012.
16. Korelitz BI, Gribetz D, Danziger I. The prognosis of ulcerative colitis with onset in childhood. I. The presteroid era. Ann Intern Med 1962; 57:592–597.

17. Korelitz BI, Wisch N. Long term therapy of ulcerative colitis with 6-mercaptopurine: a personal series. Am J Dig Dis 1972; 17:111–118.

18. Bowen GE, Irons GV Jr, Rhodes JD, Kirsner JB. Early experience with azathioprine in ulcerative colitis. JAMA 1966; 195:166–170.

19. Korelitz BI, Glass JL, Wisch N. Long-term immunosuppressive therapy of ulcerative colitis. Continuation of a personal series. Am J Dig Dis 1973; 18:317–322.

20. Present DH, Korelitz BI, Wisch N, et al. Treatment of Crohn's disease with 6-mercaptopurine. A long term, randomized, double blind study. N Engl J Med 1980; 302:981–987.

21. Summers RW, Switz DM, Sessions JT Jr, et al. National Cooperative Crohn's Disease Study: results of drug treatment. Gastroenterology 1979; 77:847–869.

22. Best WR, Becktel JM, Singleton JW, Kern F. Development of a Crohn's disease activity index. Gastroenterology 1976; 70:433–444.

23. Goldstein F, Thornton JJ, Abramson J. Comments on National Cooperation Crohn's Disease Study (NCCDS). Gastroenterology 1980; 78:1647–1648.

24. Korelitz BI, Present DH. Shortcomings of the National Cooperative Crohn's Disease Study: in the exclusion of azathioprine without adequate trial. Gastroenterology 1981; 80:193–194.

25. Korelitz BI, Present DH. Favorable effect of 6-mercaptopurine in fistulas of Crohn's disease. Dig Dis Sci 1985; 30:58–64.

26. O'Donoghue DP, Dawson AM, Powell-Tuck J, et al. Double blind withdrawal trial of azathioprine as maintenance treatment of Crohn's disease. Lancet 1978; 2:955–957.

27. Korelitz BI. Therapy of inflammatory bowel disease including use of immunosuppressive agents. Clin Gastroenterol 1980; 9:331–349.

28. Korelitz BI, Adler DJ, Mendelsohn RA, Sacknoff AL. Long-term experience with 6-mercaptopurine in the treatment of Crohn's disease. Am J Gastroenterol 1993; 88:1198–1205.

29. Present DH, Meltzer SJ, Krumholz M, et al. 6-Mercaptopurine in the management of inflammatory bowel disease: short-term and long-term toxicity. Ann Intern Med 1989; 3:641–649.

30. Haber CJ, Meltzer SJ, Present DH, Korelitz BI. Natural course of pancreatitis caused by 6-mercaptopurine in the treatment of inflammatory bowel disease. Gastroenterology 1986; 91:982–986.

31. Burke DA, Dixon MF, Axon ATR. Ulcerative colitis. Prolonged remission following azathioprine induced pancrit. J Clin Gastroenterol 1989; 11:327–330.

32. Connell WR, Kamm MA, Lennard-Jones JE, et al. Twenty-seven years experience in 739 patients of bone marrow toxicity from azathioprine in inflammatory bowel disease. Gastroenterology 1993; 102:A609.

33. Korelitz BI, Present DH, Rubin PH, Fochios SE. Desensitization to sulfasalazine after hypersensitivity reactions in patients with inflammatory bowel disease. J Clin Gastroenterol 1984; 6:27–31.

34. Greenstein AJ, Gennuso R, Sachar DD, et al. Extraintestinal cancers in inflammatory bowel disease. Cancer 1985; 56:2914–2921.

35. Lemann M, Bonhomme P, Bitoun A, et al. Traitement de la Maladie de Crohn par azathioprine ore la 6-Mercaptopurine. Gastroenterol Clin 1990; 14:548–554.

36. Connell WR, Kinlen LJ, Ritchie JK, et al. Cancer risks from azathioprine in inflammatory bowel disease. Gastroenterology 1994; 106:A667.

37. Schenk SA, Penn I. De-novo brain tumors in renal transplant recipients. Lancet 1971; 1:983–986.

38. Penn I, Hammond W, Brettschneider L, et al. Malignant lymphoma in the transplantation patients. Transplant Proc 1969; 1:106–112.

39. Glick SN, Teplick SK, Goodman LR, et al. The development of lymphoma in patient with Crohn's disease. Radiology 1984; 153:337–339.

40. Greenstein AJ, Mullin GE, Strauchen JA, et al. Lymphoma in inflammatory bowel disease. Cancer 1992; 69:1119–1123.

41. Alstead EM, Ritchie JK, Lennard-Jones JE, et al. Safety of azathioprine in pregnancy in inflammatory bowel disease. Gastroenterology 1990; 90:443–446.

42. Kozarek RA, Patterson DJ, Gelfand MD, et al. Methotrexate induces clinical and histological remission in patients with refractory inflammatory bowel disease. Ann Intern Med 1989; 110:353–356.

43. Kozarek RA, Patterson DJ, Butoman VA. Long term use of methotrexate in inflammatory bowel disease. Gastroenterology 1992; 102:648A.

44. Chamiot-Prieur C, Mesnard B, Lemann M, et al. Treatment of refractory Crohn's disease with methotrexate. Gastroenterology 1994; 106:A745.

45. Fergus B, et al. North American Crohn's Study Group. A Multicentre trial of methotrexate treatment for Crohn's disease. Gastroenterology 1994; 106:A745.

46. Brynskov J, Freund L, Rasmussen SM, et al. A placebo-controlled, double-blind randomized trial of cyclosporine, therapy in active Crohn's disease. N Engl J Med 1985; 321:845–850.

47. Hanauer SB, Smith MB. Rapid closure of Crohn's disease fistulas with continuous intravenous cyclosporine. AM J Gastroenterol 1993; 88:646–649.

48. Lobo AJ, Juby LD, Rothwell J. Long term treatment of Crohn's disease with cyclosporine; the effect of a very low dose on maintenance of remission. J Clin Gastroenterol 1991; 13:42–45. Gastroenterology 1992; 102:591A.

49. Archambault A, Feagan B, Fedorak R, et al. The Canadian Cyclosporine Crohn's Relapsed Prevention Trial. Gastroenterology 1992; 102:591A.

50. Bicks RO, Groshart KD. The current status of T lymphocyte apheresis (TLA) treatment of Crohn's disease. J Clin Gastroenterology 1989; 11:136–138.

51. Lerebours E, Bussel A, Modigliani R, et al. Treatment of Crohn's disease by lymphocyte apheresis: a randomized controlled trial. Gastroenterology 1994; 107:357–361.

52. Colonna T, Korelitz BI. The role of leukopenia in the 6-mercaptopurine induced remission of refractory Crohn's disease. Am J Gastroenterol 1994; 89:362–366.

53. Lennard L, VanLoon J, Weinshilbourn R. Pharmacogenetics of acute azathioprine toxicity relationship to thiopurine methyltransferase genetic polymorphism. Pharmacol Ther 1989; 46:149–154.

54. Lennard L, Lilleyman JS. Are children with lyumphoblastic leukaemia given enough 6-mercaptopurine? Lancet 1987; 2:785–787.

55. Bouchnik Y, Scemama G, Lemann R, et al. Effect of immunosuppressive therapy withdrawal on the course of Crohn's disease in patients successfully maintained in prolonged remission using azathioprine or 6-mercaptopurine. Gastroenterology 1994; 106:A655.

56. Van Dulleman HM, Sandes JHV, Hommes DW, et al. Treatment of Crohn's Disease with anti-Tumor Necrosis Factor chimeric monoclonol Antibody (cA2). Gastroenterology 1995; 109:129–135.

12

Treatment of Active Crohn's Disease with Salazopyrine and Derivatives of Aminosalicylic Acid (5-ASA)

Cosimo Prantera, Maria Lia Scribano, and Eva Berto   *Ospedale Nuovo Regina Margherita, Rome, Italy*

I. SALAZOPYRINE

For the past 50 years, Salazopyrine (sulfasalazine) has been regarded as the founder drug in the treatment of chronic inflammatory bowel disease (IBD). Introduced in 1940 by Nanna Svartz for the treatment of rheumatic diseases, Salazopyrine (SASP) is chemically composed of 5-aminosalicylic acid (5-ASA) and sulfapyridine (SP) linked by an azo bond.

A. Metabolism

When taken orally, 20% to 30% of the drug is absorbed at the level of the upper intestinal tract, and approximately 70% to 80% reaches the colon where the azo linkage is cleaved by the intestinal bacteria, thus liberating SP and 5-ASA (1). SP is rapidly absorbed by the colonic mucosa, metabolized by the processes of acetylation, hydroxylation, and glucuronidation, and subsequently excreted in the urine as such or in the form of metabolites (2). Traces of SP are found in the blood between three and five hours after oral intake (3). High blood levels of this molecule appear to be responsible for the majority of side effects caused by SASP, depending mainly on slow or rapid acetylator phenotype (4). Only a minimal part of 5-ASA is absorbed at the colonic level, rapidly acetylated, and excreted in the urine (2). The greater part, therefore, remains in contact with the colonic mucosa where it exerts its topical anti-inflammatory action and is then eliminated in the feces (5).

B. Mechanism of Action

One of the most likely hypotheses regarding the mechanism of action of SASP is that the 5-ASA, liberated by the cleavage of the azo bond by the colonic bacteria, represents through its anti-inflammatory action the therapeutically active part of the molecule (6). However, the efficacy of SASP demonstrated in patients with ileitis who had undergone ileostomies and in whom the substance was found in the feces in the measure of 66% to 75% would seem to suggest a therapeutic action carried out also by the unmetabolized drug (7). Recent studies have shown that SASP and its metabolites have multiple mechanisms of action that lead to an overall inhibition of the inflammatory activity mediated by cells or by chemical substances, and to a blockage of the prostaglandin metabolism (8) (Table 1).

1. Inhibition of Prostaglandin Biosynthesis

Based on the hypothesis that increase in the synthesis of prostaglandin may play an important role in the pathophysiology of IBD, several authors have evaluated the effect of SASP and its derivatives on prostanoid biosynthesis (9,10). Studies initially carried out on laboratory animals and later on the colonic mucosa of normal subjects and of patients suffering from IBD have shown that SASP and 5-ASA can inhibit the synthesis of prostaglandin E, of prostacyclin, and of thromboxane B2 (11–14). However, the therapeutic inefficacy in the treatment of IBD of other potent cyclooxygenase inhibitors such as indomethacin would seem to indicate that this mechanism is only partially involved in the pathophysiology of these diseases (15).

2. Inhibition of Lipoxygenase Product Synthesis

Many studies have been carried out on the effects of SASP and its derivatives on the formation of lipoxygenase metabolites inasmuch as the reduction of leukotriene B4 (LTB4) and other chemotactic lipid levels would appear to lead to a reduced degree of inflammation (8,16,17). These studies have led to the following observations:

> Sulfasalazine inhibits the formation at the level of human colonic mucosa of chemotactic hydroxyeicosatetraenoic acids (HETEs), of LTB4, and of sulfidopeptide-leukotrienes (LTC4, D4, E4) (18).
>
> Aminosalicylic acid reduces the production of LTB4 in the colonic mucosa both in normal subjects and in patients with Crohn's disease (CD) (12).

TABLE 1 Effects of SASP, 5-ASA, and Sulfapyridine on Various Metabolic Sites

	SASP	5-ASA	Sulfapyridine
Cyclooxygenase products			
Inhibition of prostaglandin synthesis (9,10)	Yes	Yes	No
Inhibition of prostacyclin synthesis (13,14)	Yes	Yes	Yes
Inhibition of thromboxane B2 synthesis (13,14)	Yes	Yes	Yes
Lipoxygenase products			
Inhibition of 5-HETE production (11)	Yes	No	No
Inhibition of LTB4 synthesis (12,16)	Yes	Yes	NR
Inhibition of LTC4, D4, E4 synthesis (18)	Yes	Yes	Yes
Inhibition of platelet-activating factor release (19)	Yes	Yes	No
Leukocyte functions			
Inhibition of neutrophil chemotaxis (20,21)	Yes	Yes	Yes
Inhibition of neutrophil myeloperoxydase (22)	Yes	Yes	No
Inhibition of cytotoxic effects on neutrophils	NR	Yes	No
Inhibition of cell-mediated cytotoxicity (24)	Yes	No	Yes
Inhibition of IL-1, TNF, IgA, IgG, IgM production (8,25,26)	Yes	Yes	NR
Reactive oxygen metabolites			
Scavenger action on reactive oxygen metabolites (27)	Yes	Yes	NR

NR = not reported; HETE = hydroxyeicosatetraenoic; LT = leukotriene; IL = interleukin; TNF = tumor necrosis factor.

Aminosalicylic acid and SP reduce the levels of LTC4, D4, and E4, but they are less effective than SASP in reducing the formation of 5-HETEs (11).

Aminosalicylic acid and SASP appear to inhibit platelet-activating factor release, probably through an effect on the phospholipase A2 (19).

3. Inhibition of Leukocyte Function

It has been noted that SASP, 5-ASA, and SP have several effects on neutrophils, monocytes, macrophages, platelets and mast cells. The principal effects can be summarized as follows:

Sulfasalazine and, to a certain extent, 5-ASA inhibit neutrophil chemotaxis, reduce neutrophil myeloperoxydase activity, and block bacterial or biopeptide activation of granulocytes through receptorial mechanisms, thus reducing the degree of inflammatory response (20–22).

Aminosalicylic acid inhibits the cytotoxic effects of various stimuli on human neutrophils; this could be linked to the stabilization of lysosomal membranes and reduction of enzyme release (8,20,23).

Sulfasalazine inhibits chemotaxis and phagocytosis by monocytes at therapeutic doses of the drug, as well as inhibits cell-mediated cytotoxicity (21,24).

Sulfasalazine reduces the production of interleukin 1 (IL-1), tumor necrosis factor (TNF), and the antibodies IgA, IgG, and IgM (8,25).

It can be assumed that the anti-inflammatory action of both SASP and 5-ASA is largely mediated by the effects on granulocyte and lymphocyte functions when therapeutic doses of the drugs are used (8).

4. Effects on Reactive Oxygen Metabolites

Both SASP and 5-ASA carry out a scavenger action on reactive oxygen metabolites (27). In vitro experiments, moreover, have shown that 5-ASA chelates iron, whereas SP has a much weaker action on hydroxyl radicals (28,29). In man, the stool concentration of 5-ASA after an average dose of SASP is approximately 10 times more than the concentration of the parent molecule (8). This suggests that 5-ASA is mainly responsible for the therapeutic efficacy of SASP; however, the intact molecule of SASP found at the ileal and colonic level also contributes to the anti-inflammatory action. SP, on the contrary, acts at fewer sites; it is mostly absorbed into the systemic circulation and is, therefore, less involved in the therapeutic action of SASP. It is, however, largely responsible for the side effects caused by the drug (4,30).

C. General Side Effects

The use of SASP in the treatment of IBD is hampered by side effects in a percentage of patients varying between 10% and 45% (Table 2) (4,30). Most side effects seem to be linked to high serum levels of SP found principally in patients who are of the slow acetylator phenotype (4).

There are two main groups of side effects (31–55). The first group seems to be dosage-related and is found in patients who are slow acetylators of the sulfamide molecule who tend to accumulate SP in their serum (4,56). Side effects are general and appear within the first 8 to 12 weeks of treatment, with doses of SASP varying from 4 to 8 g/day and with serum concentrations of SP greater than 50 ng/ml (4). The second group is considered

TABLE 2 Side Effects Caused by Sulfasalazine

Organ System	Side Effect	High Sulfapyridine Level	Hypersensitivity
Hematologic	Agranulocytosis (31)	No	Yes
	Hemolytic anemia (32)	Yes	No
	Megaloblastic anemia (33)	No	Yes
	Erythroid aplasia (34)	No	Yes
	Megakaryocytic aplasia (34)	No	Yes
Pulmonary	Eosinophilic pneumonitis (35)	Yes	No
	Bronchospasm (36)	Yes	No
	Fibrosing alveolitis (37)	Yes	No
Dermatologic	Maculopapular skin rash (4)	No	Yes
	Skin rash, lymphadenopathy, and fever (38)	No	Yes
	Exfoliative dermatitis (39)	No	Yes
	Stevens-Johnson syndrome (40)	No	Yes
	Lyell's syndrome (41)	No	Yes
Hepatic	Acute cholestatic hepatitis (42)	No	Yes
	Granulomatous hepatitis (43)	No	Yes
Rheumatologic	Lupus-like syndrome (44)	No	Yes
	Raynaud's phenomenon (45)	No	Yes
Gastroenterologic	Nausea, vomiting, anorexia (30,46)	Yes	No
	Abdominal pain (30)	Yes	No
	Pancreatitis (47)	No	Yes
	Bloody diarrhea (48,49)	No	Yes
Genital	Male infertility (50,51)	No	Yes
	Oligospermia (52)	No	Yes
Miscellaneous	Cyanosis (53)	Yes	No
	Neurotoxicity (54)	No	Yes
	Hair loss (55)	No	Yes

to be the idiosyncratic side effects caused by hypersensitivity reactions; they are not dose-related, are unpredictable, and generally appear at the beginning of therapy (30).

D. Desensitization

Patients who have experienced side effects during treatment with SASP may undergo desensitization therapy, which not infrequently enables them to take the drug for long periods (4). In general, when patients are likely to undergo prolonged treatment with SASP with dosages higher than 4 g/day, it is advisable to determine their acetylator phenotype and their serum levels of sulfapyridine (4,56). One of the first proposed desensitization programs suggests that after a temporary suspension of 1 to 2 weeks, the drug be reintroduced at dosages beginning with 0.5 g/day and increasing to 2 g/day. When patients have experienced serious adverse events, it is advisable to begin with a lower dosage of 0.125 g/day with frequent red and white blood cell count monitoring (4). If serious side effects such as agranulocytosis occur, then use of the drug should be suspended (4).

E. Clinical Use of SASP in Treatment of Active Crohn's Disease

About 20 years after confirmation of the usefulness of SASP in the treatment of active ulcerative colitis, the first double-blind study compared the efficacy of SASP, 3 g/day, against placebo in active CD (57). This double crossover study consisted of four one-month periods of treatment. Thirty-one patients were alternatively treated with the active drug and with placebo. The results showed that only patients who had not previously undergone operation had a symptomatic improvement.

Subsequently, in 1979, the National Cooperative Crohn's Disease Study (NCCDS) involved 74 patients with active CD, who were treated for 4 months with SASP as a single agent at a dose of 1 g per 15 kg body weight up to a maximum daily dose of 5 g (Table 3) (58). Comparison was made between this group and a group of 77 patients on placebo, a group of 85 patients on steroids, and a group of 59 patients on azathioprine. The Crohn's Disease Activity Index (CDAI) was the primary measure of efficacy, and the results were stratified according to disease sites.

The NCCDS concluded that SASP was superior to placebo to a statistically significant degree in inducing remission in patients with ileocolonic and colonic localized CD but not in ileal-localized disease. Fifty-four percent of patients being treated with SASP improved as demonstrated by the CDAI descending to less than 150 points at least once during the 17 weeks of treatment, whereas 43% maintained remission. In the placebo group, the results were respectively 50% and 30%. Previous therapy affected subsequent response to SASP; patients taking steroids before the study failed to respond to SASP. In the same year, an additional study by the NCCDS did not show any advantage of SASP plus steroid with respect to steroid alone in increasing the percentage of remission or in steroid sparing effect (59).

Although the NCCDS has become of primary importance for the treatment and future studies of CD, its study has evoked questions and criticism, especially regarding the use of the CDAI as a measure of the drug's efficacy, the drug doses used, the duration of observation, and the unusually good results of placebo treatment. The use of the CDAI as a measure of efficacy has limitations, because some of the variables contained in it (mainly pain and general well-being) are subjective factors that could be influenced by the patient's state of mind; however, the CDAI and the American study continue to be important milestones for future studies and in every day therapeutic practice.

Subsequently, a study from the Netherlands compared SASP, 6 g/day, with placebo in 26 patients followed up over 26 weeks (60). The Dutch Activity Index (AI) was the only criterion of evaluation. Sixty-two percent of patients on drug and 7.7% on placebo had a reduction of 25% of the baseline index, which, in the protocol, had been considered a criterion of success.

In 1982, the Cooperative Crohn's Disease Study in Sweden compared metronidazole with SASP in active CD (61). In this crossover study, covering two periods of four months, 78 patients with active CD were enrolled. The main evaluation criteria were the CDAI and measurement of seromucoids. SASP and metronidazole were equally effective as measured by the CDAI; metronidazole was slightly more effective when seromucoids were the criterion of efficacy.

Two years later, another important multicenter study from Germany (European Cooperative Crohn's Disease Study [ECCDS]) confirmed the usefulness of SASP in the treatment of CD in the active phase and in remission (62). The CDAI was used for evaluation of treatment outcome. A total of 452 patients were enrolled in this large trial;

TABLE 3 Clinical Trials on the Use of Sulfasalazine in Active Crohn's Disease

Author	Product	Dose (g/day)	No. of Patients	Site of Disease			Period (weeks)	Control	Therapeutic Advantage[a]	Side Effects (%)
				I	C	IC				
NCCDS (58) (1st part)	SASP	1/15 kg	151	42	17	92	17	Placebo	12%[b]	14
Singleton et al. (59)	SASP + steroid	1/15 kg + 40–60 mg/day	89	30	9	50	8	Placebo + steroid	−19%[b]	NR
van Hees et al. (60)	SASP	4–6	26	12	10	4	26	Placebo	54%[b]	61.5
CCDSS (61)	SASP	3	78	26	13	39	16	Metronidazole	20%	47.3
ECCDS (62)	SASP	3	112	26	27	59	18	Placebo	12%[b]	1.8[c]
	SASP + steroid	3 + 48 mg/day	114	32	28	54	18	Placebo	40%[b]	NR
Rijk et al. (63)	SASP + steroid	6 + 30 mg/day	60	21	20	19	16	SASP + placebo	7%	NR

[a]The therapeutic advantage is the difference between the response rate of SASP minus the control group response; if this difference is minus, then the response rate is greater with the control drug.
[b]Statistically significant.
[c]Percentage of patients withdrawn for side effects.
I = ileitis; C = colitis; IC = ileocolitis; NCCDS = National Cooperative Crohn's Disease Study; CCDSS = Cooperative Crohn's Disease Study in Sweden; ECCDS = European Cooperative Crohn's Disease Study; SASP = sulfasalazine; NR = not reported.

117 of them received SASP alone and 112 received SASP in combination with prednisolone. The study showed the superiority of the SASP-6-methylprednisolone association compared with placebo in patients with ileal, ileocolonic, and colonic disease. Significant improvement with SASP as a single drug was obtained in colonic localizations, but SASP was once again ineffective in ileal localizations.

In 1991—already the era of aminosalicylates—a new trial in the Netherlands compared SASP plus prednisone with SASP alone for treating active CD (63). Of the 71 randomized patients, statistical analysis was carried out on the 60 patients who completed the trial. During the first 6 weeks of the trial, the association of SASP (6 g/day) and steroids (30 mg/day initially) resulted in a significant improvement over SASP used alone when evaluated with the Dutch AI. This improvement continued during the period following therapy, even though at the end of 16 weeks it no longer appeared statistically significant. When evaluated with the CDAI, however, the results did not appear to be significant either at 6 weeks or at the end of the trial. The combination of SASP and steroids seemed to be more effective when the colon was in any case involved.

In this study, there was a certain difference between the baseline activity of the two treatment groups. The CDAI of the group treated with steroid was considerably higher than that treated with SASP alone. Moreover, the dose of SASP used was greater than that used in other studies and in clinical practice, and the incidence of side effects was not fully reported.

F. Side Effects of Trials

The percentage of adverse events with SASP in the previous clinical trials are listed in Table 3. As other authors have pointed out, it is difficult to differentiate between side effects of the drug and deterioration of the disease itself, especially in the presence of gastrointestinal symptoms. Percentages vary between 4.2% in Rijk's study and 61.5% in van Hees' study. Nausea, vomiting, and epigastric pain are most frequently reported. However, in these trials, treatment in only a few of the patients had to be interrupted because of the side effects.

G. Conclusions

Although SASP has been and continues to be used in the routine treatment of CD, none of these trials has provided definite evidence of this usefulness. The different doses used in these studies, the complex nature of CD, the different types and locations of lesions, and sometimes the combination with more active drugs are all factors that could have obscured its real efficacy in the treatment of active CD. From all these trials, the most that can be expected of SASP is a therapeutic advantage (defined as the response rate of drug minus the placebo response) of 10% to 11% (64).

However, some data suggest that there is a population of patients in whom the therapeutic advantage of SASP could be increased:

Sulfasalazine seems to have an effect on colonic-localized CD, but it has little or no effect when the CD is ileal localized. This effect is consistent with pharmacology in that the active compound, 5-ASA, is split in the colon.

Because 5-ASA acts locally, the response to SASP could be greater when the lesions are localized in the superficial layer of the colon, but the response may be less or nil when the inflammation is transmural. In keeping with the recent classification of CD patient subgroups, it should be the patients with the primarily inflammatory type of disease who benefit principally from the use of SASP (65).

The mild to moderate forms of CD seem to respond better than forms with severe activity, which are usually perforating.

In some studies, the subgroup of patients not previously treated with any therapy was particularly responsive to SASP. However, this is in line with the characteristics of CD, which, at the beginning, often responds well to different types of therapy.

The combination of SASP with steroid is not advisable because of increased intolerance without increased efficacy over use of steroid alone.

Doses varying between 3 and 6 g have been used in these trials. With 6 g of SASP, 2.4 g of the active moiety 5-ASA are administered. It is likely that larger doses would be more effective, but doses of 6 g of SASP are not easily tolerated. The recommended dose should, therefore, be between 3 and 5 g.

All these characteristics suggest that SASP should be the first drug to be chosen in the case of previously untreated CD patients with mild to moderate activity, with primarily inflammatory type of lesion and colonic location.

II. AMINOSALICYLATES

The appearance of systemic side effects mainly connected with SP and the need for drugs that are definitely active at the level of the small intestine have led to the elaboration of new products made up exclusively from aminosalicylates (5-ASA).

A. Pharmacokinetics of Aminosalicylates

5-Aminosalicylic acid taken orally partially undergoes an irreversible process of acetylation that determines the formation of acetyl-5-ASA (ac-5-ASA) (66). Acetylation takes place at three levels: first in the intestinal lumen and, following absorption, in the intestinal epithelium and then in the liver (67). Of the three levels of acetylation, that of the intestinal epithelium is by far the most important (67). Ac-5-ASA constitutes the principal metabolite of 5-ASA, but contrary to that of SP, the process of acetylation does not depend on the patient's acetylator phenotype (67). Both ac-5-ASA and 5-ASA are mainly eliminated through the renal filter (68). In the plasma, approximately 80% of ac-5-ASA compared with 40% of 5-ASA is linked to the plasmatic proteins. Elimination of ac-5-ASA, therefore, takes place more slowly, leading to higher plasma levels with a half-life of 6 to 9 hours, whereas 5-ASA has a half-life of 0.5 to 1.5 hours (69).

The need for a molecule that acts at the level of both ileum and colon has led to the elaboration of various release systems for 5-ASA; these will probably have an influence on future uses of the drug.

B. Formulations of 5-ASA

Various oral formulations of 5-ASA are available, each having different chemical and pharmaceutical characteristics (Table 4). The main preparations are represented by mesalazine (mesalamine). Oral administration of this molecule without delivery system is characterized by rapid absorption beginning at the level of the stomach and ending in the proximal portions of the small intestine (68). This results in scarce availability at the level

TABLE 4 Products and Sites of Release of Oral Salicylates

Product	Preparation	Solubility	Site of Release
Asacol	Mesalamine coated with Eudragit S	pH 7	Colon (terminal ileum)
Claversal Mesasal Salofalk	Mesalamine coated with Eudragit L	pH 6	Jejunum-ileum-colon
Rowasa	Mesalamine coated with Eudragit L 100	pH 6	Jejunum-ileum-colon
Pentasa	Mesalamine encapsulated in ethylcellulose microgranules	pH dependent	Jejunum-ileum-colon
Azalan	Mesalamine encapsulated in resin carrier	pH dependent	Terminal ileum Proximal colon
Dipentum	Olsalazine (5-ASA + 5-ASA)[a]	Colonic bacterial	Colon
Colazide	Balsalazide (4-aminobenzoyl-B-alanine + 5-ASA)[a]	Colonic bacterial	Colon
Ipsalazide	4-aminobenzoyl-B-glycine + 5-ASA[a]	Colonic bacterial	Colon
4-ASA	Enteric coated with Eudragit compound	pH dependent	Colon

[a]Olsalazine, balsalazide, ipsalazide deliver the 5-ASA in the colon after split of the azo bond by colonic bacterial reductase.

of the distal tracts of the ileum and of the colon, which are the sites where the action of the drug is mainly required in the treatment of CD.

It has, therefore, been necessary to produce 5-ASA preparations in the form of coated tablets that allow for the release of the active substance in the desired areas. Some oral formulations of mesalazine are coated with acrylic resins that release the active drug in different intestinal tracts according to the intraluminal pH and the bacterial flora.

Coating with Eudragit S allows for a delayed release of 5-ASA at a pH greater than 7, thus determining the liberation of the active substance in the terminal ileum and in the right colon (68,70). Highest plasma levels of the drug occur approximately 6 to 7 hours after ingestion, and maximum urinary excretion takes place within 4 to 12 hours (66). Eudragit L allows for the release of the drug at a pH greater than 6, thus rendering it active especially at the level of the small intestine (71). Maximum plasma concentrations of mesalazine coated with this resin are reached after 3 to 4 hours, with maximum urinary elimination within 4 to 12 hours (72).

Another preparation consists of mesalazine contained in microgranules of 0.7 to 1 mm in diameter, coated with a semipermeable and gastroresistant membrane of ethylcellulose. These tablets disintegrate in the stomach and liberate the microgranules. 5-Aminosalicylic acid is released by diffusion starting in the small intestine, continuing constantly and gradually in the colon without peaking, and ending in the rectum (73). Mesalazine liberation is pH dependent and relatively slow in the pH-acid conditions of the proximal intestine, but it is more rapid at the higher pH in the distal ileum and in the colon (74). The gradual release of the active substance allows for scanty absorption of the 5-ASA, which is therefore able to carry out its therapeutic action in the most distal tracts of the intestine (75).

Preparations also exist with pharmacokinetic characteristics similar to those of SASP, including olsalazine, composed of two molecules of 5-ASA, and balsalazide, in which the 5-ASA is linked by a diazo bond to an unabsorbable inert carrier (76,77). Like in SASP, the active substance in both these drugs is released in the colon by the bacterial flora (76,77).

C. Clinical Use of Aminosalicylates in the Treatment of Active Crohn's Disease

The first trials on the use of 5-ASA in the treatment of CD were carried out in Europe considerably later than those on ulcerative colitis. Initially, the dose used was fairly low, reflecting the equivalent doses of 5-ASA that were contained in SASP and used in ulcerative colitis.

The first trial on aminosalicylates was an open study from Denmark in which 18 patients with ileal or ileocolic CD were treated with 1.5 g of 5-ASA (Pentasa): 72% of these patients improved and the CDAI declined from a median of 226 to 99 points (78). The first controlled trial in 1985 (Table 5) compared 5-ASA (Salofalk) with SASP; it involved a total of 30 patients with differently localized CD. A dose of 5-ASA at 1.5 g showed a slight but not significant advantage over SASP (79).

In 1986, a British study showed a decreased fecal excretion of ^{111}In-labeled granulocytes that was greater in the six patients treated with 5-ASA (Pentasa) compared with placebo. However, owing to the small group of patients involved in the study, these interesting results were of no significance (80).

In a Danish study, 5-ASA (Pentasa) at the dose of 1.5 g was again compared with placebo. The study recorded a beneficial trend of 5-ASA in small bowel CD, whereas Pentasa at the same dose had no effect on the 40 patients in a placebo-controlled study from Oxford (81,82). In view of the uncertain efficacy of 5-ASA at the dosages used, research was oriented toward trying out higher doses.

In 1990, a German/Austrian study compared 5-ASA (Claversal) at 2 g/day with 6-methylprednisolone (starting dose of 48 mg/day) in a 24-week multicenter study (83). Insufficient efficacy was shown in 73% of 30 patients treated with Claversal and 34% of 32 patients treated with steroid. The author suggested using a higher dose of 5-ASA.

During the same year, two studies tested 5-ASA (Salofalk) at the dose of 3 g/day versus steroids at the dose of 40 mg (84,85). The drug was shown to be as effective as prednisone in inducng clinical remission. In the latter study, the concomitant treatment with steroid sullied its result. The author suggested that higher doses of 5-ASA should be given at the start of treatment to all patients and should be considered for a long treatment period of patients with more extensive disease (85).

A 16-week multicenter trial from the United States partially confirmed the initial good results (86). In this large trial, 310 patients with CD of any site were randomized to receive 5-ASA (Pentasa) at 1, 2, or 4 g/day; a fourth group received placebo. The primary criterion of efficacy was change in the CDAI. Efficacy was significantly shown only in the group treated with 4 g; remission occurred in 43% of this group and in 18% of the placebo group. Treatment with 1- or 2-g doses did not differ significantly from placebo. Pentasa was beneficial for the ileum as well as for the colon. The therapeutic advantage was 24% for Pentasa, 4 g/day, over placebo. Fifty percent of patients withdrew before completing the study period. The number of withdrawals was greater in the placebo group and in the 1- and 2-g groups. The authors' explanation was that the high dropout rate was

TABLE 5 Clinical Trials on the Use of 5-Aminosalicylic Acid in Active Crohn's Disease

| Author | Product | Dose (g/day) | No. of Patients | Site of Disease | | | Period | Control | Therapeutic Advantage[a] | Side Effects (%) |
				I	C	IC				
Maier et al. (79)	Salofalk	1.5	30	NR	NR	NR	8 weeks	SASP	7%	None
Saverymuttu et al. (80)	Pentasa	1.5	12	—	12	—	10 days	Placebo	50%[b]	None
Rasmussen et al. (81)	Pentasa	1.5	67	36	—	31	16 weeks	Placebo	10%	36.6
Mahida and Jewell (82)	Pentasa	1.5	40	22	12	6	6 weeks	Placebo	5%	15[c]
Scholmerich et al. (83)	Claversal	2	62	NR	5	NR	24 weeks	Steroid	−39%[b]	63
Maier et al. (84)	Salofalk	3	50	1	8	41	12 weeks	Steroid + SASP	−5.5%	12.5
Martin et al. (85)	Salofalk	3	50	30	—	20	12 weeks	Steroid	1%	10.5[c]
Singleton et al. (86)	Pentasa	4	310	124	64	107	16 weeks	Placebo	25%[b]	26.7
		2							6%	30.7
		1							5%	21.2

[a]The therapeutic advantage is the difference between the response rate of 5-ASA minus the control group response; if this difference is minus, then the response rate is greater with the control drug.
[b]Statistically significant.
[c]Percentage of patients withdrawn for side effects.
I = ileitis; C = colitis; IC = ileocolitis; NR = not reported; SASP = sulfasalazine.

probably related to a placebo trial design, which, for ethical reasons, allows for early withdrawal, and essentially to inefficacy of the 1- or 2-g doses (86).

One multicenter open study from the United States in 1993 reported the results of 333 patients with active disease at entry who were treated with 5-ASA (Pentasa) at less than or equal to 4 g/day (87). After a mean study time of 14 months, 42% of patients were in remission, but only 18% were able to discontinue steroid therapy permanently. The location of disease was not mentioned. In another open study, 5-ASA (Asacol) was effective in seven of nine patients intolerant or unresponsive to SASP; the authors mentioned a particularly good response in ileitis (88).

In 1992, an abstract from Canada suggested that 5-ASA (Pentasa) may be of some benefit to children with active small bowel CD (89). In one abstract from the United States, 5-ASA (Asacol) 3.2 g/day appeared to be effective therapy, in comparison with placebo, for 38 patients with Crohn's colitis or ileocolitis (90). A higher dose of 5-ASA (4.5 g) was used in a multicenter trial from Germany; the drug was as effective as 6-methylprednisolone in inducing remission in 34 cases of Crohn's ileocolitis after 8 weeks of treatment (91).

D. Side Effects

The incidence of adverse events with 5-ASA formulations is lower than that reported with SASP. As with SASP, it is difficult to differentiate between side effects related to the drug and symptoms caused by the disease itself. Furthermore, the observation period with 5-ASA is limited. Because experimentation with 5-ASAs has mainly been conducted on ulcerative colitis, the greater experience on their side effects comes from the treatment of that disease. On the other hand, recent use of considerably higher dosages in treating CD has enabled the confirmation of the relative safety of those formulations. Overall, 10% to 20% of patients who are intolerant to SASP show the same side effects when receiving 5-ASA (92). The list of more important reported adverse events with oral 5-ASA is shown in Table 6 (93–108).

Renal toxicity is an important side effect that is rarely reported, whereas diarrhea is reported with an incidence of between 4% and 6% (99). This side effect is particularly frequent, however, with Dipentum, a 5-ASA about which no trials in CD treatment have been published to date. The reported cases of pancreatitis and one case of perimyocarditis are worrying (93–96,98)

In the trials that we have reviewed, the adverse events vary between Maier's study, in which no relevant side effects are reported, and the 63% of side effects in Scholmerich's study, in which only 2 of 62 patients treated with Claversal, 2 g, withdrew from the trial on account of the side effects (83). In the large trial by Singleton et al., the total reported adverse events for the 5-ASA groups were 21.2%, 30.7%, and 26.7% for 1 g, 2 g, and 4 g, respectively, but there was a high percentage of side effects (18.8%) also reported for the placebo group (59). Nausea and vomiting were the most common side effects (7.4%), with both probably related to gastric intolerance to the drug. No sign of renal toxicity, which was monitored in all patients, was reported.

E. Conclusions

The introduction of the 5-ASAs in the therapeutic armamentarium of CD has been accepted with favor but also with a certain amount of prudent skepticism. However, within a short time, this drug has appeared to be useful in the treatment of acute phases of CD as

TABLE 6 Side Effects Caused by
5-Aminosalicylic Acid

Organ System	Side Effect
Gastroenterologic	Diarrhea (93,94)
	Pancreatitis (95,96)
	Nausea, vomiting (86)
Hepatic	Hepatotoxicity (97)
Cardiologic	Perimyocarditis (98)
Nephrologic	Nephrotic syndrome (99)
	Interstitial nephritis (100)
Hematologic	Mild neutropenia (101)
Pulmonary	Bronchospasm (101)
Dermatologic	Skin rash (102)
	Kawasaki-like syndrome (103)
	Lichen planus (104)
Rheumatologic	Lupus-like syndrome (105)
Neurologic	Peripheral neuropathy (106)
Miscellaneous	Headache (86)
	Fever (101)
	Chest pain (107)
	Hair loss (108)

well as in remission maintenance (86,109). Why has this efficacy been demonstrated in such a short period of time while, as we have seen, there are still doubts regarding the efficacy of SASP in CD?

Certain pharmacological and therapeutic differences between the 5-ASAs and SASP may provide some explanations:

The 5-ASA preparations used so far in treatment of CD deliver the active moiety to the distal small bowel and proximal colon where CD is often located, whereas SASP splits the 5-ASA in the colon.

A direct consequence of the fewer side effects expected and reported with 5-ASA has been that the doses of 5-ASA used in the latest trials are higher than those usually used with SASP; 4 g of 5-ASA corresponds to 10 g of SASP, which is the dose contained in 20 tablets of that drug. A recent editorial, however, stressed that the change of the delivery system from an azo bond to being pH dependent or mechanically released should reduce the 5-ASA delivery by approximately 50% (110).

It is likely that the action of the two drugs is linked to the contact of 5-ASA with the diseased intestinal mucosa (5). The direct consequence is that there is little or no effect on the deep lesions; efficacy is therefore greater in mild to moderate forms of CD that usually entail more superficial lesions. Compared with placebo-controlled studies in the past, those in recent years have shown a greater tendency to select patients with forms of disease in a mild to moderate rather than a severe phase. This selection has been favored by an increase in ethical motivation regarding the use of placebo; furthermore, the easier diagnosis of the disease has led to an increase in the number of patients with mild to moderate forms. In some past studies, the inclusion in a trial of patients with severe forms of CD may have obscured the efficacy of the drug tested, and it is possible that the evaluation of SASP has suffered more from this.

In conclusion, the 5-ASAs with pH or mechanically dependent delivery should be the drugs of first choice in patients with active CD localized in the ileum or in the ileum and right side of the colon, in the mild or moderate phase, and in the nonperforating form (65). Future studies should investigate the following:

Whether these drugs can also be effective in left-sided Crohn's colitis or whether 5-ASAs with azo bond (Dipentum, balsalazide) are more useful in these cases.

Whether the 5-ASAs with azo bond are effective in active phases of ileitis or in right-sided colitis.

The optimal dosage of these drugs in the active form of CD.

Whether the use of the new 5-ASAs together with steroids induces remission in a greater percentage of patients than when steroids are used alone.

The role of the 5-ASA enema in patients with left-sided Crohn's colitis.

The answers to these questions will enable a more rational use of these new products and their generating substance.

REFERENCES

1. Peppercorn MA, Goldman P. The role of intestinal bacteria in the metabolism of salicylazo-sulfapyridine. J Pharmacol Exp Ther 1972; 181:555–562.
2. Peppercorn MA, Goldman P. Distribution studies of salicylazosulfapyridine and its metabolites. Gastroenterology 1973; 64:240–245.
3. Schroeder H, Campbell DES. Absorption, metabolism and excretion of salicylazosulfapyridine in man. Clin Pharmacol Ther 1972; 13:539–551.
4. Das KM, Eastwood MA, McManus JPA, Sircus W. Adverse reactions during salicylazo-sulfapyridine therapy and the relation with drug metabolism and acetylator phenotype. N Engl J Med 1973; 289: 491–495.
5. van Hees PAM, Bakker JH, van Tongeren JHM. Effect of sulphapyridine, 5-aminosalicylic acid, and placebo in patients with idiopathic proctitis. A study to determine the active therapeutic moiety of sulphasalazine. Gut 1980; 21:632–635.
6. Azad Khan AK, Piris J, Truelove SC. An experiment to determine the active therapeutic moiety of sulphasalazine. Lancet 1977; 2:892–895.
7. Das KM, Eastwood MA, McManus JP, Sircus W. The role of the colon in the metabolism of salicylazosulfapyridine. Scand J Gastroenterol 1974; 9:137–141.
8. Gaginella TS, Walsh RE. Sulfasalazine. Multiplicity of action. Dig Dis Sci 1992; 37:801–812.
9. Collier HOJ, Francis AA, McDonald-Gibson WJ, Saeed SA. Inhibition of prostaglandin biosynthesis by sulphasalazine and its metabolites. Prostaglandins 1976; 11:219–225.
10. Hoult JRS, Moore PK. Effects of sulphasalazine and its metabolites on prostaglandin synthesis, inactivation and actions on smooth muscle. Br J Pharmacol 1980; 68:719–730.
11. Sharon P, Stenson WF. Metabolism of arachidonic acid in acetic acid colitis in rats. Similarity to human inflammatory disease. Gastroenterology 1985; 88:55–62.
12. Peskar BM, Dreyling KW, May B, et al. Possible mode of action of 5-aminosalicylic acid. Dig Dis Sci 1987; 32:51S–56S.
13. Hawkey CJ, Boughton-Smith NK, Whittle BJR. Modulation of human colonic arachidonic acid metabolism by sulfasalazine. Dig Dis Sci 1985; 30:1161–1165.

14. Boughton-Smith NK, Hawkey CJ, Whittle BJR. Sulfasalazine and the inhibition of thromboxane synthesis in human colinic mucosa. Br J Pharmacol 1983; 80:604–610.

15. Kaufman HJ, Taubin HL. Nonsteroidal antiinflammatory drugs activate quiescent inflammatory bowel disease. Ann Intern Med 1987; 107:513–516.

16. Sharon P, Stenson WF. Enhanced synthesis of LTB4 by colonic mucosa in inflammatory bowel disease. Gastroenterology 1984; 86:453–460.

17. Stenson WF, Lobos E. Sulfasalazine inhibits the synthesis of chemotactic lipids by neutrophils. J Clin Invest 1982; 69:494–497.

18. Peskar BM, Dreyling KW, Peskar BA, et al. Enhanced formation of sulfidopeptide-leukotrienes in ulcerative colitis and Crohn's disease: inhibition by sulfasalazine and 5-aminosalicylic acid. Agents Action 1986; 18:381–383.

19. Eliakim R, Karmeli F, Razin E, Rachmilewitz D. Role of platelet-activating factor in ulcerative colitis. Enhanced production during active disease and inhibition by sulfasalazine and prednisolone. Gastroenterology 1988; 95:1167–1172.

20. Molin L, Stendhal O. The effect of sulfasalazine and its active components on human polymorphonuclear leukocyte function in relation to ulcerative colitis. Acta Med Scand 1979; 206:451–457.

21. Rhodes JM, Bartholomew TC, Jewell DP. Inhibition of leucocyte motility by drugs used in ulcerative colitis. Gut 1981; 22:642–647.

22. Neal TM, Winterbourn CC, Vissers MCM. Inhibition of neutrophil degranulation and superoxide production by sulfasalazine. Comparison with 5-aminosalicylic acid, sulfapyridine, and olsalazine. Biochem Pharmacol 1987; 36:2765–2768.

23. Dull BJ, Salata K, Van Langenhove A, Goldman P. 5-aminosalicylate: oxidation by activated leukocytes and protection of cultured cells from oxidative damage. Biochem Pharmacol 1987; 36:2467–2472.

24. Kane MG, Stelli L, Stenson WF, MacDermott RP. Effects of sulfasalazine and lipoxygenase inhibitors on natural cellular cytotoxicity. Gastroenterology 1985; 88:1436.

25. Mac Dermott RP, Schloemann SR, Berotvich MJ, et al. Inhibition of antibody secretion by 5-aminosalicylic acid. Gastroenterology 1989; 96:442–448.

26. Mac Dermott RP. Current drugs (5-ASA, corticosteroids, 6-MP): mechanisms of action and minimizing toxicity. Postgraduate Course. Clinical Immunology in Gastroenterology and Hepatology. From Bench to Bedside, New Orleans, LA, May 14–15, 1994.

27. Ahnfelt-Ronne I, Nielsen OH, Christensen A, et al. Clinical evidence supporting the radical scavenger mechanism of 5-aminosalicylic acid. Gastroenterology 1990; 98:1162–1169.

28. Grisham MB. Effect of 5-aminosalicylic acid on ferrous sulfate–mediated damage to deoxyribose. Biochem Pharmacol 1990; 39:2060–2063.

29. Aruoma OI, Wasil M, Halliwell B, et al. The scavenging of oxidants by sulphasalazine and its metabolites. A possible contribution to their antiinflammatory effects? Biochem Pharmacol 1987; 36:3739–3742.

30. Taffet SL, Das KM. Sulfasalazine. Adverse effects and desensitization. Dig Dis Sci 1983; 28:833–842.

31. Cochrane P, Atkins P, Ehsanullah S. Agranulocytosis associated with sulphasalazine therapy. Postgrad Med J 1973; 49:669–672.

32. Gabor EP. Hemolytic anemia as adverse reaction to salicylazosulfapyridine. N Engl J Med 1973; 289:1372.

33. Schneider RE, Beeley L. Megaloblastic anemia associated with sulphasalazine treatment. BMJ 1977; 2:1638–1639.

34. Davies G, Palek J. Selective erythroid and megakaryocytic aplasia after sulfasalazine administration. Arch Intern med 1980; 140:1122.

35. Berliner S, Neeman A, Shoenfeld Y, et al. Salazopyrin-induced eosinophilic pneumonia, Respiration 1980; 39:119–120.

36. Jones GR, Malone DNS. Sulphasalazine-induced lung disease. Thorax 1972; 27:713–717.

37. Williams T, Eidus L, Thomas P. Fibrosing alveolitis, bronchiolitis obliterans, and sulfasalazine therapy. Chest 1982; 81:766–768.

38. Mihas AA, Goldenberg DJ, Slaughter RL. Sulfasalazine toxic reactions: hepatitis, fever, and skin rash with hypocomplementemia and immune complexes. JAMA 1978; 239:2590–2591.

39. Das KM. Sulfasalazine therapy in inflammatory bowel disease. In: Ginsberg AL, ed. Gastroenterology Clinics of North America. Management of inflammatory bowel disease. W.B. Saunders Company, Philadelphia: 1989:1–20.

40. Cameron AJ, Baron JH, Priestly BL. Erythema multiforme, drugs, and ulcerative colitis. BMJ 1966; 2:1174–1178.

41. Maddocks JL, Slater DN. Toxic epidermal necrolysis, agranulocytosis and erythroid hypoplasia associated with sulphasalazine. J R Soc Med 1980; 73:587–588.

42. Jacobs E, Pavlet P, Rahier J. Hypersensitivity reaction to sulphasalazine—another case. Gastroenterology 1978; 75:1193.

43. Namias A. Reversible sulphasalazine-induced granulomatous hepatitis. J Clin Gastroneterol 1981; 3 (2) :193–198.

44. Clementz GL, Dolin BJ. Sulfasalazine-induced lupus erythematosus. Am J Med 1988; 84:535–538.

45. Reid J, Holt S, Housley E, et al. Raynaud's phenomenon induced by sulphasalazine. Postgrad Med J 1980; 56:106–107.

46. Singleton JW, Law DH, Kelley ML Jr, et al. National Cooperative Crohn's Disease Study: adverse reactions to study drug. Gastroenterology 1979; 77:870–882.

47. Block MB, Genant HK, Kirsner JB. Pancreatitis as an adverse reaction to salicylazosulfapyridine. N Engl J Med 1970; 282:380–382.

48. Werlin S, Grand R. Bloody diarrhea—a new complication of sulfasalazine. J Pediatr 1978; 92 (3) :450–451.

49. Schwartz AG, Targan S, Saxon A, et al. Sulfasalazine-induced exacerbation of ulcerative colitis. N Engl J Med 1982; 306:409.

50. Birnie GG, McLeod TIF, Watkinson G. Incidence of sulphasalazine-induced male infertility. Gut 1981; 22:452–455.

51. Toovey S, Hudson E, Hendry WF, et al. Sulphasalazine and male infertility; reversibility and possible mechanism. Gut 1981; 22:445–451.

52. O'Morain CA, Smethurst P, Hudson E, et al. Further studies on sulfasalazine induced male infertility. Gastroenterology 1982; 82:1140.

53. Svartz N, Kallner S. Cyanosis in treatment with sulfonamide compounds. Acta Med Scan 1940; 104:309–312.

54. Wallace IW. Neurotoxicity associated with a reaction to sulphasalazine. Practitioner 1970; 204:850–851.

55. Attar A, Anuras S. Sulfasalazine and hair loss (abstr). Gastroeneterology 1981; 80:1102.

56. Das KM, Eastwood MA. Acetylation polymorphism of sulphapyridine in patients with ulcerative colitis and Crohn's disease. Clin Pharmacol Ther 1975; 18:514–520.

57. Anthonisen P, Barany F, Folkenborg O, et al. The clinical effect of salazosulphapyridine (Salazopyrin) in Crohn's disease. A controlled double-blind study. Scand J Gastroenterol 1974; 9:549–554.

58. Summers RW, Switz DM, Sessions JT Jr, et al. National Cooperative Crohn's Disease Study: results of drug treatment. Gastroenterology 1979; 77:847–869.

59. Singleton JW, Summers RW, Kern F Jr, et al. A trial of sulfasalazine as adjunctive therapy in Crohn's disease. Gastroenterology 1979; 77:887–897.

60. van Hees PAM, van Lier HJJ, van Elteren PH, et al. Effect of sulphasalazine in patients with active Crohn's disease: a controlled double-blind study. Gut 1981; 22:404–409.

61. Ursing B, Alm T, Barany F, et al. A comparative study of metronidazole and sulfasalazine for

active Crohn's disease: the Cooperative Crohn's Disease Study in Sweden. II. Result. Gastroenterology 1982; 83:550–562.

62. Malchow H, Ewe K, Brandes JW, et al. European Cooperative Crohn's Disease Study (ECCDS): results of drug treatment. Gastroenterology 1984; 86:249–266.

63. Rijk MCM, van Hogezand RA, van Lier HJJ, van Tongeren JHM. Sulphasalazine and prednisone compared with sulphasalazine for treating active Crohn's disease. A double-blind, randomized, multicenter trial. Ann Intern Med 1991; 114:445–450.

64. Salomon P, Kornbluth A, Aisenberg J, Janowitz HD. How effective are current drugs for Crohn's disease? A meta-analysis. J Clin Gastroenterol 1992; 14 (3) :211–215.

65. Sachar DB, Andrews HA, Farmer RG, et al. Proposed classification of patients subgroups in Crohn's disease. Gastroenterol Int 1992; 5:141–154.

66. Dew MJ, Ebden P, Kidwai NS, et al. Comparison of the absorption and metabolism of sulphasalazine and acrylic-coated 5-aminosalicylic acid in normal subjects and patients with colitis. Br J Clin Pharmacol 1984; 17:474–476.

67. Allgayer H, Ahnfelt NO, Kruis W, et al. Colonic N-acetylation of 5-aminosalicylic acid in inflammatory bowel disease. Gastroenterology 1989; 97:38–41.

68. Myers B, Evans DNW, Rhodes J, et al. Metabolism and urinary excretion of 5-aminosalicylic acid in healthy volunteers when given intravenously or released for absorption at different sites in the gastrointestinal tract. Gut 1987; 28: 196–200.

69. Klotz U, Maier KE. Pharmacology and pharmacokinetics of 5-aminosalicylic acid. Dig Dis Sci 1987; 32: 46S–50S.

70. Dew MJ, Hughes PJ, Lee MG, et al. An oral preparation to release drug in the human colon. Br J Clin Pharmacol 1982; 14:405–408.

71. Goebell H, Klotz U, Nehlsen B, Layer P. Oroileal transit of slow release 5-aminosalicylic acid. Gut 1993; 34:669–675.

72. Klotz U, Maier KE, Fisher C, Gauer KH. A new slow release form of 5-aminosalicylic acid for the oral treatment of inflammatory bowel disease. Arzneimittel Forschung 1985; 35: 636–639.

73. Rasmussen SN, Bondesen S, Hvidberg EF, et al. 5-aminosalicylic acid in a slow-release preparation: bioavailability, plasma level, and excretion in humans. Gastroenterology 1982; 83:1062–1070.

74. Brogden RN, Sorkin EM. Mesalazine. A review of its pharmacokinetic properties, and therapeutic potential in chronic inflammatory bowel disease. Drugs 1989; 38:500–523.

75. Christensen LA, Fallingborg J, Abildgaard K, et al. Topical and systemic availability of 5-aminosalicylate: comparisons of three controlled release preparations in man. Aliment Pharmacol Therap 1990; 4:523–533.

76. van Hogezand RA, van Hees PAM, Zwanenburg B, et al. Disposition of disodium azodisalicylate in healthy subjects. A possible new drug for inflammatory bowel disease. Gastroenterology 1985; 88:717–722.

77. Chan RP, Pope DJ, Gilbert AP, et al. Studies of two novel sulfasalazine analogues, ipsalazide and balsalazide. Dig Dis Sci 1983; 28:609–615.

78. Rasmussen SN, Binder V, Maier K, et al. Treatment of Crohn's disease with peroral 5-aminosalicylic acid. Gastroenterology 1983; 85:1350–1353.

79. Maier K, Fruhmorgen P, Bode JC, et al. Erfolgreiche Akutbehandlung chronisch-entzundlicher Darmerkrankungen mit oraler 5-aminosalicylsaure. Dtsch Med Wochenschr 1985; 10:363–368.

80. Saverymuttu SH, Gupta S, Keshavarzian A, et al. Effect of a slow-release 5'-aminosalicylic acid preparation on disease activity in Crohn's disease. Digestion 1986; 33:89–91.

81. Rasmussen SN, Lauritsen K, Tage-Jensen U, et al. 5-Aminosalicylic acid in the treatment of Crohn's disease. A 16-week double-blind, placebo-controlled, multicentre study with Pentasa. Scand J Gastroenterol 1987; 22: 877–883.

82. Mahida YR, Jewell DP. Slow-release 5-amino-salicylic acid (Pentasa) for the treatment of active Crohn's disease. Digestion 1990; 45:88–92.

83. Scholmerich J, Jenss H, Hartmann F, Dopfer H, the German 5-ASA study group. Oral 5-aminosalicylic acid versus 6-methylprednisolone in active Crohn's disease. Can J Gastroenterol 1990; 4:446–451.

84. Maier K, Frick HJ, Von Gaisberg U, et al. Clinical efficacy of oral mesalazine in Crohn's disease. Can J Gastroenterol 1990; 4:13–18.

85. Martin F, Sutherland L, Beck IT, et al. Oral 5-ASA versus prednisone in short term treatment of Crohn's disease: a multicentre controlled trial. Can J Gastroenterol 1990; 4: 452–457.

86. Singleton JW, Hanauer SB, Gitnick GL, et al. Mesalamine capsules for the treatment of active Crohn's disease: results of a 16-week trial. Gastroenterology 1993; 104:1293–1301.

87. Hanauer SB, Krawitt EL, Robinson M, et al. Long-term management of Crohn's disease with mesalamine capsules (Pentasa). Am J Gastroenterol 1993; 88:1343–1351.

88. Faber SM, Korelitz BI. Experience with Eudragit-S-coated mesalamine (Asacol) in inflammatory bowel disease. An open study. J Clin Gastroenterol 1993; 17:213–218.

89. Griffiths A, Koletzko S, Sylvester F, et al. Pentasa in active small intestinal Crohn's disease; a double-blind placebo-controlled crossover trial in children (abstr). Gastroenterology 1992; 102:A632.

90. Tremaine WJ, Schroeder KW, Harrison JW, Zinsmeister AR. A randomized, double-blind, placebo-controlled trial of oral 5-ASA (Asacol) in the treatment of symptomatic Crohn's colitis and ileocolitis (abstr). Gastroenterology 1993; 104:A792.

91. Gross V, Roth M, Fischbach W, et al. Comparison between high-dose 5-aminosalicylic acid (5-ASA) and 6-methylprednisolone (6-MP) in active Crohn's ileocolitis (abstr). Gastroenterology 1994; 106:A694.

92. Rao SS, Cann PA, Holdsworth CD. Clinical experience of the tolerance of mesalazine and olsalazine in patients intolerant of sulphasalazine. Scand J Gastroenterol 1987; 22:332–336.

93. Sandberg-Gertzen H, Jarnerot G, Kraaz W. Azodisal sodium in the treatment of ulcerative colitis. A study of tolerance and relapse—prevention properties. Gastroenterology 1986; 90:1024–1030.

94. Lauritsen K, Laursen LS, Bukhave K, Rask-Madsen J. Long-term olsalazine treatment: pharmacokinetics, tolerance and effects on local eicosanoid formation in ulcerative colitis and Crohn's colitis. Gut 1988; 29:974–982.

95. Poldermans D, van Blankenstein M. Pancreatitis induced by disodium azodisalicylate. Am J Gastroenterol 1988; 83:578–580.

96. Sachedina B, Saibil F, Cohen LB, Whittey J. Acute pancreatitis due to 5-aminosalicylate. Ann intern Med 1989; 110:490–492.

97. Hautekeete ML, Bourgeois N, Potvin P, et al. Hypersensitivity with hepatotoxicity to mesalazine after hypersensitivity to sulfasalazine. Gastroenterology 1992; 103:1925–1927.

98. Agnholt J, Sorensen HT, Rasmussen SN, et al. Cardiac hypersensitivity to 5-aminosalicylic acid (letter). Lancet 1989; 1:1135.

99. Novis BH, Korzeta Z, Chen P, Bernheim J. Nephrotic syndrome after treatment with 5-aminosalicylic acid. BMJ 1988; 1:1442.

100. Sharma BK. Safety profile of the new 5-ASA based compounds. Can J Gastroenterol 1990; 4:443–445.

101. Thomson ABR. Review article: new developments in the use of 5-aminosalicylic acid in patients with inflammatory bowel disease. Aliment Pharmacol Ther 1991; 5:449–470.

102. Fardy JM, Lloyd DA, Reynolds RPE. Adverse effects with oral 5-aminosalicylic. J Clin Gastroenterol 1988; 10:635–637.

103. Waanders H, Thompson J. Kawasaki-like syndrome after treatment with mesalazine. Am J Gastroenterol 1991; 86:219–221.

104. Alstead EM, Wilson AG McT., Farthing MJG. Lichen planus and mesalazine. J Clin Gastroenterol 1991; 13:335–337.

105. Dent MT, Ganapathy S, Holdsworth CD, Channer KC. Mesalazine induced lupus-like syndrome. BMJ 1992; 305:159.

106. Woodward DK. Peripheral neuropathy and mesalazine (letter). BMJ 1989; 299:1224.

107. Habal FM, Greenberg GR. Treatment of ulcerative colitis with oral 5-aminosalicylic acid including patients with adverse reactions to sulfasalazine. Am J Gastroenterol 1988; 83:15–19.

108. Hadjigogos K. Unusual side effects of mesalazine. Ital J Gastroenterol 1991; 23: 257.

109. Prantera C, Pallone F, Brunetti G, et al. Oral 5-aminosalicylic acid (Asacol) in the maintenance treatment of Crohn's disease. Gastroenterology 1992; 103:363–368.

110. Hayllar J, Bjarnason I. Sulphasalazine in ulcerative colitis; in memoriam? Gut 1991; 32:462–463.

13
The Role of Steroids in the Management of Crohn's Disease

Burton I. Korelitz   *Lenox Hill Hospital and New York University School of Medicine, New York, New York*

The advent of corticosteroids has favorably altered the management of many disease processes—some of known and others of unknown cause. This has been particularly true for Crohn's disease, a clinicopathological process in which the cause remains unknown 45 years after steroids became available, but, with these agents, came a degree of control over the disease, serving to convert it to a stage of inactivity or, at the very least, relieve acute symptoms. Unfortunately, the overwhelming relief that steroids provided led to relative complacency and inaction because it was believed that, with modification of dose or intermittent use of steroids, the disease could be controlled. During those early years gastroenterologists depended on sulfasalazine and the steroids for treatment of Crohn's disease until it was recognized that the steroids had no maintenance or prophylactic value either for ulcerative colitis or Crohn's disease (1–4). This has been confirmed by controlled trials (5–8). Meanwhile, the way in which steroids were used had led to less surgery and the postponement of surgery but the development of complications, some irreversible, arising from either the disease or the drugs used in its treatment (8,9).

Because there is a lack of maintenance value with steroids in the treatment of Crohn's disease and because other drugs do have such maintenance value, I believe that both forms of therapy should be used in a symbiotic manner. The "acute phase" steroids reduce the severity of the clinical manifestations of Crohn's disease and provide relief; the "chronic phase" maintenance drugs, such as the immunomodulators 6-mercaptopurine and aza-thioprine and the oral 5-aminosalicylic acid (5-ASA) products, have long periods of effectiveness, serving to both treat the disease and maintain remission after the steroids are reduced and stopped.

One study of the treatment of ulcerative colitis with steroids did show a distinction between using prednisone orally versus intravenously by demonstrating a blood level of drug that was twice as great with the latter, serving to favor the intravenous route (10). No study clarified whether the same was true for Crohn's disease. No study has empha-sized the value of higher dose over lower dose or has distinguished between corticosteroids and adrenocorticotropic hormone (ACTH) or between hydrocortisone and various syn-thetic steroids.

Patients with active Crohn's disease are usually treated with steroids. In most areas of the United States and in Europe, steroids are administered orally. In some instances, the improvement is dramatic, but, in others, the steroids fail either at the initial dose or soon after the dose is reduced. When the steroids fail, the patient is admitted to the hospital, in some cases for a trial of intravenous steroids or for surgical resection without further nonoperative treatment. Many of the patients treated with intravenous steroids respond so well that certain questions must be raised. Should oral steroids be used at all? Should the patient be admitted to the hospital for intravenous steroids much earlier, not waiting for the Crohn's disease to worsen or for irreversible complications of the disease or of the steroids themselves to occur? The latter question pertains to all indications for intravenous steroids whether there are primary bowel symptoms, partial or complete small bowel obstruction, or complex internal or external fistulas. There is no controlled study that confirms that the favorable outcome of intravenous steroids would result in a longer remission than would oral steroids or that the steroids administered either intravenously or orally have a favorable synergistic action with "chronic-phase drugs" (e.g., 5-ASA products, immunsuppressives) rather than the more "slowly active" chronic-phase drugs to be effective. One recent study did show that the combination of prednisolone and azathioprine was superiod to treatment with prednisolone alone in active Crohn's disease (11). Based on clinical observation and experience, I believe that intravenous steroids do work faster than oral steroids, that the duration of the resulting improvement is longer than that with oral steroids, and that steroids administered either way allow the time necessary for immunosuppressives or 5-ASA products, which do have prophylactic value, to take over. Perhaps there is an additional advantage to hospitalization in that patients are removed from their environment and its source of ongoing stress while full attention is given to eliminating the Crohn's disease activity.

Toxicity to steroids is a major consideration in management of Crohn's disease. However, the toxicity is a product of the dose and time. Whereas intravenous steroids are administered at high dose, their time of utilization is short; the toxicity seen with long-term oral therapy, consistent with a maintenance approach when the dose is lowered and raised, is not encountered. Therefore, intravenous steroid therapy is less likely to lead to osteoporosis, vertebral collapse, aseptic necrosis, retarded growth and development, renal stone formation, acneform eruptions, and even "moon facies," but more likely to cause early complications such as polyuria, leg edema, joint pains, and, perhaps, psychic phenomena, all of which can be more quickly and effectively dealt with in the hospital than in the outpatient situation. A discussion of the complications of corticosteroids and ACTH in inflammatory bowel disease (IBD) is presented in *Management of Inflammatory Bowel Disease* (12).

Present has favored the avoidance of steroids in the presence of abdominal masses and fistulas in Crohn's disease, with the implication that they cause worsening of these complications (13). This has not been my experience. Although Present favors the use of antibiotics under these conditions, the antibiotics are less likely to deal with the primary bowel disease, which is, after all, the causative source of the fistula and the mass. In any case, there are no controlled data that confirm one approach over the other, and there is no contraindication to using antibiotics at the same time as the steroids to cover secondary infection. My experience in using intravenous steroids in the presence of a complicating mass is that there is little difference in favorable response whether or not infection is present (14). Even when the use of intravenous steroids fails to correct, or even worsens, a fistula or mass, the systemic toxicity is usually much reduced, and surgery (drainage, diversion, or resection) can almost always be performed electively.

Using intravenous steroids might even serve as a provocative test for earlier determination of whether surgical intervention is indicated, without prolonging potentially toxic drug therapy either due to "acute-phase" or "chronic-phase" drugs—all under elective rather than urgent circumstances.

I. CHOICE OF INTRAVENOUS STEROIDS

In my experience, intravenous ACTH seems to have a more favorable effect in Crohn's disease than hydrocortisone as reported in earlier studies for ulcerative colitis (15,16). Adrenocorticotropin hormone was more effective for a first course of therapy and resulted in less dramatic responses when used for later attacks (15). Theoretically, a continuous intravenous drip of 20 U of ACTH should provide maximal adrenal stimulation; higher doses have been favored for more obvious and more rapid responses. Currently, the best dose, as determined by prolonged experience, is 120 U/day, and administration of continuous drip is more effective than divided doses (pulse therapy).

Data comparing the effect of ACTH versus hydrocortisone have come from a controlled trial in ulcerative colitis, not in Crohn's disease, and have led to the conclusion that ACTH was indeed better than hydrocortisone when the patient had not received oral steroids during the month before the initiation of intravenous therapy (17). However, when the patient received steroids until the time of intravenous introduction, the response to hydrocortisone was better. I and my colleagues submitted this therapeutic thesis to a randomized double-blind trial in Crohn's disease for which it had never been performed (18,19). Preliminary results suggest that ACTH and hydrocortisone are equally effective with or without preliminary steroid therapy.

Ulcerative colitis and Crohn's disease may differ in response to ACTH versus hydrocortisone therapy. When final calculations are available, comparison must be made in regard to rate of response and ultimate results, the severity of the illness, and the time in the course of the disease when the intravenous drug was initiated.

One disadvantage of intravenous ACTH over hydrocortisone or prednisolone therapy is the complication of adrenal hemorrhage (20,21). In most instances, this has occurred as the ACTH is being terminated and the therapy is switched to that of oral steroids. It is manifested by severe flank pain and the hemorrhage is usually confirmed by findings on computed tomography (CT) scan. The complication is reversible, except rarely, when the hemorrhage is bilateral. Whereas adrenal insufficiency has been observed infrequently after the use of ACTH intravenously, it is fairly common after rapid reduction of intravenous hydrocortisone. This has been seen most often in the postoperative period.

II. ORAL STEROIDS

If the severity of Crohn's disease is moderate, or if it is more severe but the patient refuses hospital admission for intravenous steroid therapy, then oral steroids should be initiated. Occasionally, this stage of therapy can be omitted, and management can be initiated with one of the 5-ASA products, but, if the response is slow, it is better to use the steroids early to achieve early remission, prevent irreversible damage caused by inflammatory destruction, and permit time for the 5-ASA product to become effective. Oral steroids, like intravenous steroids, should always be considered "acute-phase" drugs, not maintenance or prophylactic drugs, even if the drug must be reintroduced or the dose raised.

The initial dose of the prednisone should rarely be less than 60 mg/day. Even if the response is dramatic and a lesser dose might have been successful, it is better to smother the disease and then establish a formula for the rate of reduction according to the rate of response than to have a modest response or none at all. Raising the oral dose to more than 60 mg/day is rarely productive. Furthermore, if the disease does not respond while the dose is being reduced, then raising the dose to its last effective level or by any small increment is doomed to failure. At this point, the choices are to raise the dose to 60 mg/day once again or to admit the patient to the hospital for therapy with intravenous steroids. If steroid therapy is successful, a new and probably slower rate of steroid reduction is warranted. In either case, this maneuver should serve only to allow more time for the chosen "chronic-phase" drug to be effective, for its dose to be increased, or for a new plan of therapy to be introduced.

Whatever the total dose of oral steroids is, it should be divided into four equal parts for maximal therapeutic benefit. The drug is not being used as a maintenance drug; therefore, administering the total dose at one time or using alternate day drug therapy defeats the primary purpose of the drug. The more important decision is in choosing the "chronic-phase" program rather than oral steroids, which mask symptoms. Any prolonged use of steroids without a concomitant plan for prophylaxis is maintenance therapy in which steroids have no value and the risk of steroid complications increases.

III. INTRAMUSCULAR ADRENOCORTICOTROPIC HORMONE

Intramuscular ACTH is a compromise method of administration that has been available since Dr. Crohn's period of peak activity. There are no controlled trials to confirm whether it is better, equal to, or less effective than either intravenous ACTH or hydrocortisone, or even oral steroids. Intramuscular ACTH has the advantage of being used probably more effectively than oral steroids, in that it can be administered by the patient, and hospitalization is not required. On the other hand, by avoiding the hospitalization the patient might be deprived of the value of removal from the environment. If therapy with intramuscular ACTH fails, the patient may still require hospitalization, which might be postponed until intravenous steroids are less effective.

The customary dose of intramuscular ACTH is 80 U/day (2 ml of 40 U/ml at initiation). Then a formula is established for the rate of reduction just as with oral steroids. No advantage has been shown for the ACTH gel versus the crystalline form.

IV. INFLUENCE OF LOCATION OF CROHN'S DISEASE ON RESPONSE TO STEROIDS

According to the results of the National Cooperative Crohn's Disease Study, steroids were effective in small bowel Crohn's disease but not in Crohn's disease of the colon (22). The European Cooperative Crohn's Disease Study concluded that steroids were more effective than placebo in all segments of the bowel (23). The latter results are more in keeping with the overall experience in the every day management of Crohn's disease.

V. CORTICOSTEROID ANALOGS WITH LIMITED GLUCOCORTICOID EFFECT

The major advantage of corticosteroid analogs with limited glucocorticoid effect is the first-pass rapid metabolism in the liver that results in metabolites that provide no suppression of the hypothalamic pituitary–adrenal axis and results in reduced to absent systemic side effects.

Two major considerations arise: (a) if the corticosteroid analogs accomplish the same goal as prednisone or prednisolone without steroid toxicity, then more time can be allowed for chronic-phase drugs to be successful without steroid complications, and (b) even if they have no prophylactic value as is true of the glucocorticoids, consideration of long-term management would be altered with reference to point (a).

Much of the promise from these drugs was demonstrated by their application in enema form for the treatment of ulcerative colitis. Tixocortol pivalate, fluticasone, and budesonide all were equal, and they were a little less than equal but not clearly better than hydrocortisone, with the advantage of avoiding the systemic toxicity.

In Crohn's disease, in comparison with ulcerative colitis, oral administration would have a major advantage if these drugs were equivalent in their ability to affect small bowel disease and right-sided colonic disease by topical effect upon release.

Wright et al. and Hawthorne et al. provided data showing there were fewer (or no) side effects to fluticasone than prednisone and prednisolone but neither was as effective (24,25). Rutgeerts et al., in a European multicenter trial of controlled ileal-release budesonide vs. prednisolone for active Crohn's disease, confirmed that both were effective, but, as anticipated, the prednisolone drug was slightly more effective and the budesonide had fewer side effects (26). The differences occurring beyond 10 weeks were not evaluated in regard to maintenance of remission.

Greenberg et al., in a Canadian inflammatory bowel disease study of oral budesonide for active Crohn's disease, used the same coated capsules for targeting delivery of drug to the ileum and proximal colon. They concluded that the budesonide was effective at an optimum dose of 9 mg/day in the same number of patients as in the study above at 8 weeks. In this study, 50% of the budesonide patients had impaired adrenal function even though there were no clinically important corticosteroid-related symptoms or other toxic effects.

In general, oral budesonide has been demonstrated to be less effective than prednisolone, and probably prednisone as well, in the treatment of Crohn's disease. A major advantage of this drug would be as a prophylactic, but this has not yet been demonstrated as it has not for the glucocorticoids.

REFERENCES

1. Lennard-Jones JE, Misiewicz JJ, Connelly AM, et al. Prednisone as maintenance treatment for ulcerative colitis in remission. Lancet 1965; 1:188.
2. Jones JH, Lennard-Jones JE. Corticosteroids and corticotrophin in the treatment of Crohn's disease. Gut 1966; 7:181–187.
3. Sparberg M, Kirsner JB. Long term corticosteroid therapy for regional enteritis. Am J Dig Dis 1966; 11:865–880.
4. Cooke WT, Fielding JF. Corticosteroids or corticotrophin therapy in Crohn's disease (regional enteritis). Gut 1970; 11:921–927.
5. Bergman L, Krause U. Postoperative therapy with corticosteroids and salazosulphapyridine after radical resection for Crohn's disease. Scand J Gastroenterol 1976; 11;651–656.
6. Smith RC, Rhodes J, Healex RV, et al. Low dose steroids and clinical relapse in Crohn's disease: a controlled trial. Gut 1978; 19:606–610.
7. Mekhjan HS, Switz DM, Watts HD, et al. National Cooperative Crohn's Disease Study: factors determining recurrence of Crohn's disease after surgery. Gastroenterology 1979; 77:907–913.

8. Spencer JA, Kirsner JB, Mlynaryk P, et al. Immediate and prolonged therapeutic effects of corticotrophin and adrenal steroids in ulcerative colitis. Gastroenterology 1962; 42:111–113.

9. Korelitz BI, Lindner AE. Influence of corticotrophn and adrenal steroids on course of ulcerative colitis. Comparison with the pre-steroid ear. Gastroenterology 1964; 46:671–679.

10. Berghouse LM, Elliott PR, Lennard-Jones JE, et al. Plasma prednisolone in acute colitis. Gut 1982; 23:980–983.

11. Ewe K, Press AG, Single CC, et al. Azathioprine combined with prednisolone or monotherapy with prednisolone in active Crohn's disease. Gastroeneterology 1993; 105:367–372.

12. Felder JB, Korelitz BI. Complication of corticosteroids and adrenocorticotropic hormone in treatment of inflammatory bowel disease. In: Korelitz BI, Sohn N, eds. Management of Inflammatory Bowel Disease. St Louis: Mosby-Year Book, 1992:272–286.

13. Present DH. Crohn's disease of the small bowel. In: Bayless TM, ed. Current Therapy in Gastroenterology and Liver Disease. Philadelphia: BC Decker, 1990: 282–290.

14. Felder JB, Adler DJ, Korelitz BI. The safety of corticosteroid therapy in Crohn's disease with an abdominal mass. Am J Gastroenterol 1991; 86:1450–1455.

15. Kirsner JB, Sklar M, Palmer WC. The use of ACTH, cortisone, hydrocortisone and related compounds in the managment of ulcerative colitis. Am J Med 1957; 22:264–274.

16. Zetzel L, Atin AL. ACTH and adrenal corticosteroids in the treatment of ulcerative colitis. Am J Dig Dis 1958; 12:916–930.

17. Meyers S, Sachar DB, Goldberg JD, Janowitz HD. Corticotropin versus hydrocortisone in the intravenous treatment of severe ulcerative colitis. A randomized double-blind Gastroenterology 1983; 85:351–357.

18. Chadi RM, Felder JB, Gleim G, Korelitz BI. ACTH versus hydrocortisone in the intravenous treatment of Crohn's disease. Am J Gastroenterol 1992; 87:1312.

19. Chadi RM, Chun A, Korelitz BI, et al. Intravenous corticotropin versus ??? in the treatment of Crohn's disease. Presented at DDW, San Diego, May 16, 1995.

20. Kornbluth AA, Salomon P, Sachar DB, et al. ACTH induced adrenal hemorrhage: a complication of therapy masquerading as an acute abdomen. J Clin Gastroenterol 1990; 12:371–377.

21. Felder JB, Mendelsohn RH, Korelitz BI. Adrenocorticotropin induced adrenal hemorrhage. J Clin Gastroenterol 1991; 13:111.

22. Summers RW Jr, Swirz DH, Sessions JT, et al. National Cooperative Crohns' Disease Study. Results of drug treatment. Gastroenterology 1979; 77:847–869.

23. Malchow H, Eng K, Brandes JW, et al. European Cooperative Crohn's Disease Study (ECCDS): results of drug treatment, Gastroenterology 1984; 86:249–266.

24. Wright JB, Jarnum S, Schaffalitsky de M, et al. Oral fluticasone propionate compared with prednisolone in treatment of active Crohn's disease: a randomized double-blind multicenter study. Eur J Gastroenterol Hepatol 1993; 5:499–503.

25. Hawthorne CD, Record CO, Holdsworth CD, et al. Double blind trial of oral fluticasone propionals v. prednisolone in the treatment of active ulcerative colitis. gut 1993; 34:125–128.

26. Rutgeerts P, et al. A comparison of budesonide with prednisolone with active Crohn's disease. N Engl J Med 1994; 331:842–845.

27. Greenberg GR, Feagan BG, Martin F, et al. Oral budesonide for active Crohn's disease. N Engl J Med 1994; 331:836–841.

14

Clinical Picture of Crohn's Disease: Upper Gastrointestinal Tract

Adrian J. Greenstein and James Aisenberg   *Mount Sinai Hospital, New York, New York*

I. CROHN'S JEJUNOILEITIS

It was soon recognised that the pathologic process, while presenting its most typical aspect in the terminal ileum, was not restricted to that area; it could and did extend in a limited number of cases to the higher loops of small intestine . . . to involve the upper ileum and the lower or whole of the jejunum (1).

Crohn's jejunoileitis was first described in detail by Crohn and Yunich in 1941 (1). Seventeen of 200 patients with regional enteritis had jejunal involvement. They noted some features that differed from those of ileitis, specifically, an absence of masses, fistulas, or anorectal complications in their patients with jejunoileitis. In fact, fistulas may complicate jejunitis, but they do so less commonly than terminal ileitis. The authors also failed to observe obstructive complications, which are a feature of long-standing disease.

The radiological features of jejunitis were described in detail by Marshak et al. (2,3). They noted frequent skip areas, large inflammatory polyps, and less ulceration and fistula formation than in disease of the terminal ileum. Jejunitis could be subdivided into two phases—nonstenotic and stenotic—the former preceding the latter by four to sixteen years. Most patients with this form of granulomatous disease have long-standing disease and maintain good nutrition (until significant stenosis develops) despite extensive jejunal involvement (4). This is especially so for patients with nonstenotic jejunitis confined to the upper small bowel, presumably due to the excellent absorptive capacity of the spared ileum.

Once the stenotic phase occurs, patients demonstrate diminished oral intake. The obstructive stage is associated with crampy abdominal pain, vomiting, abdominal distention, and bacterial overgrowth in the dilated segments located between the narrowed stenotic areas (Fig. 1). Retained food and secretions are noted radiologically. The patients with advanced disease may suffer marked weight loss, inanition, weakness, and debility.

During the early phase of this disease, medical treatment may be effective. 5-aminosalicylic acid (5-ASA) agents, corticosteroids, and immunosuppressive drugs may be used. Although many clinicians advocate postoperative prophylactic medical

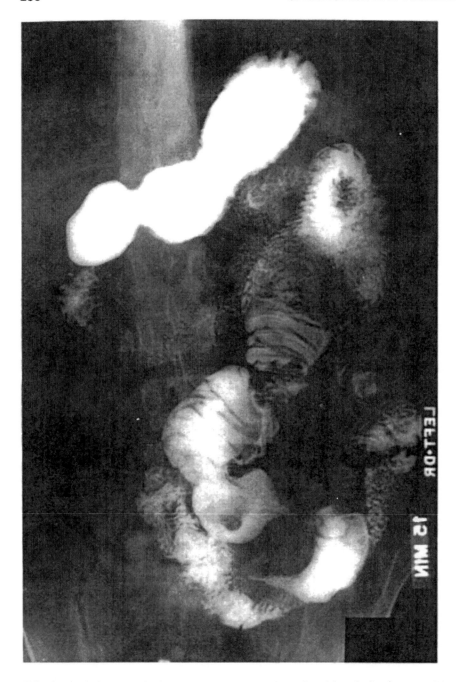

FIG. 1 Small bowel series in a man who developed multiple jejunoileal strictures, with dilated segments between.

therapy to delay recurrence of jejunal Crohn's disease, there is no proof that drugs are effective in this setting.

In earlier years, emergency surgery was common, usually for intestinal obstruction or perforation of a dilated segment. Extensive resections, especially when the ileum was also diffusely involved, often resulted in the short bowel syndrome, with severe diarrhea, steatorrhea, weight loss, fluid and electrolyte imbalance, and inability to absorb fats and fat-soluble vitamins. In this era of total parenteral nutrition, patients with short bowel syndrome can be salvaged, but at the cost of a marked deterioration in life-style and (in many instances) of life-threatening liver disease. Thus, surgery was considered a last resort for severely ill jejunitis patients. In earlier years, the mortality rate with jejunoileitis was high. Reporting on 18 (5.5%) jejunitis patients in a series of 330 patients with Crohn's disease followed up during the period of 1944 to 1970, Cooke and Swan noted six deaths, two from cancer, two from short bowel syndrome, and two from the combined effects of the complications of Crohn's disease and steroid therapy (5).

The prognosis of progressive cicatrizing jejunitis, jejunoileitis, and jejunoileocolitis has changed remarkably over the past 15 years since the original description at Oxford by EC Lee of a new operative procedure commonly known as enteroplasty or stricture-plasty (6). Since Lee's description and subsequent widespread use by Alexander-Williams, strictureplasty has become the procedure of choice for stricturing Crohn's jejunoileitis (7). Stenotic jejunal disease has become a surgical disease, with significant improvement in patient quality of life and reduced medication dependence. Operative results have become progressively better with the appreciation that all strictures must be opened simultaneously and that strictureplasty should not be carried out for acute inflammatory disease, strictures associated with fistulas, and long strictures. Some surgeons limit strictureplasty to strictures of 10 cm or less in length, whereas others put the limit at 20 to 30 cm or more (8,9). Currently, a combination of strictureplasty and resection is the most common operation, and surgery is undertaken earlier than in previous years as the excellent results of strictureplasty have become widely appreciated (7–10).

With the development of strictureplasty and of improved medical therapy, the prognosis of patients with jejunal Crohn's disease has improved considerably. In 1993, Tan and Allan reported that in 34 (5.7%) jejunitis patients in a series of 653 Crohn' disease patients, there were only two deaths, one from jejunal perforation and one from an unrelated bronchogenic carcinoma (11). The series spans three surgical eras. In the first, the 1960s, there was resection only (four operations); in the second, the 1970s, there were resection (15 operations) and bypass (5 procedures); and, in the 1980s, there were resection (30), bypass (2), and strictureplasty (37).

Strictureplasty leaves disease tissue in situ; surprisingly, however, long-term reoperative rates are not much higher than those following resection. The reoperation rate following two resections is worse than that following a single resection; yet, following multiple strictureplasties, reoperation at strictureplasty sites is rare (12,13). Reoperation is at least 10 times as frequent at nonstrictureplasty as at strictureplasty sites. There were no recurrences at strictureplasty sites in a large series from Oxford, and Greenstein has experienced only a single recurrence at a strictureplasty site in a personal series of more than 120 strictureplasties in 27 patients (10,13).

In their study of 34 patients with jejunitis (representing 537 patient-years), Tan and Allan found an operation rate of one operation per 7.3 years (0.14 operations per patient-year) (11). Reoperation was particularly high among younger patients (0.71 per patient-year) and among the patients operated on within the first year of diagnosis (0.23 per patient-year).

Jejunocolic fistulas may complicate the course of jejunoileitis, but most fistulas originate in the colon and are thus true coloileal fistulas (13). In the presence of such fistulas resection is required and strictureplasty cannot be safely carried out.

Crohn's disease of the jejunum is uncommon in children, but the few young patients with this distribution demonstrate characteristic features. As observed initially by Ginzburg et al. and later by Chrispin et al., these patients demonstrate a paucity of abdominal symptoms, making the diagnosis difficult (14,15). Diarrhea may be absent, and vomiting may also not occur even in patients with obstruction. Anorexia, fever, hypoproteinemia, gastrointestinal protein loss, clubbing, and occult blood loss with anemia were characteristic.

Jejunal adenocarcinoma is a rare but lethal complication of Crohn's jejunitis. Three of 19 patients with small bowel cancer seen at Mt. Sinai Hospital developed cancer in areas of jejunum involved by Crohn's disease (16). The mean age at onset of Crohn's disease in these three patients was 27 years, and the mean age at development of jejunal cancer was 53 years, representing an interval to onset of cancer of 26 years. Two of these three patients died within 5 years of diagnosis, and one is alive at 2 years. One patient developed two jejunal cancers in a loop of surgically excluded diseased jejunum. Malignancy in excluded loops is becoming exceedingly rare due to wider appreciation of the complications related to excluding segments of disease bowel and to the virtual disappearance of this type of operative procedure (17).

II. ESOPHAGEAL CROHN'S DISEASE

Crohn's disease of the esophagus was believed to be extremely rare, with few reported cases until recent years. This reflects the difficulty of demonstrating the often superficial lesions of Crohn's esophagitis radiologically. Reporting in 1967 on the radiological findings in several thousand patients with Crohn's disease, Marshak did not note a single case of esophageal involvement (18). By 1983, there were only 20 published cases, and the diagnosis was questionable in a number of these (19). The frequency of esophageal involvement with Crohn's disease has been appreciated during the past decade with the advent of flexible esophagogastroduodenoscopy and biopsy. A review of esophageal Crohn's disease in 1988 revealed 53 cases, noting other sites of disease in 41 cases (77%): small bowel in nine, colon in seven, ileocolitis in 17, and panintestinal in five (Fig. 2) (20). By 1992, 80 cases had been described (21).

The first three patients in whom localized stenotic esophageal Crohn's disease was suspected were described by Franklin and Taylor in 1950 (22). All three presented with dysphagia, and two required esophagectomy, one for suspected cancer. Although all three survived, in earlier years the mortality rate in patients with obstructing esophageal disease requiring surgical resection was significant. In 1954, the first case of disease involving esophagus, stomach, and jejunum was described by Heffernon et al. (23). Patients with fistulas were subsequently reported: one with multiple esophageal fistulas, perianal abscesses and fistulas, erythema nodosum, and arthritis, and two ileocolitis patients with esophageal stricture, intramural esophageal sinus tracts, and esophagobronchial or esophagogastric fistulas (24,25). These authors described in the esophagus the classical findings of regional enteritis: segmental involvement with nodular, varicoid, or cobble-

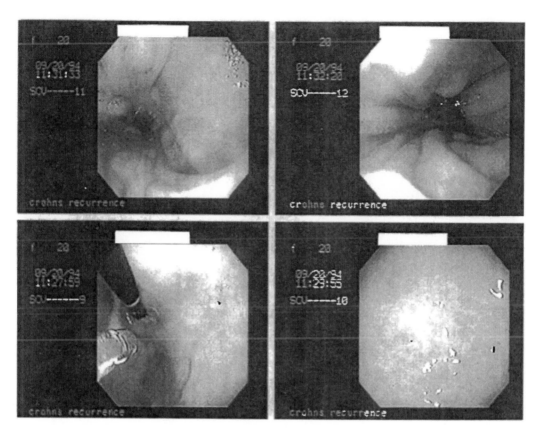

FIG. 2 Endophotographs demonstrating multiple upper gastrointestinal sites in a 21-year-old woman. This patient also had extensive small bowel and colonic disease and had been operated on several times for recurrent disease. *Top panels*, the duodenum is strictured, friable, and cobblestoned. *Lower left panel*, the cardioesophageal junction (seen in retroflex with a biopsy forceps visible) is erythematous with an aphthous ulcer. *Lower right panel*, the body of the stomach is edematous, with a mosaic pattern.

stoned mucosa; chronic ulcers; pseudomembrane formation; progressive stenosis with rigid stricture; intramural sinus tract formation; and fistulas to adjacent structures.

In 1981, Korelitz et al. performed endoscopy and biopsy of the esophagus, gastric antrum and fundus, and duodenum in 45 patients with established Crohn's disease of the small or large bowel in whom the upper gastrointestinal tract was normal radiologically (26). Gross abnormalities were found in 27 patients and histological abnormalities in 19 (including eight in whom the mucosa at the site of biopsy abnormality was endoscopically normal). In only one case, however, did the microscopic esophageal abnormality strongly suggest Crohn's esophagitis. In 1985, Schmitz-Moorman et al. carried out upper gastrointestinal endoscopy in 225 patients with lower gastrointestinal Crohn's disease (27). Endoscopic esophageal abnormalities (typically segmental erythema or aphthous ulcers) were detected in 15% of patients. Of 54 esophageal biopsies, 31 (57%) revealed nonulcerative or ulcerative inflammation, although granulomas were not detected.

In 1986, Geboes et al. reviewed 500 Crohn's disease patients seen over a period of

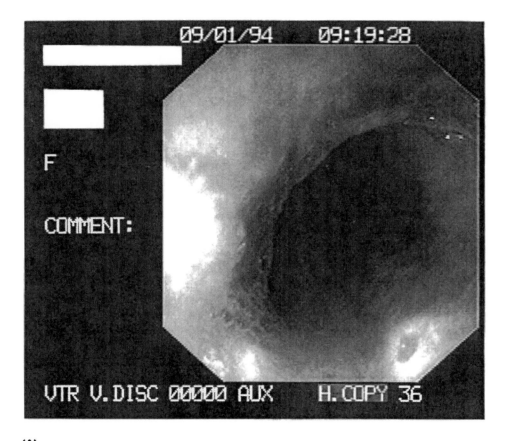

(A)

FIG. 3 A, Endophotograph of an aphthous ulcer located in the proximal esophagus of a 30-year-old black woman who presented with weight loss, diarrhea, and nausea. B, Biopsy specimen of the rim of the ulcer in the same patient demonstrating a noncaseating granuloma (lower right corner), adjacent to squamous mucosa (top) (magnification 40×). C, Noncaseating granuloma from the same case shown at a higher magnification (160×).

4 years at an outpatient clinic and noted esophageal involvement in nine (1.8%) (28). Esophageal involvement was manifested by odynophagia in eight patients and endoscopy in all nine cases revealed large, multiple, aphthoid ulcers (Fig. 3A), surrounded by normal-appearing mucosa. The most striking histologic feature was a lymphocytic infiltrate in the lamina propria with dilated lymphatics. Granulomas were noted by routine histology in only two patients, but deeper histologic sections including the lamina propria uncovered granulomas in another five (total 77%) (see Fig. 3B and C). Careful attention to biopsy technique was required to detect granulomas: multiple biopsies were made from the edge of the lesions utilizing a normal forceps with oval jaws and central spike and minimal air insufflation. The lesions could be differentiated from reflux esophagitis on both endoscopic grounds (apthae with normal intervening mucosa) and histologic grounds (absence of the epithelial alterations seen in gastroesophageal reflux disease). Esophageal involvement was apparent in critically ill patients with painful dysphagia, extraintestinal manifestations (arthritis in seven, painful aphthous stomatitis in six, vulvar lesions in four,

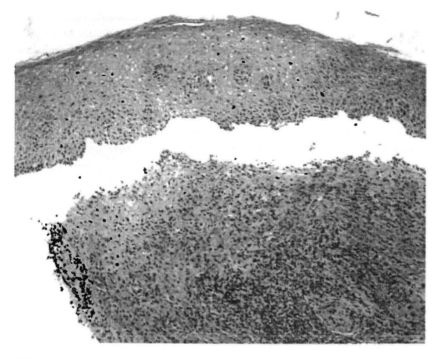

(B)

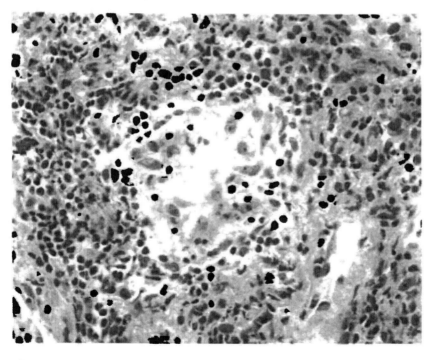

(C)

episcleritis in three, erythema nodosum in two, liver involvement in two, pericarditis in one, pyoderma in one, and multiple areas of disease (colon in nine, ileum in seven, mouth in six, anus in six, gastroduodenum in three). Corticosteroid therapy produced healing in seven of nine patients; sulfasalazine produced healing in two of nine.

In recent years, endoscopic ultrasonography has been added to the diagnostic armamentarium for esophageal Crohn's disease (21). Dancygier et al. note that endoscopic biopsies may be inadequate to characterize Crohn's esophagitis because of the transmural nature of the disease (21). Endoscopic ultrasound with high-frequency 12-MHz transducers overcomes this. In diseased areas of esophagus, irregular echo patterns at all depths of the esophagus wall are seen, and intramural echo-poor bands representing fistulous tracts may be detected. Unfortunately, these findings may also be seen in T2 carcinoma (21).

III. CROHN'S DISEASE OF THE STOMACH AND DUODENUM

Many studies do not distinguish between gastric and duodenal Crohn's disease, so these two anatomical areas are first considered together, although differentiation is made when possible.

Crohn's disease of the stomach and duodenum is a relatively uncommon form of disease occurring in 1% to 7% of patients, most frequently as continuous gastroduodenal disease involving the antrum of stomach and proximal duodenum (29). Weterman found 30 of 605 Crohn's cases had gastric and/or duodenal involvement (29). Of the 16 cases with gastric Crohn's disease, 10 (62.5%) also had duodenal involvement. These 10 gastroduodenal cases constituted 43% of the 23 patients with duodenal disease. Thirteen patients had synchronous disease elsewhere or subsequently developed ileocolitis, ileitis, or colitis. Of the eight patients with jejunal disease, four also had ileal disease and two gastroduodenal disease. Multiple sites were the rule, with at least one additional site in every single patients; one patient had six sites of disease and six had five sites. In most cases, the gastroduodenal disease was detected after the distal disease, but, in four patients, the proximal disease was detected simultaneously with the intestinal disease.

In a retrospective study of 230 patients with Crohn's disease, Lenaerts et al. noted that the diagnosis of ulcerative colitis was changed to that of Crohn's disease in five patients on the basis of gastroduodenal endoscopy (30). In this study, the gastroduodenal disease preceded the ileocolonic disease in only one patient, and none involved the stomach without evidence of disease elsewhere. However, a review of the literature by Johnson and Delaney revealed that the disease was localized to the stomach in 12 of the initial 33 cases of regional enteritis involving the stomach (31).

In 1985, Schmitz-Moorman et al. carried out upper gastrointestinal endoscopy in 225 patients with lower gastrointestinal Crohn's disease (27). Endoscopic abnormalities were found in the stomach in 49% of patients and the duodenum in 34%. Of the patients in whom biopsy specimens were taken, histopathological abnormalities were noted in 60% and 53% and granulomas in 29.4%, and 3.4%, respectively (4.9% had granulomas in both stomach and duodenum). There were significantly more gastric granulomas in young patients, in patients with ileocolic disease, and in those with short duration of disease. Endoscopic lesions included mucosal edema and redness, acute and chronic erosions, and aphthous lesions. Only chronic erosions were predictive of granulomas, diagnostic of Crohn's disease.

IV. CROHN'S DISEASE OF THE STOMACH

The first case of Crohn's disease involving the stomach was described by Gottlieb and Alpert in 1937 (32). In 1950, Comfort et al. described five patients with disease of the of the duodenum and small bowel and noted that two patients also had gastric disease (33). The classical radiological findings were well described in a series of 12 cases by Farman et al. in 1975 (34). These include the "ram's horn" sign (progressive narrowing of the antrum, funneling into the duodenum, which itself frequently involved) cobblestoning, nonspecific linear antral ulceration, antral deformity (sometimes simulating malignancy of the "linitis plastica" variety), gastric outlet obstruction, limited distensibility, and poor peristalsis. In patients with gastric Crohn's disease, the disease is almost always localized to the antrum, but the proximal stomach may also be involved (35,36). Although double-contrast barium study of the upper gastrointestinal tract may demonstrate small aphthous ulceration in more than 20% of cases, larger ulcers simulating peptic ulcer disease are less common, occurring in up to 13% of cases, with 8% found in a large series of 300 patients (4% of those for patients on steroids) (37–40).

Gray et al. described a case of esophagogastric disease involving fundus and body, simulating malignancy, and preceding the development of distal disease (36). Isolated disease involving the entire stomach, with gastrosplenic fistula requiring gastrectomy, has also been reported by Cary et al. (41). These authors discuss 13 cases of isolated Crohn's disease of the stomach, involving antrum (six cases), lower half of the stomach (one), antrum and greater curve (one), body (one), greater curve and proximal half (one), fundus and pylorus (one), and unspecified (two).

Crohn's disease of the stomach may be occult and detectable only on endoscopic examination, or it may be symptomatic. Before the endoscopic era, the diagnosis of upper gastrointestinal Crohn's disease was, in many cases, extremely difficult. Endoscopic studies in adult patients with Crohn's disease revealed gastric abnormalities in 24% to 49% of patients (26,27). The incidence of abnormalities in children is also high. Mashako et al. reported endoscopic gastric abnormalities in 13 of 31 children (42%) and granulomas on biopsy in 12 of 31 (39%) (42). In eight of the 12 patients, granulomas were found in biopsy specimens taken from macroscopically normal areas of stomach. These authors found symptoms in only five patients (16%), and radiological findings in only one (3%). The endoscopic features include mucosal nodularity, cobblestoned mucosa, multiple aphthous and linear ulcers, thickened antral folds, antral narrowing with hypoperistalsis, and duodenal stricture when the disease extends distally (43).

Overall, the incidence of symptomatic gastric Crohn's disease is probably less than 3%. The usual clinical features are chronic epigastric pain, nausea, and vomiting, with progression to outlet obstruction, including vomiting, weight loss, and weakness. These patients may also present with hemorrhage, perforation, or, rarely, fistulization (44,45). Multiple, recurrent, giant gastric ulcers with perforation have been reported (46). Rarer presentations include pernicious anemia secondary to Crohn's granulomatous gastritis, which responded dramatically to administration of intrinsic factor (47). Crohn's disease of the stomach, when mild or asymptomatic, can be treated medically (48). Treatment regimens are reviewed in detail elsewhere in this book. When severe ulceration or obstruction occurs, surgery is generally required. If the disease is localized to the distal stomach, gastrojejunostomy may be carried out, but when it is more extensive, gastrectomy (partial, subtotal, or total) is necessary. If a vagotomy is performed, it is probably advisable to elect a parietal cell, selective, or highly selective vagotomy, preserving the nerve supply of the distal bowel, so that the diarrhea of Crohn's disease is not increased. Because of the risk of fistula formation, pyloroplasty should be avoided if possible.

Cologastric fistula associated with Crohn's disease has been described in 27 cases, with three additional cases being reported with synchronous duodenocolic fistulas (49). The incidence in 1480 patients reported from the Mt. Sinai hospital was 0.6% among 907 colonic cases and 0.08% of 1211 involving the small bowel (48). Most cases originate in

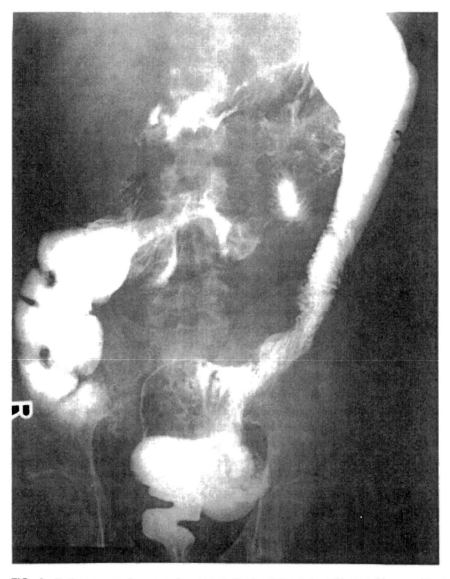

FIG. 4 Barium enema demonstrating a gastroduodenal fistula in a 31-year-old man with ulcerative colitis of 10 years' duration. Barium demonstrates filling of the stomach directly from the transverse colon. He ultimately developed fever, dehydration, 30-pound weight loss, and anemia. Barium enema revealed multiple interconnecting tracts to the stomach as well as other internal fistulas. (Courtesy of Daniel Present.)

the transverse colon and perforate into normal stomach (Fig. 4). Patients presented at a mean age of 39 years with a mean duration of disease of 16 years. Symptoms included abdominal pain, severe diarrhea, weight loss, fevers, and anemia. The diagnosis was generally made by barium enema, occasionally by upper gastrointestinal series, and rarely at laparotomy. A pathognomonic clinical manifestation in four of nine patents was feculent vomiting (48). The pathophysiology has been well summarized by Pichney et al. (49). The symptoms result from the harmful effects of colonic bacteria on the upper gastrointestinal tract and resulting atrophy of intestinal mucosa and from the cathartic effects in the colon of breakdown products of bile salts, deconjugated bile salts, and hydroxy fatty acids (49). Although two cases have been treated at least temporarily with 6-mercaptopurine, the definitive therapy is surgery (48). Initially, ileostomy, cecostomy, exclusion bypass, or diversionary colostomy were carried out to divert the fecal stream from the upper gastrointestinal tract and thus allow the severely debilitated patients to recover. Subsequently, definitive resection of the diseased colon was carried out. Currently, primary subtotal or proctocolectomy, with concomitant wedge excision of stomach is the preferred surgical approach (48). In some patients, primary ileosigmoidostomy may be carried out; in others, ileostomy with mucous fistula is the safer procedure. Most patients require a wedge excision of the stomach, but, on occasion, simple closure of the stomach is possible, as long as the gastric induration is not excessive. In patients with ileogastric fistula following previous ileocolic resection, ileocolic resection with concomitant wedge excision of the stomach and ileocolostomy is required (48).

V. CROHN'S DISEASE OF THE DUODENUM

First described in 1937 by Gottlieb and Alpert (32), Crohn's disease of the duodenum occurs in 0.5% to 4% of patients with Crohn's disease (32,50). The most common clinical presentation is duodenal obstruction (Fig. 5). A picture similar to peptic duodenal ulceration occurs not infrequently (40). Massive hemorrhage, pancreatitis, and duodenocutaneous fistula are rarer forms of presentation (44,45,51–53). A number of cases of coloduodenal fistula have been reported (49,54). As with cologastric fistulas, the site of origin is the colon in almost all cases.

The largest series reported on duodenal Crohn's disease (89 patients) came from Nugent and Roy in 1989 (50). As of that time, at least 354 patients had been reported. In 27 patients, the disease occurred synchronously in the duodenum and in distal bowel; in nine, the intestinal disease occurred years after the duodenal disease (the disease was confined to the proximal bowel for a mean of 12 years). In 60%, gastroduodenal disease was present, whereas, in 26%, ileitis was present and, in 26%, ileocolitis was present. Abdominal pain occurred in 79% of patients, weight loss in 64%, nausea and vomiting in 61%, and hemorrhage in 17%. Pancreatitis occurred in three patients in this series, although two cases were possibly related to azathioprine administration. Reflux of contrast into the pancreaticobiliary tree was also noted during upper gastrointestinal series in two cases. This phenomenon was first observed by Legge et al. (55,56). In four cases, filling of either the pancreatic and bile ducts or of the bile duct alone was demonstrated. Pancreatitis occurred in two patients and asymptomatic hyperamylasemia in a third. In a report form Zarnow et al., duodenobiliary fistula was complicated by the development of a liver abscess (57). In a report by Barthelemy, one patient suffered from recurrent pancreatitis, and filling of primary and secondary pancreatic ducts occurred during barium upper gastrointestinal study. Diffuse nodularity of the duodenum with stenosis and aphthous ulcers, as well as ileal disease, were also noted. The authors postulate a mechanism

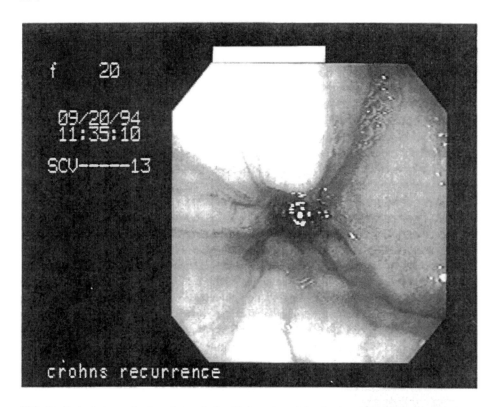

FIG. 5 Endophotograph of a stricture in the third portion of the duodenum in a 21-year-old woman with Crohn's disease involving the stomach, duodenum, jejunum, ileum, and colon (the same patient as in Fig. 2). The duodenal stricture was fibrotic and could not be traversed with the endoscope or the biopsy forceps, although it permitted the passage of barium.

in this case of "fibrosis leading to persistently open, patulous, ampulla of Vater." One of Legge's patients died of fulminating hemorrhagic pancreatitis with necrosis, but two recovered and did well for short periods of follow-up after gastroenterostomy. This operation was not curative, however, and one patient continued to have hyperamylasemia for several years.

The operative rate is high for symptomatic duodenal Crohn's disease: 37% of the cases of Nugent et al. and 91% in the series reported by Ross et al. (50,59). However, the prognosis is relatively good. In the former series, eight of 33 patients required reoperation—seven gastroenterostomy with vagotomy and one subtotal gastrectomy. Because two patients developed marginal ulcers despite vagotomy, Nugent is not enthusiastic about adding vagotomy to drainage procedures in Crohn's disease of the duodenum. On the other hand, the predominantly surgical team at the Lahey Clinical thinks that the absence of added morbidity following vagotomy justifies the continued use of this procedure, despite failure in some cases to prevent marginal ulcer (60). This attitude is supported by results from the Cleveland Clinic (59). After follow-up of 13.9 years, there is a high reoperation rate: seven of 10 patients required 10 reoperations for their duodenal Crohn's disease, and eight of the 11 required surgery for Crohn's disease elsewhere. Good to excellent results were reported in 26 of 30 surgical patients followed up for more than one year, significantly better than for distal Crohn's disease patients ($p < 0.001$) (50). Satisfactory results were reported in 11 patients as assessed by the "Karnofsky performance scale" (60).

In 1992, Pichney et al. reported a total of 52 collected cases of coloduodenal fistula, and three cases of synchronous cologastric and duodenal fistulas, to which they added a fourth (49). They stress the triad of weight loss, diarrhea, and fecal eructations, which is seen in only one-third of cases. Coloduodenal fistulas originate in the diseased colon in almost every case and may be demonstrated by barium enema or fistulogram (Fig. 6). Spirt et al. noted in a review of 46 reported cases that patients with cologastric fistulas

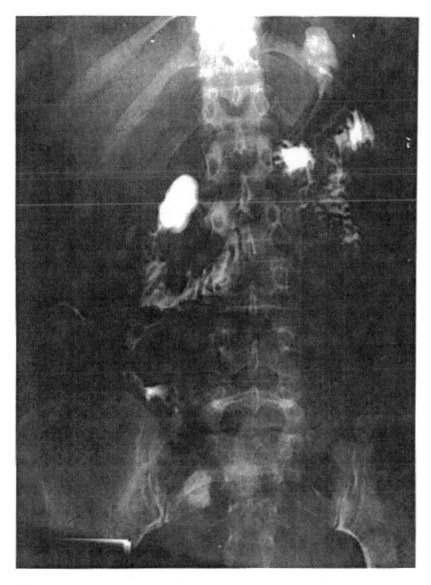

FIG. 6 Coloduodenal fistula in a 32-year-old woman with Crohn's ileocolitis of 11 years' duration, who presented with crampy abdominal pain, diarrhea, right lower quadrant fullness, and 20-pound weight loss. This fistulogram through the enterocutaneous fistula at the left of the figure confirmed the presence of the coloduodenal fistula. The patient was treated successfully by right hemicolectomy with resection of 28 cm of terminal ileum and repair of the duodenal fistula with a jejunal flap. (From Ref. 61, used with permission.)

commonly present with vomiting (39%) and with fecal eructations or frank feculent vomiting (44%), but patients with coloduodenal fistulas rarely present with vomiting (3.6%) and never have feculent vomiting or eructations. This difference is an important clue to the diagnosis and localization of upper gastrointestinal fistulas (61).

VI. CROHN'S DISEASE OF THE MOUTH

In 1969, Dudeney and Todd reported a patient with a 16-year history of small intestinal Crohn's disease who developed inflammatory lesions of the mouth related to the underlying disease (62). Since this initial report, more than 50 studies have described more than 100 patients with oral lesions in Crohn's disease (63).

The incidence of oral lesions in Crohn's disease is 6% to 20% (64). In a study of 100 patients with Crohn's disease, Basu et al. found the rate of oral lesions was significantly higher (9 in 100) than in control patients with ulcerative colitis (2 in 100) or without intestinal disease (1 in 100) (p < 0.05) (65). All nine patients had active Crohn's colitis, and one had ileocolitis. In this report, the incidence of oral lesions was related to the activity of the underlying Crohn's disease. Oral lesions in Crohn's disease are more common in younger patients, with a mean age of presentation in one review of 22 years old (63). Oral lesions in Crohn's disease are more common in the presence of other extraintestinal manifestations, such as skin or eye involvement (66).

The most common sites of oral lesions in Crohn's disease are the lips, the gingiva, and the vestibular sulci of the mouth (63). The most common macroscopic appearances of lesions are aphthous ulcers, diffuse swelling of the lips and cheek, or localized areas of linear ulceration and fissuring associated with hyperplasia of the surrounding tissue that may mimmick the "cobblestone" appearance of the intestinal lesion (64). Histologically, there is generally a dense lymphocytic infiltrate and associated lymphangiectasia, edema, and neuronal hypertrophy. Approximately 10% of oral lesions in Crohn's disease exhibit noncaseating granulomas (65). Although oral Crohn's manifestations are "extraintestinal" they are not "extraenteric" and thus they may share a common pathogenesis with Crohn's disease elsewhere in the enteric tract.

Oral lesions in Crohn's disease may also antedate the appearance of intestinal disease. In a study of 19 patients who had oral biopsies that were strongly suggestive of oral Crohn's disease, seven patients (37%) were found to have subclinical, asymptomatic evidence of underlying intestinal Crohn's disease when studied with intestinal endoscopy with biopsy and barium radiology (67). Talbot et al. reported one patient who developed intestinal Crohn's disease nine years after developing chronic noncaseating granulomatous cheilitis (swelling of the lips) (68).

Complications of oral Crohn's lesions include pain, aesthetic disfigurement from swelling, and an increased rate of dental infections (69). Both surgical treatment and treatment with antibiotics of 5-ASA agents have usually been disappointing. However, systemic immunosuppressive therapy with corticosteroids or azathioprine has been effective in approximately 50% of cases. Topical therapy, including either intralesional steroid injection or topical steroid application by ointments, pastes, or mouthwashes, has also produced remission in approximately 50% of cases (63).

VII. CONCLUSIONS

The development of routine endoscopy in recent years has revealed a remarkably high frequency of Crohn's disease of the upper gastrointestinal tract. Although most patients with microscopic involvement are asymptomatic, a number of patients with oral, esophageal, gastric, duodenal, and jejunal Crohn's disease with more severe macroscopic disease become symptomatic from the upper intestinal disease, and these symptoms may come to dominate the clinical picture. Most of these patients have distal disease as well, and it is important to assess the contribution of each site of the disease to the total clinical presentation. Frequently, the proximal disease is not diagnosed, and even when it is appreciated, its significance may be underestimated, or appropriate therapy may not be carried out. At each site, nonperforating and perforating forms of the disease occur. Obstruction, massive hemorrhage, and fistula formation may occur at these sites as in disease of the lower gastrointestinal tract. The evolution of endoscopy with gastro-duodenscopy, push enteroscopy, small bowel enteroscopy, and intraoperative endoscopy has allowed the physician to localize major sources of disease, diagnose obscure sources of bleeding, and treat complex clinical problems with increasing success. Despite the late appreciation of upper gastrointestinal Crohn's disease, manifestations of disease of the foregut are being increasingly recognized, so this important aspect of this complex disease can take its rightful place in the spectrum of granulomatous disease.

REFERENCES

1. Crohn BB, Yunich AM. Ileojejunitis. Ann Surg 1941; 113:371–380.
2. Marshak RH, Wolf BS. Chronic ulcerative jejunitis and ileojejunitis. AJR Am J Roentgenol 1953; 70:93–112.
3. Marshak RH, Lindner AE. Radiologic diagnosis of chronic ulcerative colitis and Crohn's disease. In: Kirsner JB, Shorter RG, eds. Inflammatory Bowel Disease. 2d ed. Philadelphia: Lea & Febiger, 1980:341–412.
4. Goldstein F, Abramson J, Messori DA, Szydlowski T, Thornton J. Diagnosis and treatment of diffuse ileojejunitis. Am J Gastroenterol 1977; 68:465–469.
5. Cooke T, Swan CHJ. Diffuse jejuno-ileitis of Crohn's disease. Q J Med 1974; 172:583–601.
6. Lee ECG. Aspects of treatment. Minimal surgery for chronic obstruction in patients with extensive or universal Crohn's disease. Ann R Coll Surg Engl 1982; 64:229–233.
7. Sayfan J, Wilson DAL, Allan A, Andrews H, Alexander-Williams J. Recurrence after strictureplasty or resection for Crohn's disease. Br J Surg 1989; 76:335–338.
8. Fazio VW, Tjandra JJ, Lavery IC, Church JM, Milsom JW, Oakley JR. Long-term follow-up of strictureplasty in Crohn's disease. Dis Colon Rectum 1993; 36:355–361.
9. Fazio VW, Tjandra JJ. Strictureplasty for Crohn's disease with multiple long strictures. Dis Colon Rectum 1993; 36:71–72.
10. Dehn TCB, Kettlewell MGW, Mortenson NJMcC, Lee ECG, Jewell DP. Ten year experience of strictureplasty for obstructive disease. Br J Surg 1989; 76:339–341.
11. Tan WC, Allan RN. Diffuse jejunoileitis of Crohn's disease. Gut 1993; 34:1374–1378.
12. Michelassi F, Balestracci T, Chappell R, Block GE. Primary and recurrent Crohn's disease. Experience with 1379 patients. Ann Surg 1991; 214:230–240.
13. Greenstein AJ. Personal series of 27 operated patients in preparation for publication.
14. Ginzburg L, Marshak RH, Eliasoph J. Regional jejunitis. Surg Gynecol Obstet 1960; 111:626–633.

15. Chrispin AR, Tempany E. Crohn's disease of the jejunum in children. Arch Dis Child 1967; 42:631–635.

16. Ribeiro MB, Greenstein AJ, Heimann TM, Yamazaki Y, Aufses AH Jr. Adenocarcinoma of the small intestine in Crohn's disease. Surg Gynecol Obstet 1992; 173:343–350.

17. Senay E, Keohane M, Greenstein AJ. Small bowel carcinoma in Crohn's disease: distinguishing features and risk factors. Cancer 1989; 63:360–363.

18. Marshak RH. Granulomatous disease of the intestinal tract. Radiology 1975; 114:3–22.

19. Davidson JT, Sawyers JL. Crohn's disease of the esophagus. Am Surg 1983; 49:168–172.

20. Kuboi H, Yashiro K, Shindou H, Sasaki H, Hayashi N, Nagasako K. Crohn's disease of the esophagus—report of a case. Endoscopy 1988; 20:118–121.

21. Dancygier H, Frick B. Crohn's disease of the upper gastrointestinal tract. Endoscopy 1992; 24:555–558.

22. Franklin RH, Taylor S. Nonspecific granulomatous (regional) esophagitis. J Thorac Surg 1950; 19:292–297.

23. Heffernon EW, Kepkay PH. Segmental esophagitis, gastritis and enteritis. Gastroenterology 1954; 26:83–88.

24. Achenbach H, Lynch JP, Dwight RW. Idiopathic ulcerative esophagitis—report of a case. N Engl J Med 1956; 255:456–459.

25. Ghahremani GG, Gore RM, Breuer RI, Larson RH. Esophageal manifestations of Crohn's disease. Gastrointest Radiol 1982; 7:199–203.

26. Korelitz BI, Waye JD, Kreuning J, Sommers SC, Sommers SC, Fein HD, Beeber J, Gelberg BJ. Crohn's disease in endoscopic biopsies of the gastric antrum and duodenum. Am J Gastroenterol 1981; 76:103–109.

27. Schmitz-Moorman P, Malchow H, Pittner EM. Endoscopic and bioptic study of the upper gastrointestinal tract in Crohn's disease patients. Pathol Res Pract 1985; 178:377–387.

28. Geboes K, Janssens J, Rutgeerts P, Vantrappen G. Crohn's disease of the esophagus. J Clin Gastroenterol. 1986; 8:31–37.

29. Weterman IT. Oral, oesophageal and gastroduodenal Crohn's disease. In: Allan RN, Keithley MRB, Alexander Williams J, Hawkins C, eds. Inflammatory Bowel Disease. New York: Churchill Livingstone 1983:299–306.

30. Lenaerts C, Roy CC, Vaillancourt M, Weber AM, Morin CL, Seidman E. High incidence of upper gastrointestinal involvement in children with Crohn's disease. Pediatrics 1989; 83:777–781.

31. Johnson FW, Delaney JP. Regional enteritis involving the stomach. Arch Surg 1972; 105:434–437.

32. Gottlieb C, Alpert S. Regional jejunitis. AJR Am J Roentgenol 1937; 38:881–883.

33. Comfort MW, Weber HM, Baggenstoss AH, Kiely WF. Nonspecific granulomatous inflammation of stomach and duodenum: its relation to regional enteritis. Am J Med Sci 1950; 220:616–632.

34. Farman J, Faegenburg D, Dallemand S, Chen CK. Crohn's disease of the stomach: the "rams horn" sign. Am J Roentgenol 1975; 123:242–251.

35. Finder CA, Doman DB, Steinberg WM, Lewicki AM. Crohn's disease of the proximal stomach. Am J Gastroenterol 1984; 79:494–495.

36. Gray RR, St. Louis EL, Grosman H. Crohn's disease involving the proximal stomach. Gastrointest Radiol 1985; 10:43–45.

37. Stevenson GW, Laufer I. In: Laufer I, ed. Double Contrast Gastrointestinal Radiology with Endoscopic Correlation. Philadelphia: WB Saunders 1980:356–360.

38. Chapin LE, Scudamore H, Baggenstoss AH, Bargen JA. Regioanl enteritis: associated visceral changes. Gastroenterology 1956; 30:405–415.

39. Jackson BB. Chronic regional enteritis. Ann Surg 1958; 148:81–87.

40. Fielding JF, Cooke WT. Peptic ulceration in Crohn's disease. Gut 1970; 11:998–1000.

41. Cary ER, Tremaine WJ, Banks PM, Nagorney DM. Isolated Crohn's disease of the stomach. Case report. Mayo Clin Proc 1989; 64:776–779.

42. Mashako MNL, Cezard JP, Navarro J, Mougenot JF, Sonsino E, Gargouri A, Maherzi A. Crohn's disease lesions of the upper gastrointestnal tract: correlation between clinical, radiological, endoscopic, and histologic features in adolescents and children. J Pediatr Gastroenterol Nutr 1989; 8:442–446.

43. Danzi JT, Farmer RG, Sullivan BH, Rankin GW. Endoscopic features of gastroduodenal Crohn's disease. Gastroenterology 1976; 70:9–13.

44. Kim US, Zimmerman MJ, Weiss M. Massive upper gastrointestinal hemorrhage associated with Crohn's disease of the sotmach and duodenum. Am J Gastroenterol 1973; 104:397–400.

45. Paget ET, Owens MP, Peniston WO, Mathewson C. Massive upper gastrointestinal hemorrhage. A manifestation of reignoal enteritis of the duodenum. Arch Surg 1972; 104:397–400.

46. Moonka D, Lichtenstein GR, Levine MS, Rombeau, Furth EE, Macdermott RP. Giant gastric ulcers: an unusual manifestatiom of Crohn's disease. Am J Gastroenterol 1993; 88:297–299.

47. Kraus J, Schneider R. Pernicious anemia caused by Crohn's disease of the stomach. Am J Gastroenterol 1979; 71:202–205.

48. Greenstein AJ, Present DH, Sachar DB, Slater G, Heimann T, Lachman P, Aufses AH. Gastric fistulas in Crohn's disease. Dis Colon Rectum 1989; 32:88–892.

49. Pichney LS, Fantry GT, Graham SM. Gastrocolic and duodenocolic fistulas in Crohn's disease. J Clin Gastroenterol 1992; 15:205–211.

50. Nugent FW, Roy M. Duodenal Crohn's disease: an analysis of 89 cases. Am J Gastroenterol 1989; 84:249–254.

51. Legge DA, Hoffman HN, Carlson HC. Pancreatitis as a complication of regional enteritis of the duodenum. Gastroenterology 1971; 61:834–837.

52. Altman HS, Phillips G, Bank S, Klotz H. Pancreatitis associated with duodenal Crohn's disease. Am J Gastroenterol 1983; 78:174–177.

53. Fitzgibbon TJ, Green G, Silberman H, Eliasoph J, Halls JM, Yellin AE. Management of Crohn's disease involving the duodenum, including duodenocutaneous fistula. Arch Surg 1980; 115:1022–1028.

54. Klein S, Greenstein AJ, Sachar DB. Duodenal fistula in Crohn's disease. J Clin Gastroenterol 1987; 9:46–49.

55. Legge DA, Carlson HC, Judd ES. Roentgenologic features of regional enteritis of the upper gastrointestinal tract. AJR Am J Roentgenol 1970; 110:355–360.

56. Legge DA, Hoffman HN, Carlson HC. Pancreatitis as a complication of regional enteritis of the duodenum. Gastroenterology 1971; 61:834–837.

57. Zarnow H, Grant TH, Spellberg M. Unusual complications of regional enteritis: duodenobiliary fistula and hepatic abscess. JAMA 1976; 235:1880–1881.

58. Barthelemy CR. Crohn's disease of the duodenum with spontaneous reflux into the pancreatic duct. Gastrointest Radiol 1983; 8:319–320.

59. Ross TM, Fazio VW, Farmer RG. Long-term results of surgical treatment for Crohn's disease of the duodenum. Ann Surg 1983; 197:339–406.

60. Murray JJ, Schoetz AJ, Nugent FW, Coller JA, Veidenheimer MC. Surgical management of Crohn's disease involving the duodenum. Am J Surg 1984;147(1):147:58–65.

61. Spirt M, Sachar D, Greenstein AJ. Symptomatic differentiation of duodenal from gastric fistulas in Crohn's disease. Am J Gastroenterol 1990; 85:455–458.

62. Dudeney T, Todd IP. Crohn's disease of the mouth. Proc R Soc Med 1969; 62:1237.

63. Plauth M, Jennss H, Meyle J. Oral manifestations of Crohn's disease: an analysis of 79 cases. J Clin Gastroenterol 1991; 13 (1) 29–37.

64. Basu MK, Asquith P. Oral manifestations of inflammatory bowel disease. Clin Gastroenterol 1980; 9 (2):307–321.

65. Basu MK, Asquith P, Thompson RA, Cooke WT. Oral manifestation of Crohn's disease. Gut 1975; 16:249–254.

66. Greenstein AJ, Janowitz HD, Sachar DB. The extra-intestinal complications of Crohn's disease and ulcerative colitis. A study of 700 patients. Medicine 1976: 55:401–412.

67. Scully C, Cochran K, Russell R, Ferguson MM, Ghouri MA, Lee FD, MacDonald DG, McIntyre PB. Crohn's disease of the mouth: an indicator of intestinal involvement. Gut 1982; 23:198–201.

68. Talbot T, Jewell L, Schloss E, Yakimets MD, Thompson AB. Cheilitis antedating Crohn's disease: case report and literature update of oral lesions. J Clin Gastroenterol 1984; 6:349–354.

69. Halme L, Meurman J, Laine P, von Smitten K, Syrjanen S, Lindquist C, Strand-Pettinen I. Oral findings in patients with active or inactive Crohn's disease. Oral Surg Oral Med Pathol 1993; 76:175–181.

15

Clinical Picture of Crohn's Disease: Lower Intestinal Tract

Norman Sohn *New York University School of Medicine, New York, New York*

The surgeon and the gastroenterologist work together in the patient's best interest. In many situations, operative therapy provides the patient with the optimum opportunity for correction of a problem. But, when operative and medical modalities are likely to be equally beneficial and associated with equivalent potential complications, the latter is preferred. Nevertheless, it is often the proper judgment of the surgeon and the gastroenterologist to act surgically. Several such situations are discussed in this chapter.

I. FAILURE OF MEDICAL THERAPY

Failure of medical therapy as an indication for operation in Crohn's colitis is a subjective criterion. The severe acutely ill patient who fails to respond to intensive medical therapy is occasionally seen. The exact use of corticosteroids, antibiotics, and immunosuppressive agents, as well as the duration of such therapy and the timing of operation, depend on the practice and experience of the gastroenterologist and surgeon who are caring for the patient.

Chronic anemia, malnutrition, diarrhea, and abdominal pain are all indications for operative intervention when medical therapy is not successful. Colonic strictures and fistulas are occasional indications for operation, but they are less so than in small bowel Crohn's disease, possibly because the colon is of a larger caliber and is less likely to be significantly narrowed by a stricture and because there is a lower volume and thicker consistency of colonic fistula effluent when compared with that of patients with small bowel Crohn's disease.

When the rectum in Crohn's disease is spared or only minimally involved, it can be used for an anastomosis and spare the patient, at least temporarily, a stoma. Although the long-term results of ileorectal anastomoses in Crohn's disease are less than optimum, some patients do have prolonged or permanent symptom-free intervals (1).

Laparoscopic colon surgery has been applied to patients with Crohn's disease in the performance of simple colostomy and colon resection. Its exact place in the management of Crohn's disease remains to be explored (2,3). Many cases of Crohn's disease require difficult resection due to adherence to intra-abdominal structures. This could make a laparoscopic approach particularly difficult; however, as the skill and expertise of laparoscopic surgeons increase, patients with Crohn's disease too may be benefited by this modality.

II. POUCHITIS

There are occasional reports of Crohn's disease patients adapting successfully to colectomy with an ileoanal pouch (4). There is an occasional patient suspected of having ulcerative colitis, who, after undergoing an ileal pouch operation, is determined to have had Crohn's disease from the onset. However, the operation is associated with so many potential complications in the absence of Crohn's disease that it is hard to justify its use in a patient with Crohn's disease. Many authors have counseled against such an approach (5). Others have suggested that if Crohn's disease was not clinically obvious preoperatively but only appeared in the microscopic examination of the resected specimen, then the results were similar to those patients in whom the operation was performed for chronic ulcerative colitis (6).

Pouchitis, inflammation in the ileoanal pouch, is a common complication. It occurs most commonly after operations for chronic ulcerative colitis. The importance and frequency of this problem is so great that some authors have already established a Pouchitis Disease Activity Index (7). Chronic ulcerative colitis is the most common indication for that operation. Pouchitis has also been reported after operations for familial polyposis (8). It is most vexing when the patient with Crohn's disease undergoes the ileoanal pouch operation. The cause of pouchitis is unclear. Microbiological, immunological, and ischemic factors are suspected (9–11). The most common symptom is diarrhea. Bleeding, urgency, and incontinence also occur. Treatments are variably successful and have included metronidazole, other antibiotics, and allopurinol (11,12). In some resistant cases, the pouch must be excised and a conventional ileostomy constructed.

Some of the changes that occur in pouchitis resemble those that occur in Crohn's disease, particularly that of axonal necrosis (13). The study of patients with pouchitis may reflect on the nature of Crohn's disease itself. As a result of these and other studies, it is difficult for me to understand why ileoanal pouch operations would be considered for the Crohn's disease patient.

III. CANCER

There is an increased incidence of cancer of the anus, rectum, and colon in patients with Crohn's disease. Cancers, in the Crohn's disease patient, can arise in the colon, in association with strictures, in a stoma, in a fistula, in a perineal sinus, or in a retained rectal stump. The chronic anal fistula that is difficult to evaluate and examine may harbor carcinoma. The treatment of carcinoma in this setting parallels carcinoma in the absence of Crohn's disease. Squamous and cloacogenic carcinomas are treated primarily with chemotherapy and radiation therapy, and when these therapies fail, an abdominoperineal resection is offered. Adenocarcinoma is treated surgically. However, preoperative chemotherapy and radiation therapy appear to have beneficial effect in patients in this setting (14–16). The diagnosis of carcinomas, which do occur in fistulas, is often delayed, and, in many cases, they present at a late stage, requiring this multimodal aggressive approach.

The treatment of colorectal carcinoma in Crohn's disease is the same as for other neoplasms, but diagnosis of carcinoma in Crohn's disease is difficult. Mere consideration of its diagnostic possibility does not lead to its accurate diagnosis, because, even when it is suspected, its objective documentation with an appropriate biopsy may still be difficult.

IV. INTRA-ABDOMINAL ABSCESS

Intra-abdominal abscesses occur in patients with Crohn's colitis. The development of invasive radiology has revolutionized their treatment (17). Therapy with appropriate antibiotics and corticosteroids may be effective (18). When these are inadequate, optimal treatment includes computed tomography (CT)-guided percutaneous drainage. This alone may obviate the need for operative intervention. Even if subsequent operation is indicated, after a period of drainage, it may be possible for resection with primary anastomosis to be accomplished without the need for a staged procedure.

V. APPENDIX

The occurrence of acute appendicitis in a patient with Crohn's disease is rare. Rawlinson and Hughes, in their 1985 paper, stated that there were only five such cases (19). Occasionally, histological examination of an appendectomy specimen reveals granulomatous inflammation. In this situation, there is less than a 10% risk of the patient developing Crohn's disease (20). These data support the policy of nonoperative therapy in the patient with known Crohn's disease who develops right lower quadrant pain. Initially, appropriate therapy with antibiotics or corticosteroids is indicated. Operative intervention should be deferred unless other data such as ultrasound or CT examination points to the diagnosis or the physician suspects that acute appendicitis is a likely or possible diagnosis. Laparoscopy in this type of patient, as well as in other cases of Crohn's disease, may be appropriate.

VI. COLONIC FISTULAS

Colonic fistulas are treated by resection of the primarily involved area of intestine with simple repair of the secondarily involved organ. The indication for operation in colitis should be an effort to correct the underlying physiological abnormality. The fistula per se is not an indication for operation (21). The enterovesical fistula infrequently causes significant urinary tract infections that require operation. Colovaginal or colocutaneous fistulas that cause uncontrollable skin or perineal irritation also should be resected. Ileosigmoid fistulas, unless they are a cause of uncontrollable diarrhea, need not be resected.

Enthusiasm for an operative approach to these fistulas should be tempered by the knowledge that operations for Crohn's disease fistulas can be technically trying. Furthermore, there are occasional dramatic responses to medical therapy with 6 mercaptopurine (6-MP), or cyclosporine (22).

VII. STOMAL ULCERS

Last et al. have reported on peri-ileostomy ulcers, which are difficult to heal (23). They may be a variant of pyoderma gangrenosum involving the skin around the stoma. The cases that I have seen appear to be distinct from the usual peristomal skin ulceration related to difficulty in stomal management. Treatment has included therapy with topical steroids and, most important, 6-MP.

VIII. ANORECTAL CROHN'S DISEASE

The anal and perineal complications of Crohn's disease can be a source of significant mortality; consequently, these often require therapeutic intervention. The most frequent indication for surgical intervention is persistent or recurrent pain. Continued, progressive ongoing sepsis in which pain is a minimal feature is also an indication. Other indications include the presence of feculent drainage through a perineal fistula or a rectovaginal fistula. Dyspareunia due to vulvar or vaginal complications can also indicate the need for surgery. In many cases, a trial of medical therapy consisting of metronidazole or other antibiotics is appropriate. In general, operative intervention for undrained or incompletely drained abscesses or fistulas is generally mandatory before treatment with 6-MP or cyclosporine commences.

The exact pathogenesis of anorectal infections in Crohn's disease is a matter of dispute. I believe that the chronic intersphincteric abscess, which is thought to be the basis of anal fistulas in general, not necessarily in the presence of Crohn's disease, is the common etiological factor in most anorectal Crohn's disease complications. Hughes believes that the primary lesion is a cavitating ulcer that can extend deep into the perirectal tissues or superficially to produce large ulcerations or fistulas into the perineum or vagina (24). He feels that the cavitating ulcer with aggressive ulceration and extensive burrowing through normal tissue with exuberant granulation and little frank suppuration is characteristic of Crohn's disease. Hughes also classifies anal spasm and severe pain without ulcer or sepsis as occurring in Crohn's disease. Hughes' elegant classification is an example of the lack of standardization in classification of anorectal Crohn's disease complications and exemplifies the difficulties inherent in comparing different authors' treatment of similar conditions.

Rectal pain in a patient with Crohn's disease often indicates the presence of an undrained or incompletely drained intermuscular or perirectal abscess. A few of such cases are due to anal fissures. However, the typical anal fissure in Crohn's disease is painless. There is an occasional patient who has rectal pain without any observed fistula, abscess, or ulceration.

In most cases of anal fistulas, there is a chronic intersphincteric abscess. An operative approach is most likely to be successful in alleviating the anal fistula. The site of origin of the intersphincteric abscess is sought by physical examination or by probing crypts or fistulous tracts. Computed tomography and magnetic resonance imaging (MRI) scans have been tried with varying degrees of success. The recent advances in MRI technology promise a more precise anatomical delineation of anal fistulas by this modality. Anal sphincter ultrasound has also been reported to be useful, but, in my experience, it has rarely offered more information than is available on physical examination (25).

The intersphincteric abscess is unroofed by excising a 1 cm wide portion of the overlying internal sphincter (26). This excision generally extends from the lower border of the internal sphincter up to a point approximately 3 mm proximal to the anal verge. This unroofs the intersphincteric component. The fistulous tracts can be curetted; in some cases, the fistulous tract can be cored out. In cases of complex fistulous tracts, multiple incisions are made across them and ¼-inch Penrose drains or doubled No. 5 silk or other suture material is brought through the incisions to be left in place as setons to act as chronic drains.

Setons have been found to be helpful in the treatment of anorectal Crohn's disease (27,28). Setons can be used in several ways. In most cases, they are left in place to act as a chronic drain. In some cases, the sphincter contained within the seton is incised several weeks after the seton is inserted. Theoretically, the seton will cause fibrotic adherence of the sphincter to surrounding tissues, and its subsequent division should not result in impaired continence. In a variation of this principle, the setons also can be managed by tightening them repeatedly and allowing them to cut through the sphincter contained within it. Again, the theory is that the slow division of the sphincter allows its fibrotic adherence and avoids incontinence. However, in many cases, this anticipated result is not obtained and varying degrees of incontinence can occur. This can be a serious complication in a patient with a medical condition that causes diarrhea.

Advancement flaps of anorectal mucosa or mucosa plus muscularis have also been used with varying degrees of success (29). This approach has been used in the management of rectovaginal fistulas, and this principle has been applied to other forms of anal fistulas. Gracilis muscle or other perirectal muscle flaps have also been successfully used to repair complex fistulas and postproctectomy perineal sinuses (30–32). The basic infection must be brought under control for the gracilis or other muscle flap to be effective.

Fibrin glue has been successfully used in causing adhesion in fistulous tracts with their subsequent elimination (33,34). This glue has been applied to enterocutaneous fistulas, rectal fistulas, and rectovaginal fistulas. The success rates vary with success rates as high as 60% being reported. In 1981, Slutzki et al. introduced the concept of laser obliteration of a rectal fistula (35). The beneficial effect of the laser may have been due to sterilization of the fistulous tract or to the bonding of the tissues. There are no other reports of the efficacy of laser treatment at this time. Winter et al. applied the concept of distal displacement of the internal orifice of the anal fistula in patients with Crohn's disease to eliminate the anal fistula (36).

Patients are frequently seen who, in addition to having the fistula, have extensive infection of the skin and subcutaneous tissues around the rectum. Church et al. considered this to be a variant of hidradenitis suppurativa (37). Other factors that could lead to this type of infection could be chronic persistent fistula infections with secondary infection of the skin and subcutaneous tissues. Church et al. have successfully treated this infection by excision of the affected tissue.

Anorectal strictures occur in Crohn's disease. Anal strictures in the absence of Crohn's disease are usually at the anal verge. Those in Crohn's disease are usually at the 2 to 5-cm level. A chronic intermuscular or ischiorectal abscess may be the cause of some of these. Treatment requires drainage of the abscess by a modified Parks' operation and dilatation of the stricture. If no abscess is thought to be present, simple dilatation using rigid sigmoidoscopes of increasing diameter may be adequate therapy. Such sigmoidoscopes are available in 11, 15, and 19 mm diameters. Occasionally, balloon dilatation is performed (38). Rectosigmoid balloons in diameters of 20, 30, and 40 mm are available. Usually, the 20- or 30-mm balloons are used. It is important that the diameter of the dilatation and the duration of the dilatation and application of pressures are known so that this type of therapy and its subsequent use can be properly evaluated.

Hemorrhoids are an infrequent cause of rectal pain in patients with Crohn's disease. When hemorrhoids are painful, it is because thrombosis or ulceration is present. Spontaneous resolution of the pain over a period of a few days is expected, with resolution and reabsorption of the thrombi expected over a period of a few months. Large internal hemorrhoids are not common in patients with Crohn's disease. When they do occur and are a source of symptoms, such as protrusion or bleeding, they can be treated successfully by rubber band ligation. Occasionally, treatment by infrared photocoagulation can be expected to ameliorate symptoms, particularly if the hemorrhoids are small and the bleeding can definitely be attributed to the hemorrhoids.

Anal fissure is an occasional cause of pain. A popular treatment for anal fissure is internal anal sphincterotomy. However, internal anal sphincterotomy in patients with Crohn's disease has been associated with infection at the sphincterotomy site with abscess and fistula formation. Severe abscesses have also occurred in this setting (39). Consequently, an alternative way to treat fissures, anal dilatation, is particularly applicable in patients with Crohn's disease. There are several ways to perform anal dilatation. A consistent reproducible form of dilatation is preferred (38). I prefer to use a 40-mm sausage-shaped balloon, inflated to 20 psi and maintained in position for 6 minutes. The procedure is performed under local anesthesia with conscious sedation. This has had a salutary effect on patients with painful fissures. In patients with tight strictures or in whom the risk of incontinence is extreme, a 30-mm diameter balloon can be used initially, with the 40-mm balloon reserved for failures.

Rectal prolapse is an uncommon complication of Crohn's disease. One of the theories of the occurrence of Crohn's disease proximal to the ileocecal valve or proximal to an anastomosis is that relative obstruction of the ileocecal valve or an intestinal anastomosis promotes the development of Crohn's disease by an undefined mechanism. Treatment of the prolapse either by a resection or a Ripstein operation theoretically would produce the same effect and promote the development or exacerbation of Crohn's disease. In my experience, this has happened in one case. Consequently, I depend on perineal operations to correct the prolapse. Some cases of prolapse appear to follow surgical treatment for an anal fistula, and the perirectal infection that led to the fistula must be eradicated. Thereafter, a modified Thiersch operation using stainless steel wire or Goretex can be used. The risk of infection is high; the risk of failure is also high.

The vagina is also an occasional site for involvement by Crohn's disease. Rectovaginal fistulas are not uncommon. The rectovaginal fistula, in the absence of preliminary obstetrical or surgical trauma, is often due to Crohn's disease. Rectal pain associated with the fistula is usually due to an undrained or incompletely drained intermuscular abscess, and its drainage should be attempted. Feculent drainage through the vagina can be a problem, and correction by operative approach can be offered. However, operations often require an associated proximal colostomy or ileostomy to be effective. The operations may fail and the patient must be apprised of these risks. An operation that includes a rectal advancement flap can be offered (29,40). This has been tried alone, without proximal diversion, in patients in whom the rectal mucosa appears to be in very good condition. Successes have occurred; however, failures are frequent. Successful results using a gracilis muscle or other muscle flap have also been reported (30–32). This is a meaningful approach if the patient has a rectovaginal fistula, particularly one that has recurred. Patients with Crohn's disease who undergo episiotomy as part of their obstetrical care are probably predisposed to poor healing of the episiotomy, with occasional development of anal incontinence or rectovaginal fistula.

Vulvar involvement by Crohn's disease, often due to a rectal abscess, also can occur and has been a cause of dyspareunia (41). This should be appreciated so that surgical efforts can be more profitably directed. Occasionally, the infectious process extends to the scrotum, and rectourethral and rectoejaculatory duct fistulas have been described (42).

IX. CONCLUSION

Operative therapy has much to offer many patients with Crohn's disease. It is of the utmost importance to continue medical therapy while the patient is undergoing operative therapy. Medical therapy consists of corticosteroids, 5-ASA derivatives, antibiotics, or immunosuppressive agents, alone or in combination. This combination of medical and operative therapy has the best chance of positively affecting the underlying serious medical condition of Crohn's disease patients.

REFERENCES

1. Longo WE, Oakley JR, Lavery IC, Church JM, Fazio VW. Outcome of ileorectal anastomosis for Crohn's colitis. Dis Colon Rectum 1992; 35(11):1066–1071.

2. Milsom JW, Lavery IC, Bohm B, Fazio VW. Laparoscopically assisted ileocolectomy in Crohn's disease. Surg Laparosc Endosc 1993; 3(2):77–80.

3. Romero CA, James KM, Cooperstone LM, Mishrick AS, Ger R. Laparoscopic sigmoid colostomy for perianal Crohn's diversion disease. Surg Laparosc Endosc 1992; 2(2):148–151.

4. Grobler SP, Hosie KB, Affie E, Thompson H, Keighley MR. Outcome of restorative proctocolectomy when the diagnosis is suggestive of Crohn's disease. Gut 1993; 34(10):1384–1388.

5. Handelsman JC, Gottlieb LM, Hamilton SR. Crohn's disease as a contraindication of Kock pouch (continent ileostomy). Dis Colon Rectum 1993; 36(9):840–843.

6. Hyman NH, Fazio VW, Tuckson WB, Lavery IC. Consequences of ileal pouch–anal anastomosis for Crohn's colitis. Dis Colon Rectum 1991; 34(8):653–657.

7. Sandborn WJ, Tremaine WJ, Batts KP, Pemberton JH, Phillips SF. Pouchitis after ileal pouch–anal anastomosis: a Pouchitis Disease Activity Index. Mayo Clin 1994; 69(5):409–415.

8. Kmiot WA, Williams MR, Keighley MR. Pouchitis following colectomy and ileal reservoir construction for familial adenomatous polyposis. Br J Surg 1990; 77(11):1283.

9. Gionchetti P, Campieri M, Belluzzi A, Bertinelli E, Ferretti M, Brignola C, Poggioli G, Miglioli M, Barbara L. Mucosal concentrations of interleukin-1 beta, interleukin-6, interleukin-8, and tumor necrosis factor–alpha in pelvic ileal pouches. Dig Dis Sci 1994; 39(7):1525–1531.

10. Ruseler-van Embden JG, Schouten WR, van Lieshout LM. Pouchitis: result of microbial imbalance? Gut 1994; 35(5):658–664.

11. Levin KE, Pemberton JH, Phillips SF, Zinsmeister AR, Pezim ME. Role of oxygen free radicals in the etiology of pouchitis. Dis Colon Rectum 1992; 35(5):452–456.

12. Nygaard K, Bergan T, Bjorneklett A, Hoverstad T, Lassen J, Aase S. Topical metronidazole treatment in pouchitis. Scand J Gastroenterol 1994; 29(5):462–467.

13. Dvorak, AM, Onderdonk AB, McLeod RS, Monahan-Earley RA, Cullen J, Antonioli DA, Blair JE, Morgan ES, Cisneros RL, Estrella P, et al. Axonal necrosis of enteric autonomic nerves in continent ileal pouches. Possible implications for pathogenesis of Crohn's disease. Ann Surg 1993; 217(3):260–271.

14. Picciocchi A, Coco C, Magistrelli P, Roncolini G, Netri G, Mattana C, Cellini N, Valentini V, De Franco A, Vecchio FM, et al. Concomitant preoperative radiochemotherapy in operable locally advanced rectal cancer. Dis Colon Rectum. 1994; 37(2) suppl):S69–S72.

15. Westbrook, KC, Braodwater JR. Advantages of the Papillon protocol in the preoperative treatment of rectal carcinoma. Am J Surg 1992; 164(5):433–435, discussion 436.

16. Minsky BD, Cohen AM, Kemeny N, Enker WE, Kelsen DP, Reichman B, Saltz, L, Sigurdson ER, Frankel J. Enhancement of radiation-induced downstaging of rectal cancer by fluorouracil and high-dose leucovorin chemotherapy. J Clin Oncol 1992; 10(1):79–84.

17. Cybulsky IJ, Tam P. Intra-abdominal abscesses in Crohn's disease. Am Surg 1990; 56(11):678–682.

18. Felder JB, Adler DJ, Korelitz BI. The safety of corticosteroid therapy in Crohn's disease with an abdominal mass. Am J Gastroenterol 1991; 86(1)):1450–1455.

19. Rawlinson J, Hughes RG. Acute suppurative appendicitis. A rare associate of Crohn's disease. Dis Colon Rectum 1985; 28(8):608–609.

20. Agha FP, Ghahremani GG, Panella JS, Kaufman MW. Appendicitis as the initial manifestation of Crohn's disease: radiologic features and prognosis. AJR Am J Roentgenol 1987; 149(3):515–518.

21. Margolin ML, Korelitz BI. Management of bladder fistulas in Crohn's disease. J Clin Gastroenterol 1989; 11(4):399–402.

22. Present DH, Lichtiger S. Efficacy of cyclosporine in treatment of fistula of Crohn's disease. Dig Dis Sci 1994; 39(2):374–380.

23. Last M, Fazio V, Lavery I, Jagelman D. Conservative management of paraileostomy ulcers in patients with Crohn's disease. Dis Colon Rectum 1984; 27(12):779–786.

24. Hughes LE. Clinical classification of perianal Crohn's disease. Dis Colon Rectum 1992; 35(10):928–932.

25. Van Outryve MJ, Pelckmans PA, Michielsen PP, Van Maercke YM. Value of transrectal ultrasonography in Crohn's disease. Gastroenterology 1991; 101(5):1171–1177.

26. Sohn N, Korelitz BI, Weinstein MA. Anorectal Crohn's disease: definitive surgery for fistulas and recurrent abscesses. Am J Surg 1980; 139(3):394–397.

27. Williams JG, MacLeod CA, Rothenberger DA, Goldberg SM. Seton treatment of high anal fistulae. Br J Surg 1991; 78(10):1159–1161.

28. Pearl RK, Andrews JR, Orsay CP, Weisman RI, Prasad ML, Nelson RL, Cintron JR, Abcarian H. Role of the seton in the management of anorectal fistulas. Dis Colon Rectum 1993; 36(6):573–579.

29. Jones IT, Fazio VW, Jagelman DG. The use of transanal rectal advancement flaps in the management of fistulas involving the anorectum. Dis Colon Rectum 1987; 30(12):919–923.

30. Baek SM, Greenstein A, McElhinney AJ, Aufses AH Jr. The gracilis myocutaneous flap for persistent perineal sinus after proctocolectomy. Surg Gynecol Obstet 1981; 153(5):713–716.

31. Roe AM, Mortensen NJ. Perineal reconstruction with rectus abdominis flap after resection of anal carcinoma in Crohn's disease. J R Soc Med 1989; 82(6):369–370.

32. Brough WA, Schofield PF. The value of the rectus abdominis myocutaneous flap in the treatment of complex perineal fistula. Dis Colon Rectum 1991; 34(2):148–150.

33. Kirkegaard P, Madsen PV. Perineal sinus after removal of the rectum. Occlusion with fibrin adhesive. Am J Surg 1983; 145(6):791–794.

34. Hjortrup A, Moesgaard F, Kjaergard J. Fibrin adhesive in the treatment of perineal fistulas. Dis Colon Rectum 1991; 34(9):752–754.

35. Slutzki S, Abramsohn R, Bogokowsky H. Carbon dioxide laser in the treatment of high anal fistula. Am J Surg 1981; 141(3):395–396.

36. Winter AM, Banks PA, Petros JG. Healing of transsphincteric perianal fistulas in Crohn's disease using a new technique. Am J Gastroenterol 1993; 88(12):2022–2025.

37. Church JM, Fazio VW, Lavery IC, Oakley JR, Milsom JW. The differential diagnosis and comorbidity of hidradenitis suppurativa and perianal Crohn's disease. Int J Colorectal Dis 1993; 8(3):117–119.

38. Sohn N, Eisenberg MM, Weinstein MA, Lugo RN, Ader J. Precise anorectal sphincter dilatation—its role in the therapy of anal fissures. Dis Colon Rectum 1992; 35(4):322–327.

39. Sweeney JL, Ritchie JK, Nicholls RJ. Anal fissure in Crohn's disease. Br J Surg 1988; 75(1):56–57.

40. Tuxen PA, Castro AF. Rectovaginal fistula in Crohn's disease. Dis Colon Rectum 1979; 22(1):58–62.

41. Moody G, Probert CS, Srivastava EM, Rhodes J, Mayberry JF. Sexual dysfunction amongst women with Crohn's disease: a hidden problem. Digestion 1992; 52(3–4):179–183.

42. Fazio VW, Jones IT, Jagelman DG, Weakley FL. Rectourethral fistulas in Crohn's disease. Surg Gynecol Obstet 1987; 164(2):148–150.

COMMENTARY: SURGICAL MANAGEMENT OF
CROHN'S DISEASE OF THE COLON, RECTUM, AND ANUS

John Alexander-Williams   *Edgbaston, Birmingham, England*

I. COLONIC CROHN'S DISEASE

Many patients with Crohn's disease have active disease in both large and small bowel. In three series (summarized in Table 1), 33% of 300 patients had small intestinal disease, 46% ileocolic disease, and 19% large intestinal disease alone (1–3).

The symptoms and signs of ileocolic disease are often determined by the ileal element because the involved small bowel becomes stenotic sooner than does the large-diameter colon. The symptoms of pure large bowel Crohn's disease are usually similar to those of ulcerative colitis, with persistent diarrhea, abdominal pain, and weight loss. It is often difficult to differentiate the two diseases, but two important differences have an effect on management. The first is that, in ulcerative colitis, the rectum is usually worst affected, whereas, in Crohn's disease, there is often rectal sparing, so an ileorectal reconnection is often feasible. The other difference is that if a continent pouch is created in Crohn's disease, either a Koch abdominal pouch or an ileoanal pouch, then the small bowel of or proximal to the pouch often becomes affected by acute Crohn's disease. I do not believe that colonic Crohn's disease is less likely than ulcerative colitis to undergo malignant change when the inflammation has been present for many years. I have operated on hundreds of patients with colonic, rectal, and perianal Crohn's disease, and I have compiled a few technical tips that I have learned and find valuable. Technical advice on dissection of adhesions is given in Figs. 1, 2, and 3 and on anastomoses is given in Fig. 4.

II. ILEORECTAL ANASTOMOSIS

Most patients with colonic Crohn's disease who require surgical treatment prefer to avoid a permanent stoma. I try to preserve the rectum and make an ileorectal anastomosis. However, if the rectal stump is less than 15 cm long or if it is indistensible and rigid from chronic disease, it rarely gives an adequate reservoir. Patients who have excessively frequent bowel movements after the operation think that they would have been better off with a stoma (4).

If the ends of the bowel are so severely diseased that I am worried about the healing of the anastomosis, I prefer to bring out the ends as two end-stomas, rather than make anastomosis, and protect it by a proximal diversion ileostomy. If the disease has settled after diversion for 3 months, then I reanastomose. An anastomosis in the presence of an abscess or in the presence of severe active disease at the suture line has a 30% to 40%

TABLE 1 Anatomical Location of Crohn's Disease

Series	Small Intestine	Ileocolic	Large Intestine	Other
Farmer et al., 1975	29	41	27	3
Mekhjian et al., 1979	30	55	14	1
Hellers, 1979	41	41	17	1

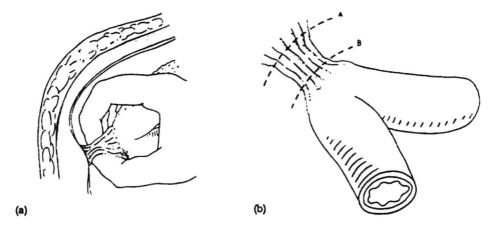

(a)   (b)

FIG. 1 a, Adherent gut is gradually encircled until it is finally attached at its most adherent point. This is then pinched off between finger tip and thumb. b, If the adhesion has to be divided because it is so firm or fibrous, it should be divided close to the parietes (A) not close to the gut (B).

chance of leakage, whereas the complications are minimal following a 12-week diversion and secondary reanastomosis.

III. SEGMENTAL COLECTOMY

In small bowel Crohn's disease, I try to preserve as much functioning gut as possible. Because small bowel disease is often segmental, I only excise short, severely diseased segments or I enlarge strictures by strictureplasty. Crohn's disease in the large bowel is also often segmental, but its preservation is not so vital to digestion or absorption as it is

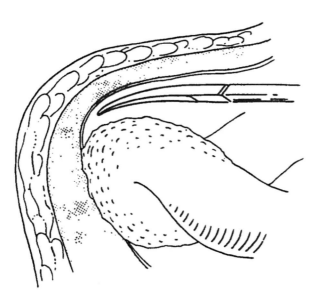

FIG. 2 "Tyre lever" maneuver, using closed scissors to create a plane of cleavage between edematous gut and abdominal wall.

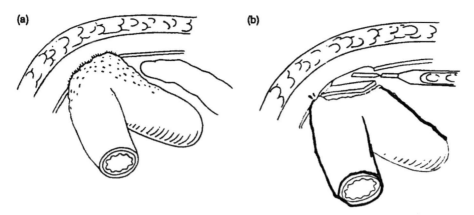

FIG. 3 **a,** The gut is so densely adherent that it may be damaged if it is levered off at the parietes. **b,** A portion of the attached parietes is cut off with diathermy: the "postage stamp" maneuver.

for the small bowel. It is important to preserve the rectum to maintain continence, but the conservation of the rest of the large bowel seems to be less important. Nevertheless, it is an attractive concept to try to preserve as much gut as possible and it seems profligate to sacrifice normal-looking bowel. Therefore, if parts of the colon look relatively normal on colonoscopy, I try to conserve them and perform segmental resection. I and my colleagues have found the complications and risks of recurrence to be no greater after segmental colectomy than after total colectomy and ileorectal anastomosis (5).

IV. PERIANAL CROHN'S DISEASE

Perianal disease is common in patients with Crohn's disease but most patients are not severely troubled by symptoms. I maintain the principle that surgical intervention should only be used to treat symptoms, not to cure the disease (6). The symptoms in perianal Crohn's disease are caused either by pus under tension, a tight fibrous stenosis, or by perianal excoriation due to discharge.

The principal reason for surgical intervention is because of pain due to pus under tension. The difficulties are to find precisely where the tension is, and how to effectively drain the pus. I ask the patient to point to the area of maximal pain and then, once the patient is anesthetized, I examine that area carefully. The place where the patient has pointed is usually the point of maximal induration, and squeezing the area often causes pus to exude from one or more skin or anal canal openings. The skin between these openings can be divided to provide drainage. This relieves tension, cures symptoms, and allows for satisfactory healing. There is no loss of continence as long as no muscle fibers are divided. In patients who become incontinent after such tracks have been widely drained, I presume that some muscle must have been divided. Furthermore, I often find it difficult to determine how much sphincter muscle is encircled by a fistula track, particularly when there is perianal scarring and deformity from recurrent sepsis. Therefore, I stress the importance of dividing tissues slowly in a bloodless field so that muscle can be identified and preserved. Whenever muscle tissue is encountered, it is not divided but simply encircled with a soft silastic seton. This seton remains in position until the induration and discomfort have subsided. It is essentially a draining seton, not a cutting

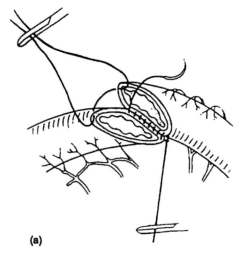

(a)

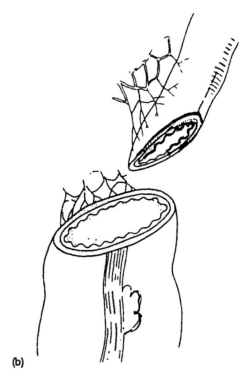

(b)

FIG. 4 a, Small bowel to small bowel anastomoses are performed by rotating the obliquely cut gut end through 180°. b, If there is still a size discrepancy between ileum and colon, a further antimesenteric incision is made.

seton. I frequently leave setons in situ for many months, so it is important that they are made of soft insert material such as silastic tubing and that the knot is reinforced with a soft nonabsorbable suture. I use soft silastic material because a stiff monofilament nylon seton knot often causes a patient some discomfort. I have seen patients who have had such severe complex perianal sepsis that they have to be advised to have a proctectomy before they were referred to me. In some of these, I have left draining setons through tracks around sphincters for years, with satisfactory control of symptoms.

Anal and low rectal strictures are often difficult to manage, particularly when associated with fistulas. However, it always surprises me that patients experience little trouble despite a stricture that barely admits my little finger on examination. I have found that the most successful management of symptomatic stricture is a gentle (one index finger) dilatation under anesthesia, repeated every one or two months if needed. Perseverance is necessary; in some patients, five or six such dilatations were performed before long-term success in control of symptoms was achieved.

These practical tips in surgical management are not all orthodox surgical maneuvers; they have been acquired by repeated analysis of mistakes. Most are peculiar to the management of Crohn's disease, a disease that most surgeons deal with only infrequently.

REFERENCES

1. Farmer RG, Hawk WA, Turnbull RB. Clinical patterns in Crohn's disease: a statistical study of 615 cases. Gastroenterology 1975; 71:245–250.
2. Hellers G. Crohn's disease in Stockholm county 1955–1974—a study of epidemiology results of surgical treatment and longterm prognosis. Acta Chir Scand Suppl 1979; 490:1–84.
3. Mekhjian HS, Switz DM, Melnyk CS, Rankin GB, Brooks RK. Clinical features and natural history of Crohn's disease. Gastroenterology 1979; 77:898–906.
4. Ambrose NS, Keighley, MRB, Alexander-Williams J, Allan RN. Clinical impact of colectomy and ileorectal anastomosis in the management of Crohn's disease. Gut 1984; 25:223–227.
5. Allan A, Andrews H, Hilton, CJ, Keighley MRB, Allan RN, Alexander-Williams J. Segmental colonic resection is an appropriate operation for short skip lesions due to Crohn's disease in the colon. World J Surg 1989; 13:611–616.
6. Alexander-Williams J, Buchmann P. Perianal Crohn's Disease. World J Surg 1980; 4:203–208.

16
Prevention of Relapse and Recurrence

Cosimo Prantera and Arnaldo Andreoli   *Ospedale Nuovo Regina Margherita, Rome, Italy*

I. INTRODUCTION

Crohn's disease is a chronic inflammatory process characterized by recurrent inflammatory states. In the natural history of this disease, there is an alternation of flare-ups (relapse phases) and of phases in which the disease is almost or completely asymptomatic (remission phases). According to various case studies, approximately 25% to 50% of patients relapse per year and approximately 70% relapse within 2 years (1–5). Approximately 70% of patients undergo surgery at least once during their lives for Crohn's disease complications (6–10). After complete resection of all the diseased gut, the lesion reappears endoscopically (recurrence) within 1 year in 70% to 90% of patients, and, within 3 years, approximately 90% of patients are symptomatic (11,12).

Maintenance of remission and prevention of recurrence after resection are two of the three main goals in the treatment of Crohn's disease. Although they have often been considered together in various studies, remission maintenance and recurrence prevention are two different situations in the natural history of this disease: induced medical remission is quite often not concomitant with a complete healing of lesions (1,13,14), whereas, with surgery, all the diseased macroscopic lesions are nearly always removed. Consequently, the timing of the flare-up of symptoms is different in the two situations, with maintenance of clinical remission usually being longer after surgery. Another possible source of bias in studies is in the length of follow-up, which must last for at least 12 to 14 months, because there is a high maintenance of remission rate for placebo at 3 months and even at 6 and 9 months (15).

When different studies are grouped together as in metaanalysis, confusion can occur concerning the definition of recurrence, which can be an endoscopic or radiological recurrence, a clinical recurrence, or a surgical recurrence when the patient is again in need of surgery. These different types of recurrence vary in timing as well as in clinical importance. Recurrence of Crohn's disease has also been related to other variables such as age at diagnosis, extent of disease, site of disease, time interval between onset of symptoms and surgery, and presence of perforating disease (16–22). All these variables can be confounding factors in the evaluation of trials.

Cigarette smoking is a risk factor for the development of Crohn's disease (23–28). A univariate analysis showed that, after 10 years, the recurrence rate, defined as the need for repeat surgery, was 70% in smokers and 41% in nonsmokers (29).

A multivariate study to evaluate the role of smoking in postoperative clinical, surgical, and endoscopic recurrence of Crohn's disease has recently been performed (30). In this study, the cumulative 6-year recurrence rate showed that 60% of nonsmokers, 41% of ex-smokers, and 27% of smokers were symptom-free; the endoscopic recurrence observed 1 year after surgery was 35%, 27%, and 70% for nonsmokers, ex-smokers, and smokers, respectively. This study, therefore, suggests that smoking habits could play a significant role in Crohn's disease recurrence.

All these factors can have an influence on relapse and recurrence, as well as on the severity of symptoms, meaning that the efficacy of drugs in improving the natural history of Crohn's disease must be judged carefully.

II. USE OF SULFASALAZINE IN RELAPSE AND RECURRENCE PREVENTION

Most random clinical trials on the efficacy of sulfasalazine (SASP) as maintenance therapy of Crohn's disease have given negative results (1–3,31,32). The National Cooperative Crohn's Disease Study (NCCDS) and the successive European Cooperative Crohn's Disease Study (ECCDS), which used a similar study design, both came to negative conclusions (1,2). These two landmark studies would seem to advise against any further attempt to use SASP for remission maintenance.

Several criticisms have been made concerning the methodology of these studies (33–35). The main criticism regards the low dose of SASP used in the NCCDS study. The patients in maintenance phase received an average dose of 2 g of SASP, which several authors consider to be inadequate (33). This dosing was the same as that usually used in the maintenance treatment of ulcerative colitis, but a higher dose requirement of 5-aminosalicylic (5-ASA) compounds in the treatment of Crohn's disease as compared with ulcerative colitis was recently observed by some authors (36–38). This higher dose may be necessary because inflammation in Crohn's disease is transmural rather than mucosal as in ulcerative colitis. Some authors have suggested that, in Crohn's disease, the full therapeutic dosage of 3 to 4 g/day of SASP must be continued to maintain remissions (39).

The ECCDS used a dosage of 3 g/day of SASP, but it did not distinguish between the distribution among patients for whom the goal of therapy was prevention of recurrence after surgery and for whom the goal was maintenance of remission induced by medical therapy. From the natural history of the disease, it is known that the percentage of postoperative symptomatic recurrence in nontreated patients is approximately 20% after 2 years, lower than the percentage of relapses observed after an induced medical remission (2,4,10).

Another variable that could have contributed to the negative result of the studies on maintenance with SASP is the different localizations of Crohn's disease. Sulfasalazine is split to release the active moiety 5-ASA by bacterial action in the colon (40). The concentration of the active agent is therefore unlikely to influence ileal disease (41).

The only controlled study to give an opposite result on the prophylactic effect of SASP extended for 2 years on primary resected patients came from Germany (42). Unfortunately, the subdivision of patients according to the completeness of resection gave somewhat contrasting results that are difficult to understand. Some authors have, however, reported a trend toward a beneficial effect on recurrence and relapse prevention in patients treated with SASP (35,43–46).

Despite these controversial results, randomized clinical trials have failed to demonstrate a clinically important effect of medical therapy with SASP in Crohn's disease remission maintenance.

These studies have also failed to address completely many of the important questions regarding the selection of patients for therapy and dosing (47). Because of its pharmacological characteristics, SASP could probably be favorably used in the remission maintenance of colitis, although further studies should be carried out on this topic, and the exact dosage has still to be established.

III. USE OF 5-AMINOSALICYLIC ACID IN RELAPSE PREVENTION

Data on the efficacy of 5-ASA in relapse prevention are more easily interpreted because the studies are more recent than those on SASP, and they are more homogeneous concerning distinction between relapse and recurrence, type of recurrence being considered (clinical or endoscopic), length of follow-up, and dosage used. The "Cape Town classification" has defined relapse/recurrence as reappearance of symptoms (Crohn's Disease Activity Index [CDAI] > 150) and/or of alteration in laboratory findings confirmed by objective means (endoscopically or radiologically) (48). However, in most studies, relapse was essentially considered as the reappearance of symptoms, that is, an increase in the CDAI of more than 150.

Controlled studies on 5-ASA that take into account only patients in whom remission has been medically induced indicate that 5-ASA is effective in reducing the risk of relapse for up to 12 months in patients whose disease is in clinical remission: 23% to 38% of relapses in patients treated with 5-ASA versus 36% to 94% in the placebo group at 12 months, with a relative risk (95% of confidence interval) ranging between 0.40 and 0.81 (41,49–52).

Two studies that have not yet been published in full report contrasting results. One open trial from Israel confirms the efficacy of oral 5-ASA in remission maintenance, and the interim report of a large placebo-controlled trial from Italy showed that 5-ASA at 3 g/day was no better than placebo in delaying relapse when administered immediately after achieved remission (53,54). The 5-ASA products used in these studies were Asacol, Pentasa, Claversal, and Salofalk, all of which deliver the active drug in the small bowel and proximal colon (41,50,52,54–56).

The dosages ranged from 1.5 to 2.4 g/day, and all were effective, so it is difficult to determine the optimal dosage of 5-ASA for maintenance therapy. In active Crohn's disease, the minimally effective dosage seems to be 4 g/day; if Crohn's disease were like ulcerative colitis in that for maintenance, approximately half of the daily dose is used in the active phase, then the dosage of 5-ASA sufficient for maintenance of remission in Crohn's disease would be approximately 2 g/day (57).

Subgroup analysis by site of disease indicates that the types of 5-ASA used in these studies are effective in ileal and possibly in ileocolic disease but apparently not in colonic disease. In one study, which included a large number of patients with ileitis, 2.4 g of 5-ASA (Asacol) showed a notable therapeutic advantage (defined as the response rate of drug minus the placebo response) of 21% (41). In this trial, the favorable response in patients with ileal disease was probably related to a more effective control of the inflammatory process in the ileum by the drug, which is released in the distal small intestine and proximal colon.

A recent study indicates that the cost for preventing each relapse is between $4000 and $10,000, which is comparable to the average cost for treating a relapse (58). On one hand, these studies suggest treatment with 5-ASA for all patients—or at least for those with ileal lesions—on the other hand, problems of cost and of possible side effects suggest treatment for selected populations. One study indicates that patients with short duration of remission (less than 3 months) are at "high relapse risk" and suggests that the role of maintenance therapy should focus on this high-risk population (52). But rigid adherence to this guideline would start all patients who have had a recent flare-up on maintenance therapy, resulting in the unnecessary treatment of a proportion of patients who, even without therapy, would not have had an early relapse. It would be better to look at the patient's previous clinical course as an indicator of "risk status" and to consider at high risk those patients who have had two or more relapses in the last year.

Other authors have suggested treating patients whose laboratory test alterations show them to be at high risk of relapse (59). However, not all patients with raised laboratory tests of inflammation have a relapse of symptoms within 2 years (60). In this case also, a certain percentage of patients would receive unnecessary therapy. Moreover, when this indication was followed, patients with abnormally high laboratory test results did not show any evident advantage from treatment with 2 g of 5-ASA (61).

The efficacy of 5-ASA in preventing symptomatic relapse is greater than that observed with SASP. One explanation for this efficacy, apart from the fact that the split location of active substance is the distal small bowel and proximal colon for the new formulation and the colon for SASP, could be that the dose of 2.4 g of 5-ASA is equivalent to 6 g of SASP, which has never been used in remission maintenance trials (41) (see Table 1).

TABLE 1 Controlled Trials on Efficacy of Salazopyrin (SASP) and Aminosalicylic Acid (5-ASA) in the Prevention of Clinical (C) and Endoscopic (E) Relapse (Rl) and Recurrence (Rc)

Ref.	Year	Drug	Dose (g)	Control	Pt	Rl/Rc	C/E	TA %
(3)	1977	SASP	3	P	43	Rl + Rc	C	–26
(31)	1978	SASP	3	P	66	Rc	C	+31
(1)	1979	SASP	0.5/15K	P	159	Rl + Rc	C	–9
(2)	1984	SASP	3	P	115	Rl + Rc	C	+6
(42)	1989	SASP	2	P	86	Rc	C	+8
(53)	1994	5-ASA	1	P	59	Rl	C	+15
(41)	1992	ASACOL	2.4	P	125	Rl	C	+23
(65)	1994	ASACOL	2.4	NT	110	Rc	E	+24
(50)	1990	CLAVERSAL	1.5	P	206	Rl	C	+16
(54)	1994	CLAVERSAL	3	P	106	Rl	C	–3
(52)	1993	PENTASA	2.0	P	161	Rl	C	+16
(55)	1995	PENTASA	3.0	P	87	Rc	E	—
(49)	1988	SALOFALK	1.5	P	64	Rl	C	+12
(56)	1995	SALOFALK	3.0	P	163	Rc	C	+19

P, placebo; NT, no treatment; TA, therapeutic advantage; Pt, number of patients. All results are at 12 months except those of (55) which are at 6 months, and those of (56) which are at 3 years.

IV.   USE OF 5-AMINOSALICYLIC ACID
IN PREVENTION OF RECURRENCE AFTER SURGERY

Postoperative recurrence of lesions is endoscopically present in 70% to 90% of cases within 1 year after surgery and is already in 63% to 75% of cases after 3 months (11,12,62,63,64). Recurrence begins with the appearance of aphthae, which usually become worse with time and form ulcers and stenosis (11,12). Ninety percent of patients with endoscopic recurrence become symptomatic within 3 years, and the more severe the endoscopic recurrence, the earlier the symptomatic recurrence (11).

These data have prompted studies to find out whether treatment initiated immediately after surgery prevents or delays endoscopic and subsequent clinical recurrence. Furthermore, because almost all endoscopic recurrences after ileocolic resection for ileitis are located in the anastomosis, researchers have used a drug such as 5-ASA whose pharmacological characteristics make it suitable for use in that site without relevant side effects (12). A recent prospective randomized open trial has shown that 2.4 g/day of 5-ASA (Asacol) is effective in preventing endoscopic recurrence in patients who have undergone operation for Crohn's ileitis; at 24 months, the cumulative proportion of recurrence was 0.52 in the 5-ASA group compared with 0.85 in the control group (65). Even symptomatic recurrence was reduced by treatment. The results of this study, however, are partially impugned by two possible biases: the lack of a placebo-controlled group and the fact that the endoscopists were aware of the treatment assigned to the patients. Only 4.4% of patients reported adverse events.

A recent article reported the results of a one-year placebo-controlled trial of 5-ASA 3 g (Pentasa) in the prevention of endoscopic recurrence after intestinal resection for Crohn's disease (55). The 87 patients in the two groups were homogeneous in respect to pre-trial clinical characteristics including smoking. The authors concluded that 5-ASA is effective in reducing the grade of endoscopic activity of disease recurrence, but only a small difference concerning clinical relapse was observed. Another more recent multicenter study (56) involved 87 patients and 76 controls. The active group received 5-ASA 3 g (Salofalk) for three years; the therapeutic advantage of the active drug over placebo was of 19% at three years. Surprisingly for a drug which is split in the small bowel, the least treatment effect was observed in patients with Crohn's ileitis. One case of pancreatitis was attributed to 5-ASA.

V.   USE OF STEROIDS IN THE PREVENTION OF
RECURRENCE AND ACUTE FLARES

Corticosteroids are beneficial in the management of active Crohn's disease and induce remission of symptoms in a high percentage of patients, possibly 80% (1). On the contrary, the failure of corticosteroids to maintain remission or prevent postoperative recurrence has been repeatedly confirmed (1,66–69). The ECCDS, however, showed that patients with active disease who responded to 6-methylprednisolone and achieved a clinical remission were subsequently well managed with low dosages of 6-methylprednisolone (8 mg/day) for 2 years (2). Thus, maintenance therapy with steroids was beneficial in this group, which probably included a certain number of patients with steroid-dependent disease. Steroid-dependent patients are not responsive to maintenance therapy with 5-ASA and need long-term treatment with steroids to control their symptoms. In these patients, a clinical relapse can often be expected when the dose of prednisone is reduced to less than

15 mg/day (67). The dosage of steroid used in the trials for the maintenance phase was often lower than 15 mg/day, so it is possible that higher dosages could be successful.

Contrary to the results of negative studies, in clinical practice, patients with aggressive forms of disease are managed well with long-term treatment using various doses of steroid, although these long-term therapies are accompanied by unacceptable side effects. Among the most serious consequences are complications such as osteopenia and osteonecrosis, myopathy, infections, diabetes, glaucoma, cataracts, hypertension, adverse cosmetic effects, and temporary or permanent loss of adrenocortical function (70,71). Since 1963, alternate-day prednisolone administration has been suggested to counteract these unacceptable side effects (72).

It is generally agreed that, to reduce side effects, it is preferable to use short-acting steroids such as prednisolone and to give them on alternate mornings (73). The main benefit is that the low plasma steroid levels on the off-day permit recovery of the hypothalamic-pituitary-adrenal–axis (74). Alternate-day steroid administration permits continued growth and development in adolescents, prevents the effects of steroids on the development of diabetes, and reduces the need for potassium replacement (75). The prevention of osteoporosis and fractures by the alternate-day administration of steroids, however, is not clearly established (76,77). In a recent study, Bello et al. treated 55 patients with alternate-day prednisone at the average dose of 25 mg every other morning, for a mean duration of 6.6 years, and showed a favorable response in 33 (78). The most frequent side effects were a moon face in almost all patients and acne-type rashes in young patients; no patient developed osteonecrosis or fractures (see Table 2).

Considering the relatively high effectiveness of long-term alternate-day prednisone treatment in Crohn's disease and the low rate of side effects reported, such treatment appears to be a valid option for selected patients with Crohn's disease. Results are awaited of two trials on maintenance remission with the topically acting corticosteroid (budesonide), which appears to be effective in acute Crohn's disease (79–82). A recent abstract from Europe (83) seems to confirm that oral budesonide at the dosage of 6 mg/day is significantly more effective than placebo in delaying relapse of ileocecal Crohn's disease, with minor side effects. The potentially minor side effects of this new steroid are particularly interesting in the long-term treatment of Crohn's disease.

TABLE 2 Trials on Efficacy of Immunosuppressive Drugs in the Prevention of Relapse (Rl) and Recurrence (Rc)

Ref.	Year	Drug	Dose	Control	FU (yr)	Rc/Rl	Pt	RFR
(2)	1984	MTP	8mg/day	P	2	Rl	130	47%–35%
(78)	1991	PRD	25mg/on alternate day	—	6.6	Rl	55	60%
(86)	1978	AZA	2mg/kg/day	P	2	Rl	51	95%–59%
(87)	1990	6-MP	1.5mg/kg/day	—	2	Rl	36	63%
(89)	1993	6-MP	50mg/day	—	2.8	Rl	49	79%
(89)	1993	6-MP	50mg/day	—	3.4	Rc	10	90%
(108)	1991	Cyc	2mg/kg/day	—	0.9	Rl	14	14%
(109)	1994	Cyc	5mg/kg/day	P	1.6	Rl	205	35%–50%

MTP, methylprednisolone; PRD, prednisone; AZA, azathioprine; 6-MP, 6-mercaptopurine; Cyc, cyclosporine; P, placebo; FU, follow-up; RFR, relapse free rate; Pt, number of patients

VI. IMMUNOSUPPRESSIVE THERAPIES FOR REMISSION MAINTENANCE AND PREVENTION OF POSTOPERATIVE RECURRENCE

A. Azathioprine and 6-Mercaptopurine

6-Mercaptopurine (6-MP) which is split off the azathioprine (AZA) molecule by cleavage of an imidazolyl ring, appears to be the active moiety of this compound. The two drugs seem to have identical therapeutic effects but at different dosages. The molecular weight of AZA is almost twice that of 6-MP; hence, the dose of 6-MP represents about 55% of the dose of AZA needed to produce comparable therapeutic and toxic effects (84). The upper limit of relative safety of AZA is approximately 2 mg/kg per day, corresponding to 1.1 mg/kg per day of 6-MP (35).

Although these drugs should not be used in the maintenance treatment of Crohn's disease until sulphasalazine and other 5-ASA compounds have failed, there is a role for immunosuppressive agents in approximately 20% of patients—those with refractory or steroid-dependent disease.

The key study of 6-MP in Crohn's disease is a 2-year double-blind randomized crossover study that demonstrated the effectiveness of 6-MP compared with placebo in permitting discontinuation or reduction of steroids and in closing fistulas (85). The authors noted a delay of response to therapy (> 3 months) in 32% of the 83 patients involved in the study; in 19% of patients, response took longer than 4 months. In accordance with these results, a bias against 6-MP, which has a slow onset of action, could have influenced the negative results of the NCCDS, which experimented with AZA for a relatively short period.

The efficacy of AZA in maintaining remission was first shown in a 1978 study in which patients who were in remission while taking AZA for at least 6 months were randomized to one group, which continued with AZA therapy, and to another group, which was treated with placebo (86). The cumulative probability of relapse was nil versus 25% at 6 months and 5% versus 41% at 12 months with AZA and placebo, respectively.

Another positive report on the use of 6-MP in long-term treatment of adolescents was published in 1990. Thirty-six young Crohn's disease patients with intractable symptoms were treated for at least 6 months with a maximum daily dose of 75 mg of 6-MP (87). In a follow-up beyond 1 year, 23 of the patients showed continued remission, and no serious complications were seen. Conversely, 6-MP in pediatric inflammatory bowel disease, at the dose of 1.3 mg/kg, showed good clinical efficacy in refractory disease, but at the price of a high incidence of hepatitis (88).

In some of the studies, the efficacy of 6-MP was controlled through achievement of therapeutic goals. The most common goal was the steroid-sparing effect. Steroids were discontinued in 55% to 66% of patients (85,89). Seventy-nine percent of patients in whom steroids could be stopped and for whom long-term follow-up data were available were able to remain steroid-free for a mean time of 2.8 years (89).

A recent study demonstrated a correlation between induced leukopenia (below 5000) and the achievement of remission (90). The success rate for eliminating or markedly reducing steroids by 6-MP was 77% in all patients, but success was achieved in 97% of patients who developed leukopenia.

In approximately 60% of patients of different series, internal fistulas were successfully healed (85, 89, 91). No other drugs besides 6-MP and AZA, including steroids, SASP, and metronidazole, have proved to be effective in closing the internal fistulas of Crohn's disease. Whereas total parenteral nutrition sometimes allows a transient closure, the fistulous tract often reopens when enteral feeding is resumed (92). Another reported result is that 88% of patients with Crohn's disease–related arthritis had resolution of joint symptoms on 6-MP without concomitant use of steroids (89).

No observations have been published on the prophylactic value of either 6-MP or AZA after surgical resection except in one study concerning only 10 patients, nine of whom remained disease-free after a mean follow-up of 41 months (89).

Of particular concern are the possible side effects related to long-term use of 6-MP, but the reported side effects in another long-term study were surprisingly low. Of the 396 patients with inflammatory bowel disease (IBD) treated for a mean period of 60.3 months, 3.3% had pancreatitis, 2% bone marrow depression, 2% allergic reactions, and one patient had toxic hepatitis; all these complications were reversible. Infectious complications were seen in 7.4% patients, 1.8% of whom had severe cases. One case of diffuse histiocytic lymphoma of the brain was observed (93). In another report, 78 patients were treated with 6-MP or AZA for a mean period of 1.6 years (94). Four major side effects (three serious cases of infections, one case of pancreatitis) and 16 minor side effects were observed. Therapy was discontinued in eight subjects. Only one case of colonic cancer was observed during the follow-up (94).

It is suspected that long-term treatment with AZA or 6-MP increases the risk for various neoplasms including colon cancer in IBD patients (95,96). A recent study from England, however, did not find any increased risk in 755 IBD patients treated with 2 mg/kg of AZA for a median of 12.5 months. After a median follow-up of 9 years, the authors found 31 cases of cancer compared with 24.3 expected in the general population (97).

Although long-term follow-up studies suggest that the incidence of side effects associated with antimetabolite therapy is low and that these are usually reversible, a withdrawal of the drugs for adverse events has been reported in 17% of patients (93). Moreover, 6-MP and AZA act slowly, and the long latency period limits the usefulness of these drugs in some patients.

B. Cyclosporine

Cyclosporine is a potent immunosuppressive agent, acting predominantly on T lymphocytes (98). Some anecdotal reports and a single randomized controlled trial have shown encouraging but not impressive results in the use of this drug for active Crohn's disease refractory to conventional agents (99–104). Cyclosporine acts more rapidly than AZA and 6-MP (usually within days or weeks) (103–107). The risk of a recurrence after discontinuation of cyclosporine treatment warrants that the drug should be tapered slowly if improvement is achieved (99). This should reduce the incidence of flare-ups (104). However, the scant long-term efficacy of a short course of cyclosporine in Crohn's disease has also suggested that the drug must be given continuously to maintain remission (104). Unfortunately, recent studies on long-term therapy with cyclosporine in Crohn's disease have given disappointing results. An open study showed that a dosage of 2 mg/kg per day did not seem to maintain remission; this datum has been confirmed by the results of an 18-month, placebo-controlled trial in Canadian patients (108,109). The 151 patients who received a mean oral dosage of cyclosporine of approximately 5 mg/kg per day experienced exacerbation of disease in a higher percentage than the 154 patients in the placebo group. The mean blood cyclosporine level in this study was 182 ± 61 ng/ml, which is considered by some authors to be lower than efficacy level (110). In the study on the acute phase, patients who showed improvement received an average dosage of 7.8 mg/kg per day, producing higher blood cyclosporine levels (425 ng/ml) than those of unresponsive patients (103).

In the open study by Lobo et al., more than 80% of the patients who gained remission with cyclosporine had a relapse at the dosage of 3 mg/kg per day when a tapering regimen was used to reach the maintenance dosage of 2 mg/kg per day (108). This suggests that the minimum dosage necessary for maintenance in Crohn's disease could be approximately 5 mg/kg per day, or, as shown in ulcerative colitis, a continuous intravenous administration at the start of therapy could be advisable (107). The intravenous route, followed by oral administration, was used in the first days of therapy in the long-term treatment of 21 patients with Crohn's disease fistulas in two different American hospitals (110,111). In the first study, five patients were treated for a mean of 6.2 months; two out of three treatments were successful (110). In the second study, 88% of success was reported; but, whereas seven of 16 patients had closure of fistula, another seven had only a moderate improvement (111). The mean duration of follow-up was 12.2 months. Both studies registered various side effects only in the maintenance phase. Discontinuation of the drug often caused perianal disease relapse.

The risk of chronic cyclosporine nephrotoxicity is dose dependent, increasing with a daily dose of more than 5 mg/kg (112). It has been shown that cyclosporine at a dosage of 5 mg/kg per day is associated with a decrease in effective renal plasma flow (ERPF) and glomerular filtration rate after 6 weeks of therapy and that, after reducing the dose of cyclosporine, the ERPF does not return to baseline levels (113). However, this side effect was not confirmed in a recent study that reports the follow-up (median 36 months) of 1663 patients who received renal allografts and who were treated with cyclosporine at dosages of between 3 and 6 mg/kg per day (114). Only 30 of these patients discontinued the drug because of nephrotoxicity.

A long-term Canadian study also reported few adverse events (109). Seven of 151 patients were withdrawn because of increased serum creatinine levels or because of hypertension; paresthesia, headache, and hypertrichosis were the causes of withdrawal for eight other patients.

In conclusion, as can be seen from published studies and from everyday practice, the results of using cyclosporine in Crohn's disease are nowhere near the notable efficacy shown in a preliminary study on ulcerative colitis (107). Because of the probable narrow limits between efficacy and toxicity and because of the high relapse rate after discontinuation or reduction of the drug, the use of cyclosporine in remission maintenance of Crohn's disease is not advisable except in randomized, controlled clinical trials (115).

NOTE ADDED IN PROOF: After this chapter had been prepared, a randomized controlled trial on cyclosporine for remission maintenance has been published (Stange E, Modigliani R, Pena AS, et al. European trial of cyclosporine in chronic active Crohn's disease: a 12-month study. Gastroenterology 1995; 109:774–782). This European study enrolled 182 patients with different values of activity for a period of 12 months. The patients received low doses of steroid plus cyclosporine (5 mg/kg/day by mouth) or placebo. No differences were observed between the two groups; one case of renal dysfunction, one of depression, and a case of septicemia were observed on cyclosporine.

VII. ANTIBIOTICS FOR REMISSION MAINTENANCE

On the assumption that bacteria in the gut lumen may play a role in the origin, symptoms, and/or complications of Crohn's disease, various antibacterial drugs have been used in affected patients (116,117). Few controlled trials of antibiotics have been conducted in Crohn's disease, and the results have been conflicting and sometimes disappointing (118–120).

A. Metronidazole

Metronidazole is the most used antibiotic in the treatment of active Crohn's disease. This nitromidazole compound was first reported to be effective in active disease in 1975, at the dosage of 20 mg/kg per day (121). Another study suggested that it would be especially beneficial to patients with colonic disease in whom diarrhea was a particular problem (122).

Following these reports, a series of controlled clinical trials on metronidazole were carried out as treatment for active Crohn's disease. Some of them showed no significant differences between metronidazole and placebo, but the patient populations were heterogeneous for disease location and/or concomitant therapy with steroids or SASP (118,121). Other authors suggested that metronidazole was more effective than placebo in patients with colitis or ileocolitis and slightly more effective than sulphasalazine (119,120). A very recent trial from Belgium studied the effect of metronidazole on Crohn's disease recurrence. 60 patients resected for ileal Crohn's disease were randomizedly assigned to receive metronidazole (20 mg/kg) or identical placebo. After 3 months of therapy, the severity of endoscopic lesions and the clinical recurrence in the antibiotic group were significantly reduced. Gastrointestinal intolerance, paraesthesias and one case of polyneuropathy were observed with the active drug (64).

Metronidazole has also been used in the long-term treatment (at least 12 months) of perianal Crohn's disease (123,124). More than 50% of patients had a complete healing of lesions, and nearly 100% showed improvement. However, suspension or dosage reduction of the drug was often associated with exacerbation of perianal symptoms.

The more frequent adverse reactions from therapy with metronidazole include minor gastrointestinal disturbance, metallic taste, glossitis, furry tongue, urticaria, vaginal and urethral burning, dark urine, and reversible neutropenia. A disulfiram-like side effect has been reported in patients on metronidazole who drink alcoholic beverages. Nervous system side effects include headache, ataxia, vertigo, encephalopathy, and peripheral neuropathy.

The most significant side effect encountered with metronidazole therapy was paresthesias. These occurred in approximately 50% of the patients, especially young patients, and developed approximately 6 months after the initiation of drug therapy. Side effects appeared to be dose related and tended to persist for prolonged periods after discontinuation of the drug (124–125).

B. Ciprofloxacin

In one anecdotal report, four patients with active Crohn's ileitis showed an improvement in abdominal pain and diarrhea when treated with ciprofloxacin, a quinolone antibiotic, despite the absence of any obvious enteric infection, suggesting that ciprofloxacin could have a place as primary therapy in Crohn's disease (126).

In one long-term study, 10 patients with severe perianal Crohn's disease, refractory to other forms of therapy, were treated with ciprofloxacin for a minimum of 3 months at the dosage of 1000 to 1500 mg/day (127). Healing of perianal lesions occurred in two patients for more than 2 years. Five patients, who were followed up for 4 years, had from one to frequent recurrences, but the symptoms repeatedly subsided on 1- to 3-month courses of ciprofloxacin. Two patients did not achieve complete remission and were mildly symptomatic on continuous ciprofloxacin.

A brief report on the efficacy of the combination of metronidazole (250 mg four times a day) and ciprofloxacin (500 mg twice a day) in 31 patients with refractory or steroid-dependent active Crohn's disease has recently been published (128). It showed an achievement of complete clinical remission in 51.6% of patients, a reduction of CDAI to below 170 in 61.3%, and a failure rate of only 19.4% after 3 months of therapy. Significant side effects were experienced by 12.9% of 31 patients, but disappeared after the therapy was stopped. No similar experience has been published as long-term therapy.

C. Antimyobacterials

Several recent reports have suggested that one or more mycobacteria may be associated with Crohn's disease, although others have not found any evidence to support their pathogenic role (129–134). In the last 15 years, there have also been studies suggesting some clinical benefit from various antimycobacterial drugs in Crohn's disease (135–138).

The only controlled trial with rifampicin and ethambutol was negative, but the high number of patients withdrawn for side effects (9 of 27) and the use of only two drugs partially reduces the significance of its results (139). In fact, the atypical mycobacteria identified in patients with Crohn's disease show high resistance to antibiotics, and multiple drug therapy would seem to be advisable to eradicate these organisms (140).

A 9-month open trial with a multiple drug regimen (rifampicin, ethambutol, isoniazid, and pyrazinamide or clofazimine) showed inconclusive results of these drugs as maintenance therapy (141). Another controlled trial of antituberculous therapy used rifampicin, ethambutol, and isoniazid in 126 British patients (142). During the 2 years of study, no significant differences in radiological assessment, CDAI, laboratory tests, or need of steroid or surgery were found between active and placebo groups.

Clofazimine, a powerful antimycobacterial and anti-inflammatory drug, was used as a single agent in a placebo-controlled trial on remission maintenance (143). Twenty-eight patients went into disease remission with steroid (16 on clofazimine group and 12 on placebo). After 8 months of therapy with clofazimine or placebo, 12 patients maintained remission on active drug in comparison with six on placebo (p = ns).

A recent double-blind, placebo-controlled trial with a multiple antibiotic regimen was performed on 40 patients with refractory, steroid-dependent Crohn's disease (144). The patients in the active group received 600 mg of rifampicin only once, on the day of entry into the trial, and ethambutol, dapsone, clofazimine. The result of this study showed that 15 of 19 patients with severe, steroid-dependent Crohn's disease maintained a good quality of life for 7 months without steroids, compared with 6 of 17 on placebo. The trial registered a high relapse rate on placebo (52.9% overall at 3 months and 64.7% at 9 months). The authors suggested that the positive result of this study could be explained by the partial suppression of the intestinal flora similar to that obtained with antibiotics or with elemental diets (145,146).

A new rifamycin derivative (rifabutin) was tested in a small placebo-controlled trial (147). The effect on remission maintenance was negative, but the limited patient sample reduces its statistical significance. The same drug was used together with streptomycin as maintenance treatment in six patients with severe refractory Crohn's disease (148). The authors concluded that this antimycobacterial therapy was effective in moderating the course of Crohn's disease (see Table 3).

TABLE 3 Trials on Efficacy of Antibiotics in the Prevention of Clinical (C) and Endoscopic (E) Relapse (Rl) and Recurrence (Rc)

Ref.	Year	Drug	Control	Rc/Rl	C/E	FU	Pt	RFR	TA
(141)	1989	E + R + I + Py	—	Rl	C	9 months	20	50%	NR
(147)	1989	Rifabutin	P	Rl	C	6 months	24		ND
(143)	1991	Clofazimine	P	Rl	C	12 months	28		+25%
(64)	1995	Metronidazole	P	Rc	E	3 months	60		+23%
(64)	1995	Metronidazole	P	Rc	C	36 months	60		+19%
(142)	1994	E + R + I	P	Rl	C	24 months	126		ND
(144)	1994	E + D + C + R	P	Rl	C	7 months	36		+34%

C, clofazimine; D, dapsone; E, ethambutol; I, isoniazide; Py, pyrazinamide; R, rifampicin; ND, no difference; P, placebo; Pt, number of patients; RFR, recurrence free rate; TA, therapeutic advantage; NR, not reported.

VIII. CONCLUSION

The prevention of symptoms in patients in remission because of surgery or medical therapy is one of the major goals in Crohn's disease treatment. The cost of this prevention must be evaluated according to side effects of the drugs used and advantage of lack of symptoms. The fact that many flare-ups clear up rapidly after a short course of medical therapy should also be considered.

There are, however, certain situations in which medical preventive therapy is suggested:

Patients with short bowel after surgery in whom it is necessary, if possible, to avoid new intestinal resections. In these patients, the use of maintenance therapy with drugs such as 6-MP is advisable.

Patients with aggressive type of Crohn's disease, either because of recurrent severe flare-ups or because of pathological lesions such as the "primarily fistulizing form." However, medical therapies are not usually able to modify the course of these types of Crohn's disease.

Patients with complications not related to Crohn's disease but whose general condition makes it inadvisable to wait for acute phases.

Patients in whom, when there are new flare-ups, it is impossible or inadvisable to use stronger drugs (steroid, 6-MP) because of intolerance, side effects, or general pathological situation.

Patients who are planning a pregnancy.

As far as the drugs to be used are concerned, the choice is not wide:

Aminosalicylates for ileal and SASP for colonic location are the drugs of choice for a good cost–benefit relation between side effects and efficacy. Unfortunately, their efficacy is fairly limited, showing a 10% to 24% therapeutic advantage defined as the difference between drug and placebo response (15,41,57). However, these two drugs can be safely used in pregnancy (149). The dose varies between 2 and 4 g. Higher doses probably could increase the therapeutic advantage, but at the risk of a higher percentage of side effects. Establishing the optimal dosage balanced between efficacy and adverse events will be one of the major goals of Crohn's disease treatment.

6-MP and azathioprine can be used in more aggressive forms of the disease.

Alternate-day steroids are a good alternative in young patients in whom the use of 6-MP/AZA is not indicated for motives of fertility or intolerance; the alternate-day steroids ensure lower side-effects.

Antibiotics used as a single agent or in a multiple regimen could be a possible alternative in refractory cases, particularly in Crohn's colitis with perianal disease. Their real usefulness, however, has still to be fully confirmed.

Finally, every patient with Crohn's disease should be informed about the risk of smoking in increasing the probability of symptoms relapse, recurrence after surgery, and severity of symptoms.

Many more controlled clinical trials are needed to confirm or deny the efficacy of drugs in remission maintenance and recurrence prevention. It is important, however, for future trials to differentiate between the various types of Crohn's disease, and, in the treatment groups, to balance the factors that can negatively influence the natural history of the disease. The approach of splitting up rather than gathering together could be more useful if effective therapies are to be found.

REFERENCES

1. Summers RW, Switz DM, Session JT Jr, et al. National Cooperative Crohn's Disease Study: results of drug treatment. Gastroenterology 1979; 77:847–869.

2. Malchow H, Ewe K, Brandes JW, et al. European Cooperative Crohn's Disease Study (ECCDS). Gastroenterology 1984; 86:249–266.

3. Lennard-Jones JE. Sulphasalazine in asymptomatic Crohn's disease. A multicentre trial. Gut 1977; 18:69–72.

4. Meyers S, Janowitz HD. Natural history of Crohn's disease. An analytic review of the placebo lesson. Gastroenterology 1984; 87:1189–1192.

5. Landi B, Anh TN, Cortot A, Groupe d'Etudes Therapeutiques Des Affections Inflammatoires Digestives. Endoscopic monitoring of Crohn's disease treatment: a prospective, randomized clinical trial. Gastroenterology 1992; 102:1647–1653.

6. Mekhijan HS, Switz DM, Watts HD, et al. National Cooperative Crohn's Disease Study: factors determining recurrence of Crohn's disease after surgery. Gastroenterology 1979; 77:907–913.

7. Farmer RG, Hawak WA, Turnbull RB. Clinical patterns in Crohn's disease: a statistical study of 615 cases. Gastroenterology 1975; 68:627–636.

8. Farmer RG, Whelan G, Fazio VW. Long-term follow-up of patients with Crohn's disease. Relationship between the clinical pattern and prognosis. Gastroenterology 1985; 88:1818–1825.

9. Whelan G, Farmer RG, Fazio VW, Goormastic M. Recurrence after surgery in Crohn's disease. Relationship to location of disease (clinical pattern) and surgical indication. Gastroenterology 1985; 88:1826–1833.

10. Sachar DB. The problem of postoperative recurrence of Crohn's disease. Med Clin North Am 1990; 74:183–188.

11. Rutgeerts P, Geboes K, Vantrappen G, et al. Predictability of the postoperative course of Crohn's disease. Gastroenterology 1990; 99:956–963.

12. Olaison G, Smedj K, Sjodahl R. Natural course of Crohn's disease after ileocolic resection: endoscopically visualized ileal ulcers preceding symptoms. Gut 1992; 33:331–335.

13. Olaison G, Sjodal R, Tagesson C. Glucocorticoid treatment in ileal Crohn's disease: relief of symptoms but not of endoscopically viewed inflammation. Gut 1990; 31:325–328.

14. Modigliani R, Mary JY, Simon JF, et al. Clinical, biological and endoscopic picture of attack of Crohn's disease: evolution on prednisone. Gastroenterology 1990; 98:811–818.

15. Salomon P, Kornbluth A, Aisemberg J, Janowitz HD. How effective are current drugs for Crohn's disease? A meta-analysis. J Clin Gastroenterol 1992; 14(3):211–215.

16. Kyle J. Prognosis after ileal resection for Crohn's disease. Br J Surg 1971; 58:735–737.

17. Schoefield PF. The natural history and treatment of Crohn's disease. Ann R Coll Surg Engl 1965; 36:258–259.

18. deDombal FT, Burton I, Goligher JC. Recurrence of Crohn's disease after primary excisional surgery. Gut 1971; 12:519–527.

19. Lock MR, Farmer RG, Fazio VW, et al. Recurrence and reoperation for Crohn's disease: the role of disease location in prognosis. N Engl J Med 1981; 304:1586–1589.

20. Fricker MJ, Segall MM. The resectional reoperation rate for Crohn's disease in a general community hospital. Dis Colon Rectum 1983; 26:305–309.

21. Steinberg DM, Allan RN, Thompson H, et al. Excisional surgery with ileostomy for Crohn's disease colitis with particular reference to factors affecting recurrence. Gut 1974; 15:845–851.

22. Greenstein AJ, Lachman P, Sachar DB, et al. Perforating and nonperforating indications for repeated operations in Crohn's disease: evidence for two clinical forms. Gut 1988; 29:588–592.

23. Franceschi S, Panza E, La Vecchia C, et al. Non specific inflammatory bowel disease and smoking. Am J Epidemiol 1987; 125:455–452.

24. Lindberg E, Tysk C, Andersson K, Janerot G. Smoking and inflammatory bowel disease. Gut 1988; 352–357.

25. Parsson PG, Ahlbom A, Hellers G. Inflammatory bowel disease and tobacco smoke. A case control-study. Gut 1990; 31:1377–1381.

26. Silverstein M, Lashner B, Hanauer SB, et al. Cigarette smoking in Crohn's disease: Am J Gastroenterol 1989; 84:31–33.

27. Tobin MV, Logan RFA, Langman MJS, et al. Cigarette smoking and inflammatory bowel disease. Gastroenterology 1987; 93:316–321.

28. Sommerville KW, Logan RFA, Edmond M, Langman MJS. Smoking and Crohn's disease. BMJ 1984; 289–954–956.

29. Sutherland LR, Ramcharan S, Bryant H, Fick G. Effect of cigarette smoking on recurrence of Crohn's disease. Gastroenterology 1990; 98:1123–1128.

30. Cottone M, Rosselli M, Orlando A, et al. Smoking habits and recurrence in Crohn's disease. Gastroenterology 1994; 106:643–648.

31. Wenkert A, Kristensen M, Eklund AE. The long-term prophylactic effect of salazosulpha-pyridine (Salazopyrin) in primarily resected patients with Crohn's disease: a controlled double-blind trial. Scand J Gastroenterol 1978; 13:161–167.

32. Bergman L, Krause U. Postoperative treatment with corticosteroids and salazosulphapyrid-ine (Salazopyrin) after radical resection for Crohn's disease. Scand J Gastroenterol 1976; 11:651–656.

33. Goldstein F, Thornton JJ, Abramson J. Comments on National Cooperative Crohn's Disease Study (NCCDS). Gastroenterology 1980; 78:1647–1648.

34. Korelitz BI, Present DH. Shortcomings of the National Crohn's Disease Study: the exclusion of azathioprine without adequate trial. Gastroenterology 1981; 80:193–194.

35. Goldstein F. Maintenance treatment for Crohn's disease: has the time arrived? Am J Gastro-enterol 1992; 87:551–556.

36. Dissanayake AS, Truelove SC. A controlled therapeutic trial of long-term maintenance treatment of ulcerative colitis with sulphasalazine (Salazopyrine). Gut 1973; 14:923–926.

37. Hanauer SB. The role of mesalazine in Crohn's disease. Scand J Gastroenterol 1990; (suppl 172):56–59.

38. Scholmerich J, Jenss H, Hartmann F, et al. Oral 5-aminosalicylic acid versus 6-methylpred-nisolone in active Crohn's disease. Can J Gastroenterol 1990; 4:445–457.

39. Goldstein F, Farquhar S, Thornton JJ, et al. Favorable effects of sulfasalazine on small bowel Crohn's disease: a long-term study. Am J Gastroenterol 1987; 82:848–853.

40. Peppercorn MA, Golman P. Distribution studies of salicylazosulfapyridine and its metabolites. Gastroenterology 1973; 64:240–245.

41. Prantera C, Pallone F, Brunetti G, Italian IBD Study Group. Oral 5-aminosalicylic acid (As-acol) in the maintenance treatment of Crohn's disease. Gastroenterology 1992; 103:363–368.

42. Ewe K, Herfarth C, Malchow H, Jesdinsky HJ. Postoperative recurrence of Crohn's disease in relation to radicality of operation and sulfasalazine prophylaxis: a multicenter trial. Digestion 1989; 42:224–232.

43. Goldstein F, Murdock MG. Clinical and radiologic improvement of regional enteritis and enterocolitis after treatment with salicylazosulfapyridine. Am J Dig Dis 1971; 16:421–431.

44. Goldstein F, Thornton JJ, Abramsom J. Anti-inflammatory drug treatment in Crohn's disease. Am J Gastroenterol 1976; 66:251–258.

45. Goldstein F, Menduke H, Thornton JJ, et al. Anti-inflammatory drug treatment of Crohn's disease: a prospective evaluation of 100 consecutively treated patients. J Clin Gastroenterol 1980; 2:77–85.

46. Goldstein F. Current status of medical treatment for inflammatory bowel disease. Am J Gastroenterol 1983; 78:841–844.

47. Lashner BA. Incorporating randomized clinical trials into clinical practice: maintenance treatment for Crohn's disease. Am J Gastroenterol 1992; 87:549–550.

48. Lee CG, Papaioannou N. Recurrences following surgery for Crohn's disease. J Clin Gastro-enterol 1980; 9:419–438.

49. Wellman W, Schroder U. New oral preparations for maintenance therapy in Crohn's disease (abstr). Can J Gastroenterol 1988; 2A:71A–72A.

50. International Mesalazine Study Group. Coated oral 5-aminosalicylic acid versus placebo in maintaining remission of inactive Crohn's disease. Aliment Pharmacol Ther 1990; 4:55–64.

51. Bresci G, Petrucci A, Banti S. 5-Aminosalicylic-acid in the prevention of relapses of Crohn's disease in remission: a long-term study. Int J Clin Pharma Res 1991; 11:200–202.

52. Gendre JP, Mary JY, Florent C, et al. Oral mesalamine (Pentasa) as maintenance treat-ment in Crohn's disease: a multicenter placebo-controlled study. Gastroenterology 1993; 104:435–439.

53. Aber N, Odes SH, Fireman Z, et al. A controlled double blind multicenter study of the effectiveness of 5-aminosalicylic acid in patients with Crohn's disease in remission (abstr). Gastroenterology 1994; 106(4 part 2):A646.

54. de Franchis R, Brignola C, Del Piano M, a multicenter study group. Oral 5-aminosalicylic acide (5-ASA) in the prevention of early relapse of Crohn's disease. Interim analysis of a multicenter double blind randomized placebo-controlled trial (abstr). Gastroenterology 1994; 106(4 part 2):A670.

55. Brignola C, Cottone M, Pera A, et al. Mesalamine in the prevention of endoscopic recurrence after resection for Crohn's disease. Gastroenterology 1995; 108:345–349.

56. McLeod RS, Wolff BG, Steinart H, et al. Prophylactic mesalamine treatment decreases postoperative recurrence of Crohn's disease. Gastroenterology 1995; 109:401–413.

57. Singleton JW, Hanauer SB, Gitnick GL, et al. Mesalamine capsules for the treatment of active Crohn's disease: results of a 16-week trial. Pentasa Crohn's Disease Study Group. Gastro-enterology 1993; 104:1293–1301.

58. Messori A, Brignola C, Trallori G, et al. Effectiveness of 5-aminosalicylic acid for maintaining remission in patients with Crohn's disease. A meta-analysis. Am J Gastroenterol 1994; 89:692–698.

59. Brignola C, Campieri M, Farruggia P, et al. A laboratory index for predicting relapse in asymptomatic patients with Crohn's disease. Gastroenterology 1986; 91:1490–1494.

60. Boirivant M, Leoni M, Tariciotti D, et al. The clinical significance of serum C reactive protein levels in Crohn's disease: results of a prospective longitudinal study. J Clin Gastroenterol 1988; 10(4):401–405.

61. Brignola C, Iannone P, Pasquali S, et al. Placebo-controlled trial of oral 5-ASA in relapse prevention of Crohn's disease. Dig Dis Sci 1992; 37(1):29–32.

62. Tytgat GNJ, Mulder CJJ, Brummelkamp WH. Endoscopic lesions in Crohn's disease early after ileocecal resection. Endoscopy 1988; 20:260–262.

63. Florent C, Cortot A, Quandale P, GETAID, et al. Placebo controlled trial of Claversal in the prevention of early endoscopic relapse after "curative" resection for Crohn's disease (CD). Gastroenterology 1992; 102:A623.

64. Rutgeerts P, Hiele M, Geboes K, et al. Controlled trial of metronidazole for prevention of Crohn's recurrence after ileal resection. Gastroenterology 1995; 108:1617–1621.

65. Caprilli R, Andreoli A, Capurso L, et al. Oral mesalazine (5-aminosalicylic acid; Asacol) for the prevention of post-operative recurrence of Crohn's disease. Aliment Pharmacol Ther 1994; 8:35–43.

66. Jones JH, Lennard-Jones JE: Corticosteroids and corticotrophin in the treatment of Crohn's disease. Gut 1966; 7:181–186.

67. Sparberg N, Kirsner JB. Long term corticosteroid therapy for regional enteritis: an analysis of 58 courses in 54 patients. Am J Dig Dis 1966; 11:865–880.

68. Cooke WT, Fielding JF. Corticosteroid or corticotrophin therapy in Crohn's disease (regional enteritis). Gut 1970; 11:921–927.

69. Bergman L, Krause V. Postoperative treatment with corticosteroids and salazosulphapyridine (Salazopyrin) after radical resection for Crohn's disease. Scand J Gastroenterol 1976; II:651.

70. Lukert BP, Raisz LG. Glucocorticoid-induced osteoporosis, pathogenesis and management. Ann Intern Med 1990; 112:352–364.

71. Zizic TM, Marcoux C, Hungersford DS, et al. Corticosteroid therapy associated with ischemic necrosis of bone in systemic lupus erythematosus. Am J Med 1985; 79:596–641.

72. Horter JG, Reddy WJ, Thorn GW. Studies on intermittent corticosteroid dosage regimen. N Engl J Med 1963; 269:591–596.

73. Claman HN. Anti-inflammatory effects of corticosteroids. Clin Immun Allergy 1984; 4:317–329.

74. Shurmeyer TH, Tsokos GC, Avgerinos PC, et al. Pituitary adrenal responsiveness to corticotropin-releasing–hormone in patients receiving chronic, alternate-day glucocorticoid therapy. J Clin Endocrinol Metab 1985; 61:22–27.

75. Whittington PF, Barnes HV, Bayless TM. Medical management of Crohn's disease in adolescence. Gastroenterology 1977; 72:1338–1344.

76. Gluck OS, Murphy WA, Hahan TS, et al. Bone loss in adults receiving alternate-day glucocorticoid therapy. A comparison with daily therapy. Arthritis Rheum 1981; 24:892–898.

77. Sheagran JM, Jowsay J, Bird DDC, et al. Effect on bone growth of daily versus alternate-day corticosteroid administration. An experimental study. J Lab Clin Med 1977; 89:120–130.

78. Bello C, Goldstein F, Thorton J. Alternate-day prednisone treatment and treatment maintenance in Crohn's disease. Am J Gastroenterol 1991; 4:460–466.

79. Inflammatory Bowel Disease Study Group. Budesonide 9 or 15 mg rapidly improves quality of life (QOL) in active Crohn's disease (abstr). Gut 1993; 34(suppl 4):F210.

80. Rutgeerts P, Lofberg R, Malchow H, European Budesonide Study Group. Budesonide versus prednisolone for the treatment of active ileocecal Crohn's disease (abstr). Gastroenterology 1993; 104(4):A772.

81. Wolman SL, Greenberg GR. Oral budesonide in active Crohn's disease: an initial experience (abstr). Gastroenterology 1991; 100(5 part 2):A263.

82. Lofberg R, Danielsson A, Salde L. Oral budesonide in active Crohn's disease. Aliment Pharmacol Ther 1993; 7:611–616.

83. Lofberg R, Rutgeerts P, Malchow H, European Budesonide Study Group. Budesonide CID

for maintenance of remission in ileocecal Crohn's disease. A European multicenter placebo controlled trial for 12 months (abstr). DDW 1994; A:2299.

84. Windholz M. The Merck Index. 10th ed. Rahway, NJ: Merk and Co. 1983.

85. Present DH, Korelitz BI, Wisch N, et al. Treatment of Crohn's disease with 6-mercaptopurine. A long-term randomized double blind study. N Engl J Med 1980; 302:981–987.

86. O'Donoghue DP, Dowson AM, Powell-Tuck J, et al. Double-blind withdrawal trial of azathioprine as maintenance treatment for Crohn's disease. Lancet 1978; 2:955–957.

87. Markowitz J, Rosa J, Grancher K, et al. Long-term 6-mercaptopurine treatment in adolescents with Crohn's disease. Gastroenterology 1990; 99:1347–1351.

88. Gold D, Pettei M, Kessler B, Levine J. 6-Mercaptopurine (6-MP) in pediatric inflammatory bowel disease (IBD) (abstr). Am J Gastroenterol 1992; 87(2):A320.

89. Korelitz BI, Adler DJ, Mendelsohn RA, Sacknoff A. Long-term experience with 6-mercaptopurine in the treatment of Crohn's disease. Am J Gastroenterol 1993; 88:1198–1205.

90. Colonna T, Korelitz BI. The role of leukopenia in the 6-mercaptopurine–induced remission of refractory Crohn's disease. Am J Gastroenterol 1994; 89:362–366.

91. Korelitz BI, Present DH. Favorable effect of 6-mercaptopurine on the fistulae of Crohn's disease. Dig Dis Sci 1985; 30:58–64.

92. Elson CO, Layden TJ, Nemchausky BA, et al. An evaluation of total parenteral nutrition in the management of inflammatory bowel disease. Dig Dis Sci 1980; 25:42–48.

93. Present DH, Meltzer SJ, Krumholz MP, et al. 6-Mercaptopurine in the management of inflammatory bowel disease: short- and long-term toxicity. Ann Intern Med 1989; 111:641–649.

94. O'Brien J, Bayless TM, Bayless JA. Use of azathioprine or 6-mercaptopurine in the treatment of Crohn's disease. Gastroenterology 1991; 101:39–46.

95. Zelig M, Choi P. Azathioprine or 6-mercaptopurine therapy and colon carcinoma in Crohn's disease (letter). Gastroenterology 1992; 102:1448.

96. Meyers S. The use of 6-mercaptopurine in adolescents (letter). Gastroenterology 1991; 100:1156.

97. Connell WR, Kamm MA, Dickson M, Balkwill AM, Ritchie JK, Lennard-Jones JE. Long-term neoplasia risk after azathioprine treatment in inflammatory bowel disease. Lancet 1994; 343:1249–1252.

98. Hess AD, Esa AH, Colombani PM. Mechanism of action of cyclosporine: effect on cells of the immune system and on subcellular events in T cell activation. Transplant Proc 1988; 2(suppl 2):29–39.

99. Allison MC, Pounder RE. Cyclosporin for Crohn's disease. Aliment Pharmacol Ther 1987; 1:39–43.

100. Peltekian KM, Williams CN, MacDonald AS, et al. Open study of cyclosporine in patients with severe active Crohn's disease refractory to conventional therapy. Can J Gastroenterol 1988; 2:5–11.

101. Allam BF, Tillman JE, Thomson TJ, et al. Effective intravenous cyclosporin therapy in a patient with severe Crohn's disease on parenteral nutrition. Gut 1987; 28:1166–1169.

102. Brynskov J, Binder V, Riis P, et al. Low-dose cyclosporin for Crohn's disease: implications for clinical trials. Aliment Pharmacol Ther 1989; 3:135–142.

103. Brynskov J, Freund L, Norby Rasmussen S, et al. A placebo-controlled, double-blind randomized trial of cyclosporine therapy in active, chronic Crohn's disease. N Engl J Med 1989; 321:845–850.

104. Brynskov J, Freund L, Norby Rasmussen S, et al. Final report on a placebo-controlled, double-blind, randomized, multicentre trial of cyclosporine treatment in active chronic Crohn's disease. Scand J Gastroenterol 1991; 26:689–695.

105. Lichtiger S, Present DH. Preliminary report: cyclosporin in treatment of severe ulcerative colitis in children. J Pediatr 1991; 119:994–997.

106. Actis GC, Ottobrelli A, Barletti A, et al. Cyclosporin controls severe acute ulcerative colitis by abolishing the acute phase response (abstr). Gastroenterology 1993; 104:A658.

107. Lichtiger S, Present DH, Kornbluth A, et al. Cyclosporine in severe ulcerative colitis refractory to steroid therapy. N Engl J Med 1994; 330(26):1841–1845.

108. Lobo AJ, Juby LD, Rothwell J, et al. Long-term treatment of Crohn's disease with cyclosporin: the effect of a very low dose on maintenance of remission. J Clin Gastroenterol 1991; 13:42–45.

109. Feagan BG, McDonald JWD, Rochon J, et al. Low-dose cyclosporine for the treatment of Crohn's disease. N Engl J Med 1994; 330(26):1846–1851.

110. Hanauer SB, Smith MB. Rapid closure of Crohn's disease fistulas with continuous intravenous cyclosporin A. Am J Gastroenterol 1993; 88:646–649.

111. Present DH, Lichtiger S. Efficacy of cyclosporine in treatment of fistula of Crohn's disease. Dig Dis Sci 1994; 39(2):374–380.

112. Feutren G, Mihatsch MJ. Risk factors for cyclosporine-induced nephropathy in patients with autoimmune disease. N Engl J Med 1992; 326:1654–1660.

113. Lobo AJ, Juby LD, Rothwell J, et al. The effect of oral cyclosporin on renal function in Crohn's disease. Gut 1989; 30:A1480.

114. Burke JF, Pirsch JD, Ramos EL, et al. Long-term efficacy and safety of cyclosporine in renal-transplant recipients. N Engl J Med 1994; 331(6):358–363.

115. Sartor RB. Cyclosporine therapy for inflammatory bowel disease. N Engl J Med 1994; 330(26):1897–1898.

116. Moss AA, Carbone JV, Kressel HY. Radiological and clinical assessment of broad-spectrum antibiotic therapy in Crohn's disease. Am J Roentgenol 1978; 131:787–790.

117. Keighley MRB. Infection and the use of antibiotics in Crohn's disease. Can J Surg 1984; 27: 438–441.

118. Ambrose NS, Allan RN, Keighley MRB, et al. Antibiotic therapy for treatment in relapse of intestinal Crohn's disease. Dis Colon Rectum 1985; 28:81–85.

119. Ursing B, Alm T, Barany F, et al. A comparative study of metronidazole and sulfasalazine for active Crohn's disease: the Cooperative Crohn's Disease Study in Sweden. II. Result. Gastroenterology 1982; 83:550–562.

120. Sutherland L, Singleton J, Sessions J, et al. Double blind, placebo controlled trial of metronidazole in Crohn's disease. Gut 1991; 32:1071–1075.

121. Ursing B, Kamme G. Metronidazole for Crohn's disease. Lancet 1975; i:775–777.

122. Allan RN, Cooke WT. Evaluation of metronidazole in the management of Crohn's disease (abstr). Gut 1977; 18:A422.

123. Bernstein LH, Frank MS, Brandt LJ, Boley SJ. Healing of perianal Crohn's disease with metronidazole. Gastroenterology 1980; 79:357–365.

124. Brandt LJ, Bernstein LH, Boley SJ, Frank MS. Metronidazole therapy for perineal Crohn's disease: a follow-up study. Gastroenterology 1982; 83:383–387.

125. Duffy LF, Daum F, Fischer SE, et al. Peripheral neuropathy in Crohn's disease patients treated with metronidazole. Gastroenterology 1985; 88:681–684.

126. Peppercorn MA. Is there a role for antibiotics as primary therapy in Crohn's ileitis? J Clin Gastroenterol 1993; 17(3):235–237.

127. Turunen U, Farkkila V, Valtonen V, Seppala K. Long-term outcome of ciprofloxacin treatment in severe perianal or fistulous Crohn's disease (abstr). Gastroenterology 1993; 104:A793.

128. Prantera C, Kohn A, Zannoni F, et al. Metronidazole plus ciprofloxacin in the treatment of active, refractory Crohn's disease: results of an open study. J Clin Gastroenterol 1994; 19(1):79–80.

129. Burnham WR, Lennard-Jones JE. Mycobacteria as a possible cause of inflammatory bowel disease. Lancet 1978; 2:693–696.

130. Chiodini RJ, Van Kruningen HJ, Thayer WR, et al. Possible role of mycobacteria in inflammatory bowel disease. I. An unclassified mycobacterium species isolated from patients with Crohn's disease. Dig Dis Sci 1984; 29:1073–1079.

131. Gitnick G, Coolins J, Beaman B, et al. Preliminary report on isolation of mycobacteria from patients with Crohn's disease. Dig Dis Sci 1989; 34:925–932.

132. Graham DY, Markesich DC, Yoshimura HH. Mycobacteria and inflammatory bowel disease. Results of culture. Gastroenterology 1978; 92:436–442.

133. Kobayashi K, Brown WR, Brennan PJ, et al. Serum antibodies to mycobacterial antigens in active Crohn's disease. Gastroenterology 1988; 94:1404–1411.

134. Butcher PD, McFadden JJ, Hermon-Taylor J. Investigation of mycobacteria in Crohn's disease tissue by Southern blotting and DNA hybridisation with cloned mycobacterial genomic DNA probes from Crohn's disease isolated mycobacteria. Gut 1988; 9:1222–1228.

135. Ward M, McManus JPS. Dapsone in Crohn's disease. Lancet 1975; 1:1236–1237.

136. Warren JB, Rees HC, Cox TM. Remission of Crohn's disease with tuberculosis chemotherapy (letter). N Engl J Med 1986; 314:182.

137. Prantera C, Bothamley G, Levenstein S, et al. Crohn's disease and mycobacteria: two cases of Crohn's disease with high antimycobacterial antibody levels cured by dapsone therapy. Biomed Pharmacother 1989; 43:295–299.

138. Parker MC, Hampson SJ, Saverymuttu SH, et al. Combination antimycobacterial chemotherapy with major clinical response in established Crohn's disease (abstr). Gut 1987; 28:A1390.

139. Shaffer JL, Hughes S, Linaker BD, et al. Controlled trial of rifampicin and ethambutol in Crohn's disease. Gut 1984; 25:103–105.

140. Grange JM. Mycobacterial and Human Disease. London: Arnold E, 1988.

141. Hampson SJ, Parker MC, Saverymuttu AEJ, et al. Quadruple antimycobacterial chemotherapy in Crohn's disease: results at 9 months of a pilot study in 20 patients. Aliment Pharmacol Ther 1989; 343–352.

142. Swift GL, Srivastava ED, Stone R, et al. Controlled trial of antituberculous chemotherapy for two years in Crohn's disease. Gut 1994; 35:363–368.

143. Afdhal NH, Long A, Lennon J, et al. Controlled trial of antimycobacterial therapy in Crohn's disease. Clofazimine versus placebo. Dig Dig Sci 1991; 36(4):449–453.

144. Prantera C, Kohn A, Mangiarotti R, et al. Antimycobacterial therapy in Crohn's disease: results of a controlled, double-blind trial with a multiple antibiotic regimen. Am J Gastroenterol 1994; 4:513–518.

145. Sartor RB. Role of intestinal microflora in initiation and perpetuation of inflammatory bowel disease. Can J Gastroenterol 1990; 4:271–277.

146. Saverymuttu S, Hodgson HJF, Chadwick VS. Controlled trial comparing prednisolone with an elemental diet plus non-absorbable antibiotics in active Crohn's disease. Gut 1985; 26:994–998.

147. Basilisco G, Ranzi T, Campanini MC, et al. Controlled trial of rifabutin in Crohn's disease. Curr Ther Res 1989; 46(2):245–250.

148. Thayer WR, Coutu JA, Chiodini RJ, Van Kruininger HJ. Use of rifabutin and streptomycin in the therapy of Crohn's disease (abstr). Gastroenterology 1988; 94(5 part 2):A458.

149. Habal FM, Hui G, Greenberg GR. Oral 5-aminosalicylic acid for inflammatory bowel disease in pregnancy: safety and clinical course. Gastroenterology 1993; 105:1057–1060.

COMMENTARY

David B. Sachar   *Mount Sinai Medical Center, New York, New York*

A computer can retrieve 149 references on the prevention of relapse and recurrence in Crohn's disease, but only the keenest and most perceptive minds could analyze all the data as cogently and critically as Drs. Prantera and Andreoli have done in this chapter. They have brought at least six of the most pivotal issues into sharp focus.

First, the authors have clearly distinguished between maintenance of medically induced or spontaneous remissions on the one hand and prevention of postoperative recurrence on the other. Moreover, they have carefully pointed out those studies that failed to draw this crucial distinction within their patient populations, such as the ECCDS (2).

We could, in fact, carry the issue even further by noting that the concept of "maintenance of remission" actually embraces at least five different approaches. One might be called "continued active therapy," in which a particular treatment that has already brought the disease into remission is either continued or withdrawn; this was, for example, the maintenance design of the classic O'Donoghue study of azathioprine and of the ECCDS trial of 6-methylprednisolone (2,86). A second approach is newly introduced therapy, "out of the blue," so to speak, as in the recent French study of Pentasa (52). A third design entails the temporary or "bridging" use of an agent for short-term maintenance, which is then switched over to another drug for the long term, as in the transition from oral cyclosporine to 6-mercaptopurine for treating ulcerative colitis (107). The fourth method is to monitor clinical or laboratory indicators prospectively, seeking an early warning of impending relapse, which is then aborted by the initiation of treatment, as Brignola et al. have attempted to do with the preemptive use of steroids (J Clin Gastroenterol 1988; 10:631). Fifth, there are purely postoperative trials like those of Caprilli et al. and McLeod et al. (56,65). As this chapter emphasizes, no study of maintenance therapy should be reviewed without specifying the particular design it uses.

Besides their careful attention to different study designs, the second strength of Prantera and Andreoli's analysis is their concern with various definitions of relapse or recurrence. The possibility of subjectivity in determining these events, even by endoscopic criteria, represents a potential criticism of unblinded studies (e.g., reference 65).

The third pillar of this chapter is its recognition of the importance of dosage in assessing and comparing results. They are, for example, correct in observing that the most effective maintenance therapy with 5-ASA appears to require at least 2 g/day of active drug. On the other hand, their recommendation of 1.1 mg/kg per day of 6-mercaptopurine as "the upper limit of relative safety" is out of accord with my own clinical experience, which sets 1.5 mg/kg per day as a minimum effective dosage and 2.5, or occasionally even 3.0, mg/kg per day as necessary upper limits (unless leukopenia supervenes at a lower dose). Also, the authors seem more optimistic about the efficacy and safety of alternate-day steroids than are many of the rest of us who treat adults.

The fourth strong point of Prantera and Andreoli's review is their emphasis on the need for long durations of follow-up in view of the high maintenance of remission rate on placebo (15), a fact often overlooked in less critical studies.

Fifth, the authors focus intently on the role of confounding factors (e.g., smoking [30] or disease location [41]) and of different "risk strata" (e.g., duration of prior remission, [52]) in influencing the results of clinical trials. This point cannot be overemphasized. To the many potential confounding factors and risk strata inherent in postoperative studies, for example, we might also add operative history (i.e., primary versus repeated resection), choice of surgical procedure (e.g., anastomosis versus ileostomy), and indication for surgery (e.g., short-duration fistulizing disease versus long-duration fibrostenotic disease). A heterogeneous mixture of cases (e.g., reference 56) can impede easy interpretation of results.

Finally, Prantera and Andreoli are to be commended for their pragmatic balance between, on the one hand, a richly documented and critically analyzed review of the literature and, on the other hand, a willingness to depart from strictly charted territory to make specific recommendations (e.g., using 6-mercaptopurine postoperatively for high-risk patients) on the basis of clinical instinct and experience. Therapeutic restraint, confined to what published studies and meta-analyses justify, is generally admirable, but a little courage and imagination are sometimes necessary in the management of this baffling disease.

17
Nutrition and Special Diets

John E. Lennard-Jones *St. Mark's Hospital, London, England*

Nutritional repletion in Crohn's disease is a positive aspect of treatment that is often neglected. Depletion of nutrients leads to growth failure in young people and weakness and wasting at all ages. Dietary modification can relieve symptoms, and there is evidence that it can also reduce inflammation. Although these three aspects of nutritional therapy are not independent, they are discussed separately.

I. NUTRITIONAL DEPLETION

Chronic nutritional depletion in normal people leads to functional and psychological changes, as well as to loss of body tissue. Muscle weakness is manifested by loss of strength and rapid fatigability. Psychological changes include depression, apathy, and loss of sociability. In a patient with Crohn's disease, these changes due to malnutrition may be added to the effects of past or present inflammation. Nutritional depletion can often be reversed by simple, safe, inexpensive treatments so that the patient's quality of life is improved even though Crohn's disease persists.

A. Growth Retardation

Pediatricians record the height and weight of children regularly; gastroenterologists, physicians, and surgeons who care for children and young people with Crohn's disease tend to neglect this important aspect of supervision (1). If growth retardation is to be recognized early, not only must height and weight be compared with normal standards at diagnosis but regular measurements must also be made thereafter to assess growth velocity (2,3). A rate of growth that is slower than normal because of disease can be succeeded by a period of "catch up" growth that is as great as the maximum normal rate or more, if treatment is successful and if the epiphyses have not fused.

The usual cause for growth retardation is a poor appetite with decreased calorie intake. In one series, the intake was 50% to 70% of that recommended for children of the same age and sex. The mean growth rate increased more than threefold when an increase in daily energy intake from a mean of 1535 to 2493 kCal was achieved by oral supplementation in five growth-retarded adolescents (4). The poor appetite is often associated with active inflammation or an exacerbation of symptoms, such as abdominal pain or diarrhea, by food. Treatment of active disease must therefore accompany measures to increase food intake. The role of corticosteroids in this regard is complex, and the major factor leading to growth retardation appears to be the activity of inflammation rather than steroid therapy (5). A short course of treatment with a corticosteroid may improve appetite and growth. Long-continued daily treatment retards growth but a single dose of glucocorticoid on alternate days may not do so (3).

To improve food intake, simple explanation and the use of appetizing snacks may be effective, but often it is not. In one study, a dietary assessment was made and a caloric goal appropriate for the person's current height was set. A liquid supplement to normal food was then given with either an elemental or polymeric diet, according to taste preference, which supplied an extra 600 to 1200 kCal daily for up to 1 year until caloric requirements were met by food alone. Satisfactory growth was achieved in five patients but all were at or below the 15th percentile at the end of the follow-up period (4). The most effective way of improving nutrient consumption is for the child or young person to pass a fine nasogastric tube each night, through which 1 to 1.5 L (1000–1500 kCal) of liquid proprietary feed is infused during sleep. Eight adolescents who did so gained a mean of 11.75 kg in weight and 6.98 cm in height over 1 year compared with minimal growth in six subjects who rejected this treatment and relied on supplementation of food by day (6). In this study, results obtained with a simpler, cheaper polymeric diet were as good as those obtained with an elemental diet reported by other investigators (7). When an increased dietary intake is impossible due to abdominal pain, or when there is severe malabsorption, parenteral nutrition at home should be considered.

B. Nutritional Repletion in Adults with Chronic Crohn's Disease

As in young people, nutritional depletion in adults is usually due to poor food intake rather than a raised metabolic rate or malabsorption. A group of 13 patients with Crohn's disease who experienced a mean weight loss of 15% differed from 11 patients without weight loss by taking an average of 700 kCal less energy daily and by scores showing evidence of poor appetite and depression. No differences were found in disease activity, energy expenditure, or fecal energy loss (8).

Thus, the main aim of nutritional treatment is to increase calorie intake. A controlled crossover trial showed the marked benefit that occurred when outpatients with Crohn's disease increased their nutrient intake by approximately 500 kCal daily through drinking a liquid polymeric supplement that supplied approximately 1.5 kCal per milliliter (9). Thus, a relatively small volume of a liquid supplement taken between meals or at bedtime can be recommended to improve the nutrition of adults with chronic Crohn's disease.

C. Nutritional Repletion in Acute or Complicated Crohn's Disease

When patients are acutely ill, severe loss of body weight and lean body mass occur, accompanied by muscle weakness demonstrable by respiratory function tests, grip strength tests, and other measures (10). Nutritional repletion can improve muscle function within a few days, before changes in weight or body protein are demonstrable (10). Food plus liquid nutritional supplements may be adequate to increase food intake to a satisfactory level, but, more commonly, a nasogastric infusion of a liquid complete nutritional supplement overnight or throughout the 24 hours may be needed to improve nutrition. If severe inflammation or sepsis is present, anabolism is depressed and gain in lean body mass or serum proteins may not occur although further deterioration in nutritional state is prevented. Parenteral nutrition is indicated if there is likely to be a period of starvation, for example, after major surgery, or if the gut cannot be used for nutritional support such as during ileus or in the presence of a high small bowel fistula.

D. Nutritional Repletion in Intestinal Failure

Treatment of intestinal failure when the gut is unable to absorb sufficient electrolytes or nutrients from normal food to maintain health has recently been reviewed elsewhere by Lennard-Jones (11). Severe malabsorption of this type can occur after resection of a major part of the small intestine for Crohn's disease. In general, nutritional problems do not arise unless the length of small gut remaining is less than 200 cm. There are two major types of shortened small intestines: (a) a major resection of jejunum, ileum, and the whole large intestine, leaving a proximal length of jejunum ending at a stoma, or (b) a major resection of small bowel, leaving the residual small intestine in continuity with a length of functional colon.

1. Shortened Small Intestine Ending at a Terminal Stoma

The major problem of a patient with a high jejunostomy is sodium loss with corresponding fluid depletion. A potentially dangerous situation (with hypotension and prerenal uremia) requiring urgent intravenous replacement may develop over a few days. Less easily recognized is chronic sodium depletion with low plasma volume, minimal sodium excretion in the urine, and increased plasma aldosterone. Most patients with a jejunostomy need a supplement of water and sodium. Use can be made of coupled sodium and glucose absorption in the jejunum, but a sodium concentration of 90 mmol/L or more in the lumen is necessary because the jejunum can maintain only a small concentration gradient between the intestinal lumen and plasma. Conversely, the presence of water or more dilute sodium solutions in the lumen lead to sodium secretion. In health, the sodium secreted is absorbed by the ileum and colon. When a high jejunostomy is present, the sodium is lost from the body. Thus, patients with a high jejunostomy are helped by sipping a glucose–electrolyte solution through the day and by not drinking large volumes of water or other low-sodium drinks. Each liter of suitable replacement solution contains 60 mmol (3.5 g) of sodium chloride, 30 mmol (2.5 or 2.9 g) of sodium bicarbonate or citrate, and 110 mmol (20 g) of glucose.

Measurements of the difference between the total energy value of food consumed and the energy content of the jejunostomy effluent show, as expected, that there is malabsorption. Many patients absorb approximately two-thirds as much energy as normal and thus have to increase their daily energy intake by one-half to maintain weight (12). This can be done by eating larger and more frequent meals, supplemented by snacks between meals and at bedtime. The snacks can be ordinary food or a specially prepared liquid or semisolid supplement. There is no evidence that an elemental or hydrolyzed diet offers clinical benefit over ordinary food (13). Patients with a jejunostomy do not need to restrict fat in their diet. A constant proportion of the fat is absorbed; thus, the more that is eaten, the more of this high-energy source is absorbed. The resulting increase in fat content of the jejunostomy effluent does not appear to have any adverse metabolic effect, such as increased loss of divalent cations, nor does it make the effluent socially unpleasant (13,14).

2. Shortened Small Intestine in Continuity with a Functional Length of Large Intestine

The colon absorbs sodium efficiently and patients with a shortened small intestine do not usually suffer from sodium deficiency. In health, some carbohydrate enters the colon from the ileum. Most of this carbohydrate is fermented by colonic bacteria to short-chain fatty acids, which are absorbed by the colonic mucosa. After a major resection of small intestine, more unabsorbed carbohydrate than normal enters the colon; absorption of the resulting short-chain fatty acids provides an energy source as great as 500 kCal (15).

After major intestinal resection, excess fat enters the colon. Long-chain unsaturated fatty acids inhibit water absorption by the colon and increase transit rate causing liquid diarrhea. Steatorrhea leads to increased colonic oxalate absorption and hyperoxaluria, which, on precipitation, forms calcium oxalate renal stones.

Patients with a short gut in continuity with colon thus need to eat more energy-rich foods than normal and to favor a diet high in carbohydrate but low in fat and oxalate. However, fat is a good energy source and adds to the palatability of food. In practice, patients adjust their diet when they can see clinical benefit. Fat reduction is accepted as long as there is an improvement in diarrhea with decreased frequency, more solid consistency of the stools, or less unpleasant smell. A strict low-oxalate diet is accepted if renal stones are troublesome.

II. POSSIBLE MECHANISMS BY WHICH DIETARY MODIFICATION COULD INFLUENCE SYMPTOMS OR REDUCE INFLAMMATION

A. Food Antigens

The cause of Crohn's disease is unknown. An immune response to one or more antigens in food might induce inflammation or, as a secondary phenomenon, aggravate inflammation when food antigens pass through an abnormally permeable mucosa.

B. Altered Immunity

Malnutrition leads to diminished cellular immunity and, conversely, nutritional repletion could alter the imune response and so affect inflammation (16).

C. Inflammatory Mediators

Derivatives of arachidonic acid play a major role in the inflammatory cascade. Partial replacement of arachidonic acid by other polyunsaturated fatty acids alters the metabolic pathway, with the formation of altered eicosanoids, such as less active leukotriene B5 rather than leukotriene B4. Modification of fatty acids in the diet may thus affect inflammation.

Antioxidants in the diet could alter the activity of free oxygen radicals and thus improve inflammation.

D. Metabolic Substrates and Growth Factors

Glutamine is an essential metabolic substrate for enterocytes, and depletion may affect their function or viability; conversely, repletion could diminish intestinal permeability and improve function. Colonocytes depend for part of their metabolic fuel on short-chain fatty acids in the gut lumen. The integrity of the epithelium is thus adversely affected by absence of fermentable carbohydrate in the colon.

E. Digestive Enzymes

Tryptic activity is demonstrable in ileostomy effluent. Decreased secretion of digestive enzymes could reduce inflammation of diseased mucosa.

F. Motility

Partial obstruction leads to increased motor activity proximally, which is the basis of colic and distention. Solid or semisolid food residues can cause hold-up at a site of intestinal narrowing and so lead to abdominal symptoms.

G. Altered Bacterial Flora

The colonic bacterial flora depends for its metabolism on substrates derived from food residues. Alteration of the substrate by withholding food or altering its composition could affect the number of bacteria present or the relative frequency of different types of bacteria. Free flow of liquid intestinal contents when an intestinal stricture is present could reduce the bacterial overgrowth associated with stasis. These alterations could affect inflammation by reducing pathogenic bacteria or potentially harmful bacterial cell products, such as formyl-methionyl-leucyl-phenylalanine (FMLP), in the lumen.

III. DIFFICULTIES IN DISTINGUISHING BETWEEN RELIEF OF SYMPTOMS AND REDUCED INFLAMMATION

The clinical assessment of Crohn's disease depends on recording symptoms; on assessment of structural changes by endoscopy, radiology, or biopsy; and on assessment of functional changes, such as intestinal permeability, leucocyte migration across the mucosa into the gut lumen, protein loss into the gut, increased synthesis of acute phase proteins, and decreased serum albumin (17–20).

Most therapeutic trials of dietary therapy rely for quantification on one or more of the published indices, many of which depend largely on rating symptoms. Rather than mix symptoms and biochemical or other measurements in one index, it would be better if alteration in symptoms, changes in structure, and different measures of inflammation were assessed and recorded separately. In this way, changes in symptoms could be distinguished from altered inflammation, because the two do not necessarily improve together or at the same rate. Even a measure such as stool weight can be confusing because it reflects changes in diet, absorption, and exudation from the gut wall.

Many therapeutic trials of dietary therapy have been published. The results are difficult to interpret because the numbers of patients in each trial are often small, with the possibility of detecting apparent change that is due to chance or failing to detect real change. The types of patient included may be specially selected, groups may be unbalanced due to heterogeneity of the disease, methods of assessment vary from trial to trial, and the results can be confounded by drug or other treatments. The following discussion reviews the published trials and categorizes them by their overall aim.

IV. DELETIONS FROM DIET

A. Removal of All Oral Nutrients

Theoretically, the effect of removing all nutrients from the gut lumen could be beneficial as a possible treatment for Crohn's disease because aggravating factors are reduced.

Conversely, it could be deleterious because essential substrates for epithelial cell metabolism are removed.

Uncontrolled clinical reports of replacing oral nutrient intake by parenteral nutrition suggest that this is an effective treatment for many patients with Crohn's disease. One of the most persuasive reports is one in which total parenteral nutrition was given as sole therapy for 12 weeks to 30 consecutive patients with complicated Crohn's disease referred for surgical treatment (21). No medication or oral intake was allowed. In 25 cases, there was prompt improvement. Abdominal pains ceased, stools returned to normal, and body weight increased. There was a decrease in the Crohn's Disease Activity Index (CDAI) and the blood sedimentation rate; the serum albumin increased. Within 1 month of completing treatment, all 25 patients returned to work or household activities, ate normal meals, and had no evidence of active Crohn's disease. One-third of the patients relapsed during the next year, and 80% relapsed within 3 years. The parenteral nutrition was associated with a complication in nine patients. The authors draw an unfavorable comparison between the cumulative relapse rate after parenteral nutrition and the relapse rate after surgery.

It is generally accepted that total bowel rest can reduce inflammation in Crohn's disease, but the treatment is difficult for the patient, expensive, and potentially dangerous. A review of 18 published papers shows that a clinical remission of at least 1 year's duration occurs in approximately 60% of patients, independent of site of disease, given parenteral nutrition over 4 to 6 weeks as the only form of nourishment (22). However, the treatment does not influence the subsequent natural course of the disease.

Why does parenteral nutrition work and is it better than other treatments? Two controlled trials investigated the role of "bowel rest." In the first study (see Table 1), 20 patients with Crohn's disease whose body weight was less than 80% of ideal and/or whose CDAI showed evidence of disease activity, were randomized into two groups, both given identical parenteral nutrition (23). One group of 10 patients was allowed to drink a formula diet or eat a low residue diet, the other group took nothing by mouth. Three and two patients, respectively, required surgery, the other patients improved to a similar extent as judged by the CDAI. Note the small size of the trial and that the group allowed to eat did not take a normal diet.

The second trial was similar in design but contained three groups of patients (24). The

TABLE 1 Controlled Trials of Parenteral Nutrition Alone Versus Oral Nutrients

Reference	Diet	No. Entered	No. Completed	Duration (days)	Remission
23	PN	10	8	20–60	8
	PN + PD	10	7		7
24	PN	17	12	21	12
	PN + food	15	12		9
24	PN	17	12	21	12
	PD	19	17		11
26	PN	19	16	9 ± 3	14
	ED	17	13		12
TOTAL	PN	63	48		46
	Oral diet	61	49		39

PN = parenteral nutrition; PD = polymeric diet; ED = elemental diet.

patients entered were unresponsive to medical management and were taking between 15 and 45 mg of prednisone daily. Randomization resulted in 17 patients who received a full parenteral nutrition regimen without nutrients by mouth for 3 weeks for comparison with 15 patients who were given approximately one-third of the nutrients parenterally and encouraged to eat full palatable meals (1160–2950 Cal daily in patients who responded to treatment). A significant ($p < 0.01$) and equivalent decrease in the CDAI occurred in both groups, and the remission rates were similar, 71% and 60%, respectively. The results in the 17 patients given nothing by mouth were also compared with those in 19 who were given a whole protein liquid nutrient solution by nasogastric tube. The outcome at the end of 3 weeks was similar in these two groups. Note that, in this trial, patients in all three groups took prednisone daily for more than 4 weeks before entering the study, and they continued it at a mean dose of 21 to 24 mg daily during the trial. The response to prednisolone continues for 8 to 12 weeks (25).

A randomized comparison of treatment between an oral elemental diet and complete bowel rest using parenteral nutrition, both without drug treatment, was performed in 36 patients with active Crohn's disease over a mean of 9 days (26). Evaluable results in 13 and 16 patients, respectively, showed that all but two patients in each group entered clinical remission. No differences were detected in the success rate, speed of achieving remission, or decline in the CDAI in the two groups.

These three trials all suggest that "bowel rest" gives no advantage over enteral nutrition. A fourth trial with discordant results was undertaken in 25 patients with acute attacks of Crohn's colitis, nine of whom were treated with parenteral nutrition, eight with an elemental diet, and eight with a polymeric liquid diet during 4 to 6 weeks. There was significant improvement in all three groups, but the response to parenteral nutrition was greater in regard to reduction in stool weight ($p < 0.02$), decrease in CDAI ($p < 0.05$), decrease in alpha-1-antitrypsin clearance ($p < 0.05$), and endoscopic appearance of the colon ($p < 0.05$), although colonic ulceration persisted in one-half to three-fourths of the patients in all groups (27).

In conclusion, there is much evidence that bowel rest, made possible by parenteral nutrition, improves both the symptoms and the inflammation in Crohn's disease. The reason for the improvement is uncertain but could be due to improvement in the patient's general nutritional state. The three trials described, each of which based results mainly on a disease activity index depending mainly on symptoms, suggested that the response is no better than when patients take an elemental diet, a whole protein liquid diet or a low residue diet, and even normal food supplemented by parenteral nutrition (23,24,26). The fourth trial, published as an abstract, is the only one that used a measure of bowel protein loss and an endoscopic assessment (27). This trial is small, but it is the most sophisticated and suggests an advantage for parenteral nutrition. The debate continues and awaits larger, well-controlled trials, without the confounding effects of drug treatment, using good measures of inflammation. Until then, the disadvantages of parenteral nutrition compared with its doubtful extra benefit have persuaded most clinicians to abandon it as a primary treatment of active Crohn's disease in favor of enteral regimes. There has been no controlled comparison of parenteral nutrition and standard drug therapy.

B. Removal of Large Molecules

Theoreticaly, an elemental diet (a solution of amino acids, glucose, and little fat, with minerals and vitamins) or a partially hydrolyzed "peptide" diet (peptides, oligosaccharides, medium-chain length triglycerides) might be expected to reduce inflammation. To test this hypothesis, such diets need comparison with liquidized normal food or with a polymeric diet, defined as one containing whole protein, polysaccharides, and fat. An elemental diet can also be compared with a hydrolyzed diet.

1. Evidence that Treatment with an Elemental Hydrolyzed or Polymeric Liquid Diet Is Associated with Reduced Inflammation

Several reports describe objective measurements made before and after treatment with an elemental diet or hydrolyzed diet. Seven patients with extensive jejunoileal Crohn's disease with low serum proteins associated with gastrointestinal protein loss in the stools (measured by appearance of an intravenous dose of $^{51}CrCl_3$, which binds to serum proteins) were given an elemental diet (Vivonex HN) for 28 to 56 days. Serum proteins rose ($p < 0.05$) and gastrointestinal protein loss decreased ($p < 0.05$) during treatment, although neither returned to normal (20) (Fig. 1). Other investigators studied the effect of two elemental diets on urinary excretion of orally administered ^{51}Cr EDTA (ethylenediaminetetraacetic acid) as a measure of intestinal permeability and on fecal excretion of ^{111}In-labeled leukocytes as a measure of inflammation (19). Twenty-seven of 34 patients with active Crohn's disease went into clinical remission, usually within 1 week of starting treatment. After treatment for 4 weeks, there was a significant improvement in intestinal permeability ($p < 0.01$), and 12 of 20 patients tested had a result within the normal range. There was also a significant ($p < 0.01$) decrease in fecal leukocyte secretion, but not to normal values, and in the serum C-reactive protein level ($p < 0.05$).

Two similar studies have been performed before and after treatment with a hydrolyzed diet. Intestinal permeability in 14 children with active Crohn's disease was studied after oral administration of lactulose and rhamnose followed by measurement of urinary excretion; the result was expressed as a ratio of recovery of the two sugars (17). All the

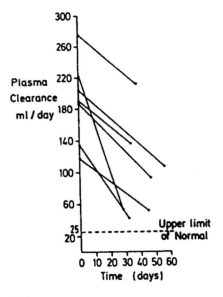

FIG. 1 Gastrointestinal protein loss in seven patients with extensive jejunoileal Crohn's disease treated with elemental diet (Vivonex HN). (From Ref. 20.)

children showed an improvement in the ratio after treatment with Flexical and half showed values within the normal range after treatment for 6 weeks.

There appears to have been only one comparison of an elemental and a hydrolyzed diet. Eight patients with active Crohn's disease were studied before and after treatment for 4 to 8 weeks with a diet containing chemically defined amino acids, dextrin as carbohydrate, and 0.636% soya bean oil as lipid, and five patients were given a diet composed of egg-white hydrolysate (85% amino acids, dipeptides or tripeptides), dextrin as in the elemental diet, and 5% fat as soybean or corn oil (18). Before treatment, all patients had abnormal ratios of the lactose–rhamnose excretion ratio as a measure of intestinal permeability. The urinary ratio returned to normal in all eight patients treated with the elemental diet but remained abnormal in three of five patients after treatment for 8 weeks with the hydrolyzed diet, suggesting that the peptides or fat diminished improvement.

In a comparison of an elemental and a polymeric diet, four and six patients, respectively, completed treatment for 28 days. Improvements were seen in both groups studied by fecal protein loss and indium-leukocyte scanning (28). Similarly, in another trial, improvement in alpha-1-antitrypsin clearance and colonoscopic evidence of ulceration occurred equally among 24 and 12 patients, respectively, given one of these two types of diet (29).

Ten patients with active Crohn's disease, given an elemental diet for 6 weeks, were examined by double-contrast radiography of the small and large intestine before and after treatment (30). The radiographs were assessed under blinded conditions in regard to time sequence. Strictures in two patients were unchanged, but cobblestoning or ulceration was improved in every case. These changes were associated with improved symptoms and a decrease in erythrocyte sedimentation rate (ESR), C-reactive protein, and alpha-2-globulin.

Seven children with predominantly ileal disease took a polymeric liquid diet rich in transforming growth factor (TGF-β_2) as the only treatment for 8 weeks. The C-reactive protein levels and ESR decreased to normal, the serum albumin rose, and six of seven paired ileal biopsies showed improvement after treatment (Fig. 2) (31).

2. Controlled Trial Comparing a Hydrolyzed Diet with Blended Normal Food

Only one randomized trial has been reported in which a hydrolyzed diet (10% to 30% free amino acids, 70% to 90% short-chain peptides, with a chain length not exceeding six amino acids, dextrin-maltose, and fat as 50% medium-or-long-chain fatty acids) has been compared with pureed normal hospital food (Fig. 3). The relative distribution of protein, carbohydrate, and fat as energy sources was similar in the two diets, which were given for 2 weeks. Although 19 patients, almost all with slight or moderately active Crohn's disease, were entered, seven patients dropped out because they could not tolerate the diets, leaving six patients in each group. There was a tendency toward a decreased activity index in both groups, and a significant ($p < 0.05$) decrease in daily bowel frequency with the pureed diet. This pilot trial illustrates the need to study the consistency as well as the chemical composition of the diet.

3. Controlled Trials Comparing an Elemental and a Polymeric Diet

There have been four controlled trials in which an elemental diet has been compared with a polymeric diet (Table 2) (28,29,33,34).

Two trials give an equivalent result and one each favored an elemental or a poly-

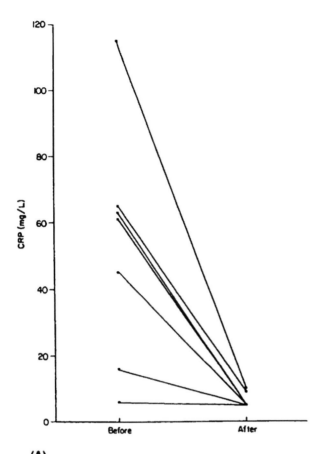

(A)

FIG. 2   (A) C-Reactive protein (B) erythrocyte sedimentation rate in seven children with predominantly ileal Crohn's disease treated with a polymeric diet (casein-based, rich in transforming growth factor) for 8 weeks as the sole source of nutrition. (From Ref. 31.)

meric diet (Fig. 4). A meta-analysis of these four trials showed no difference between the two types of diet (35). The pooled odds ratio for whole protein compared with amino acid–based diets was 1.77 (95% CI 0.65–4.81) after excluding one trial, which caused heterogeneity.

4.   Controlled Trials Comparing an Elemental and a Hydrolyzed Diet

There have been three randomized comparisons of an elemental diet and a hydrolyzed diet (36–38). None showed a significantly different result in regard to clinical remission, although one trial suggested a greater improvement in acute-phase proteins with the elemental diet (Fig. 5) (Table 3).

5.   Conclusion

In conclusion, there is no convincing evidence that an elemental diet is therapeutically better than a hydrolyzed or polymeric diet. However, further comparative studies are needed using sophisticated tests of intestinal function in larger numbers of patients so

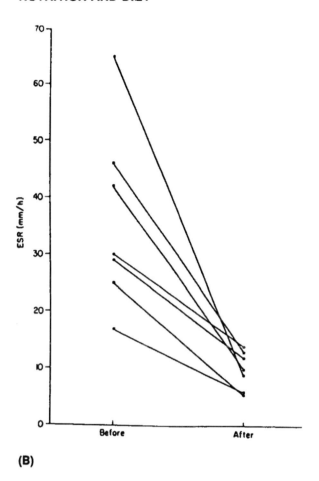

(B)

that improvement in symptoms can be distinguished clearly from changes in the severity of inflammation.

C. Removal of Fat

A review of liquid diets used as treatment for Crohn's disease has suggested that the use of diets with a very low fat content (0.6%–1.3% of total calories) has been associated with a good outcome, whereas the use of diets containing high quantities of fat (12%–30% of total calories) was associated with less favorable results (18,37,39,40). In particular, when large amounts of linoleic acid were present, the outcome was poor (33,41). The result of treatment with diets containing intermediate or large amounts of fat, a large proportion of which was monounsaturated fatty acid, was more favorable (28,42). The authors suggest that clinical benefit may follow when insufficient substrate is provided for two-series eicosanoid synthesis and, conversely, supplying such a substrate may aggravate inflammation. In a comparative trial, a lower remission rate was observed after treatment with a liquid diet yielding 36.8% of calories as long-chain triglycerides than with three other diets containing less long-chain fatty acids (43). The authors reviewed the literature and found a negative correlation between remission rate and long-chain fatty acid content of the diet $(r = -0.761, p = 0.009)$.

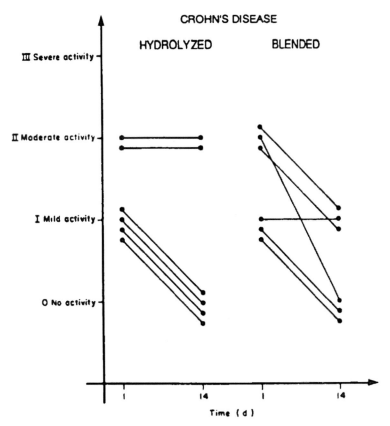

FIG. 3 Change in Crohn's disease activity on treatment with a hydrolyzed liquid diet or blended normal ward diet (From Ref. 32.)

TABLE 2 Controlled Trials of Elemental Versus Polymeric Diet in Active Crohn's Disease

Reference	Diet	No. Entered	No. Completed	Duration (days)	Diet	Remission
28	ED	7	4	28	EO28 (T)	2
	PD	7	6		Enteral 400 (T)	5
33	ED	16	14	28	Vivonex (T)	12
	PD	14	12		Fortison (T)	5
29	ED	15	14	20–43	Vivonex HN (T)	10[a]
	PD	15	15		Realmentyl/Nutrison (T)	11[a]
34	ED	13	12	21	EO28 (O)	9
	PD	11	11		Trisorbon (O)	8
TOTAL	ED	51	44			33
	PD	47	44			29

[a]Equal and significant improvement in fecal weight, erythrocyte sedimentation rate, and serum alpha-2-globulin, alpha-1 antitrypsin clearance, and colonoscopic appearance.
ED = elemental diet; PD = polymeric diet; (T) = tube feed; (O) = oral feed.

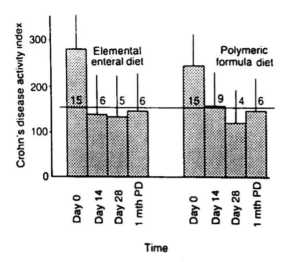

FIG. 4 Mean values of Crohn's disease activity index (CDAI) in a group of 15 patients treated with an elemental diet and 15 patients treated with a polymeric formula diet. Results are shown before, during (14 and 28 days), and 1 month after treatment. The numbers above the line indicate the numbers of patients with CDAI > 150 at each time. (From Ref. 29.)

There are two main series of fatty acids that are not interconvertible. Some fatty acids have a double bond at the n-6 position and others at the n-3 position. Linoleic acid (C18:2, n-6) is a precursor of arachidonic acid (C20:4, n-6), which is found in all membranes and is the source of two-series eicosanoids, which have two double bonds in the side chains of the five-membered ring. These eicosanoids include leukotriene B4 (LTB4), prostaglandin E_2 and thromboxane A_2. Gamma-linolenic acid (GLA,C18:3, n-6) is a precursor of dihomogamma-linolenic acid (DGLA,C20:3, n-6), which competes with arachidonic acid for the cyclooxygenase enzymes, leads to the production of one-series

TABLE 3 Controlled Trials of Elemental Versus Hydrolysed Diet in Active Crohn's Disease

Reference	Diet	No. Entered	No. Completed	Duration (days)	Diet	Remission
36	ED	14	11	14	EO28	11[a]
	HD	15	12		Pepdite 2+	11[a]
37	ED	19	16	21	Vivonex (T)	16[b]
	HD	21	15		Peptamen (T)	15[b]
38	ED	19	17	28	EO28	8
	HD	16	12		Pepti-2000	5
TOTAL	ED	52	44			35
	HD	52	39			31

[a]Significant falls in alpha-1 antichymotrypsin, erythrocyte sedimentation rate and C-reactive protein occurred only with ED.
[b]Significant reductions in Crohn's Disease Activity Index and alpha-1 acid glycoprotein in both groups.
ED = elemental diet; HD = hydrolysed diet; (T) = tube feed.

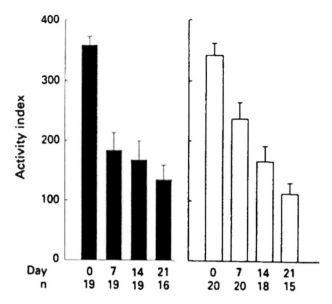

FIG. 5 Changes in Crohn's disease activity index over 3 weeks in 19 patients treated with an amino acid (solid bars) and 20 patients treated with a peptide based (open bars) diet. (From Ref. 37.)

eicosanoids with one double bond in the side chains, and decreases production of LTB4. Alpha-linolenic acid is a precursor of eicosapentaenoic acid (EPA,C20:5, n-3), which can replace arachidonic acid in cell membranes, and favors the production of three-series eicosanoids with three double bonds in the side chain, which have less proinflammatory effects than the two-series eicosanoids.

Modification of fatty acid ingestion may thus affect the inflammatory cascade. The effects of fat on the immune system are complex and have been reviewed by several authors (16). For example, a low-fat diet slows the progression of inherited autoimmune disease in animals. Future dietary research in Crohn's disease might be directed to the use of liquid diets differing only in the quantity and composition of fat that they contain.

D. Removal of Sugar and Refined Carbohydrate

Epidemiological studies have suggested that patients with Crohn's disease eat more sugar then healthy control subjects. The clinical course of 32 patients treated with a fiber-rich, unrefined carbohydrate diet for a mean of more than 4 years has been compared retrospectively with that of 32 matched patients who received no dietary instruction. The patients treated with the diet spent fewer days in the hospital and appeared to need surgery less frequently (44).

As a result of this experience, a large, multicenter trial included 352 patients with inactive or mildly active Crohn's disease who were randomized into two groups, one of which took, for 2 years, a diet high in unrefined carbohydrate with little or no sugar, and the other a diet unrestricted in sugar but low in fiber. Patient compliance, as judged by formal dietary assessment was good. No clear difference in clinical course was detected among patients who accepted either type of dietary advice (45).

E. Removal of Solid Residues

The evidence so far suggests that liquid diets are beneficial and that their effectiveness may vary with their lipid content. Because therapeutic results were similar when pureed normal food was compared with a liquid diet, the hypothesis that the consistency of the diet is an important feature is supported (32). The relative merits of normal versus pureed food requires formal testing.

One patient with extensive stricturing of the small bowel became well on an amino acid–based feed (Vivonex) (34). Subsequently, he was given two whole-protein feeds (Ensure Plus followed by Triosorbon) and continued to improve in terms of weight and serum albumin. Over the next 4 years, during which he took mainly Triosorbon as his source of nourishment, a series of challenges, each lasting 1 or 2 months, was performed. Substances tested without clinical deterioration included carrageenan, three other permitted emulsifiers, sucrose, and then normal food components including bread, potatoes, oranges, a variety of meats, dairy products, flour, and rice. When vegetables were added, there was prompt symptomatic relapse and deterioration in blood test results. Remission was achieved only by using the liquid diet and not with the previous successful low-residue diet. After surgical treatment by six strictureplasties, the patient was able to take a normal diet. It seems likely that, in this case, undigestible fiber led to intestinal stasis because of the strictures. Thus, in some patients, solid food may cause a degree of bolus obstruction which aggravates inflammation.

A controlled trial among 70 patients without strictures has shown no difference in outcome between patients advised to take a low-residue diet and a group who took a normal diet (46). There was a significant threefold difference in fiber-containing foods eaten by the two groups.

F. Elimination of Specific Foods: Exclusion Diets

The topic of exclusion diets is controversial because investigation of food intolerance largely depends on assessment of symptoms. To study food intolerance in Crohn's disease, the prevalence of food-related symptoms in the general population should be considered first and then their prevalence in patients with noninflammatory bowel symptoms.

1. Prevalence of Food-Related Symptoms in the General Population

In a carefully planned survey among 15,000 randomly selected households in Great Britain, approximately one in five people perceived a connection between food and various physical and psychological symptoms (47). Among the 18,880 persons questioned, 1576 (8.3%) related gut symptoms to the type of food eaten.

A selected group of 93 subjects, who all considered that some symptom developed after taking one or more of eight foods, was tested under double-blind conditions. Each food was compared with a placebo, both included in a specially designed vehicle to disguise the taste of the test food. Blinding was confirmed by tasting panels. Symptoms were assessed by a diary card scoring system as test substances were taken in random order during 3-day periods separated by 4 rest days. The foods were cow's milk, hen's eggs, wheat, soya, oranges, prawns, nuts, and chocolate. Eighteen subjects (19.4%) developed one or more symptoms and five (5.4%) developed intestinal symptoms while taking one or more of the foods as compared with the control.

Thus, in the general population, approximately one in 12 persons regard certain foods as causing gut upset, which can be confirmed in some by careful double-blind challenge.

2. *Food Intolerance Is Common Among Patients with Nonspecific Gut Symptoms*

Patients diagnosed as suffering from irritable bowel with negative investigations have been treated with an exclusion diet (48). Over 3 weeks, 189 such patients excluded dairy products, cereals, citrus fruits, potatoes, tea, coffee, alcohol, additives, and preservatives. Symptoms in almost half (48%) of the patients improved. These patients then reintroduced foods singly and in a specified order, each over a period of 2 days. If symptoms recurred, the food was again avoided and reintroduced at the end of the introduction phase, which lasted approximately 2 months. Seventy-three (81.3%) of 91 patients were able to identify foods that caused symptoms; more than half the patients identified two to five such foods. Dairy products, chocolate, eggs, and wheat products were each frequently regarded as a cause of symptom, followed by nuts, tea, coffee, citrus fruits, and potatoes.

Thus, approximately half of a series of patients with noninflammatory gut complaints improved when a range of foods was excluded from the diet, and the majority of such people, when they then added foods one at a time, perceived certain foods as a cause of symptoms. In this study, one or more of 33 various foods were identified by patients in this way.

3. *Patients with Crohn's Disease Tend to Restrict Their Diet*

Thirty-four patients without a stoma, who had been treated surgically for Crohn's disease and who passed an average of five stools daily, were questioned in a standardized manner about their diet, and the results were compared with those of 27 healthy people interviewed in the same way (49). The patients restricted their diet significantly ($p < 0.001$) more often than the control subjects. Only approximately one-fourth of the patients had been seen by a dietitian, and it is unlikely that this difference was due to dietary advice. From a detailed checklist of individual foods, patients listed 23 that upset them more often than the controls, although cabbage/broccoli (approximately 40%) and chocolate (30%) affected both groups equally. The greater frequency of upset in patients compared wtih controls was significant ($p < 0.01$) for nuts, raw fruits, tomatoes, and alcohol. Other foods with marked, but not statistically significant, differences included corn, dairy products, spices, onions, lettuce, citrus fruits, coffee, and tea.

Conversely, patients did not regard themselves as upset by poultry, white fish, lamb, white bread, cooked fruit, or potatoes. Thus, many patients with Crohn's disease avoid certain foods by self-selection. There was also a consensus in this small group of surgically treated patients as to foods that did not cause trouble and could thus form the basis for exploration of a more varied diet.

4. *Formal Study of Exclusion Diets in Crohn's Disease*
Suggests that They Relieve Symptoms in Some Patients

Investigations of exclusion diets in Crohn's disease have been based on study of patients whose symptoms were absent or greatly improved after a preliminary period of treatment with total parenteral nutrition, elemental diet, or, in a few cases, an exclusion diet. Foods have then been reintroduced one at a time and patients have noted the effects on gut symptoms. Details vary from study to study.

In assessing results of this type, it must be remembered that some healthy volunteers develop diarrhea, abdominal wind, cramps, and light-headedness after finishing a period on an elemental diet and starting normal food (50).

One group of investigators started introduction of a single food each day after a 2-week period of "bowel rest" or dietary treatment had induced remission (CDAI < 150)

(51,52). The first foods introduced were those regarded as unlikely to cause symptoms, such as chicken or fish, leaving until later foods such as cereals or dairy products. A food that apparently provoked symptoms was subsequently avoided until it was reintroduced later to confirm that it did aggravate symptoms. By this means, 64 of 77 patients identified 27 foods or groups of foods, one or more of which upset them. There were many similarities to the list of foods described by patients in the dietary survey already discussed. Among all patients who started on the diet, there was a relapse rate of 22% in the first 6 months; thereafter, the rate decreased and was approximately 40% at 3 years (52). In a controlled trial, the relapse rate among 40 patients who adopted an individualized diet in this way was 62% at 2 years (53).

Another group of investigators studied 20 patients whose Crohn's disease was in remission (withdrawal of steroids and CDAI < 150 or simple index < 3) after treatment with an elemental or polymeric diet for 4 weeks (54). Thereafter, one new food was added daily, except for wheat, which was introduced over 5 days. Six patients relapsed during the early stages of food reintroduction and did not improve when the most recently added food was stopped. Five patients remained well and did not identify any aggravating food. Nine patients (45%) were apparently intolerant to at least one of 15 foods, the most common being dairy products and bananas. Four of these nine underwent double-blind rechallenge with suspect foods, but no test gave a positive result.

A third study involved 42 patients who had responded satisfactorily to 4 to 8 weeks of treatment with an elemental diet (55). The patient's own normal diet was discussed, with particular attention paid to personally suspected food intolerance. An individualized reintroduction program was then devised so that each successive addition was made over 5 days and suspect foods were reintroduced last. When symptoms developed, the most recently introduced food was stopped and tried again later; further symptoms with this second challenge led to the offer of a double-blind trial assessment. Eight of the 42 patients withdrew because of disease relapse that could not be related to food and six others withdrew because the dietary restrictions were too severe. Of the remaining 28 patients, eight remained symptom free and 20 identified one or more foods as causing symptoms when reintroduced into the diet. Three of the 20 declined a second challenge; of the remainder seven remained well when the suspect food was taken again and 10 patients complained of symptoms elicited by a total of 11 foods. Double-blind challenges were undertaken in five of the 10 patients who developed symptoms twice with one or more foods; four of five tests were positive for wheat, milk (lactose tolerance test normal), peanuts, and salicylate.

Thus, all groups of investigators have shown that many patients with Crohn's disease attribute symptoms to certain foods. One group failed to demonstrate recurrence of symptoms when suspect foods were reintroduced under double-blind conditions, but another group succeeded in doing so in four of five patients. The analogy between the findings in irritable bowel symdrome and those in Crohn's disease is striking. It seems likely that inflammation alters the visceral sensibility or motility of the gut so that various stimuli, including food, can cause gut symptoms. The evidence that an exclusion diet improved inflammation depends largely on the relapse rate because patients were in remission when they started the test procedures to detect food intolerance. Whether the relapse rate was less than expected is undecided. Regrettably, the only trials that could have answered the point used a steroid-treated group or patients taking a high fiber diet as the controls (52,53).

5. Food Sensitivity During the Use of Liquid Diets

Specific sensitivities to carbohydrate of maize origin but not of potato origin have been described in two patients on an elemental diet (55).

In one case report, a patient with extensive jejunoileal Crohn's disease had been steroid dependent for approximately 12 years (56). Complete remission of symptoms, return to normal of blood tests, improvement of radiographic appearances, and weaning from steroids occurred on treatment with a liquid polymeric milk-free diet (Ensure Plus) over 18 months. A lactose tolerance test was normal. This patient developed severe recurrent symptoms within 6 hours of taking milk. This was confirmed on double-blind challenge 1 year after remission had occurred with as little as 5 ml of milk added to the liquid diet. On further open challenge with milk 6 months later, there was no adverse reaction. Temporary sensitivity to milk in this patient seems to have been proved.

6. Conclusion

The variety of foods alleged to cause symptoms by different patients argues against a limited number of food components that aggravate symptoms in most cases. However, a small proportion of patients have a specific sensitivity demonstrable by blinded challenge.

Many patients with Crohn's disease take a near-normal diet but find out for themselves that modest dietary restriction helps. For those patients with intractable troublesome symptoms, a simple diet (see p. 326) is likely to give the least symptoms. Patients can use this bland diet as a basis, and, if it helps, they can widen the variety of foods taken so as to take as normal a nutritious diet as possible. Only in the most severely affected patients does a formal exclusion diet with successive reintroductions of different foods appear indicated. Occasional patients are found to have specific food sensitivities in this way.

V. THERAPEUTIC ADDITIONS TO THE DIET

A. Mucosal Trophic Factors

Additions to the diet might provide trophic factors that decrease mucosal permeability or favor the metabolism of epithelial cells. Enterocytes are dependent on glutamine for their metabolism. The addition of glutamine to an elemental diet prolonged survival and reduced bacterial translocation in methotrexate-induced enterocolitis in rats (57). A possible role for glutamine in the treatment of Crohn's disease does not appear to have been studied. A polymeric diet rich in TGF-β_2 given as sole treatment over 8 weeks to seven children with newly diagnosed ileal Crohn's disease resulted in clinical, biochemical, and histological improvement in all of them; two ileal biopsies showed inflammation to have returned to normal (31).

Colonocytes are dependent for their metabolism on short-chain fatty acids, particularly butyric acid, in the bowel lumen. These are derived from bacterial fermentation of carbohydrate unabsorbed by the small bowel. As described, a preliminary trial of a diet high in unrefined carbohydrate, which would tend to increase the carbohydrate available for fermentation by colonic bacteria, suggested that it might be beneficial in Crohn's disease, but this was not confirmed by a larger multicenter controlled trial (44,45).

B. Effect of Nutrition on Immune Response

A comparison of some measures of immune function has been made between two groups of patients with Crohn's disease, one that was undernourished and the other well nourished, as judged by a midarm circumference below or above 90% of an ideal standard and confirmed by other measurements (58). The undernourished patients had significantly reduced total lymphocyte and T-lymphocyte counts and a reduced proportion of monocytes that ingested latex particles. Serum orosomucoid levels were significantly higher ($p < 0.001$) in the undernourished patients, and there was a trend towards higher clinical activity scores. An oral enteral supplement of 550 kCal daily was given to 21 undernourished patients over 2 to 4 months without change in drug treatment. During this time, there was a significant improvement not only in measures of nutritional status but also in total ($p < 0.01$) and T-lymphocyte ($p < 0.01$) counts, and significant decrease in orosomucoid levels ($p < 0.01$). These studies thus suggest that nutritional therapy may not only reverse undernutrition but also affect the severity of inflammation and improve immunological function.

Besides protein–calorie malnutrition, a wide range of specific nutrients may influence the immune response under experimental conditions (16). Examples are vitamins A, C, D, and E; arginine; metals such as iron, zinc, copper, and selenium; and fatty acids. The field of immune modulation by dietary means in all types of disease is at an early stage and is likely to be an area of research in Crohn's disease. A controlled trial of vitamin A supplementation of the diet in Crohn's disease has not shown benefit over a period of 9 to 23 months (59). Supplementation of the diet with zinc did not alter immune function but Vitamin C supplements improved lymphocyte transformation in well-nourished patients with Crohn's disease (60).

C. Eicosanoid Precursors and Antioxidants

As discussed, unsaturated fatty acids act as precursors for the one, two, and three series of prostaglandins. The metabolic paths are separate so that Gamma-linolenic acid leads to dihomogammalinolenic acid, precursor of the one series, and arachidonic acid, precursor of the two series. Alpha-linolenic acid leads to eicosapentaenoic acid, precursor of the three series. Eicosapentaenoic acid and docosahexaenoic acid (DCHA C22:6n-3) are a major components of fish oils; the latter is a strong competitive inhibitor of the synthesis from arachidonic acid of prostaglandins but has little effect on the leukotriene pathway.

Experimental observations in rats have shown that the course of experimental colitis induced by trinitrobenzene sulphonic acid was mitigated and shortened by addition of cod liver oil (omega-3) to the diet as compared with sunflower oil (omega-6). There was an associated decreased liberation of thromboxane B_2 into the colonic lumen 20 and 30 days after induction of the colitis (61). Feeding eicosapentaenoic acid, approximately 1 to 8 g daily, and docosahexaenoic acid, approximately 1 to 3 g daily, in the form of fish oil to 29 patients with Crohn's disease resulted in a trend to decreased formation of LTB4 by ionophore-stimulated leukocytes (62). There was no demonstrable change in clinical activity of the disease, but the patients studied appear to have been in remission already. The choice of olive oil stabilized with vitamin E as the control may not have been an inactive preparation.

Production of damaging oxygen species by leukocytes and other cells may play a role in the inflammatory response. Antioxidants such as ascorbic acid, alpha-tocopherol, beta-carotene, selenium, and methonine could decrease inflammation. Experimentally, oral vitamin E reduced inflammation in chemically induced colitis (63). There has been a small pilot trial of a mixture of all these compounds in ulcerative colitis but not in Crohn's disease (64). The absence of benefit in a controlled trial of vitamin A acetate, 100,000 U daily, for 9 to 15 months in 86 patients with stable moderately active Crohn's disease on disease activity or relapse rate has previously been discussed (59).

VI. COMPARISON OF DIETARY MODIFICATION WITH DRUG THERAPY

A. Elemental Diet Versus Corticosteroid Drugs

There have been four controlled trials of an elemental diet against corticosteroid therapy (Table 4). The first trial to be published included only patients with newly diagnosed acute Crohn's disease who had no previous treatment (40). There was convincing similarity between the results with the two forms of treatment over 4 weeks, by which time, eight of 10 steroid-treated and nine of 11 dietetically treated patients were in remission. Two subsequent trials have been conducted on patients who had no previous treatment, one in children with newly diagnosed Crohn's disease and another in adults (30,65). The latter trial was not randomized but was characterized by serial measurements of acute-phase reactants and by radiological examination by a double-contrast technique of the small and large bowel before and after treatment for 6 weeks. There was greater improvement in the radiographic appearances after the elemental diet than after steroid treatment. Crossover from steroids to elemental diet was associated with improvement in radiological appearance and a rapid decrease in C-reactive protein. In general, these results have confirmed the results of the initial trial that clinical improvement during the first few weeks of treatment is similar whether elemental diet or prednisolone is given.

The fourth trial was conducted among adults with both newly diagnosed and established disease, some of whom had had previous treatment (Fig. 6) (66). Nine of 22 patients could not tolerate the elemental diet, whether given orally or by nasogastric tube. Thus, on an intention-to-treat basis, the results in this trial were better for prednisolone than the diet; for those who completed the treatments, the results were similar, although the relapse rate after prednisolone was significantly less ($p < 0.05$) than after the elemental diet over 1 year.

A trial in which an elemental diet combined with antibacterial drugs was compared

TABLE 4 Controlled Trials of Elemental Diet Versus Corticosteroid Drug

Reference	Treatment	No. Entered	No. Completed	Duration (days)	Remission
40	ED	11	9	28	9
	Steroids	10	8		8
65	ED	9	9	21	7
	Steroids	9	9		6
30	ED	10[a]	10	42	8
	Steroids	10	10		3
66	ED	22	11[b]	28	10
	Steroids	20	19		17
TOTAL	ED	52			34
	Steroids	49			34

[a]Nonrandomized trial.

[b]Nine patients could not tolerate the diet.

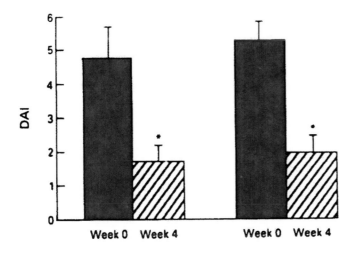

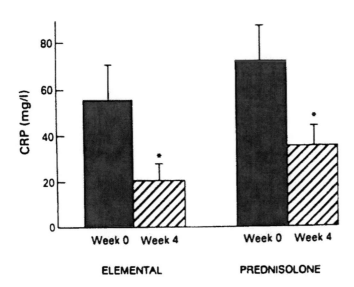

FIG. 6 Changes in Crohn's disease activity (Harvey-Bradshaw index) and C-reactive protein before and after treatment in 13 of 22 patients who were able to tolerate an elemental diet and 20 patients treated with prednisolone. *Week 4 compared with week 0 result, $p < 0.05$. (From Ref. 66.)

with prednisolone gave very good results in both groups, but it is not possible to dissociate the effect of the diet and the drugs (67).

B. Hydrolyzed Diet Versus Drug Therapy

In a preliminary study (Table 5), a European Cooperative Study group randomized 99 patients to a hydrolyzed protein and carbohydrate liquid diet, containing sunflower oil (Survimed) or to sulfasalazine and 6-methylprednisolone. Diet treatment was given over 3 to 6 weeks depending on the rate of improvement. There were 20 (40%) withdrawals

TABLE 5 Controlled Trials of Hydrolysed or Polymeric Liquid Diet Versus
Corticosteroid ± Sulfasalazine Therapy

Reference	Treatment	No. Entered	No. Completed	Duration (days)	Remission
68	HD	51	31[a]	21–42	21
	Drug	44	41		32
41	HD	55	48	< 28	29
	Drug	52	48		41
69	HD	8	7	42	7
	Drug	7	6		6
70	HD	34	NS	35–56	26
	Drug	34	NS		31
71	HD	9	5	< 28	3
	Drug	10	8		7
42	PD	15	14	28	12
	Drug	17	15		15
TOTAL	Diet	172			98
	Drug	164			132

[a]Twenty patients were noncompliant.
HD = hydrolyzed diet; PD = polymeric diet; NS = not stated.

from the diet group because of unpalatability of the diet. The results in the patients who completed treatment for 3 weeks were similar in the two test groups, except that, in the third week, the frequency of soft stools per week was about twice as high in the diet as in the drug group.

To avoid loss of patients taking an oral liquid diet, the same cooperative study group performed a second trial in which continuous nasogastric infusion was used to give an oligopeptide diet (Peptisorb) for at least 4 weeks (Fig. 7) (41). Randomization resulted in 55 patients receiving this enteral regimen as the only treatment and 52 patients receiving a combination of 6-methylprednisolone in reducing doses and sulfasalazine, 3 g daily, over 6 weeks. Disease activity was assessed by the CDAI. In this trial, seven of 55 patients (13%) in the diet group withdrew due to noncompliance and were regarded as treatment failures; four patients withdrew from the drug treatment group. The number of patients reaching remission (29 of 55) was significantly fewer (p < 0.01) among the diet group than the drug-treated group (41 of 52). The rate at which remission was achieved was also slower in the diet than the drug-treated group.

A trial among 15 children with active Crohn's disease compared a hydrolyzed diet (Flexical) given by nasogastric tube to eight patients over 6 weeks with a regimen in 7 others of corticotrophin, followed by prednisolone and sulfasalazine (69). The therapeutic results were equal in regard to improvement measured by activity index and biochemical markers of inflammation. Linear growth over 6 months was significantly greater (p < 0.05) among children who received the diet. A larger trial in 68 patients, all prepubertal and all with active Crohn's disease, showed a similar remission rate between prednisone and diet (Vital NH) in newly diagnosed cases (94% and 86%, respectively), but a lower remission rate in recurrent disease among the diet-treated patients (83% and 50%) due to

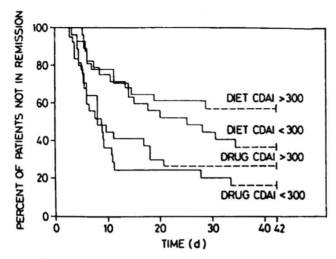

FIG. 7 Percentage of patients in remission (CDAI decreased by 40% or at least 100 points) among 55 patients treated with a hydrolyzed liquid diet (Peptisorb) or 55 patients treated with 6-methylpred-nisolone and sulfasalazine. The results are divided into patients with severe (CDAI > 300) or less severe Crohn's disease at entry. The proportion of patients was less and the rate of remission was slower among the patients treated with diet for up to 42 days when analyzed overall (p < 0.01). (From Ref. 41).

the effect of persistent loose stools on the Activity Index (70). Times to remission were similar (11.3 and 11.1 days).

A small randomized trial compared results of treatment in three groups of patients, one treated with prednisone, another with a hydrolyzed diet (Vital HN), and a third with both. Four of nine patients given the diet alone were unable to complete the trial, leaving three of five who responded. The two groups of patients who received prednisone responded better, with a remission rate of 70% to 75%.

C. Polymeric Diet Versus Corticosteroid Therapy

In a randomized trial among 32 patients admitted to a hospital with clinically symptomatic Crohn's disease, one group was treated with a polymeric diet given by continuous nasogastric infusion for up to 4 weeks and the other with 1 mg/kg per day of prednisone initially and then with a reducing dose (42). Remission rates were similar, 88% and 80%, respectively, and the times to achieve remission were similar. Tolerance of the diet was good, and no patient had diarrhea attributable to diet intolerance. Four patients in the steroid group developed drug-related side effects.

D. Elemental Diet in Steroid-Dependent and Steroid-Refractory Disease

Patients with Crohn's disease whose symptoms are uncontrolled by high doses of steroids or whose symptoms reappear on reduction of the dose present a therapeutic problem. Among 16 such patients, remission was induced, and it was possible to withdraw all drug therapy in 10 patients by treatment with an elemental diet (Vivonex) given by continuous nasogastric infusion over 4 weeks; six patients failed to improve (72). Seven patients remained well for 6 months or more (six on an exclusion diet) without drug treatment.

E. Conclusion

All trials suggest that enteral diets give results greater than expected with placebo (73). All reports have shown a similar response with an elemental diet or steroids, as long as patients can tolerate the diet. The largest trial, conducted wtih previous experience of a similar trial, showed that the results of treatment with a hydrolyzed diet were inferior to those of a combination of prednisolone and sulphasalazine, with regard to both the rate and proportion of patients entering remission. The most recent trial suggests that a polymeric diet and steroid therapy appear to be equivalent.

However, a detailed meta-analysis on an intention-to-treat basis has shown that overall liquid diets result in a lower remission rate than steroids (pooled odds ratio 0.35; 95% CI 0.23–0.54), and a similar difference persists even if patients withdrawn because of noncompliance with the diet are excluded (35). For this reason, and because of the unpalatability of most enteral diets or the inconvenience of nasogastric infusion therapy, most clinicians and patients are likely to prefer drug therapy initially. However, in children who need a growth spurt or in patients resistant to or dependent on steroid therapy, enteral diets offer an effective alternative to this drug treatment. Evidence suggests that a polymeric diet can be tried first and only if it fails is an elemental or hydrolyzed diet indicated.

VII. FUTURE RESEARCH

There is a large body of evidence that liquid enteral diets are an effective treatment, but the reason is still uncertain. Consistency of the diet could be tested by comparing a normal diet with the same diet after it has been blended to a semisolid consistency. The chemical composition of liquid diets could be varied by using an elemental diet of exactly known composition as the reference diet and comparing its effectiveness with the same diet to which fat, glutamine, or other components are added. The possible role of n-3 fatty acids, antioxidants, and glutamine as treatments need further study.

VIII. PRACTICAL RECOMMENDATIONS

A. Nutritional Support

1. Nutritional depletion retards growth, impairs muscle function, affects the immune response, and leads to loss of morale and depression.

2. Growth must be monitored in young people with Crohn's disease. Retardation of growth is largely due to inadequate food intake. Supplementation of normal diet with a nasogastric liquid tube feed at night can be the most effective method of repletion.

3. Adults with chronic Crohn's disease are often malnourished due to inadequate food intake. A supplement to be taken as a drink between meals is often beneficial.

4. Patients with acute Crohn's disease are often severely nutritionally depleted and a short period of replacement can lead to functional improvement of muscle strength and other features before structural changes are detectable.

5. Intestinal failure due to malabsorption after a major small bowel resection may require use of sodium–glucose drinks and appropriate nutritional replacement.

B. Reduction of Inflammation

1. Bowel rest achieved by total parenteral nutrition can reduce inflammation in Crohn's disease but is not used for this purpose because it is potentially dangerous and expensive, and liquid diets are often as effective.

2. Elemental, hydrolyzed, and polymeric liquid diets appear to give equivalent results in reducing inflammation. A polymeric diet is the most palatable and inexpensive; it should, therefore, be the first choice. It is possible that the composition of hydrolyzed or polymeric diets affects therapeutic outcome. Until more information is available, a diet relatively low in fat should be used.

3. Liquid diets can be used as a first line of treatment instead of a corticosteroid drug, to wean steroid-dependent patients from the drug, or to treat steroid-resistant disease. In general, on an intention-to-treat basis, liquid diets do not give as good results as drug therapy, but part of this difference is due to the inability of some patients to take the diet. Nutritional therapy is particularly helpful for young people because growth is enhanced and inflammation reduced.

C. Symptom Relief

1. Patients with Crohn's disease often voluntarily restrict their diet to relieve symptoms. Most patients can take a bland diet, which includes poultry, white fish, lamb, white bread, cooked fruit, and potatoes. If they wish to try such a diet, they should be encouraged to add sequentially as many other foods as possible until they are taking a normal or near-normal diet. Many patients find that certain foods upset them, and, in this, they resemble patients with noninflammatory bowel symptoms. Trial of a strict exclusion diet is not indicated for most patients but may help some with intractable symptoms.

D. The Future

Of interest are reports in which diets of different composition are compared to test the effect of reducing or increasing intake of specific nutrients on the inflammatory response.

REFERENCES

1. Barton JR, Ferguson A. Failure to record variables of growth and development in children with inflammatory bowel disease. BMJ 1989; 298:865–866.
2. Kirschner BS, Voinchet O, Rosenberg IH. Growth retardation in inflammatory bowel disease. Gastroenterology 1978; 75:504–511.
3. Markowitz J, Daum F. Growth impairment in pediatric inflammatory bowel disease. Am J Gastroenterol 1994; 89:319–326.
4. Kirschner, BS, Klich JR, Kalman SS, et al. Reversal of growth retardation in Crohn's disease with therapy emphasizing oral nutritional restitution. Gastroenterology 1981; 80:10–15.
5. Motil KJ, Grand RJ, Davis-Kraft L, et al. Growth failure in children with inflammatory bowel disease: a prospective study. Gastroenterology 1993; 105:681–691.
6. Aiges H, Markowitz J, Rosa J, et al. Home nocturnal supplemental nasogastric feedings in growth-retarded adolescents with Crohn's disease. Gastroenterology 1989; 97:905–910.

7. Morin CL, Roulet M, Roy CC, et al. Continuous elemental enteral alimentation in children with Crohn's disease and growth failure. Gastroenterology 1980; 79:1205–1210.

8. Rigaud D, Angel L, Melchior JC, et al. Weight loss in Crohn's disease (CD): acute attacks and increased energy expenditure are not the major factors. Gastroenterology 1989; 96:A416.

9. Harries AD, Danis V, Heatley RV, et al. Controlled trial of supplemented oral nutrition in Crohn's disease. Lancet 1983; 1:887–890.

10. Christie PM, Hill GL. Effect of intravenous nutrition on nutrition and function in acute attacks of inflammatory bowel disease. Gastroenterology 1990; 99:730–736.

11. Lennard-Jones JE. Practical management of the short bowel. Aliment Pharmacol Ther 1994; 8:563–577.

12. Messing B, Pigot F, Rongier M, et al. Intestinal absorption of free oral hyperalimentation in the very short bowel syndrome. Gastroenterology 1991; 100:1502–1508.

13. McIntyre PB, Fitchew M, Lennard-Jones JE. Patients with a jejunostomy do not need a special diet. Gastroenterology 1986; 91:25–33.

14. Woolf GM, Miller C, Kurian R, et al. Diet for patients with a short bowel: high fat or high carbohydrate? Gastroenterology 1983; 84:823–828.

15. Nordgaard I, Hansen BS, Mortensen PB. Colon as a digestive organ in patients with short bowel. Lancet 1994; 343:373–376.

16. Cunningham-Rundles S, Nutrient Modulation of the Immune Response. New York: Marcel Dekker, 1992.

17. Sanderson IR, Boulton P, Menzies I, et al. Improvement of abnormal lactulose/rhamnose permeability in active Crohn's disease of the small bowel by an elemental diet. Gut 1987; 28:1073–1076.

18. Ito K, Hiwatashi N, Kinouchi Y, et al. Improvement of abnormal intestinal permeability in active Crohn's disease by an elemental diet. Gastroenterology 1992; 102:A641.

19. Teahon K, Smethurst P, Pearson M, et al. The effect of elemental diet on intestinal permeability and inflammation in Crohn's disease. Gastroenterology 1991; 101:84–89.

20. Logan RFA, Gillon J, Ferrington C, et al. Reduction of gastrointestinal protein loss by elemental diet in Crohn's disease of the small bowel. Gut 1981; 22:383–387.

21. Müller JM, Keller HW, Erasmi H, et al. Total parenteral nutrition as the sole therapy in Crohn's disease—a prospective study. Br J Surg 1983; 70:40–43.

22. Matuchansky C. Parenteral nutrition in inflammatory bowel disease. Gut 1986; 27S1:81–84.

23. Lochs H, Meryn S, Marosi L, et al. Has total bowel rest a beneficial effect in the treatment of Crohn's disease? Clin Nutr 1983; 2:61–64.

24. Greenberg GR, Fleming CR, Jeejeebhoy KN, et al. Controlled trial of bowel rest and nutritional support in the management of Crohn's disease. Gut 1988; 29:1309–1315.

25. Landi B, N'Guyen Anh T, Cortot A, et al. Endoscopic monitoring of Crohn's disease treatment: a prospective, randomized clinical trial. Gastroenterology 1992; 102:1647–1653.

26. Jones V, Alun. Comparison of total parenteral nutrition and elemental diet in induction of remission of Crohn's disease: long-term maintenance of remission by personalized food exclusion diets. Dig Dis Sci 1987; 32(suppl):100S–107S

27. Rigaud D, Cerf M, Melchior JC, et al. Nutritional assistance (NA) and acute attacks of Crohn's disease (CD): efficacy of total parenteral nutrition (TPN), as compared with elemental (EEN) and polymeric (PEN) enteral nutrition. Gastroenterology 1989; 96:A416.

28. Park RHR, Galloway A, Danesh BJZ et al. Double-blind controlled trial of elemental and polymeric diets as primary therapy in active Crohn's disease. Eur J Gastroenterol Hepatol 1991; 3:483–490.

29. Rigaud D, Cosnes J, Le Quintrec Y, et al. Controlled trial comparing two types of enteral nutrition in treatment of active Crohn's disease: elemental v polymeric diet. Gut 1991; 32:1492–1497.

30. Okada M, Yao T, Yamamoto T, et al. Controlled trial comparing an elemental diet with prednisolone in the treatment of active Crohn's disease. Hepatogastroenterology 1990; 37:72–80.

31. Beattie RM, Schiffrin EJ, Donnet-Hughes A, et al. Polymeric nutrition as the primary therapy in children with small bowel Crohn's disease. Aliment Pharmacol Ther 1994; 8:609–615.

32. Larsen P, Munkholm, Rasmussen D, Rønn B, et al. Elemental diet: a therapeutic approach in chronic inflammatory bowel disease. J. Intern Med 1989; 225:325–331.

33. Giaffer MH, North G, Holdsworth CD. Controlled trial of polymeric versus elemental diet in treatment of active Crohn's disease. Lancet 1990; 1:816–818.

34. Raouf AH, Hildrey V, Daniel J, et al. Enteral feeding as sole treatment for Crohn's disease: controlled trial of whole protein v amino acid based feed and a case study of dietary challenge. Gut 1991; 32:702–707.

35. Fernández-Bañares F, Cabré E, Esteve-Comas M, et al. How effective is enteral nutrition in inducing clinical remission in active Crohn's disease? A meta-analysis of the randomized clinical trials. Gastroenterology 1994; 106:A679.

36. Middleton SJ, Riordan AM, Hunter JO. Peptide based diet: an alternative to elemental diet in the treatment of acute Crohn's disease. Gut 1991; 32:A578–A579.

37. Royall D, Jeejeebhoy KN, Baker JP, et al. Comparison of amino acid v peptide based enteral diets in active Crohn's disease: clinical and nutritional outcome. Gut 1994; 35:783–787.

38. Mansfield JC, Giaffer MH, Holdsworth CD. Amino-acid versus oligopeptide based enteral feeds in active Crohn's disease. Gut 1992; 33(suppl 2):S3.

39. Fernández-Bañares F, Cabré E, González-Huix F, et al. Enteral nutrition as primary therapy in Crohn's disease. Gut 1994; 35(suppl 1):S55–S59.

40. Ó'Morain C, Segal AW, Levi AJ. Elemental diet as primary treatment of acute Crohn's disease; a controlled trial. BMJ 1984; 288:1859–1862.

41. Lochs H, Steinhardt HJ, Klaus-Wentz B, et al. Comparison of enteral nutrition and drug treatment in active Crohn's disease. Gastroenterology 1991; 101:881–888.

42. González-Huix F, de Léon R, Fernández-Bañares F, et al. Polymeric enteral diets as primary treatment of active Crohn's disease: a prospective steroid controlled trial. Gut 1993; 34:778–782.

43. Middleton SJ, Rucker JT, Kirby GA, et al. Long chain triglycerides adversely affect dietary treatment of active Crohn's disease. Gastroenterology 1994; 106:A734.

44. Heaton KW, Thornton JR, Emmett PM. Treatment of Crohn's disease with an unrefined-carbohydrate, fibre-rich diet. BMJ 1979; 2:764–766.

45. Ritchie JK, Wadsworth J, Lennard-Jones JE, et al. Controlled multicentre therapeutic trial of an unrefined carbohydrate, fibre rich diet in Crohn's disease. BMJ 1987; 295:517–520.

46. Levenstein S, Prantera C, Luzi C, et al. Low residue or normal diet in Crohn's disease: a prospective controlled study in Italian patients. Gut 1985; 26:989–993.

47. Young E, Stoneham MD, Petruckevitch A, et al. A population study of food intolerance. Lancet 1994; 343:1127–1130.

48. Nanda R, James R, Smith H, et al. Food intolerance and the irritable bowel syndrome. Gut 1989; 30:1099–1104.

49. McDonald PJ, Fazio VW. What can Crohn's patients eat? Eur J Clin Nutr 1988; 42:703–708.

50. McCamman S, Beyer PL, Rhodes JB. A comparison of three defined formula diets in normal volunteers. Am J Clin Nutr 1977; 30:1655–1660.

51. Workman EM, Jones V, Alun, Wilson AJ, et al. Diet in the management of Crohn's disease. Hum Nutr Appl Nutr 1984; 38A:469–473.

52. Jones V, Alun, Dickinson RJ, Workman E, et al. Crohn's disease: maintenance of remission by diet. Lancet 1985; 2:177–180.

53. Riordan AM, Hunter JO, Cowan RE, et al. Treatment of active Crohn's disease by exclusion diet: East Anglian multicentre controlled trial. Lancet 1993; 342:1131–1134.

54. Giaffer MH, Cann P, Holdsworth CD. Long-term effects of elemental and exclusion diets for Crohn's disease. Aliment Pharmacol Ther 1994; 5:115–125.

55. Pearson M, Teahon K, Levi AJ, et al. Food intolerance and Crohn's disease. Gut 1993; 34:783–787.

56. Ginsberg AL, Albert MB. Treatment of patient with severe steroid-dependent Crohn's disease with nonelemental formula diet: identification of possible etiologic dietary factor. Dig Dis Sci 1989; 34:1624–1628.

57. Fox AD, Kripke SA, Paula J de, et al. Effect of a glutamine-supplemented enteral diet on methotrexate-induced enterocolitis. J Parenter Enter Nutr 1988; 12:325–331.

58. Harries AD, Danis VA, Heatley RV. Influence of nutritional status on immune functions in patients with Crohn's disease. Gut 1984; 25:465–472.

59. Wright JP, Mee AS, Parfitt A, et al. Vitamin A therapy in patients with Crohn's disease. Gastroenterology 1985; 88:512–514.

60. Animashaun A, Kelleher J, Heatley RV, et al. The effect of zinc and vitamin C supplementation on the immune status of patients with Crohn's disease. Clin Nutr 1990; 9:137–146.

61. Vilaseca J, Salas A, Guarner F, et al. Dietary fish oil reduces progression of chronic inflammatory lesions in a rat model of granulomatous colitis. Gut 1990; 31:539–544.

62. Lorenz R, Weber PC, Szimnau P, et al. Supplementation with n-3 fatty acids from fish oil in chronic inflammatory bowel disease—a randomized placebo-controlled, double-blind crossover trial. J Intern Med 1989; 225(suppl 1):225–232.

63. Blumenstein BJ, Ma CK, Zhang X, et al. Orally administered oxygen radical scavenger (vitamin E) reduces mucosal damage in a rat model of inflammatory colitis. Gastroenterology 1994; 106:A1018.

64. Millar AD, Blake DR, Rampton DS. An open trial of antioxidant nutrient therapy in active ulcerative colitis. Gut 1994; 35(suppl 5):S29.

65. Seidman EG, Bouthillier L, Weber AM, et al. Elemental diet versus prednisone as primary treatment of Crohn's disease. Gastroenterology 1986; 90:A1625.

66. Gorard DA, Hunt JB, Payne-James JJ, et al. Initial response and subsequent course of Crohn's disease treated with elemental diet or prednisolone. Gut 1993; 34:1198–1202.

67. Saverymuttu S, Hodgson HJF, Chadwick VS. Controlled trial comparing prednisolone with an elemental diet plus non-absorbable antibiotics in active Crohn's disease. Gut 1985; 26:994–998.

68. Malchow H, Steinhardt HJ, Lorenz-Meyer H, et al. Feasibility and effectiveness of a defined-formula diet regimen in treating active Crohn's diseae. Scand J Gastroenterol 1990; 25:235–244.

69. Sanderson IR, Udeen S, Davies PSW, et al. Remission induced by an elemental diet in small bowel Crohn's disease. Arch Dis Child 1987; 62:123–127.

70. Seidman E, Griffiths A, Jones A, et al. Semi-elemental (S-E) diet vs prednisone in pediatric Crohn's disease. Gastroenteroloy 1993; 104:A778.

71. Lindor KD, Fleming CR, Burnes JU, et al. A randomized prospective trial comparing a defined formula diet, corticosteroids, and a defined formula diet plus corticosteroids in active Crohn's disease. Mayo Clin Proc 1992; 67:328–333.

72. O'Brien CJ, Giaffer MH, Cann PA, et al. Elemental diet in steroid-dependent and steroid-refractory Crohn's disease. Am J Gastroenterol 1991; 86:1614–1618.

73. Salomon P, Kornbluth A, Aisenberg J, et al. How effective are current drugs for Crohn's disease? A meta-analysis. J Clin Gastroenterol 1992; 14:211–215.

COMMENTARY

Arthur D. Heller   *New York Hospital–Cornell Medical Center, New York, New York*

Professor Lennard-Jones chapter on nutrition and special diets in Crohn's disease is comprehensive in scope, attentive to theoretical rationale in pathophysiology, and pragmatic in approach to patient care.

Appropriate emphasis is placed on general nutritional screening and the functional consequences of inadequate nutrition, that is, weight loss, debility, and weakness. Micronutrient deficiencies (e.g., folate, cobalamin, cations, iron) that may require attention in this high-risk population are not particularly addressed. Nutritional repletion in Crohn's disease requires specific supplementation of vitamins and minerals in amounts greater than ordinarily provided by proprietary formulas; for example, patients with chronic diarrhea or fistula losses have increased zinc losses that may have to be treated to allow an increase in lean body mass. Unless this is done, providing macronutrients (carbohydrate, protein, fat calories) may preferentially increase fat stores.

The approach to patients with nutritional failure is very practical, including the formula for an effective oral rehydration solution. Important distinctions in therapy for patients with jejunostomy versus short bowel in continuity with the colon are highlighted.

An overview of *potential* or *hypothetical* mechanisms by which dietary modification could influence symptoms or reduce inflammation is presented. Unlike the rest of the chapter, which is amply referenced, this section has a relative paucity of cited work, which reflects our relative ignorance. Given this lack of supporting clinical data, the tantalizing conclusions stated should be conditional, for example, "antioxidants in the diet [might] alter the activity of free oxygen radicals and [possibly] improve inflammation." The paragraph does not mention whether the statements are accrued from in vitro, in vivo animal, or human data. This criticism does not detract from the nicely presented theoretical constructs upon which rational therapy might be based.

Lennard-Jones' critique of studies mixing symptoms and biochemical measurements as an index of efficacy is well-taken. Symptom relief and reduction of inflammation are not necessarily one and the same. This is further elaborated upon in the section on exclusion diet studies. The difficulties inherent in interpreting data on food intolerance in patients with functional as well as organic bowel disease are cogently presented.

A systematic approach to therapy is evident in the "Deletions from Diet" section. The discussion regarding fat content of diets is especially engaging regarding future directions in research. As mentioned by the author, "Antioxidants such as ascorbic acid, alpha-tocopherol, beta-carotene, selenium, and methionine could [or might] decrease inflammation."

Comparisons of dietary modification with drug therapy (with helpful summary figures) were useful. Problems with tolerability and a lesser efficacy of dietary therapy limit its use, but it remains an effective option for patients.

I found the recommendations at the end of the chapter to be practical. Overall, the chapter is a valuable contribution to our knowledge of nutrition in inflammatory bowel disease.

18
Crohn's Disease in Childhood and Adolescence

Jay A. Barth and Richard J. Grand   *New England Medical Center,*
Tufts University School of Medicine, Boston, Massachusetts

This chapter discusses Crohn's disease in the pediatric population and focuses on the distinguishing features of the disorder in this age group. Although there are many similarities with the disease as it occurs in adults, various aspects of diagnosis and management differ in childhood Crohn's disease. A foremost concern, and one that is unique in the management of children, is the effect of the disease and its treatment on growth. This issue is considered in detail. Various treatment modalities and their possible toxicities are reviewed, with special attention given to the goals of therapy in the pediatric age group.

Crohn's disease occurs throughout the alimentary tract in children, as it does in adults. The site of disease is ileocolonic in 50% to 60% of patients; in 30% to 35%, it is confined to the small bowel, and, in 10% to 15%, to the large intestine (1–3). Gastroduodenal involvement is generally thought to be rare, but evidence of disease can be found on biopsy in as many as 30% to 40% of patients with known Crohn's disease of the lower gastrointestinal tract (4,5).*

I. EPIDEMIOLOGY

The peak incidence of Crohn's disease is the second and third decades of life, and 25% of new cases occur in patients younger than 20 years old (6). Most pediatric cases occur between ages 16 and 20 years; in less than 5%, the onset of disease is younger than age 5 years (7,8). There are rare reports of Crohn's disease occurring in infants (Table 1) (9,10).

The incidence of Crohn's disease in children has increased over time, making it more common than ulcerative colitis in this age group (11). The incidence of Crohn's disease among children 16 years old and younger in Scotland rose from 0.6 to 2.3 per 100,000 over the period 1968 to 1983; the incidence of ulcerative colitis did not change significantly during that time (12). A study in Baltimore showed an incidence of 3.5 per 100,000 children ages 10 to 19 years (11). The incidence among Scandinavian children younger

---

Editor's note: In my own experience, gross gastric and duodenal involvement in Crohn's disease is fairly common in young people, particularly in adolescents.—B.K.

TABLE 1   Age at Time
of Diagnosis of Crohn's
Disease in Children and
Adolescents

Age	Percent
0–10	5
11–15	35
16–20	60

Source: Ref. 7.

than 15 years is 2.5 and, between ages 15 and 19 years, it is 5.3 per 100,000 (13). The prevalence of Crohn's disease in children age 16 years old and younger is 10 per 100,000 in Britain and in Sweden (14,15).

II. GENETICS

It is well established that there is a genetic basis of Crohn's disease, as is evident by the increased prevalance of the disease in patients' families. Family history is positive for inflammatory bowel disease in 21% of newly diagnosed inflammatory bowel disease patients, especially for those with Crohn's disease (6). Inflammatory bowel disease is found in 5% to 25% of first degree relatives of patients with Crohn's disease or ulcerative colitis (16–18). The parents of a child with Crohn's disease are at 35 to 70 times the risk of the general population of developing the disease, and siblings are similarly at greatly increased risk, estimated at 17 to 35 times that of unrelated persons (19). A report of monozygotic twins showed that seven of eight pairs were concordant for Crohn's disease (20). Children of parents with Crohn's disease have a 9% risk of developing the disease (16).

Crohn's disease does not follow a simple mendelian inheritance pattern. Investigators have identified a variety of human leukocyte antigens (HLA) that are found more frequently in patients with Crohn's disease compared with those with ulcerative colitis and normal controls. These include HLA B44 and Cw5, HLA-B27 in association with ankylosing spondylitis, HLA B12, Cw5, and/or DR7, and the combination of DR1 and DQw5 (21–23). Despite these advances, no specific genetic marker of Crohn's disease has been found. As yet unidentified environmental, or possibly infectious, factors may be necessary for the development of clinical disease in a genetically predisposed individual.

III. CLINICAL FEATURES

A. Gastrointestinal

There are several modes of presentation of Crohn's disease in childhood, and, on average, there is a delay of 13 months between the onset of symptoms and diagnosis (24). In some cases, children experience growth retardation for months to years before the gastrointestinal symptoms develop (25,26). If intestinal inflammation is mild, the patient may have only subtle suggestions of gastrointestinal disease, such as early satiety or anorexia, delaying the diagnosis until the development of more obvious symptoms, most commonly abdominal pain or diarrhea (Table 2).

The specific gastrointestinal symptoms a patient experiences tend to correspond to the site of disease involvement. Abdominal pain is the most common complaint on presentation. The pain is most frequently periumbilical and may indicate diffuse small bowel or large intestinal disease (1,27). When the terminal ileum is involved, pain typically occurs in the right lower quadrant, but may also be experienced in the periumbilical or epigastric regions (1). Palpation of the abdomen, however, will likely elicit tenderness in the right lower quadrant (28). Seventy percent of patients with gastroduodenal Crohn's disease suffer from epigastric pain (29). In the rare cases of esophageal involvement, the patient may complain of odynophagia (30).

Abdominal pain can be explained by several pathophysiological mechanisms. A variety of mediators, such as bradykinin, histamine, serotonin, and substance P, are released by inflamed mucosa, which stimulate afferent pain fibers. Transmural disease can irritate the serosa and cause pain. In cases of complete or partial obstruction, there is proximal distention and stretching of the intestinal wall, stimulating painful sensation. Finally, diseased intestine may have disordered motility, resulting in cramping (31,32).

Diarrhea is due to a variety of causes, which depend on the site of disease. In small bowel disease, stools are typically loose and gross blood is absent. When mucosal ulceration occurs, bleeding may ensue. In cases of extensive jejunal or ileal disease, malabsorption results in osmotic diarrhea. Protein, fat, and carbohydrate malabsorption may occur (33). Malabsorbed fatty acids or bile salts stimulate colonic secretion of water and electrolytes (34,35). Extensive terminal ileal disease may cause bile acid pool depletion, contributing to steatorrhea (36). Inflammation of the colon interferes with the normal absorption of water and electrolytes, and, if colonic disease is severe, blood and proteins are lost through the mucosa, contributing to net secretion (37).

Crohn's disease in children is often associated with the presence of perianal disease. This can take the form of fissures, which also occur in less serious disorders such as constipation, and skin tags, which, if small, can be found in normal children. Perianal fistulas or abscesses are almost pathognomonic of Crohn's disease. These findings may precede the onset of gastrointestinal symptoms or vary in appearance with the level of activity of intestinal inflammation (38,39).

TABLE 2 Clinical Features on Presentation in Children with Crohn's Disease

Feature	Range (%)	n = 144 (%)
Weight loss	80–92	87
Abdominal pain	62–86	72
Diarrhea	66–72	69
Fever	26–83	49
Rectal bleeding	14–29	23
Joint complaints	18–25	21
Growth retardation	30–33	30

Source: Refs. 1 and 24.

B. Extraintestinal

Crohn's disease is characterized by the frequent occurrence of extraintestinal symptoms. Fever occurs in 50% to 80% of patients and may precede or accompany the onset of gastrointestinal symptoms. The fever may be constant and lowgrade, or have an intermittent or daily spiking pattern, with temperatures as high as 104°F (1,24). Joint complaints are common; arthritis or arthralgia have been reported, in 18% of patients in one series, in some cases years before any gastrointestinal symptoms (1). The arthritis is usually monoarticular, often affecting the knee or ankle, but any joint may be involved, and migratory polyarthritis also occurs. In either case, the arthritis is transient, asymmetric, and nondeforming (1.40). It tends to parallel the activity of intestinal disease and is more common in cases of colonic or ileocolonic inflammation (41). Two percent to 6% of patients have ankylosing spondylitis, which occurs independently of gastrointestinal disease (42). In one study, clubbing due to hypertrophic osteoarthropathy occurred in 30% of children with Crohn's disease, especially in those with small bowel disease (1).

The most common cutaneous manifestations of Crohn's disease are erythema nodosum and pyoderma gangrenosum, which complicate 1% to 4% of cases of pediatric Crohn's disease (43,44). Erythema nodosum occurs more frequently in Crohn's disease than in ulcerative colitis and tends to resolve with improvement in bowel disease, especially the colonic type (45). Pyoderma gangrenosum is reported to be more common in ulcerative colitis than in Crohn's disease and is associated with trauma and surgical sites in 0.1% of cases (46). Other skin manifestations are polyarteritis nodosa and "metastatic Crohn's disease," or granulomatous dermatitis, a rare complication in children (47).

Children with Crohn's disease may also suffer musculoskeletal complications. Granulomatous myositis has occurred in the setting of Crohn's disease of the colon (48). Osteopenia may be found in pediatric patients as a result of long-term steroid therapy, and has also been observed at the time of diagnosis (49,50). Avascular necrosis of the femoral heads may be due to steroid use, but it has been reported as a complication of Crohn's disease itself (51,52).

Ocular disease is a relatively frequent complication of Crohn's disease. Symptomatic uveitis occurs in 3% of pediatric patients, whereas it is present without symptoms in up to 30% (53). Other eye manifestations of Crohn's disease are iritis and episcleritis (54). Orbital pseudotumor has been reported in pediatric Crohn's disease (55).

The oral mucosa may be affected by canker sores or aphthous stomatitis. Oral involvement tends to follow the activity of intestinal disease (56).

Renal disease also complicates pediatric Crohn's disease. Nephrolithiasis occurs in 5% of children with Crohn's disease, primarily those with ileal disease (1). Calcium oxalate stones develop as result of increased oxalate absorption (45). Urate and phosphate stones also occur (57). Enterovesicular fistulas can cause pneumaturia and urinary tract infections (58). Inflamed bowel may, by mass effect, cause obstructive hydroureter and hydronephrosis (59). Amyloidosis is a rare complication of pediatric Crohn's disease (60,61).

There are a number of hepatobiliary complications of Crohn's disease, including steatosis, chronic active hepatitis, and even cirrhosis (62). Crohn's disease in children may rarely present with liver disease (63). Among adults 10% of cases of sclerosing cholangitis are due to Crohn's disease (64), and this complication has been reported in young patients with Crohn's disease (65,66). Cholelithiasis and acalculous cholecystitis are recognized complications although the pathogenesis of gallstones in Crohn's disease is not fully understood (67,68). The increased risk of cholesterol stones has been explained on the basis of ileal disease or resection, leading to depletion of the bile acid pool and bile supersaturation (69). Recent studies have shown that neither site of disease nor history of resection is associated with increased incidence; rather, the risk of gallstones increases with duration of disease, number of laparotomies, and other factors, such as gallbladder stasis, which are necessary for stone formation (70,71).

Pacreatitis occurs with increased frequency in children with Crohn's disease. When the duodenum is affected, inflammation of the ampulla of Vater may obstruct the pancreatic duct, leading to pancreatitis (72). In cases in which the duodenum is not involved, the cause may be gallstones or biliary sludge, an immunological process, or, in cases of ileal disease, dilatation of the small bowel proximal to the stenotic ileum (72,73).

Pulmonary disease is a rare manifestation of Crohn's disease. There is a report of a 3-year-old with intestinal Crohn's disease who was found to have multiple noncaseating granulomas of the lungs (74).

There are also hematological and vascular complications of Crohn's disease. A hypercoagulable state is described, associated with thrombocytosis, increased levels of fibrin, factor V, and factor VIII, and decreased antithrombin III (75). There have been reports of pediatric patients with neurovascular and other thromboembolic events (76).

C. Undernutrition and Growth Failure

Of particular concern in pediatric Crohn's disease is the effect of the illness on nutrition and growth. Both weight and height are affected, often years before any overt gastrointestinal symptoms develop (26). Weight loss before diagnosis occurs in as many as 80% to 87% of children (24,77). Linear growth failure is also common and has been found on presentation in 30% of patients (1,24). The incidence of attenuated growth rate before diagnosis is considerably higher, approaching 90% of patients in one study, and approximately half of these children had reduced height velocity before any weight loss (25). Some data indicate that growth retardation is more common in patients with colitis or ileocolitis than in those with small bowel disease alone (1), but others have not found such a difference between these groups (7).

Growth failure is defined as cessation of growth or decreased growth velocity over 6 to 12 months, a decline of 1 standard deviation (SD) in height percentile, and/or retardation of bone age more than 2 years or 2 SD (78). To determine whether a patient has growth failure, previous growth data must be obtained from the history and from pediatrician's records. Often, these critical data are incomplete or unavailable (79). Patients also may suffer from delay in sexual maturation.

Malnutrition that persists over a long period of time can cause "nutritional dwarfism": short stature, normal weight for height, and delayed puberty (26). Although most adult patients with Crohn's disease since childhood have heights that are within the normal range, studies of pediatric patients who were followed to physical maturity have revealed a significant number whose growth is permanently affected. One study revealed that 17% of patients had growth failure (80). Another group demonstrated that 37% of patients had deficits in adult heights that were predicted at the time of diagnosis (81). Steroid use has been cited as a contributing factor in growth delay, but the major cause appears to be uncontrolled inflammation (82).

Several other factors also account for the growth impairment seen in Crohn's disease; the most important of these is malnutrition. This results primarily from inadequate caloric intake (26). In one study, growth-impaired patients were shown to ingest 54% of the recommended number of calories for their height–age (83). Anorexia can result from early satiety, and delayed gastric emptying has been documented in some patients (84,85). The taste of food may also be adversely affected, and meal-related cramps and postprandial diarrhea further discourage appetite (86). Studies of tumor necrosis factor (TNF), which is associated with disturbance in appetite, have yielded conflicting results: whereas one study showed elevation of TNF in children with inflammatory bowel disease, another failed to show this abnormality (87,88).

Malabsorption is another cause of malnutrition and is primarily due to mucosal inflammation (24,33). Protein-losing enteropathy, as a result of intestinal inflammation, is found in up to 70% of patients (89,90). Abnormal xylose absorption has been found in 16% of patients and may be due to mucosal disease or bacterial overgrowth (33). Although lactose intolerance has been found in 30% of children with Crohn's disease, it is no more common among these patients than in a control group of children with recurrent abdominal pain (91). The presence of lactose intolerance suggests that the patient may have diffuse small bowel disease or bacterial overgrowth. Maldigestion of fat, leading to steatorrhea, has been reported in one study to occur in 30% of patients. This may be due to depletion of bile acids from ileal inflammation or ileal resection (33). Malabsorption of various macronutrients and micronutrients may lead to deficiencies of folate, iron, vitamin K, vitamin B_{12}, vitamin D, calcium, magnesium, and zinc (92–96).

Malnutrition may also be a result of increased energy requirement in Crohn's disease. Energy expenditure is elevated in the presence of fever, which may complicate Crohn's disease, but it is not clear if the disease itself has this effect (97). Studies of adolescents and adults have demonstrated similar basal metabolic rates in those with and without Crohn's disease, except adult patients who are less than 90% of ideal body weight do have increased energy expenditure per unit body mass (98–100).

There is little evidence that growth retardation in Crohn's disease is based on endocrine abnormalities. Studies have demonstrated that patients with growth failure have normal levels of pituitary, thyroid, and adrenal hormones, and, in most studies, growth hormone (98,101–103). Occasional studies have shown reduced growth hormone levels, both spontaneous and stimulated, but, in one of these studies, there was no correlation between the growth hormone level and severity of growth retardation, and administration of growth hormone to three patients in another study had no effect on their growth (104–106). Depressed levels of somatomedin C, a growth hormone–dependent growth factor, have also been found in some of these children, but this is likely due to malnutrition and is not a primary abnormality, because these levels normalize with improved nutrition (101). Similarly, delays in bone age improve with nutritional rehabilitation (101).

Steroid treatment is a well-recognized cause of growth retardation (107). Because Crohn's disease itself can cause growth retardation, steroid therapy, by controlling disease activity, may permit growth (108). In this circumstance, growth may proceed at a "normal" rate, but not at the increased rate needed for "catch-up" growth (45). The use of low-dose, alternate-day steroid, if sufficient to suppress inflammation, interferes with growth less than daily dosing (109–111).

D. Psychological

Studies in adults have shown that psychiatric disorders, primarily depression, are more frequent in Crohn's disease patients (112,113). There are conflicting findings both of the relationship of psychiatric problems to disease severity, and of the association of stress with onset and exacerbations of Crohn's disease (113–117).

Children with Crohn's disease experience increased prevalence of depression (118, 119). One study found that depression correlated not with disease severity, but with life events and family conflicts, whereas another study demonstrated an association of internalizing psychological styles with disease activity (120,121). Another risk factor for psychopathology, in one study, is growth retardation (122). No correlation has been found between stress and the onset or relapses of Crohn's disease in children (118,123).

IV. GASTROINTESTINAL COMPLICATIONS

Crohn's disease in children, as in adults, is associated with a number of potential gastrointestinal complications. Obstruction is usually caused by stricture, abscess, or adhesions from prior surgery. Severe inflammation can cause symptomatic narrowing of the intestinal lumen. Complete obstruction occurs acutely or subacutely, often with bilious vomiting, whereas partial obstruction may, over time, lead to bacterial overgrowth.

Fistulas most commonly are perianal or perirectal, but may also be enteroenteric, enterovesicular, enterovaginal, or enterocutaneous. Enterocolic fistulas can result in malabsorption of nutrients and small bowel bacterial overgrowth. In children, fistulas are generaly associated with inflammation, independent of stenosis, in contrast to adult patients, whose fistulas are frequently associated with stenosis (124).

Abscesses occur in the presence of transmural inflammation, secondary to perforation or fistula. The principal symptoms of abscess, fever, and localized pain or tenderness may be difficult to distinguish from those of a flare of disease in a segment of bowel and may be indistinguishable from those of a phlegmon (125).

Free perforation is unusual; in adults, it tends to occur in the ileum. It is not directly correlated with disease duration, steroid use, obstruction, or toxic dilatation (126). Pediatric cases have been reported (125). Toxic megacolon complicated 12% of cases of Crohn's colitis in one pediatric series, but this seems to be a higher than expected frequency of this complication (7). Frank hemorrhage is likewise a rare complication (127).

The risk of intestinal malignancy is increased in Crohn's disease (128). Cancer of the small bowel occurs 16 to 85 times more frequently in patients with Crohn's disease than in an age-and-sex-matched population (129,130). The risk of developing colorectal cancer in two older studies was estimated at 7 to 20 times that of the general population (128,130). Two recent studies have more discrepant findings. One demonstrated a risk of colorectal cancer in extensive Crohn's colitis of approximately 20 times that of the general population, with a cumulative risk at 22 years after onset of symptoms of 8%, about the same risk as in extensive ulcerative colitis, and another showed no increased risk (129,131). Early age at onset may be an independent risk factor for malignancy (128,131,132). Patients with long-standing disease that began in childhood should undergo surveillance for dysplasia, but prophylactic colectomy is not recommended (45,131). For further information on cancer in patients with Crohn's disease, see Chapter 28 of this volume.

V. DIAGNOSIS

The diagnosis of Crohn's disease in children is based on the history of illness, physical examination, laboratory data, radiological findings, and, ultimately, on endoscopic appearance and histology. In reviewing the history, careful attention should be given to any extraintestinal symptoms, growth velocity, rate of sexual maturation, and family history of inflammatory bowel disease. It is important to obtain accurate measurements of height and weight, and to plot these on appropriate growth curves and compare them with previous data. The abdomen must be examined for areas of tenderness or fullness, masses, and, in the case of acute abdominal complaints, for peritoneal signs. Extraintestinal manifestations detectable on examination include stomatitis, clubbing, arthritis, rash, and perianal disease. Often overlooked, but critical, is evaluation of the patient's nutritional status, which is made by measurements of midarm circumference and triceps skinfold thickness (Table 3).

The laboratory values most often abnormal on presentation are elevated erythrocyte sedimentation rate (ESR) in 80% to 90% of patients, anemia in 50% to 70%, hypoalbuminemia in 45% to 60%, leukocytosis in 40% to 70%, hyperglobulinemia and guaiac postive stool, each in about 35% (Table 4) (133). Low levels of calcium, magnesium, phosphorus, and zinc are also found due to decreased nutritional intake, malabsorption, bleeding, and sloughing of epithelium. The mean corpuscular volume (MCV) may be low, secondary to blood loss or dietary iron deficiency, or elevated, because of folate or vitamin B_{12} deficiency. Levels of fat soluble vitamins may be decreased in cases of severe ileal disease. Multiple stool samples must be taken on presentation for culture for bacterial pathogens, *Clostridium difficile,* and ova and parasites.

Testing for antineutrophil cytoplasmic antibodies (ANCA), is useful in adults in distinguishing ulcerative colitis from Crohn's disease (134). Two studies have examined the role of ANCA in pediatric patients and have arrived at slightly different findings (135,136). One group found ANCA to be 83% sensitive and 90% specific, and perinuclear fluorescence pattern (p-ANCA) to be 62% sensitive and 97% specific in diagnosing ulcerative colitis, similar to the findings in adult patients (134). Twenty-two percent of the Crohn's disease patients were positive for ANCA, but at significantly lower titers than those with ulcerative colitis. Of the Crohn's disease patients positive for ANCA, 70% had c-ANCA and 30% p-ANCA, essentially the opposite ratio found in the ulcerative patients (135). Another study found ANCA to be only 66% sensitive and 84% specific and p-ANCA to be 46% sensitive and 79% specific for the diagnosis of ulcerative colitis. Twenty percent of the patients with Crohn's disease were positive for ANCA, all had p-ANCA, and all had colonic disease; none with only small bowel involvement had ANCA (136).

There are numerous radiological studies available, and the clinician must prudently select those most appropriate for a particular patient. An upper gastrointestinal series with small bowel follow through (UGI/SBFT) is indicated for all patients at the time of presentation to define the presence and extent of upper gastrointestinal disease. Enteroclysis is usually not needed for this purpose but may be useful if the findings on UGI/SBFT are uncertain. The role of the barium enema has changed over the years. Colonoscopy has replaced it for routine diagnostic purposes, but it is valuable in the evaluation of colonic fistulas. If physical examination reveals an abdominal mass or if focal tenderness is accompanied by fever, an abdominal ultrasound or computed tomography (CT) scan is indicated to evaluate for abscess or lymphoma (137).

Another diagnostic modality to consider is nuclear medicine study. The poor sensitivity and specificity of the ^{111}In-tagged leukocyte scan in children limits its usefulness, although it may have a role in the investigation of occult small bowel disease (138,139). Technetium-99m hexamethyl propylene amine oxime (HMPAO)-labeled leukocyte scintigraphy has been shown in adults to be accurate in assessing the extent and activity of Crohn's disease of the small intestine and colon (140,141). A study of pediatric patients

TABLE 3 Clinical and Laboratory Evaluation of the Child with Suspected Crohn's Disease

History
  Abdominal pain, appetite
  Stool frequency, consistency, rectal bleeding
  Family history
  Growth data
  Activity level
  Psychosocial history
Physical examination
  Height, weight
  Abdominal tenderness, mass
  Rectal examination; perianal disease
  Rash, arthritis, clubbing, oral lesions
  Anthropometrics
  Tanner stage
Laboratory tests
  Complete blood count and differential, platelets, reticulocyte count
  Erythrocyte sedimentation rate
  Serum total protein, albumin, immunoglobulins, iron studies, calcium, magnesium, folate, vitamins A, E, D, B_{12}, zinc
  Stool guaiac, leukocytes
  Stool bacterial culture, parasite examination, *Clostridium difficile* toxin test
  If indicated:
    Antineutrophil cytoplasmic antibodies
    Lactose breath test
    Glucose breath test for bacterial overgrowth
    72-hour fecal fat
    Stool alpha-1-antitrypsin
Radiographic studies
  Upper gastrointestinal and small bowel series
  Bone age
  If indicated:
    Abdominal films: flat plate and upright
    Enteroclysis
    Barium enema, fistulogram
    Ultrasound, computed tomography
Nuclear medicine
  99mTc-hexamethyl propylene amine oxime
Endoscopic studies
  Colonoscopy and terminal ileoscopy with biopsies
  If indicated:
    Upper endoscopy with biopsies
    Endoscopic retrograde cholangiopancreatography

Source: Ref. 45.

TABLE 4 Common Laboratory Abnormalities
in Children with Crohn's Disease

Feature	Percentage
Elevated erythrocyte sedimentation rate	80–90
Anemia	50–70
Hypoalbuminenia	45–60
Leukocytosis	40–70
Hyperglobulinemia	37

Source: Refs. 1, 24, 133.

using this technique yielded similar results (142). Measuring the bone age is important in the evaluation of growth retardation and assessment of growth potential.

The diagnosis of Crohn's disease is made definitively based on endoscopic and histological findings. Colonoscopy with multiple biopsies is essential, and it is important to intubate the terminal ileum, although it may be difficult in young patients, because biopsies of this site are the most sensitive and specific test for Crohn's disease (143,144). Although it is usually possible to perform colonoscopy with terminal ileoscopy in children under conscious sedation, the use of general anesthesia should be considered in specific cases. Biopsies should be taken of representative areas throughout the colon, even if the endoscopic appearance is normal, because grossly normal mucosa may reveal abnormalities on pathologic examination (145). Noncaseating granuloms are found in the lamina propria or submucosa in one-third of cases, and the yield improves with an increasing number of biopsies (146,147). The presence of granulomas varies with the severity of disease, and they are found more frequently in children than in adults (148).

Upper gastrointestinal endoscopy is more sensitive than upper gastrointestinal series for the diagnosis of gastroduodenal Crohn's disease, but it is generally performed only when clinically indicated by symptoms (149,150). In a small minority of cases when the site of disease is inaccessible endoscopically, the diagnosis rests on characteristic radiological findings in the context of clinical and laboratory abnormalities.

VI. DIFFERENTIAL DIAGNOSIS

A large number of disorders must be considered in the differential diagnosis of Crohn's disease in children, but the investigation should be focused based on the particular presentation of the patient. The child with poor intake and weight loss may be suffering from psychological illness, such as anorexia nervosa. Cases of Crohn's disease have been misdiagnosed as anorexia nervosa in adolescent females, and anorexia nervosa has accompanied Crohn's disease (1,151). Short stature may be due to endocrine disease, such as growth hormone deficiency. If growth failure is accompanied by delayed sexual maturation, hypopituitarism is possible. These pathological conditions must be distinguished from constitutional growth delay and genetic short stature by appropriate hormone measurements and bone age determination.

The diagnostic considerations in the child with diarrhea depend on whether it is accompanied by gross blood. Bloody diarrhea is most often due to bacterial infection, and potential pathogens include *Salmonella, Shigella, Yersinia, Campylobacter, Aeromonas,*

Clostridium difficile, and enterotoxigenic and enterohemorrhagic *Escherichia coli* (152, 153). Other possibilities include hemolytic uremic syndrome, which is usually associated with infection by *E. coli* 0157:H7 (154). Henoch-Schönlein purpura, before the appearance of the characteristic rash, can mimic Crohn's disease with intermittent, sometimes severe, abdominal pain and joint symptoms accompanying diarrhea (155). The incidence of acquired immunodeficiency syndrome has increased in the pediatric population and may be the underlying process in a child with colitis and weight loss, or perianal disease, due to herpes simplex virus or chlamydia infection. In human immunodeficiency virus (HIV) disease, routine bacterial cultures may be negative, because the infection may be due to an opportunistic pathogen, such as *Cryptosporidium, Microsporidium, Isospora belli,* cytomegalovirus, and *Mycobacterium avium* (156).

Non-bloody diarrhea in children is usually due to viral infection and its duration may be from 1 to 2 weeks. Persistent diarrhea may be due to malabsorption syndromes such as lactase deficiency, which is unusual before age 5 years, celiac disease, or excessive dietary intake of poorly absorbed sugars, such as sorbitol. Infectious causes of chronic diarrhea include parasites, primarily *Entamoeba histolytica, Giardia* or *Cryptosporidium,* which are not uncommon in the day-care setting (157). Irritable bowel syndrome causes diarrhea less frequently in children than in adults, but is is a consideration, especially in an adolescent with persistent diarrhea (158).

Rectal bleeding without diarrhea may be due to a number of causes. Meckel's diverticulum has a peak incidence in the first 2 years of life, but it can occur throughout childhood. Bleeding from this source is usually painless, although abdominal pain occurs in some cases (159). The presence of colonic polyps should be considered if there is bleeding without pain. A common cause of rectal bleeding in children is fissures due to constipation and associated straining. These are usually evident on examination, and they occur in the absence of perianal disease, such as skin tags or inflammation. Hemolytic uremic syndrome, mentioned previously, is another cause of rectal bleeding.

Perianal disease, especially with fistula or abscess, should raise the suspicion of Crohn's disease in any child, but other perianal abnormalities may have different causes. Perianal erythema may be due to streptococcal infection. Perianal condylomata acuminata, caused by papilloma virus infection, may be confused with the perianal lesions of Crohn's disease. When perianal disease is present without obvious evidence of colitis, sexual abuse may merit consideration.

Chronic abdominal pain is common in children and has numerous causes. The syndrome of recurrent abdominal pain occurs in up to 10% of 7- to 11-year-olds (160). Characteristically, the pain is periumbilical or epigastric, although it may also be so in Crohn's disease (1). Constipation is another common cause of abdominal pain in children, and it may be present despite a regular defecation pattern. Lactose intolerance occurs after age 5 years, and it may cause episodes of pain that patients do not associate with ingestion of lactose. Other causes of persistent abdominal pain are peptic ulcer disease, esophagitis, parasitic infections, urinary tract disease, pancreatitis, and lymphoma. Given the frequency with which children have abdominal pain, the decision to investigate for a serious cause, such as Crohn's disease, should be made selectively. If the pain is not associated with diarrhea, nausea, vomiting, fever, weight loss, growth failure, or any extraintestinal manifestations, and if it does not awaken the child from sleep, then Crohn's disease is less likely.

Pain that predominates in the right lower quadrant may be due to Crohn's disease involving the terminal ileum or cecum, but other causes must be considered, especially if the pain is of acute onset. Appendicitis may be the presentation of Crohn's disease or can occur during the course of the disease (161). *Yersinia* infection can also localize to the right lower quadrant and may further mimic Crohn's disease with its associated arthritis and erythema nodosum. Other causes of pain that occur in this region are intussusception, more common in infants and young children, and ovarian cysts or torsion.

Cystic fibrosis may resemble Crohn's disease, with weight loss, growth failure, anemia, and bulky stools due to steatorrhea. Both cystic fibrosis and celiac disease may occur with Crohn's disease (162,163). The prevalence of Crohn's disease in cystic fibrosis is estimated to be 17 times that of age-matched controls, but this finding requires further study and confirmation (163).

Patients with arthritis, unexplained fever, or rash may have juvenile rheumatoid arthritis, which, like Crohn's disease, is often subtle in its presentation. In all such cases, the physician should explore carefully for any gastrointestinal signs or symptoms, which may predate or accompany the presenting complaint.

VII. THERAPY

The management of Crohn's disease in children may be divided into three categories: medical, nutritional, and surgical treatments. The patient may benefit from a combination of these modalities. Because there is no cure, the goal of therapy is to control symptoms while minimizing toxicity. Treatment decisions should not be based on laboratory data alone, and these data do not always correlate with findings on colonoscopy (164). Ultimately, management should be guided by the patient's clinical condition and other available information. Growth is an important consideration in the treatment of children, both in terms of growth retardation as a symptom of the disease and the impact of therapy on growth. In children, most studies of therapeutic modalities use the Pediatric Crohn's Disease Activity Index (PCDAI) to assess clinical efficacy of a particular intervention. This scoring system is divided into five categories: general activity, physical examination and clinical complications, nutrition, x-ray findings, and laboratory data. The PCDAI is straightforward to perform and results are reproducible (165).

A. Medical

1. Steroids

Much of the treatment of pediatric Crohn's disease (Table 5) is derived from studies in adults because no large-scale, controlled trial of medical therapies has been conducted in children. Several adult trials have shown that steroids are effective in inducing remission of disease and are ineffective in preventing relapse when given daily at low dose (166–168). Use of steroids is indicated when there is acute disease that is unresponsive to other treatment, extensive small bowel inflammation, severe systemic symptoms or extraintestinal manifestations, and postoperative recurrence of disease.

The dosage of prednisone or methylprednisolone is 1 to 2 mg/kg per day and rarely is as high as 3 mg/kg per day (maximum 60 to 90 mg/day), it is given orally or parenterally, once daily or in two divided doses. The dose and route of administration depend on the severity of the disease. The intravenous route is used in severe disease when the patient needs to be hospitalized. When the patient shows a response to intravenous steroid, a comparable dose is given orally, and then tapered to 1 mg/kg per day, given once daily, as the patient improves. After 3 to 4 weeks, the dose is lowered by 5 mg per day each week,

TABLE 5 Medical Therapy of Crohn's Disease in Children

Indication	Dose
Severe inflammation	
Prednisone or methylprednisolone	1–2 (rarely 3) mg/kg/day, divided bid, maximum rarely exceeds 90 mg/day. Taper to 1 mg/kg/day qd, and then by 5 mg/day every week to qod or off therapy
Mild to moderate inflammation and maintenance of remission	
Sulfasalazine	50–75 mg/kg/day, divided bid to tid, maximum 3–4 g/day
Asacol	40–50 mg/kg/day, divided tid, maximum 4.8 g/day
Dipentum	25–50 mg/kg/day, divided bid, maximum 1 g/day
Pentasa	Adult dose, 2–4 g/day, divided qid
Also for perianal disease	
Metronidazole	15 mg/kg/day, divided tid, maximum 1.5 g/day
Refractory disease/immunosuppressives	
Azathioprine	2 mg/kg/day, qd or divided bid
6-Mercaptopurine	1.5 mg/kg/day, qd or divided bid

bid = twice a day; qd = every day; qod = every other day; tid = three times a day; qid = four times a day.

or by 2.5-mg increments if the starting dose was low. Over the next 4 to 6 weeks, the steroid is either tapered at this rate until it is discontinued, or tapered to an alternate day regimen when the daily dose is 10 to 20 mg. The former schedule is generally used in the newly diagnosed patient who has responded well to treatment, whereas the latter is the preferred schedule in other patients, especially when inflammatory activity has been slow to respond to therapy. Patients on alternate-day dosing are weaned off steroid therapy entirely when remission is achieved.

Despite the efficacy of steroids, their use may be limited by side effects. Children, like adults, are at risk of developing hypertension, osteoporosis, avascular necrosis, glaucoma and posterior subcapsular cataracts, diabetes, and pseudotumor cerebri. Adolescents are particularly sensitive to changes in their appearance, particularly weight gain, hirsutism, striae, acne, and "moon facies." Psychological effects of steroids are not uncommon, in particular, mood changes, such as depression, and hyperactivity. These problems may interfere with school performance, which can be distressing to both patient and parents.

The effect of steroids on growth is a critical issue in the treatment of pediatric disease, but persistent disease activity has an even more profound impact on growth (82). As discussed, some patients grow only if their disease is controlled with steroids. Alternate-day steroid therapy is preferable to daily dosing in this regard if disease activity is suppressed on this regimen (109,111). Alternate-day steroid therapy also appears not to interfere with normal bone mineralization (110). The extent to which an alternate-day schedule permits growth is not known; this issue has yet to be determined by a large, controlled trial. During puberty, patients should have periodic bone age measurements to assess growth potential, which may guide management decisions. To minimize their undesirable effects, steroids should be discontinued as soon as disease remission is achieved.

2. Sulfasalazine and 5-Amino Salicylates

Sulfasalazine (SAS) and salicylate preparations have a role in the treatment of mild to moderately active disease and, more importantly, in the maintenance of remission. Studies conducted in adults have demonstrated that SAS is effective in Crohn's colitis, and some studies have shown an effect on small bowel disease as well and recommend its use in this setting, generally at a dose higher than that usually used for colitis (111,166,167,169,170). The dose should be increased gradually to full dose over 7 days to miminize side effects at the initiation of treatment. If a genetic predisposition is likely, glucose-6-phosphate dehydrogenase (G6PD) screening should precede the use of SAS. The most frequently observed side effects are headache, nausea, vomiting, abdominal pain, and bloody diarrhea. If such a reaction occurs, the dosage should be lowered or the medication discontinued until the reaction resolves, then the dose should be increased more slowly from a lower starting dose as tolerated. Serious side effects include neutropenia, pancreatitis, and reversible oligospermia (171). Because SAS may impair folate absorption, patients on this medication must either receive supplemental folate or have serum folic acid levels measured at regular intervals.

The 5-aminosalicylic acid (5-ASA) preparations, Asacol and Pentasa, may be more valuable than SAS in the treatment of small bowel disease (172). Asacol can be used to treat terminal ileal disease, and Pentasa theoretically has more effect proximally, because it can be released in the jejunum, although altered motility may delay transit of Pentasa. A small, double-blind study in children with proximal and distal small bowel disease showed improvement in those taking Pentasa compared with placebo-treated patients. The only side effect observed, mild hair loss in one patient, was reversible (173). Although no controlled trials are available in pediatric Crohn's disease, Dipentum, which is split by colonic bacteria, may be useful in patients with Crohn's colitis who are allergic to sulfa compounds or who have persistent side effects of SAS.

There is a range of doses for each of these medications, and the appropriate dose for each patient depends on the level of disease activity and tolerance of any side effects. The dosage of SAS for active disease is 50 to 75 mg/kg per day, with a maximum of 3 to 4 g/day divided in two to three doses. The medication is available in 500-mg tablets, but a suspension preparation may be made for young patients who require lower doses or cannot take tablets. Folate supplementation is 1 mg/day for all patients. The dosage of Asacol is 40 to 50 mg/kg per day divided in three doses, with a maximum of 4.8 g/day. It is available as a 400-mg tablet, which cannot be crushed or suspended. Pentasa is available in 250-mg tablets; the adult dosage is 2 to 4 g/day divided in four doses. The dose of Dipentum is 25 to 50 mg/kg per day, with a maximum of 1 g/day, given in 2 divided doses. The capsule may be opened and sprinkled onto food for children too young to take intact capsules.

3. Antibiotics

Antibiotics have several roles in the management of Crohn's disease. Broad-spectrum intravenous antibiotic coverage, typically with ampicillin, gentamicin, and clindamycin or metronidazole, is used in the treatment of abscesses. These antibiotics may also be indicated in the patient with fever and localized tenderness but without a proven abscess when microperforation is suspected.

Metronidazole is effective in the treatment of Crohn's colitis, but is less effective in small intestinal disease (174). It is not commonly used in pediatric therapy as a first line agent in primary treatment, although it may be more effective than SAS in this role (175).

Metronidazole is used more frequently as an adjunct to steroids or salicylate when there is inadequate improvement on these medications (176). Metronidazole is also used in the treatment of perianal disease. Although it is effective in this role, the recurrence rate is as high as 75% when it is discontinued (177). Ciprofloxacin, a quinolone antibiotic, is also used to treat perianal disease, and there is a small series suggesting that it may have a role in the primary treatment of ileitis (178). Ciprofloxacin is not recommended for use in children younger than 12 years of age. Metronidazole is also commonly used in the treatment of bacterial overgrowth, to which some patients are predisposed. Other antibiotics, for example oral kanamycin, can be alternated wtih metronidazole if needed to treat this process.

Metronidazole may cause reversible, peripheral neuropathy, especially when used for long periods. In one study, a majority of children treated for a mean of 7 months developed sensory neuropathy or decreased nerve conduction (179). Other side effects, of which the patient should be warned, include metallic taste and an disulfiram-type effect. The dosage is 15 mg/kg per day divided in 3 doses, with a maximum of 1.5 g/day. Treatment generally should not exceed 6 months because there is a risk of side effects with cumulative high doses (45).

4. Immunosuppressives

Immunosuppressive agents are used in a variety of settings in the management of pediatric Crohn's disease, although there have been no prospective, controlled trials conducted in children. Immunosuppressives function primarily as steroid-sparing agents in patients who are dependent on high-dose steroids or those who have, or are at risk of developing, serious complications of prolonged steroid use. To maintain remission achieved with steroids, immunosuppressives are also used in patients with flare-ups of disease that are recurrent and difficult to control. These agents may have a role in treating disease refractory to standard medical therapy and not amenable to surgical treatment.

Azathioprine (AZA) and its metabolite, 6-mercaptopurine (6-MP), are the most commonly used immunosuppressants, although there are minimal data on their use in pediatric patients. An open trial of AZA in 12 steroid-dependent children demonstrated a complete response in six and partial response in three as measured by ther ability to discontinue or lower the dose of steroids, respectively (180). 6-Mercaptopurine was shown to be effective in an unblinded trial of 36 adolescents with refractory symptoms, based on clinical improvement, decreased steroid use, and improvement of perianal disease. Of the 30 patients treated for more than 1 year, 80% were off steroids and just more than 20% required surgical resection (181). In adults, 6-MP is effective in the treatment of gastroduodenal disease, internal fistulas, and perianal disease (182).

The dosage of AZA is 2 mg/kg per day and that of 6-MP is 1.5 mg/kg per day. Each is given once daily or in divided doses. The starting dose should be low and increased to the full dose over 5 days to minimize gastrointestinal discomfort. The highest tolerated dose should be used, the limitation being development of leukopenia or lymphopenia, because the medication may not be fully effective unless leukopenia is achieved (183). The only toxicities observed in the pediatric trials were decline in white blood cell (WBC) count, which may be useful clinically as an indicator of drug effect, and mild elevation of liver enzymes (180,181). The WBC count and differential, bilirubin, transaminases, and amylase should be monitored weekly for 1 month after initiating treatment, then monthly for 3 months, and then every 3 to 6 months thereafter. The optimal duration of therapy is not known; in adults, some advocate lowering the dosage to 1 mg/kg per day after 1 year if the patient is doing well (184). The risk of malignancy remains a concern, but, in adults, it is a rare complication (185). There were no malignancies in the aformentioned pediatric studies, but the number of patients was small and follow-up was only 1 to 2 years.

There are few reports on the use of cyclosporin (CSA) in children with inflammatory bowel disease, and most of these patients had ulcerative colitis (186–191). In these studies, CSA was either started orally or administered parenterally then changed to oral form. Desired blood levels ranged from 100 to 300 ng/ml. Based on these trials and larger ones in adults, it appears that, in many cases, CSA is effective in inducing remission of active disease unresponsive to standard therapy, including intravenous steroids (192,193). The duration of remission, though, is variable, and relapse is common when CSA is withdrawn. One group has shown that, in children, CSA-induced remission may be prolonged with the adjunctive use of AZA or 6-MP (194). The main benefit of CSA, if it does maintain prolonged remission, may be in the postponement of surgery in the ill patient receiving high-dose steroid, allowing time for reduction of the steroid dose and for nutritional rehabilitation. There are no reports on the use of methotrexate in children with Crohn's disease.

5. Other Agents

Some patients with frequent diarrhea may benefit from an antimotility agent, such as loperamide. The dosage is 0.1 mg/kg per dose given 2 to 3 times a day, with a maximum daily dose of 4–6 g. Antimotility medications must be used cautiously and stopped if the patient develops any symptoms suggestive of obstruction, megacolon, or perforation. Some care givers recommend against the use of these agents to avoid masking symptoms of active disease (111). Patients with choleretic diarrhea from extensive ileal disease or resection may benefit from cholestyramine. There has been limited study of the use of growth hormone in patients with short stature and normal growth hormone levels. An early report of three such patients showed no benefit in such therapy (106).

B. Nutritional

The role of nutritional intervention in Crohn's disease is a dual one, serving as supplementation or as primary therapy. Every child with Crohn's disease must undergo full nutritional assessment at the time of diagnosis and at intervals thereafter. The evaluation includes determination of height, weight, growth velocity, triceps skin fold thickness, midarm circumference, and the following laboratory tests: serum protein and albumin, and mineral and vitamin levels, particularly iron, magnesium, calcium, zinc, folate, and vitamin B_{12}. The patient's diet should also be reviewed to assess intake of calories and protein. This may be performed by recall of intake or more reliably with a 3-day diet diary.

The goals of supplementation are to correct deficiencies of macronutrients and micronutrients, to compensate for persistent losses from inflamed bowel, to provide sufficient protein and calories for positive nitrogen balance, to promote catch-up growth to premorbid percentiles, and to promote sexual maturation. Supplementation reverses growth retardation in most patients (86). Growth velocity has been shown to increase from 1.8 to 6.2 cm per year if caloric intake within 90% of recommended is achieved (83). Such improvement depends on the patient's growth potential, and supplementation must be administered before bone maturation is complete (78). The general guideline for supplementation is provision of at least 140% to 150% of recommended daily allowance (RDA) for protein and calories based on height–age, but this may vary for each patient.

Nutritional supplementation may be provided in various ways. Growth improves with the administration of total parenteral nutrition, but the gastrointestinal tract should be used when possible (195,196). Exceptions are in patients with severe inflammation, who have significant malabsorption, and in patients who have short bowel syndrome due to resection. In such cases, parenteral nutrition is needed to provide adequate calories (92). When the alimentary tract is used, oral supplementation alone is rarely successful, because it is difficult for patients to maintain an increased oral intake consistently on a long-term basis. Generally, patients require continuous overnight nasogastric feedings, alone or in combination with daytime oral supplements. There is a variety of formulas from which to choose. They fall into two categories: elemental and intact protein formulas (197). Although there are theoretical advantages of an elemental formula, such as minimizing malabsorption in patients with significant small bowel disease, its superiority to whole protein formula as a supplement has not been established. A low-residue diet is indicated in patients with symptomatic intestinal narrowing or stricture, but it appears to be of no benefit to patients without these complications (92).

The efficacy of nutritional therapy as primary treatment of Crohn's disease has been demonstrated in pediatric trials but is not widely used in clinical practice, probably because there are practical difficulties in administering an elemental diet and problems with patient compliance. This mode of therapy has been best studied in the setting of acute disease, either on initial presentation or at relapse. Several studies in adults have shown similar remission rates for elemental diet and steroids for patients who remained on the formula for the entire study period (198,199). Two pediatric trials with small numbers of patients have demonstrated the same results (200,201). In most patients, the formula was administered via nasogastric tube, although some adult patients took a portion or even all of the formula by mouth. Better compliance was achieved in the patients in whom the diet was administered by tube continuously overnight while allowing only clear liquids by mouth during the day. The studies also suggest that completely elemental formulas, in which the protein source is free amino acids, are more effective than semielemental preparations, which consist of oligopeptides (202). There is some evidence that elemental diet is more effective in small bowel disease than in colonic disease (203). Remission is usually achieved within several weeks, but the rate of relapse is high when the diet is stopped. The treatment may be more effective if moderate-dosage steroid, 0.3 to 0.5 mg/kg per day of prednisone, is started before resuming a normal diet (204).

Studies in growth-impaired children with Crohn's disease have shown that administering an elemental diet for 1 out of 4 months, followed by a gradual reintroduction of a regular diet, leads to increased growth velocity (205,206). It is not clear, however, how much of this effect is due to the composition of the formula rather than to increased caloric intake. Although it has not been studied in children, an elemental diet may be useful in treating disease refractory to standard medical therapy. A small trial in adults showed that elemental diet was effective in steroid-resistant and steroid-dependent patients in achieving remission and allowing tapering of steroids during a 6-month to 1-year follow-up period (207). Patients with strictures, fistulas, or severe perianal disease may also benefit from the very low residue elemental formulas.

The mechanism of action of the elemental diet is not well understood. Part of the benefit is due to enhanced nutritional status, but at least one study demonstrated an effect beyond that achieved with whole protein diets providing the same number of calories (208). One possibility is that the elemental diet acts by creating a state of bowel rest. Studies show that complete bowel rest is effective in active disease but this may be due to the concurrent administration of total parenteral nutrition (209–211). There may also be a benefit of decreased antigenic stimulation of abnormally permeable gut, thereby diminishing the immune response of inflamed intestine and improving permeability (212,213). Bacterial antigens may be involved in the inflammation of Crohn's disease, and an elemental diet alters the bowel flora, perhaps thereby modifying the immune response (214,215).

C. Surgical

Surgical treatment has an important role in the management of pediatric Crohn's disease. In one long-term study of children and adolescents with Crohn's disease, surgery was performed in 69% of all patients within 7.7 years of diagnosis; 63% of those patients had small bowel disease and 71% colonic disease (7). In another such study, with a follow-up period of 15 years, 95% of patients with ileocolonic, 83% with colonic and 56% with small bowel disease underwent surgery; the mean interval between diagnosis and surgery was 1.7 years and 4 years in the first 2 groups, respectively (216). The indications for surgery vary with the site of disease. The most common indications in small intestinal disease, accounting for nearly 80% of operations in one study, were obstruction and internal fistulas (7). In colonic disease, there is a wider variety of indications, including persistent bleeding, toxic megacolon, obstruction, perforation, abscess, fistula, and perianal disease (1,7,217). Patients may also undergo surgery for refractory symptoms, including growth failure, despite maximal medical and nutritional therapy. Steroid dependency and toxicity have been considered reasons to operate, but the use of immunosuppressives may offer an alternative to such patients.

Small bowel resection is performed for localized disease or stricture. Strictureplasty has been performed successfully in many adult patients (218). A report of a small number of pediatric patients who have undergone this procedure, either alone or with resection, demonstrated clinical improvement over a 19-month follow-up period (219). When disease involves one part of the colon, limited resection with a colostomy is a viable option, whereas patients with diffuse colitis should undergo total proctocolectomy or, if the rectum is spared of disease, colectomy with ileorectal anastomosis (217). An endorectal pull-through procedure should not be performed because of the risk of recurrence and development of postoperative fistula or abscess.

The indications for local surgical treatment of perianal disease include painful abscess or draining fistula (220). When a child has severe perianal disease, some caregivers advocate fecal diversionary procedures, whereas others have not found it helpful (221–223).

Although surgery is not curative, resection often provides the patient with a disease-free period. The outcome is best for disease limited to the small intestine or ileocecal region (224). In one study, 80% of children who underwent resection for terminal ileal disease were in remission 4 years postoperatively (223). Results are poor for segmental resection of colonic disease, for which the rate of relapse is as high as 70% within 5 years (223). Recurrence of disease after total proctocolectomy depends on whether the terminal ileum is involved at the time of surgery. Seventy percent of patients with terminal ileal disease experience relapse within 5 to 10 years of surgery compared with 15% of patients with disease limited to the colon (225). The risk of recurrence also increases with disease duration before surgery, and relapse occurs earlier in patients who undergo surgery for failure of medical therapy compared with those operated on for specific complications, such as obstruction or abscess (226). Rates of reoperation are high and depend on the site of disease, varying from 50% at 10 years for disease limited to the small bowel to 65% when the colon is also involved (227).

Patients with growth failure despite intensive medical therapy and nutritional intervention may benefit from surgery. The data are conflicting in this regard, with some studies demonstrating a greater effect of surgery than others (1,227–231). For example, one group demonstrated catch-up growth in 10 of 16 children who underwent surgery, eight of 12 with ileocolonic disease and two of four with colonic involvement, whereas, in another study, only two of 14 children had catch-up growth after surgery (216,231). Optimizing postoperative growth appears to depend on several factors: the patient must be prepubertal or in early puberty, all active disease must be resected, and the patient must have a prolonged period of remission after surgery (231,232). Any gains in growth postoperatively also depend on maintaining adequate nutritional status and on discontinuing steroid therapy or tapering such therapy to alternate-day dosing.

VIII. PROGNOSIS

The prognosis of Crohn's disease with onset in childhood has been the subject of several studies, with follow-up periods of various lengths (1,7,216,227). Clinical disease severity does not appear to correlate with age at onset, but does depend on the site of disease (7). In general, patients with colonic disease alone or with small bowel involvement have poorer outcomes than those with only small bowel disease; they have more extraintestinal symptoms, greater number of operations, longer steroid requirement, and higher mortality rate (1,7). Mortality rates vary among studies. One group following up 177 children reported a mortality rate of 2% at 5 years and 11% at 20 years after onset (227). Another found a 13% mortality rate at 15-year follow-up among 67 patients, and a third investigator reported no deaths in a group of 200 patients over approximately a 10-year period (28,216). The largest long-term pediatric study, one of 522 patients diagnosed before age 21 years reported a mortality rate of 2.4% at a mean follow-up of 7.7 years (7). Recent mortality data are not available. The common causes of death include postoperative complications, perforation, obstruction, and hemorrhage (216,227).

Long-term data regarding disease activity and quality of life for children with Crohn's disease are encouraging. In a 15-year follow-up study of children with onset of Crohn's disease by age 16 years, two of three had no evidence or residual disease, one of four were clinically well, although they had radiological findings of residual or recurrent disease, and 1 of 10 were symptomatic (216). A study of adults, whose mean duration of illness was 9 years, measured quality of life based on the parameters of education, marital and parental status, employment, and physical activity, and found no differences between Crohn's disease patients and controls. Nevertheless, more than half of those with Crohn's disease felt that their disease interfered with their professional and personal lives (232). There are similar discrepancies in the self-assessment of patients diagnosed in childhood. In one study that had a 7.7-year follow-up, only 23% of patients rated their quality of life as good (7). There was no difference between patients who had and had not undergone surgery. Another study, with a follow-up period of 9 years, found that 80% of patients considered their state of health to be good or excellent, and 71% felt that they were not limited in their routine daily activity by their disease (233).

The management of Crohn's disease in children, because of its complexities, should be coordinated by the gastroenterologist but requires the combined efforts of the pediatrician or primary care physician, nutritionist, nurse, and, frequently, social worker or mental health professional. The patient and family must participate in treatment decisions, and, for this, they must be fully informed and educated. The patient's ability to understand depends on the child's age, but any effort to involve the patient is rewarded with enhanced cooperation and compliance. Careful, regular evaluation of clinical and nutritional status, growth and sexual maturation, psychological adjustment, and compliance with therapy is essential, and, even when the disease is quiescent, follow-up should be at intervals of no longer than 6 months. Despite the potential for intermittent disease activity and the regular monitoring that it requires, the child with Crohn's disease should expect to lead a full, normal life.

REFERENCES

1. Gryboski JD, Spiro HM. Prognosis in children with Crohn's disease. Gastro 1978; 74:807–817.
2. Kelts DG, Grand RJ. Inflammatory bowel disease in children and adolescents. Curr Probl Pediatr 1980; 10:1–40.
3. Motil K, Grand RJ, Ulcerative colitis and Crohn's disease in children. Pediatr Rev 1987; 9:109–120.
4. Lenaerts C, Roy CC,Vaillancourt M, et al. High incidence of upper gastrointestinal tract involvement in children with Crohn's disease. Pediatrics 1989; 83:777–781.
5. Mashako MNL, Cezard JP, Navarro J, et al. Crohn's disease lesions in the upper gastrointestinal tract: correlation between clinical, radiological, endoscopic, and histological features in adolescents and children. J Pediatr Gastroenterol Nutr 1989; 8:442–446.
6. Mendeloff AI. The epidemiology of inflammatory bowel disease. Clin Gastro 1980; 9:259–270.
7. Farmer RG, Michener WM. Prognosis of Crohn's disease with onset in childhood or adolescence. Dig Dis Sci 1979; 24:752–757.
8. Grand RJ, Homer DR. Approaches to inflammatory bowel disease in childhood and adolescents. Pediatr Clin North Am 1975; 22:835–850.
9. Miller RC, Jackson M, Larson E. Regional enteritis in early infancy. Am J Dis Child 1971; 122:301–311.
10. Chong SKF, Blackshaw AJ, Morson BC, et al. Prospective study of colitis in infancy and early childhood. J Pediatr Gastroenterol Nutr 1986; 5:352–358.
11. Calkins BM, Lillienfeld AM, Garland CF, et al. Trends in incidence rates of ulcerative colitic and Crohn's disease. Dig Dis Sci 1984; 29:913–920.
12. Barton JR, Gillon S, Ferguson A. Incidence of inflammatory bowel disease in Scottish children between 1968 and 1983; marginal fall in ulcerative colitis, three-fold rise in Crohn's disease. Gut 1989; 30:618–622.
13. Olafsdottir EJ, Gjermund F, Haug K. Chronic inflammatory bowel disease in children in western Norway. J Pediatr Gastroenterol Nutr. 1989; 8:454–458.
14. Ferguson A. Crohn's disease in children and adolescents. J R Soc Med 1984; 77(suppl 3):30–34.
15. Ekbom A, Helmick C, Zack M, Adami HO. The epidemiology of inflammatory bowel disease: a large, population based study in Sweden. Gastroenterology 1991; 100:350–358.
16. Farmer RG, Michener WM, Mortimer EA. Studies of family history among patients with inflammatory bowel disease. Clin Gastroenterol 1980; 9:271–277.
17. Lashner BA, Evans AA, Kirsner JB, et al. Prevalence and incidence of inflammatory bowel disease in family members. Gastroenterology 1986; 91:1396–1400.
18. Meucci G, Vecchi M, Torgano G, et al. Familial aggregation of inflammatory bowel disease in Northern Italy. Gastroenterology 1992; 103:514–519.
19. Fielding JF. The relative risk of inflammatory bowel disease among parents and siblings of Crohn's disease patients. J Clin Gastroenterol 1986; 8:655–657.
20. McConnell RB. Genetic aspects of idiopathic inflammatory bowel disease. In: Kirsner JB, Shorter RG, eds. Inflammatory Bowel Disease. 3rd ed. Philadelphia: Lea & Febiger, 1988:87–95.

21. Purrmann J, Bertrams J, Knapp M, et al. Gene and haplotype frequencies of HLA antigens in 269 patients with Crohn's disease. Scand J Gastroenterol 1990; 25:981–985.

22. Smolen JS, Gangl A, Polterauer P, et al. HLA antigens in inflammatory bowel disease. Gastroenterology 1982; 82:34–38.

23. Toyoda H, Wang SJ, Yang HY, et al. Distinct associations of HLA class II genes with inflammatory bowel disease. Gastroenterology 1993; 104:741–748.

24. Burbidge FJ, Huang S, Bayless TM. Clinical manifestations of Crohn's disease in children and adolescents. Pediatrics 1975; 55:866–871.

25. Kanof ME, Lake AM, Bayless TM. Decreased height velocity in children and adolescents before the diagnosis of Crohn's disease. Gastroenterology 1988; 95:1523–1527.

26. Kirschner BS, Voinchet O, Rosenberg IH. Growth retardation in inflammatory bowel disease. Gastroenterology 1978; 75:504–511.

27. Hyams JS. Crohn's disease. In: Wyllie R, Hyams JS, eds. Pediatric Gastrointestinal Disease. Philadelphia: WB Saunders, 1993:742–764.

28. Kirschner BS. Inflammatory bowel disease in children. Pediatr Clin North Am 1988; 35:189–208.

29. Griffiths AM, Alemayehu E, Sherman P. Clinical features of gastroduodenal disease in adolescents. J Pediatr Gastroenterol Nutr 1989; 8:166–171.

30. Treem WR, Ragsdale BD. Crohn's disease of the esophagus: a case report and review of the literature. J Pediatr Gastroenterol Nutr 1988; 7:451–455.

31. Ridge JA, Wayu LW. Abdominal pain. In: Sleisenger MH, Fordtran JS, eds. Gastrointestinal Disease. Philadelphia: WB Saunders, 1993:150–161.

32. Sandborn WJ, Phillips SF. Pathophysiology of symptoms and clinical features of inflammatory bowel disease. In: Kirsner JB, Shorter RG, eds. Inflammatory Bowel Disease. 4th ed. Baltimore: Williams & Wilkins, 1995;407–428.

33. Beeken WL. Absorptive defects in young people with regional enteritis. Pediatrics 1973; 52:69–74.

34. Rhoads JM, Powell DW. Diarrhea. In: Walker WA, Durie PR, Hamilton JR, et al, eds. Pediatric Gastrointestinal Disease. Philadelphia: BC Decker, 1991:62–78.

35. Phillips SF, Gaginella TS. Intestinal secretion as a mechanism in diarrheal disease. In: Jerzy Glass GB, ed. Progress in Gastroenterology. Vol. III. New York: Grune & Stratton, 1977:481–504.

36. Hofman AF. Bile acid malabsorption caused by ileal resection. Arch Intern Med 1972; 130:597–605.

37. Head LH, Heaton JW, Kivel RM. Absorption of water and electrolytes in Crohn's disease of the colon. Gastroenterology 1969; 56:571–579.

38. Markowitz J, Daum F, Aiges H, et al. Perianal disease in children and adolescents with Crohn's disease. Gastroenterology 1984; 86:829–833.

39. Palder SB, Shandling B, Bilik R. Perianal complications of pediatric Crohn's disease. J Pediatr Surg 1991; 26:513–515.

40. Lindsley CB, Schaller JG. Arthritis associated with inflammatory bowel disease. J Pediatr 1974; 84:16–20.

41. Danzi JT. Extraintestinal manifestations of idiopathic inflammatory bowel disease. Arch Intern Med 1988; 148:297–302.

42. Moll JM. Inflammatory bowel disease. In: Panayi GS, ed. Clinics in Rheumatic Disease. Philadelphia: WB Saunders, 1985:87–105.

43. Paller AS. Cutaneous changes associated with inflammatroy bowel disease. Pediatr Dermatol 1986; 3:439–445.

44. Levitt MD, Ritchie JK, Lennard-Jones JE, et al. Pyoderma gangrenosum in inflammatory bowel disease. Br J Surg 1991; 78:676–678.

45. Jackson WD, Grand RJ. In: Walker WA, Durie PR, Hamilton JR, et al, eds. Pediatric Gastrointestinal Disease. Philadelphia: BC Decker, 1991:592–608.

46. Klein JD, Biller JA, Leape L, Grand RJ. Pyoderma gangrenosum occurring at multiple incision sites. Gastroenterology 1987; 92:810–813.

47. Sutphen JL, Cooper PH, Mackel SE, Nelson DL. Metastic cutaneous Crohn's disease. Gastroenterology 1984; 86:941–944.

48. Menard D, Haddad H, Blain JG, et al. Granulomatous myositis and myopathy associated with Crohn's colitis. N Engl J Med 1976; 295:818–819.

49. Jackson WD, Dawson-Hughes B, Grand RJ. Effects of Crohn's disease on bone mineral density in children (abstr). Gastroenterology 1988; 94:A203.

50. Ghosh S, Cowen S, Hannan WJ, Ferguson A. Low bone mineral density in Crohn's disease, but not in ulcerative colitis, at diagnosis. Gastroenterology 1994; 107:1031–1039.

51. Vakil N, Sparberg M. Steroid-related osteonecrosis in inflammatory bowel disease. Gastroenterology 1989; 96:62–67.

52. Freeman HJ, Kwan WC. Non-corticosteroid associated osteonecrosis of the femoral heads in two patients with inflammatory bowel disease. N Engl J Med 1993; 329:1314–1316.

53. Daum F, Gould HB, Gold D, et al. Asymptomatic transient uveitis in children with inflammatory bowel disease. Am J Dis Child 1979; 133:170–171.

54. Salmon JF, Wright JP, Murray ADN. Ocular inflammation in Crohn's disease. Ophthalmology 1991; 98:480–484.

55. Young RSK, Hodes BL, Cruse RP, et al. Orbital pseudotumor and Crohn's disease. J Pediatr 1981; 99:250–252.

56. Plauth M, Jenss H, Meyle J. Oral manifestations of Crohn's disease: an analysis of 79 cases. J Clin Gastroenterol 1991; 13:29–37.

57. Deren JJ, Porush JG, Levitt MF, Khilnani MT. Nephrolithiasis as a complication of ulcerative colitis and regional enteritis. Ann Intern Med 1962; 56:843–853.

58. Greenstein AJ, Janowitz MD, Sachar DB. The extraintestinal complications of Crohn's disease and ulcerative colitis: a study of 700 patients. Medicine 1976; 55:401–412.

59. Present DH, Rabinowitz JG, Banks PA, Janowitz HD. Obstructive hydronephrosis—a frequent but seldom recognized complication of granulomatous disease on the bowel. N Engl J Med 1969; 280:523–528.

60. Kahn E, Markowitz J, Simpser E, et al. Amyloidosis in children with inflammatory bowel disease. J Pediatr Gastroenterol Nutr 1989; 8:447–453.

61. Kirschner BS, Samowitz W. Secondary amyloidosis in Crohn's disease of childhood. J Pediatr Gastroenterol Nutr 1986; 5:816–821.

62. Dew MJ, Thompson H, Allan RN. The spectrum of hepatic dysfunction in inflammatory bowel disease. Q J Med 1979; 189;113–135.

63. Kane W, Miller K, Sharp HL. Inflammatory bowel disease presenting as liver disease during childhood. J Pediatr 1980; 97:775–778.

64. Porayko MK, Wiesner RH, LaRusso NF, et al. Patients with asymptomatic primary sclerosing cholangitis frequently have progressive disease. Gastroenterology 1990; 98:1594–1602.

65. Ramelli GP, Tonz O, Zimmerman A, Lentze MJ. Crohn's disease with sclerosing cholangitis and liver cirrhosis in adolescence. Eur J Pediatr 1991; 150:557–559.

66. Ong JC, O'Loughlin EV, Kamath KR, et al. Sclerosing cholangitis in children with inflammatory bowel disease. Aust N Z J Med 1994; 24:149–153.

67. Cohen S, Kaplan M, Gottleib L, Patterson J. Liver disease and gallstones in regional enteritis. Gastroenterology 1971; 60:237–245.

68. Hyams JS, Baker E, Schwartz AN, et al. Acalculous cholecystitis in Crohn's disease. J Adolesc Health Care 1988; 10:151–154.

69. Heaton KW. Disturbances of bile acid metabolism in intestinal disease. Clin Gastroenterol 1976; 6:69–89.

70. Huthcinson R, Tyrrell PNM, Kumar C, et al. Pathogenesis of gallstones in Crohn's disease: an alternative explanation. Gut 1994; 35:94–97.

71. Baumgartner G, Sauerbruch T. Gallstones: pathogenesis. Lancet 1991; 338:1117–1121.

72. Eisner TD, Goldman IS, McKinley MJ. Crohn's disease and pancreatitis. Am J Gastroenterol 1993; 88(4):583–586.

73. Eisner, 1993; Scully RE, Mark EJ, Mcneely WF, et al. Case Records of the MGH. N Engl J Med 1994; 330:196–201.

74. Calder CJ, Lacy D, Raafat F, et al. Crohn's disease with pulmonary involvement in a 3 year old boy. Gut 1993; 34:1636–1638.

75. Lam A, Borda IT, Inwood MJ, Thompson S. Coagulation studies in ulcerative colitis and Crohn's disease. Gastroenterology 1975; 68:245–251.

76. Lloyd-Still JD, Tomasi L. Neurovascular and thromboembolic complications of inflammatory bowel disease in childhood. J Pediatr Gastroenterol Nutr 1989; 9:461–466.

77. Kirschner BS. Crohn's disease in children and adolescents. In: Bayless TM, ed. Current Management of Inflammatory Bowel Disease. Toronto: BC Decker, 1989:244–247.

78. Grand RJ. Growth in children and adolescents. In: Bayless TM, ed. Current Management of Inflammatory Bowel Disease. Toronto: BC Decker, 1989:237–244.

79. Barton JR, Ferguson A. Failure to record variables of growth and development in children with inflammatory bowel disease. BMJ 1989; 298:865–866.

80. Kirschner BS. Growth and development in chronic inflammatory bowel disease. Acta Pediatr Scand 1990; 366(suppl):98–104.

81. Markowitz JM, Grancher K, Rosa J, et al. Growth failure in pediatric inflammatory bowel disease. J Pediatr Gastroenterol Nutr 1993; 16:373–380.

82. Motil KJ, Grand RJ, Davis-Kraft L, et al. Growth failure in children with inflammatory bowel disease: a prospective study. Gastroenterology 1993; 105:681–691.

83. Kirschner BS, Klich JR, Kalman SS, et al. Reversal of growth retardation in Crohn's disease with therapy emphasizing oral nutritional restitution. Gastroenterology 1981; 80:10–15.

84. Grill BB, Lange R, Markowitz R, et al. Delayed gastric emptying in children with Crohn's disease. J Clin Gastroenterol 1985; 7:216–226.

85. Grybowski JD, Burger J, McCallum R, Lange R. Gastric emptying in childhood inflammatory bowel disease. Am J Gastroenterol 1992; 87:1148–1153.

86. Kelts DG, Grand RJ, Shen G, et al. Nutritional basis of growth failure in children and adolescents with Crohn's disease. Gastroenterology 1979; 76:720–727.

87. Murch SH, Lamkin VA, Savage MO, et al. Serum concentrations of tumor necrosis factor alpha in childhood chronic inflammatory bowel disease. Gut 1991; 32:913–917.

88. Hyams JS, Treem WR, Eddy E, et al. Tumor necrosis factor alpha not elevated in children with inflammatory bowel disease. J Pediatr Gastroenterol Nutr 1991; 12:439–447.

89. Thomas DW, Sinatra FR, Merritt RJ. Fecal alpha-1-antitrypsin excretion in young people with Crohn's disease. J Pediatr Gastroenterol Nutr 1983; 2:491–496.

90. Beeken WL, Bush HJ, Sylvester DL. Intestinal protein loss in Crohn's disease. Gastroenterology 1972; 62:207–215.

91. Kirschner BS, DeFavaro MV, Jenson W. Lactose malabsorption in children and adolescents with inflammatory bowel disease. Gastroenterology 1981; 8:829–832.

92. Motil KJ, Grand RJ. Nutritional management of inflammatory bowel disease. Pediatr Clin North Am 1985; 32:447–469.

93. Driscoll RH Jr, Meredith SC, Sitrin M, et al. Vitamin D deficiency and bone disease in patients wtih Crohn's disease. Gastroenterology; 83:1252–1258.

94. Krawitt EL, Beeken WL, Janney Crohn's disease. Calcium absorption in Crohn's disease. Gastroenterology 1976; 71:251–254.

95. McClain C, Soutor C, Zieve L. Zinc deficiency: a complication of Crohn's disease. Gastroenterology 1980; 78:272–279.

96. Gerlach K, Morowitz DA, Kirsner JB. Symptomatic hypomagnesemia complicating regional enteritis. Gastroenterology 1970; 59:567–574.

97. Beisel WR, Wannemacher RW, Neufeld HA. Relation of fever to energy expenditure.

In: Kinney JM, Leuse E, eds. Assessment of Energy Metabolism in Health and Disease. Columbus, OH: Ross Laboratories, 1980:144.

98. Kelts DG, Grand RJ, Shem G, et al. Nutritional basis of growth failure in children and adolescents with Crohn's disease. Gastroenterology 1979; 76:720–727.

99. Barot LR, Rombeau JL, Steinberg JJ, et al. Energy expenditure in patients with inflammatory bowel disease. Arch Surg 1981; 116:460–462.

100. Kuschner RF, Schoeller DA. Resting and total energy expenditure in patients with inflammatory bowel disease. Am J Clin Nutr 1991; 53:161–165.

101. Kirschner BS, Sutton MM. Somatomedin-C levels in growth impaired children and adolescents with chronic inflammatory bowel disease. Gastroenterology 1986; 91:803–806.

102. Tenore A, Berman WF, Parks JS, Bongiovanni AM. Basal and stimulated growth hormone concentrations in inflammatory bowel disease. J Clin Endocrinol Metab 1977; 44:622–628.

103. Braeger CP, Torresani T, Murch SH, et al. Urinary growth hormone in growth-impaired children with chronic inflammatory bowel disease. J Pediatr Gastroenterol Nutr 1993; 16:49–52.

104. Farthing MJG, Campbell CA, Walker-Smith J, et al. Nocturnal growth hormone and gonadotropin secretion in growth retarded children with Crohn's disease. Gut 1981; 22:933–938.

105. McCaffrey TD Jr, Nasr K, Lawrence AM, Kirsner JB. Severe growth retardation in children with inflammatory bowel disease. Pediatrics 1970; 45:386–393.

106. McCaffrey TD Jr, Nasr K, Lawrence AM, Kirsner JB. Effect of administered human growth hormone on growth retardation in inflammatory bowel disease. Dig Dis 1974; 19:411–416.

107. Friedman M, Strang LB. Effect of long-term corticosteroids and corticotrophin on the growth of children. Lancet 1966; 2:568–572.

108. Berger M, Gribetz D, Korelitz B. Growth retardation in children with ulcerative colitis: the effect of medical and surgical therapy. Pediatrics 1975; 55:459–467.

109. Hyams JS, Moore RE, Leichtner AM, et al. Relationship of type-1 procollagen to corticosteroid therapy in children with inflammatory bowel disease. J Pediatr 1988; 112:893–898.

110. Issenman RM, Atkinson SA, Radoja C, Fraher L. Longitudinal assessment of growth, mineral metabolism, and bone mass in pediatric Crohn's disease. J Pediatr Gastroenterol Nutr 1993; 17:401–406.

111. Whittington PF, Barnes HV, Bayless TM. Medical management of Crohn's disease in adolescence. Gastroenterology 1977; 72:1338–1344.

112. Whybrow PC, Kane FJ, Lipton MA. Regional ileitis and psychiatric disorder. Psychosom Med 1968; 30:209–221.

113. Helzer JE, Chammas S, Norland C, Stillings WA, Alpers DH. A study of the association between Crohn's disease and psychiatric illness. Gastroenterology 19w. 84; 86:324–330.

114. McKegney FP, Gordon RO, Levine SM. A psychosomatic comparison of patients with ulcerative colitis and Crohn's disease. Psychosom Med 1970; 32:153–166.

115. Gerbert B. Psychological aspects of Crohn's disease. J Behav Med 1980; 3:41–58.

116. North CS, Alpers DH, Helzer JE, et ral. Do life events or depression exacerbate inflammatory bowel disease? Ann Intern Med 1991; 114:381–386.

117. Garrett VD, Brantley PJ, Jones GN, McKnight GT. The relation between daily stress and Crohn's disease. J Behav Med 1991; 14:87–96.

118. Burke PM, Meyer V, Kocoshis SA, et al. Depression and anxiety in pediatric inflammatory bowel disease. J Am Acad Child Adolesc Psychiatry 1989; 28:948–951.

119. Raymer D, Weininger O, Hamilton JR. Psychological problems in children with abdominal pain. Lancet 1984; 1(8374):439–440.

120. Burke P, Kocoshis SA, Chandra R, et al. Determinants of depression in recent onset of pediatric inflammatory bowel disease. J Am Acad Child Adolesc Psychiatry 1990; 29:608–610.

121. Wood B, Watkins JB, Boyle JT, et al. Psychological functioning in children with Crohn's disease and ulcerative colitis: implications for models of psychobiological interaction. J Am Acad Child Adolesc Psychiatry 1987; 26:774–781.

122. Steinhausen H, Kies H. Comparative studies of ulcerative colitis and Crohn's disease in children and adolescents. J Child Psychol Psychiatry 1982; 23:33–42.

123. Gilat T, Hacohen D, Lilos P, Langman MJ. Childhood factors in ulcerative colitis and Crohn's disease. An international cooperative study. Scand J Gastroenterol 1987; 22:1009–1024.

124. Kahn E, Markowitz J, Blomquist K, Daum F. The morphologic relationship of sinus and fistula formation to intestinal stenoses in children with Crohn's disease. Am J Gastroenterol 1993; 88:1395–1398.

125. Biller JA, Grand RJ, Harris BH. Abdominal abscesses in adolescents with Crohn's disease. J Pediatr Surg 1987; 22:873–876.

126. Katz S, Shulman N, Levin L. Free perforation in Crohn's disease. A report of 33 cases and review of the literature. Am J Gastroenterol 1986; 81:38–43.

127. Bernstein L. Complications of inflammatory bowel disease. Pract Gastro 1987; 11:35–39.

128. Weedon DD, Shorter RG, Ilstrup DM, et al. Crohn's disease and cancer. N Engl J Med 1973; 289:1099–1103.

129. Persson PG, Karlen P, Bernell O, et al. Crohn's disease and cancer: a population based cohort study. Gastroenterol 1994; 107:1675–1679.

130. Greenstein AJ, Sachar DB, Smith H, et al. A comparison of cancer risk in Crohn's disease and ulcerative colitis. Cancer 1981; 48:2742–2745.

131. Gillen CD, Walmsley RS, Prior P, et al. Ulcerative colitis and Crohn's disease: a comparison of the colorectal cancer risk in extensive colitis. Gut 1994; 35:1590–1592.

132. Sachar DB. Cancer in Crohn's disease: dispelling the myths. Gut 1994; 35:1507–1508.

133. Thomas DW, Sinatra FR. Screening laboratory tests for Crohn's disease. West J Med 1989; 150:163–164.

134. Duerr RH, Targan SR, Landers CJ, et al. Anti-neutrophil cytoplasmic antibodies in ulcerative colitis. Gastroenterology 1991; 100:1590–1596.

135. Winter HS, Landers CJ, Winkelstein A, et al. Anti-neutrophil cytoplasmic antibodies in children with ulcerative colitis. J Pediatr 1994; 125:707–711.

136. Proujansky R, Fawcett PT, Gibney KM, et al. Examination of anti-neutrophil cytoplasmic antibodies in childhood inflammatory bowel disease. J Pediatr Gastroenterol Nutr 1993; 17:193–197.

137. Jabra AA, Fishman EK, Taylor GA. Crohn's disease in the pediatric patient: CT evaluation. Radiology 1991; 179:495–498.

138. Tolia V, Kuhns LR, Chang CH, Slovit TL. Comparison of indium-111 scintigraphy and colonoscopy with histologic study in children for evaluation of colonic chronic inflammatory bowel disease. J Pediatr Gastroenterol Nutr 1991; 12:336–339.

139. Gordon I, Vivian G. Radiolabeled leukocytes: a new diagnostic test in occult infection/inflammation. Arch Dis Child 1984; 59:62–66.

140. Sciarretta G, Furno A, Mazzoni M, et al. Tc-99m hexamethyl propylene amine oxime granulocyte scintigraphy in Crohn's disease: diagnostic and clinical relevance. Gut 1993; 34:1364–1369.

141. Spinelli F, Milella M, Sara R, Banfi F, et al. The 99mTc-HMPAO leukocyte scan: an alternative to radiology and endoscopy in evaluating the extent and activity of inflammatory bowel disease. J Nucl Biol Med 1991; 35:82–87.

142. Charron M, Orenstein SR, Bhargava S. Detection of inflammatory bowel disease in pediatric patients with technetium-99m-HMPAO-labeled leukocytes. J Nucl Med 1994; 35:451–455.

143. Williams CB, Laage NJ, Campbell CA, et al. Total colonoscopy in childhood. Arch Dis Child 1982; 57:49–53.

144. Hassall E, Barclay GN, Ament ME. Colonoscopy in childhood. Pediatrics 1984; 73:594–599.

145. Goodman MJ, Skinner JM, Truelove SC. Abnormalities in apparently normal bowel mucosa in Crohn's disease. Lancet 1976; 1:275–278.

146. Riddell RH. Pathology of idiopathic inflammatory bowel disease. In: Kirsner JB, Shorter RG, eds. Inflammatory Bowel Disease. 4th ed. Baltimore: Williams & Wilkins, 1995:517–552.

147. Chong SKF, Blackshaw AJ, Boyle S, et al. Histologic diagnosis of chronic inflammatory bowel disease in childhood. Gut 1985; 26:55–59.

148. Schmitz-Moormann P, Schag M. Histology of the lower intestinal tract in Crohn's disease of children and adolescents. Pathol Res Pract 1990; 186:479–484.

149. Mashako MNL, Cezard JP, Navarro J, et al. Crohn's disease lesions in the upper gastrointestinal tract: correlation between clinical, radiological, endoscopic, and histological features in adolescents and children. J Pediatr Gastroenterol Nutr 1989; 8:442–446.

150. Rutgeers P, Onette E, Vantrappan G, et al. Crohn's disease of the stomach and duodenum: a clinical study with emphasis on the value of endoscopy and endoscopic biopsies. Endoscopy 1980; 12:288–294.

151. Mallett P, Murch S. Anorexia nervosa complicating inflammatory bowel disease. Arch Dis Child 1990; 65:298–300.

152. San Joaquin VH. *Aeromonas, Yersinia,* and miscellaneous bacterial enteropathogens. Pediatr Ann 1994; 23:544–548.

153. Afghani B, Stutman HR. Toxin-related diarrheas. Pediatr Ann 1994; 23:549–555.

154. Neill MA, Tarr PI, Clausen CR, et al. *Escherichia coli* 0157:H7 as a predominant pathogen associated with the hemolytic uremic syndrome: a prospective study of the Pacific Northwest. Pediatrics 1987; 80:37–40.

155. Glasier CM, Siegel MJ, McAlister WH, Shackelford GD. Henoch-Schönlein syndrome in children: gastrointestinal manifestations. AJR Am J Roentgenol 1981; 136:1081–1085.

156. Powell KP. Approach to gastrointestinal manifestations in infants and children with HIV infection. J Pediatr 1991; 119:S34–40.

157. Kenney RT. Parasitic causes of diarrhea. Pediatr Ann 1994; 23:414–422.

158. Everhart JE, Renault PF. Irritable bowel syndrome in office based practice in the US. Gastroenterology 1991; 100:998–1015.

159. Rutheford RB, Akers DR. Meckel's diverticulum: a review of 148 patients. Surgery 1966; 59:818–826.

160. Apley J, Naish N. Recurrent abdominal pains: a field survey of 1,000 school children. Arch Dis Child 1958; 33:165–170.

161. Yang SS, Gibson P, McCaughey RS, et al. Primary Crohn's disease of the appendix: a report of 14 cases and review of the literature. Ann Surg 1979; 189:334–339.

162. Euler AR, Ament ME. Celiac sprue and Crohn's disease: an association causing severe growth retardation. Gastroenterology 1977; 72(4 Pt 1):729–731.

163. Lloyd-Still JD. Crohn's disease and cystic fobrosis. Dig Dis Sci 1994; 39:880–885.

164. Holmquist L, Ahren C, Fallstrom SP. Relationship between results of laboratory tests and inflammatory activity assessed by colonoscopy in children and adolescents wtih ulcerative colitis and Crohn's colitis. J Pediatr Gastroenterol Nutr 1989; 9:187–193.

165. Lloyd-Still JD, Green OC. A clinical scoring system for chronic inflammatory bowel disease in children. Dig Dis Sci 1979; 24:620–624.

166. Summers RW, Switz DM, Sessions JT, et al. National Cooperative Crohn's Disease Study: results of drug treatment. Gastroenterology 1979; 77:847–869.

167. Malchow H, Ewe K, Brandes JW, et al. European Cooperative Crohn's Disease Study: results of drug treatment. Gastroenterology 1984; 86:249–266.

168. Smith RC, Rhodes J, Heatley RV, et al. Low dose steroids and clinical relapse in Crohn's disease: a controlled trial. Gut 1978; 19:606–610.

169. Van Hees PAM, Van Lier HJJ, et al. Effect of sulfasalazine in patients with active Crohn's disease: a controlled double-blind study. Gut 1981; 22:404–409.

170. Wenckert A, Kristensen M, et al. The long-term prophylactic effect of salazosulphapyridine in primarily resected patients with Crohn's disease. Scand J Gastroenterol 1978; 13:161–167.

171. Peppercorn M. Advances in drug therapy for inflammatory bowel disease. Ann Intern Med 1990; 112:50–60.

172. Prantera C, Pallone F, Brunetti G, et al. Oral 5-aminosalicylic acid (Asacol) in the maintenance treatment of Crohn's disease. Gastroenterology 1992; 103:363–368.

173. Griffiths A, Koletzko S, Sylvester F, et al. Slow-release 5-aminosalicylic acid therapy in children with small intestinal Crohn's disease. J Pediatr Gastroenterol Nutr 1993; 17:186–192.

174. Sutherland I, Singleton J, Sessions J, et al. Double-blind, placebo-controlled trial of metronidazole in Crohn's disease. Gut 1991; 32:1071–1075.

175. Ursing B, Alm T, Barany F, et al. A comparative study of metronidazole and sulfasalazine for active Crohn's disease: the Cooperative Crohn's Disease Study in Sweden. II. Result. Gastroenterology 1982; 83:550–562.

176. Hildenbrand H, Berg NO, Hoevels J, Ursing B. Treatment of Crohn's disease with metronidazole in childhood and adolescence. Gastroenterol Clin Biol 1980; 21:19–25.

177. Brandt LJ, Bernstein LH, Boley SJ, Frank MS. Metronidazole therapy for perianal Crohn's disease: a follow-up study. Gastroenterology 1982; 83:383–387.

178. Peppercorn MA. Is there a role for antibiotics as primary therapy of Crohn's ileitis? J Clin Gastroenterol 1993; 17:235–237.

179. Duffy LF, Daum F, Fisher SE, et al. Peripheral neuropathy in Crohn's disease patients treated with metronidazole. Gastroenterology 1985; 88:681–684.

180. Verhave M, Winter HS, Grand RJ. Azathioprine in the treatment of children wtih inflammatory bowel disease. J Pediatr 1990; 117:809–814.

181. Markowtiz J, Rosa J, Grancher K, et al. Long-term 6-mercaptopurine treatment in adolescents with Crohn's disease. Gastroenterology 1990; 99:1347–1351.

182. Korelitz BI, Adler DJ, Mendelsohn RA, Sacknoff AL. Long-term experience with 6-mercaptopurine in the treatment of Crohn's disease. Am J Gastroenterol 1992; 88:1198–1205.

183. Colonna T, Korelitz BI. The role of leukopenia in the 6-mercaptopurine–induced remission of refractory Crohn's disease. Am J Gastroenterol 1994; 89:362–366.

184. Korelitz BI. Immunosuppressive therapy. In: Bayless TM, ed. Current Management of Inflammatory Bowel Disease. Toronto: BC Decker, 1989:252–257.

185. Present DH, Meltzer SJ, Krumholz MP, et al. 6-Mercaptopurine in the management of inflammatory bowel disease: short-and long-term toxicity. Ann Intern Med 1989; 111:641–649.

186. Benkov KJ, Rosh JR, Schwersenz AH, et al. Cyclosporine as an alternative to surgery in children with inflammatory bowel disease. J Pediatr Gastroenterol Nutr 1994; 19:290–294.

187. Kirschner BS, Whitington PF, Malfeo-Klein R. Experience with cyclosporine A in severe non-specific ulcerative colitis (abstr). Pediatr Res 1989; 25:117A.

188. LaTulippe Naccarini DA, Minor ML. Cyclosporine and 6-mercaptopurine in pediatric inflammatory bowel disease. Gastro Nursing 1994; 16:169–175.

189. Dannecker G, Malchow H, Hiessen KH, Ranke MB. Crohn's disease: initial experience with CSA in an adolescent girl. Deutsche Mediz Wochen 1985; 110:339–343.

190. Sandborn WJ, Goldman DH, Lawson GM, Perrault J. Measurement of colonic tissue cyclosporine concentration in children with severe ulcerative colitis. J Pediatr Gastroenterol Nutr 1992; 15:125–129.

191. Treem WR, Davis PM, Hyams JS. Cyclosporine treatment of severe ulcerative colitis in children. J Pediatr 1991; 119:994–997.

192. Brynskov J, Freund L, Rasmussen SN, et al. A placebo-controlled, double-blind, randomized trial of cyclosporine therapy in active chronic Crohn's disease. N Engl J Med 1989; 321:845–850.

193. Lichtiger S, Present DH, Kornbluth A, et al. Cyclosporine in severe ulcerative colitis refractory to steroid therapy. N Engl J Med 1994; 330:1841–1845.

194. Ramakrishna J, Langhans N, Calenda K, et al. Combined use of cyclosporine A and azathioprine in pediatric inflammatory bowel disease. Gastroenterology 1994; 106:A23.

195. Layden T, Rosenberg J, Nemchansky B, et al. Reversal of growth arrest in adolescents with Crohn's disease after parenteral alimentation. Gastroenterology 1976; 70:1017–1021.

196. Strobel CT, Byrne WJ, Ament ME. Home parenteral nutrition in children with Crohn's disease: an effective management alternative. Gastroenterology 1979; 77:272–279.

197. Aiges H, Markowitz J, Rosa J, Daum F. Home nocturnal supplemental nasogastric feedings in growth-retarded adolescents with Crohn's disease. Gastroenterology 1989; 97:904–910.

198. Saverymuttu S, Hodgson HJF, Chadwick VS. Controlled trial comparing prednisolone with an elemental diet plus non-absorbable antibiotics in active Crohn's disease. Gut 1985; 26:994–998.

199. Gorad DA, Hunt JB, Payne-James JJ, et al. Initial response and subsequent course of Crohn's disease treated with elemental diet or prednisolone. Gut 1993; 34:1198–1202.

200. Seidman EG, Bouthillier L, Weber AM, et al. Elemental diet versus prednisone as primary treatment of Crohn's disease. Gastroenterology 1986; 90:1625A.

201. Sanderson IR, Udeen S, Davies PSW, et al. Remission induced by an elemental diet in small bowel Crohn's disease. Arch Dis Child 1987; 61:123–127.

202. Lochs H, Steinhardt HJ, Klaus-Wentz B, et al. Comparison of enteral nutrition and drug treatment in active Crohn's disease. Gastroenterology 1991; 101:881–888.

203. Teahon K, Bjarnason I, Pearson M, Levi AJ. Ten years' experience with an elemental diet in the management of Crohn's disease. Gut 1990; 31:1133–1137.

204. Sabbah SJ, Seidman EG. Dietary management of Crohn's disease in children and adolescents. In: Bayless TM, ed. Current Management of Inflammatory Bowel Disease. Toronto: BC Decker, 1989:230–236.

205. Belli DC, Sediman E, Bouthillier L, et al. Chronic intermittent elemental diet improves growth failure in children with Crohn's disease. Gastroenterology 1988; 94:603–610.

206. Polk DB, Hattner JA, Kerner JA. Improved growth and disease activity after intermittent administration of a defined formula diet in children with Crohn's disease. J Pediatr Gastroenterol Nutr 1992; 16:499–504.

207. O'Brien CJ, Giaffer MH, Cann PA, et al. Elemental diet in steroid-dependent and steroid-refractory Crohn's disease. Am J Gastroenterol 1991; 86:1614–1618.

208. Giaffer MH, North G, Holdsworth Crohn's disease. Controlled trial of polymeric versus elemental diet in the treatment of active Crohn's disease. Lancet 1990; 335:816–819.

209. Muller JM, Keller HW, Erasmi H, Pichmaier H. Total parenteral nutrition as the sole therapy in Crohn's disease. Br J Surg 1983; 70:40–43.

210. McIntyre PB, Powell-Tuck J, Wood SR, et al. Controlled trial of bowel rest in the treatment of severe acute colitis. Gut 1986; 27:481–485.

211. Greenberg GR, Fleming CR, Jeejeebhoy KN et al. Controlled trial of bowel rest and nutritional support in the management of Crohn's disease. Gut 1988; 29:1309–1315.

212. Sanderson JR, Boulton P, Menzies I, Walker-Smith JA. Improvement of abnormal lactulise/rhamnose permeability in active Crohn's disease of the small bowel by an elemental diet. Gut 1987; 28:1073–1076.

213. Teahon K, Smethurst P, Pearson M, et al. The effect of elemental diet on intestinal permeability and inflammation in Crohn's disease. Gastroenterology 1991; 101:84–89.

214. Shorter RG, Huizenga KA, Spencer RJ. A working hypothesis for the etiology and pathogenesis of non-specific inflammatory bowel disease. Am J Dig Dis 1972; 17:1024–1030.

215. Crowther JS, Drasar BS, Goddard P, et al. The effect of a chemically defined diet on the faecal flora and faecal steroid concentration. Gut 1973; 14:790–793.

216. Puntis J, McNeish AS, Allan RN. Long term prognosis of Crohn's disease with onset of childhood and adolescence. Gut 1984; 35:329–336.

217. Telander RL. Crohn's disease. In: Welch KJ, Randolph JG, Ravitch MM, et al, eds. Pediatric Surgery. Ed 4. Chicago: Year Book, 1986:958–968.

218. Pritchard TJ, Scoetz DJ, Filler PC, et al. Strictureplasty of the small bowel in patients with Crohn's disease: an effective surgical option. Arch Surg 1990; 125:715–717.

219. Oliva L, Wylie R, Alexander F, et al. The results of strictureplasty in pediatric patients with multifocal Crohn's disease. J Pediatr Gastroenterol Nutr 1994; 18:306–310.

220. Palder SB, Shandling B, Bilik R. Perianal complications of pediatric Crohn's disease. J Pediatr Surg 1991; 26:513–515.

221. Orking BA, Telander RL. The effect of intraabdominal resection or fecal diversion on perianal disease in pediatric Crohn's disease. J Pediatr Surg 1985; 20:343–347.

222. Statter MB, Hirschl RB, Coran AC. Inflammatory bowel disease. Pediatr Clin North Am 1993; 40:1213–1231.

223. Davies G, Evans CM, Whand WS, Walker-Smith JA. Surgery for Crohn's disease in childhood: influence of site of disease and operative procedure on outcome. Br J Surg 1990; 77:891–894.

224. Coran AC, Klein MD, Sarahan TM. The surgical management of terminal ileal and right colon Crohn's disease in children. J Pediatr Surg. 1983; 18:592–594.

225. Hyams JS, Grand RJ, Colodny AH, et al. Course and prognosis after colectomy and ileostomy for inflammatory bowel disease in childhood and adolescence. J Pediatr Surg 1982; 17:400–405.

226. Griffiths AM, Wesson DE, Shandling B, et al. Factors influencing postoperative recurrence of Crohn's disease in childhood. Gut 1991; 32:491–495.

227. Castille RG, Telander RL, Cooney DR, et al. Crohn's disease in children: assessment of the progression of disease, growth, and prognosis. J Pediatr Surg 1980; 15:462–469.

228. Frey CF. Colectomy in children with ulcerative and granulomatous colitis. Arch Surg 1972; 104:416–423.

229. Vionchet O, Kirsner JB, Rosenberg IH. Growth retardation in inflammatory bowel disease: the impact of surgery on subsequent growth and development (abstr). Gastroenterology 1973; 64:816.

230. Guttman FJ. Granulomatous enterocolitis in childhood and adolescence. J Pediatr Surg 1974; 9:115–121.

231. Homer DR, Grand RJ, Colodny AH. Growth, course, and prognosis after surgery for Crohn's disease in children and adolescents. Pediatrics 1977; 59:717–725.

232. Lipson AB, Savage MO, Davies PS, et al. Acceleration of linear growth following intestinal resection for Crohn's disease. Eur J Pediatr 1990; 149:687–690.

233. Sorenson VZ, Olsen BG, Binder V. Life prospects and quality of life in patients with Crohn's disease. Gut 1987; 28:382–385.

COMMENTARY

Fredric Daum   *North Shore University Hospital–Cornell University Medical College, Manhasset, and New York University–Bellevue Hospital, New York, New York*

The chapter on Crohn's disease in childhood and adolescence by Barth and Grand reflects a significant effort to summarize what is presently known about pediatric Crohn's disease. The authors have also included 233 references to provide data.

I. EPIDEMIOLOGY

Although the literature suggests that the first peak incidence of Crohn's disease occurs in adolescents between 16 and 20 years of age, Crohn's disease is also an illness of younger children. The experience at North Shore University Hospital-Cornell University Medical College indicates that 40% to 50% of the children with Crohn's disease at the time of presentation are 12 years of age or younger.

II. CLINICAL FEATURES

A. Extraintestinal

In an excellent review by Hyams (Hyams JS. Pediatr Gastroenterol Nutr 1994; 7–21), the author provides an extensive review of complications involving virtually every organ system of the body. In the adult population, it is estimated that at least one extraintestinal manifestation is seen in approximately 25% to 35% of patients with inflammatory bowel disease. It is clear that Crohn's disease is a systemic disease, not just an intestinal illness.

B. Undernutrition and Growth Failure

The pathogenesis of growth failure in children with Crohn's disease is usually attributed to malnutrition, corticosteroid therapy, and uncontrolled inflammation or disease activity. Significant malabsorption of fat with loss of calories and associated growth failure is uncommon in children, even in the patient who has undergone an ileal resection. On occasion, bile salts may stimulate diarrhea in the patient who has not only had an ileal resection but also is experiencing extensive disease proximal to an ileal–colonic anastomosis. In such patients, cholestyramine an anion-exchange resin may be helpful in alleviating these symptoms.

Steroid therapy may interfere with linear bone growth in the face of adequate dietary intake (Hyams J, Carey DE. J Pediatr 1988; 113:249–254). Prednisone taken daily for only 7 to 10 days in commonly prescribed dosages (0.3–1.0 mg/kg per day) had been shown to impair serum procollagen levels, a biochemical marker of linear bone growth (Ref. 109).

There are also data that suggest that increased cytokine production may suppress linear bone growth. Rats with colitis induced by TNBS enemas exhibit decreased tibial bone growth unrelated to nutritional deficiencies (Chawla A, Koniaris S, Katz R, Fisher SE. Pediatr Res 1993; 33(4):99A). This observation may explain why even well-nourished children with Crohn's disease often do not experience adequate linear bone growth.

III. GASTROINTESTINAL COMPLICATIONS

The potential for malignancy of the small intestine and/or colon in children with Crohn's disease is unclear. Recent data (Markowitz J, McKinley M, Kahn E, Stiel L, Rosa J, Grancher BS, Daum F. Am J Gastroenterol 1994; 89:1694) indicate that flow cytometry from biopsy specimens obtained from the colon in adolescents or young adults with Crohn's disease of more than 10 years duration may reveal abnormalities consistent with premalignant change. This study is being undertaken at North Shore University Hospital-Cornell University Medical College because of the recent deaths of two patients younger than 25 years of age, one with Crohn's disease and the other with ulcerative colitis. The young adult with Crohn's disease at the time of surgery had an undifferentiated adenocarcinoma within a stricture in the transverse colon and eventually died of metastatic disease. Because colectomy in Crohn's disease is not curative, it is seldom recommended prophylactically, no matter what the duration of disease. Colectomy in long-standing Crohn's colitis in the presence of a colonic stricture may be warranted.

IV. DIAGNOSIS

Upper gastrointestinal series with small bowel follow-through (UGI/SBFT) still remains the only feasible method by which jejunal, proximal, and midileal Crohn's disease can be diagnosed. Esophageal, gastric, and proximal duodenal Crohn's disease is best evaluated by upper endoscopy and biopsies. Enteroclysis may be useful, especially when partial small bowel obstruction is suspected and the site of stenosis is not well delineated by an UGI/SBFT. An air contrast barium enema may reveal early Crohn's disease of the colon, but colonscopy with biopsies remains the approach of choice for most pediatric gastroenterologists. A computed tomography (CT) scan with contrast may be the best diagnostic study when either the small bowel or colon is evaluated for a fistula. A CT scan may also allow the differentiation of an abscess from thickened loops of bowel secondary to inflammation.

Indications for upper gastrointestinal endoscopy include symptoms of upper gastrointestinal disease such as epigastric pain and heartburn, among others. In the child with growth failure and early satiety for solids, an upper gastrointestinal endoscopy may reveal significant inflammation of the stomach and duodenum when the upper gastrointestinal series has failed to demonstrate such condition. Biopsies of the antrum to determine the presence of *Helicobacter pylori* should also be done at the same time. Determining the presence and extent of upper gastrointestinal disease often affects the choice of medical therapy and perhaps influences the route for nutritional supplementation.

V. DIFFERENTIAL DIAGNOSIS

In differentiating functional chronic abdominal pain from that of Crohn's disease, several factors should be taken into consideration. Functional pain tends to be periumbilical or to migrate in association with shifts of intraluminal gas. Functional pain also tends to be relieved by the passage of gas or stool. Finally, functional pain rarely awakens the patient unless the patient reacts with intolerance to a carbohydrate load within a few hours of going to sleep.

Although Crohn's disease may be isolated to the appendix and present with right lower quadrant pain, acute suppurative appendicitis is uncommon in Crohn's diseae (Kahn E, Markowtiz J, Daum F. Mod Pathol 1992; 5:380–382).

VI. THERAPY

While the goal of some clinicians is to suppress inflammation completely, most pediatric gastroenterologists use medications primarily to alleviate symptoms, paying less attention to specific laboratory data, colonoscopic appearance, and histologic data. This approach reflects an attempt to improve the patient's quality of life without causing significant drug toxicity.

A. Medical

1. Steroids

Steroids not only can be used orally or parenterally but are also often effective when given rectally to treat left-sided Crohn's colitis. Cortisone can be given in a foam preparation or in an enema solution. There are no data as to what extent these medications spread proximally from the anus based on body size. It may well be that, in smaller children, steroid given in this fashion reaches the transverse colon or even the right colon. In children with Crohn's disease primarily involving the left colon, the intrarectal steroid preparation may also be tapered over a period of time. Whether the relapse rate is diminished by maintaining the patient on an intrarectal preparation once or twice each week (as has been suggested with the use of 5-ASA enemas in patients with left-sided ulcerative colitis) is not yet known.

The side effects of steroids that tend to be of greatest concern in the pediatric population are adverse cosmetic changes and suppression of linear bone growth. Compliance may be a problem, and, in the adolescent who does not become cushingoid on an appropriate dose of steroid, noncompliance should be suspected. Avascular necrosis is extremely uncommon in the pediatric population. Although psychological effects of steroids are thought to be common in children, there are no data to suggest the frequency of these psychological complications or their specific nature in children who often receive less corticosteroid per body weight than their adult counterparts.

2. Sulfasalazine and 5-Aminosalicylates

Although there are no data to suggest whether sulfasalazine is effective in the treatment of pediatric Crohn's diseae and, if so, in what dosage, the dosage prescribed is usually similar to that in ulcerative colitis. Except for possible sulfa allergy, which is idiosyncratic, other side effects noted by Barth and Grand tend to be unusual with this dosage.

The use of Pentasa for upper gastrointestinal Crohn's disease has not yet been evaluated in children. A question that remains unresolved is whether delaying gastric and proximal small bowel motility might result in the release of Pentasa in the stomach and proximal small bowel for the treatment of gastric and duodenal Crohn's disease. The number of Pentasa tablets required for a therapeutic effect in adults with Crohn's disease may preclude its use in children and adolescents. It is doubtful that Dipentum is effective in acute Crohn's colitis, and there are no data as to whether Dipentum should be used for maintenance therapy. There are no data to indicate that 5-ASA enemas are effective in Crohn's colitis.

3. Antibiotics

Although metronidazole may be the antibiotic of choice for the treatment of bacterial overgrowth, its potential disulfiram effect may limit its use in adolescents who drink alcohol. In this situation, a variety of broad-spectrum antibiotics such as amoxicillin and tetracycline (in children older than age 7 years) can be used. Long-term treatment with metronidazole warrants that a history be taken regarding symptoms of peripheral neuropathy and that a sensory examination be done periodically. To limit its use to less than 6 months may not be in the patient's best interest.

4. Immunosuppressives

The starting dosages of azathioprine (AZA) and 6-mercaptopurine (6-MP) are arbitrary. Most commonly, the dosages prescribed modulate the immune system but do not suppress it. A dosage of 2 mg/kg per day of AZA or 1.25 to 1.5 mg/kg per day of 6-MP is commonly prescribed for children. However, if after using these dosages for 3 to 4 months, there is little improvement, higher dosages should be used until leukopenia is observed. Even in patients who do not respond within 3 to 4 months, if the immunomodulator is continued for another 6 to 8 months, another 30% of patients experience a steroid-sparing effect (Ref. 181).

B. Nutritional

Not only have there been studies to suggest that elemental diet may be as effective as steroid therapy in the treatment of acute Crohn's disease but a recent study has also demonstrated similar efficacy with an exclusive whole protein enteral diet compared with prednisolone treatment (Ruuska T, Savilahti E, Maki M, Ormala T, Visakorpi JK. J Pediatr Gastroenterol Nutr 1994; 19:175–180).

Enteral supplementation can be given orally, via nasogastric tube, or, on occasion, through a gastrostomy tube. If a percutaneous gastrostomy is contemplated, the patient should undergo endoscopy and biopsy specimens should be obtained from the fundus and antrum of the stomach. If there is evidence of gastric inflammation, a gastrostomy tube should not be placed to avoid a possible gastric cutaneous fistula.

C. Surgical

Surgical resection of the colon in patients with intractable colonic symptoms or dependency on growth-suppressive doses of steroids may substantially improve a child's quality of life, despite the concern for disease recurrence in the small bowel. My experience indicates that such patients rarely undergo significant small bowel disease recurrence, and, when recurrence occurs, symptoms can usually be treated with medical therapy. Quality of life in these patients is markedly improved with patients able to continue their education, seek employment, and establish independent lives.

19
Crohn's Disease in the Elderly

Geetanjali A. Akerkar and Mark A. Peppercorn *Beth Israel Hospital and Harvard Medical School, Boston, Massachusetts*

Although Crohn's disease was described initially in young adults, it has become increasingly apparent that Crohn's disease may affect the elderly, with the new onset of disease occurring well into the seventh and eighth decades of life. Early reports of Crohn's disease in the elderly suggested that it was a distinct entity with a severe course and a bad outcome. More recent studies have tended to blur any differences between the young and old with this disorder. This chapter emphasizes the differences that do exist as it reviews the epidemiology, clinical presentation, differential diagnosis, treatment options, and outcome of the older patient with Crohn's disease.

I. EPIDEMIOLOGY

The reported proportion of elderly patients with Crohn's disease has varied over time. In 1958, Crohn and Yarnis reported that 4.3% of their 530 patients had the onset of illness after age 50 years (1). Whereas, Smith et al. described the incidence of Crohn's disease in the elderly populaiton in Clydesdale, United Kingdom, to be as high as 31% (2). Subsequent studies have shown much lower rates. Shapiro et al. reported an incidence of 5% after age 60 years, and Fabricus et al. reviewed cases of 600 Crohn's disease patients over a period of 40 years and found that 8% of these patients were diagnosed at an age older than 60 years (3,4). In 1988, Rose et al. showed an increasing incidence in patients older than age 50 years in Wales from .18/10^5 cases in the 1930s to 8.3/10^5 cases in 1988, with a peak age-specific incidence in the eighth decade of life (5). Although this study was population based and reports an age-specific incidence rate, most studies have been retrospective analyses of patients seen at large referral centers and may not truly give an accurate incidence of Crohn's disease in the elderly population.

Many older studies further complicate the statistics by failing to make a crucial distinction in patient selection; they include patients whose disease began well before and well after 50 years of age (6). The importance of this distinction was shown in 1980. Rusch and Simonowitz reviewed 141 patients with Crohn's disease and separated the patients into three groups (7). Group A had 126 patients younger than age 50 years, Group B had nine patients aged 50 to 65 years diagnosed before age 49 years, and Group C had six patients aged 50 to 60 years diagnosed after age 49 years. They found that patients older than 50 years but diagnosed before age 49 years behaved much like younger patients, whereas patients both diagnosed when they were older than age 50 years had a short duration of symptoms and a severe course. More recent papers refer to diagnosis of Crohn's disease at a specific age (3,4,8–13).

Although it is no longer disputed that Crohn's disease may have its onset in the elderly, it remains less clear whether there is a bimodal incidence with a peak age of onset in the third decade and a second peak in later life, in the seventh or eighth decade (5,8,14,15). The data from Rose et al. argue strongly for a biomodal distribution and a new onset of disease in patients older than age 50 years (5). It is unclear whether the second peak represents a different disease or the same disease influenced and changed by age-related factors. For example, elderly patients tend to differ from their younger counterparts in the major sites of disease involvement. This observation may support the theory that Crohn's disease is altered by ischemic disease. However, the distribution differences may also support the concept of a different disease.

With regard to sex differences, most studies show a female predominance of Crohn's disease in the elderly (3,6,8,9,14,16). Several recent studies, however, document either no sex predominance or a male predominance (4,7,10,11).

II. CLINICAL PRESENTATION AND EVALUATION

The clinical features of elderly Crohn's disease patients differ little from their younger counterparts (3,10,12). Patients typically report diarrhea, weight loss, abdominal pain, change in bowel habits, and rectal bleeding. Many studies show that older patients have a gradual onset of disease (4,16). Surprisingly, a significant number of elderly patients with ileal involvement were noted to present acutely. Fabricus et al. reviewed the course of Crohn's disease in 47 patients and found that, of 22 patients with small bowel disease, 14 presented acutely with peritonitis and obstructive symptoms; in contrast, only one of 22 patients with large bowel disease presented acutely (4). Similarly, another study reported six of 33 patients with ileitis or ileocolitis presented acutely with a small bowel obstruction (3).

With regard to the distribution of disease, an early study reported that Crohn's disease in the elderly tends to more frequently involve the colon, especially in women (17). A decade later, other investigators observed that, in a mixed population, the incidence of large bowel involvement was 16%. When patients older than age 50 years were isolated in that same group of individuals, the incidence of large bowel disease increased to 40%. Women outnumbered men by 8 to 1 (2). More recent series also report that, in older patients, Crohn's disease has a propensity to affect the large bowel (10,11,13,14,18). In contrast, there have been a few reports of ileal disease predominance in the elderly Crohn's disease patient (3,12,16).

In 1985, Fabricus et al. compared the site of involvement between young and old patients and noted that distal colonic disease was most common in the older group of patients, whereas extensive colonic disease was noted in younger patients (4). Distal colonic disease was noted in 40% of patients older than age 60 years as opposed to only 6% of patients younger than 60 years. Twenty-seven percent of patients younger than 60 years demonstrated extensive colonic involvement as opposed to 4% in the older group (4). Thus, it can be concluded that elderly Crohn's patients are more likely to have distal colonic involvement.

Esophageal, gastroduodenal, and proximal small bowel involvement with Crohn's disease have been described in previous studies, but no age-specific incidence has been reported. One report reviewed 47 patients who were 60 years of age or older at diagnosis. Three patients were noted to have disease in the stomach, jejunum, and midileum (4).

The evaluation of the elderly patient with Crohn's disease includes obtaining routine laboratory tests. Common findings include anemia, leukocytosis, hypoalbuminemia, and an elevated sedimentation rate. In addition, one study reported that patients diagnosed when they were older than age 50 years were more likely to be anemic, to be hypoalbuminemic, and to have liver abnormalities when compared with younger patients (7). As with younger patients, the diagnosis of Crohn's colitis in the older patient usually rests on historical features coupled with findings on endoscopy or barium enema. These findings include aphthous ulcerations, cobblestoned mucosa, skip lesions, and asymmetric involvement of the bowel, findings similar to those in younger patients. Biopsies showing granulomas may be highly suggestive of the diagnosis if certain infections and foreign bodies are excluded. However, granulomas are present in only approximately 30% of patients. For patients with small bowel disease, an x-ray film of the small intestine is usually required to make the diagnosis. There does not appear to be any difference in the radiological characteristics between younger and older Crohn's disease patients (11).

III. DIFFERENTIAL DIAGNOSIS

Elderly patients with Crohn's disease can be difficult to diagnose on presentation. They present with nonspecific symptoms and often are misdiagnosed because of the higher incidence of other gastrointestinal disorders in this age group. Feczko et al. examined the clinical and radiological findings of 99 patients older than 50 years with the diagnosis of Crohn's disease (11). They observed that the presenting symptoms and radiographic appearance in older patients may be mimicked by infectious colitis, ischemic bowel disease, and diverticulitis (11).

Infectious colitis occurs commonly in the elderly. Well-known etiologic agents include *Salmonella*, *Shigella*, and *Campylobacter*. *Yersinia* and *Vibrio* species are infrequent agents. In the elderly, special attention needs to be paid to *Clostridium difficile* colitis and to *Escherichia coli* serotype 0157:H7, both of which may cause significant morbidity (6).

Ischemic colitis is predominantly a disorder of the elderly and may coexist with Crohn's disease. Although patients with ischemic colitis usually have an abrupt onset of symptoms, the course of ischemic bowel disease in some patients may be indolent, making its differentiation from Crohn's disease difficult (6).

Because diverticulitis involves the colon segmentally and presents with evidence of localized peritonitis and obstruction, its distinction from Crohn's colitis may be problematic. Similarly, carcinoma of the colon, especially left-sided cancers that tend to obstruct and may perforate, have to be distinguished from Crohn's colitis in a similar fashion.

Drug-associated colitis, especially that related to the use of nonsteroidal anti-inflammatory agents, radiation bowel disease, and segmental colitis associated with diverticula are additional entities occurring in the elderly that need to be distinguished from Crohn's disease (19,20).

Evaluation of the elderly patient who may have Crohn's disease should include a detailed history (including recent antibiotic and other drug use, radiation exposure), stool cultures for bacterial pathogens, stool examination for *C. difficile* toxin, radiographic evaluation with special consideration given to computed tomography (CT) scanning to help exclude diverticulitis, and endoscopic examination with biopsies.

IV. COMPLICATIONS

A. Intestinal

In 1976, Truelove and Peña described several local intestinal complications in Crohn's disease patients of all ages, including acute dilation of the colon, fistulas, anal fissures, abscesses, obstruction, hemorrhage, and carcinoma of the colon (21). Systemic complications were listed as analgesic nephropathy, perforated duodenal ulcer, and nephrotic syndrome (21). A later study observed that 58% of elderly patients with Crohn's disease required surgery because of one of these complications (3). Similarly, Carr and Schofield noted that elderly patients with large bowel disease frequently suffered hemorrhage and colonic perforation (9).

Tchirkow et al. found that elderly patients were vulnerable to complications of comorbid conditions, including congestive heart failure, wound infections, and post-operative seizures (16). In particular, elderly patients who presented with severe diarrhea and malnutrition had a high risk of complications and death from surgery (16). The overall prognosis and complication risk are influenced by the site and extent of disease. In a series with a 13-year follow-up, Farmer et al. examined 592 patients of all ages with Crohn's disease and reported site specific complications; obstruction was noted in small bowel disease, fistula and abscess were observed in ileocolic disease, and megacolon was reported in large bowel disease (22). The most frequent complication was perianal disease, with fistula found in 35% of patients.

B. Extraintestinal

The incidence of extraintestinal manifestations in Crohn's disease patients of all ages has been reported to be 1.4% (2). A study in 1981 reviewed 33 patients diagnosed with Crohn's disease after age 60 years and noted that one patient with colitis presented with pyoderma gangrenosum and one patient with ileitis had erythema nodosum (3). Carr and Schofield examined 64 elderly patients and reported that one patient with left-sided Crohn's colitis had erythema nodosum (9). Similarly, another study observed that three of 15 patients with colorectal Crohn's disease demonstrated extraintestinal manifestations (pyoderma gangrenosum in two and arthritis in one). No extraintestinal manifestations were noted in 10 patients with small bowel disease (16). Given the small size of these studies, it is difficult to determine the rate of extraintestinal manifestations in the older patient with Crohn's disease.

C. Colorectal Cancer

Carcinoma of the colon is one of the most dreaded complications of inflammatory bowel disease. Patients with extensive ulcerative colitis begin to have an increased risk of colon cancer 7 to 8 years after the onset of disease activity. The risk in ulcerative colitis probably increases by 0.5% per year. Recently, it has been suggested that older patients wtih ulcerative colitis may be at even greater risk because of their advanced age (23).

The awareness of the risk of colon cancer in Crohn's disease has lagged that in ulcerative colitis, and the reported incidence has varied greatly. In 1985, Binder et al. described only one case of colon cancer in 185 Crohn's disease patients, corresponding to an annual risk of 0.06% and a cumulative risk after 10 years of .56% (24). In the same year, another report suggested that carcinomas in Crohn's disease are found primarily in bypassed loops of small bowel (22).

Other studies have suggested a higher incidence of colorectal cancer in Crohn's disease, although not at the higher frequency described in most studies of ulcerative colitis (25). Furthermore, in a large retrospective cohort study examining the occurence of colorectal cancer in 1655 patients with Crohn's disease, 12 colorectal cancers were diagnosed, yielding an increased overall risk of 2.5. Patients in whom Crohn's disease was diangosed before age 30 years and who had any colonic disease at diagnosis entailed a higher relative risk, 20.9 compared with 2.2 in those diagnosed after age 30 years (26). The issue of increased risk of colorectal cancer in Crohn's disease may have come full circle with the recent report that, given the same disease extent and duration, there may be no differences in colon cancer between patients with ulcerative colitis and Crohn's disease (27).

Finally, there have been several large retrospective studies that have examined the risk of extracolonic malignancy in Crohn's disease. Ekbom et al. observed an increase in squamous skin cancers in Crohn's disease patients (28). Similarly, Greenstein et al. showed that, of 1227 patients with Crohn's disease, 28 had extraintestinal cancer, with a predominance of squamous cell and reticuloendothelial neoplasms (29).

V. TREATMENT

A. Medical

Early studies report conservative general measures for treatment of Crohn's disease, including therapy with vitamins, opiates to control diarrhea, and measures to maintain nutrition. Corticosteroids and sulfasalazine were introduced into Crohn's disease therapy in the 1940s, with the hope that symptoms and clinical status, would improve and surgery would be deterred. Review of the early literature, however, shows disappointing results; lack of efficacy of medical treatment in Crohn's disease was apparent when the number of patients requiring surgery was so high (16,17,30). In one study, only 26% of new cases and 7% of referred cases had escaped a surgical operation in the Radcliffe Infirmary (21). Others report a more favorable outcome with medical treatment. One study reported that 16 of 25 patients responded well to a medical regimen (3). In addition, several investigators note that elderly patients with left-sided disease showed a good response to medical treatment and required few surgical interventions (4,9,12). Specifically, one recent study found that 15 of 22 patients with large bowel disease responded to medical treatment, in contrast to 22 patients with distal ileal disease who presented acutely and required surgery (4). Harper et al. compared 24 elderly patients with a younger group matched for sex and duration of disease. Elderly patients were less frequently treated with prednisone and sulfasalazine, but there was no difference in the response to medical treatment or need for surgery (18).

Medical treatment for the elderly patient should follow the same principles as in the younger patient, with careful recognition of comorbid conditions in the older patients. In patients with mild to moderate Crohn's colitis and ileocolitis, treatment should include sulfasalazine or one of the new oral 5-aminosalicylic acids (5-ASA). In patients with Crohn's ileitis, the new slow-release forms of 5-ASA (Asacol or Pentasa) should be used because sulfasalazine has not been shown to be useful in ileitis alone. The slow-release forms also have been shown to decrease relapse rates by approximately 40% when administered long term to patients wtih inactive Crohn's disease. This benefit has been most marked in patients with ileitis and in those with prior bowel resections (31).

In patients in whom aminosalicylates are poorly tolerated or fail to achieve improvement, antibiotics should be considered; metronidazole for colonic disease and ciprofloxacin or, alternatively, tetracycline, amoxicillin, or cephalexin for small bowel disease.

If 5-ASA agents and antibiotics fail to achieve effective treatment in patients wtih mild to moderate disease or if the patient is severely ill, corticosteroids should be used. Old age is not a contraindication to steroid therapy. However, prolonged use of corticosteroids in the elderly may exacerbate diabetes, hypertension, congestive heart failure, and osteoporosis or cause paradoxical depression (6). Appropriate surveillance for bone disease and use of supplementary calcium and vitamin D must be considered. Thomas reviewed complications of long-term corticosteroid use in 100 elderly patients and found that dose-related side effects were noted in 40% of patients, including osteoporosis in 16% and hypertension in 12% (32).

If a response is not achieved with aminosalicylates, antibiotics, or steroids or if the patient is steroid dependent then the immunomodulators, 6-mercaptopurine (6-MP) and azathioprine should be considered as they would be in younger patients. The two agents can be used interchangeably and both are effective in the treatment of active Crohn's disease in reducing steroid requirements and in maintaining remission in the disorder (33–35). The safety of long-term treatment with 6-MP and azathioprine in the elderly population has not been well studied. However, current literture shows a low incidence of side effects, and most investigators conclude that elderly patients deserve a trial of intensive treatment (36–38).

For patients refractory to the aforementioned treatments, methotrexate may be especially useful for patients dependent on a moderate dose of steroids (> 20 mg/day) (39). Although methotrexate has not been specifically studied in the elderly, there is wide use of this agent in older patients with rheumatoid arthritis and psoriasis. Finally, oral cyclosporin in high doses may include remission in active disease, but relapse rates are high on withdrawal of therapy (40). Low-dose cyclosporin has not been shown to maintain remission (41).

B. Surgery

Surgical intervention always has had a prominent role in the treatment of the Crohn's disease patient. Indications for surgery in the elderly are not different from their younger counterparts and include the following: unresponsiveness to medical therapy, perforation, obstruction, fistula, and malignancy. Comparison of operative rates between the older and younger patients yields mixed results. Fochios reported that 69% of patients younger than 50 years of age required surgical procedures compared with 43% of patients older than 50 years of age (12). In contrast, Rusch and Simonowitz noted that the incidence of emergent surgery increased with age (7). This older age group of patients also was noted to have an increased number of postoperative complications. Interestingly, Tchirkow et al. observed that elderly patients requiring surgery were more debilitated from severe malnutrition, which may explain the higher postoperative complication rate (16).

When surgical data on elderly patients and their younger counterparts were compared, there was no difference in the recurrence rate, which was approximately 80% in both groups (18). Other reports on the rates of recurrence, however, have been variable.

Goligher noted a lower recurrence rate in older patients, that is, 13% in patients older than 40 years of age compared with 47% in patients younger than age 40 years (42). Similarly, another study reported clinical recurrence in the elderly to be 21% at 9 years after initial surgery (3). Because there is still significant postoperative recurrence of disease in the elderly population, it is important to note that recent studies have shown a delay in or prevention of postoperative recurrence with the use of 5-ASA agents and metronidazole (43).

VI. OUTCOME

Early reports concluded that elderly patients with Crohn's disease had a higher incidence of complications and mortality over younger patients (7,9). Simpson et al. reported a significant perioperative mortality rate: 58% in the group of patients older than 60 years as compared with only 7% in younger patients (44). In 1988, Prior et al. looked at mortality in the elderly population with Crohn's disease and by applying a correction for age to a previous paper from Oxford, concluded that the relative risk of dying from Crohn's disease as a direct cause and to associated complications within the digestive system decreased over time (45). This contrasts with the findings of Truelove and Pona who reported an increased risk (21). More recent reports find that elderly patients have a benign course and have the same mortality rate as their younger counterparts (11,46). Gupta et al. estimate a 14% mortality rate in the older population (10). Softley et al. report the death rate in the elderly to be 2.4% as compared with 0.8% in younger patients (13). Both groups conclude that the course of Crohn's disease is more favorable in elderly patients than had been previously suspected.

VII. SUMMARY

In approximately 5% of patients with Crohn's disease, the onset of disease occurs after age 50 years, and there is likely a bimodal distribution with a second incidence peak in the seventh or eight decade of life. Although the clinical presentation of Crohn's disease in the elderly is similar to that of younger patients, Crohn's disease in the elderly has a female predominance with distal colonic disease being frequently reported. The diagnosis of Crohn's disease in the older patient may be difficult because it can be easily confused with infectious, ischemic, and drug-related processes, as well as with diverticulitis and carcinoma. Complications in the elderly seem to be related to the site of involvement, with a propensity for ileal disease–related problems. Treatment in the elderly varies little from that in younger patients, but special caution should be exercised in the use of steroids in the older patient. Finally, whereas mortality rates were initially felt to be extremely high in the older patient, subsequent studies support the notion of similar course of complications and mortality in older patients as compared with their younger counterparts.

REFERENCES

1. Crohn BB, Yarnis H. Regional Ileitis. Philadelphia: Grune & Stratton, 1958:26.
2. Smith IS, Young S, Gillespie G, et al. Epidemiological aspects of Crohn's disease in Clydesdale, 1961–1970. Gut 1975; 16:62–67.
3. Shapiro P, Peppercorn M, Antonioli D, et al. Crohn's disease in the elderly. Am J Gastroenterol 1981; 76:132–137.

4. Fabricus PJ, Gyde SN, Shouler P, et al. Crohn's disease in the elderly. Gut 1985; 26:461–465.
5. Rose JD, Roberts GM, Williams G, et al. Cardiff Crohn's disease jubilee: the incidence over 50 years. Gut 1988; 29:346–351.
6. Brandt LJ. Colitis in the elderly. Hosp Pract 1987; 22:165–188.
7. Rusch V, Simonowitz D. Crohn's disease in the older patient. Surg Gynecol Obstet 1980; 150:184–186.
8. Garland C, Lilienfeld A, Mendeloff A, et al. Incidence rates of ulcerative colitis and Crohn's disease in fifteen areas of the United States. Gastroenterology 1981; 81:1115–1124.
9. Carr N, Schofield F. Inflammatory bowel disease in the elder patient. Br J Surg 1982; 69:223–225.
10. Gupta S, Saverymuttu S, Keshavarazian A, et al. Is the pattern of inflammatory bowel disease different in the elderly? Age Ageing 1985; 14:366–370.
11. Feczko P, Barbour J, Halpert R, et al. Crohn's disease in the elderly. Radiology 1985; 157:303–304.
12. Fochios S. Inflammatory bowel disease in the elderly. In: Korelitz BI, Sohn N, eds. Inflammatory Bowel Disease. Philadelphia: Grune & Stratton, 1985:31–34.
13. Softley A, Myren J, Clamp E, et al. Inflammatory bowel disease in the elderly patient. Scand J Gastroenterol 1988; 23(suppl44):27–30.
14. Lee FI, Costello FT. Crohn's disease in Blackpool-incidence and prevalence 1968–80. Gut 1985; 26:274–278.
15. Fireman Z, Grossman A, Lilos P, et al. Epidemiology of Crohn's disease in the Jewish population of central Israel, 1970–1980. Am J Gastroenterol 1989; 84(3):255–258.
16. Tchirkow G, Lavery IC, Fazio VW, et al. Crohn's disease in the elderly. Dis Colon Rectum 1983; 26:177–181.
17. Comes JS, Stetcher M. Primary Crohn's disease of the colon and rectum. Gut 1961; 189:189–200.
18. Harper P, McAuliffe T, Beeken W. Crohn's disease in the elderly. A statistical comparison with younger patients matched for sex and duration of disease. Arch Intern Med 1986; 146:753–755.
19. Kaufmann HJ, Taubin HL. Nonsteroidals activate quiescent inflammatory bowel disease. Ann Intern Med 1987; 107:513–516.
20. Peppercorn MA. Drug-responsive chronic segmental colitis associated with diverticula: clinical syndrome in the elderly. Am J Gastroenterol 1992; 87:609–611.
21. Truelove SC, Peña AS. Course and prognosis of Crohn's disease. Gut 1976; 17:192–201.
22. Farmer R, Whelan G, Fazio VW, et al. Long-term follow-up of patients with Crohn's disease. Gastroenterology 1985; 88:1818–1825.
23. Grimm I, Friedman L. Inflammatory bowel disease in the elderly. Gastroenterol Clin North Am 1990; 1:361–389.
24. Binder V, Hendriksen C, Kreiner S. Prognosis in Crohn's disease—based on results from the country of Copenhagen 1985; 26:146–150.
25. Yardley JH, Ranohoff DF, Riddell RH, et al. Cancer in inflammatory bowel disease: how serious is the problem and what should be done about it? Gastroenterology 1983; 85:197–200.
26. Ekbom A, Helmick C, Zack M, et al. Increased risk of large-bowel cancer in Crohn's disease with colonic involvement. Lancet 1990; 336:357–359.
27. Choi PM, Zelig MP. Similarity of colorectal cancer in Crohn's disease and ulcerative colitis: implications for carcinogenesis and prevention. Gut 1994; 35:950–954.
28. Ekbom A, Helmick C, Zack M, et al. Extracolonic malignancies in inflammatory bowel disease. Cancer 1991; 67:2015–2019.
29. Greenstein A, Gennuso R, Sachar D, et al. Extraintestinal cancers in inflammatory bowel disease. Cancer 1985; 56:2914–2921.
30. Cooke WT, Mallas E, Prior P, et al. Crohn's disease: course, treatment and long-term prognosis. QJ Med 1980; 49:363–384.

31. Thomson ABR. International Mesalazine Study Group. Coated oral 5-ASA vs placebo in maintaining remission of inactive Crohn's disease. Pharmacol Ther 1990; 4:55–64.
32. Thomas TPL. The complications of systemic corticosteroid therapy in the elderly. Gerontology 1984; 30:60–65.
33. Present DH, Korelitz BI, Wisch N, et al. Treatment of Crohn's disease with 6-mercaptopurine. A long-term, randomized, double-blind study. N Engl J Med 1980; 302(18):981–987.
34. Present DH. 6-Mercaptopurine and other immunosuppressive agents in the treatment of Crohn's disease and ulcerative colitis. Gastroenterol Clin North Am 1989; 18(1); 57–71.
35. O'Donaghue DP, Dawson AW, Powell-Tuck J, et al. Double-blind withdrawal trial of azathioprine in maintenance treatment of Crohn's disease. Lancet 1978; 2:955–957.
36. Wade JF, King TE. Infiltrative and interstitial lung disease in the elderly patient. Clin Chest Med 1993; 14(3); 501–521.
37. Ito T, Yamamoto K, Kinoshita T, et al. The continuous-DCMP therapy for acute non-lymphocytic leukemia in elderly patients. Rinsho Ketsueki 1989; 30(4); 421–428.
38. Ruutu T, Almqvist A, Hallman H, et al. Treatment of acute myeloid leukemia in elderly patients. Haematologica 1991; 97:91.
39. North American Crohn's Study Group Investigators. A Multicentre trial of methotrexate treatment for chronically active Crohn's disease. Gastroenterology 1994; 106(4).
40. Brynskov J, Freund L, Rasmussen SN, et al. A placebo-controlled, double-blind, randomized trial of cyclosporine therapy in active chronic Crohn's disease. N Engl J Med 1989; 321:845–850.
41. Feagan B, et al. Low dose cyclosporine for the treatment of Crohn's disease. N Engl J Med 1994; 330:1846–1851.
42. Goligher JC. Inflammatory disease of the bowel: results of resection for Crohn's disease. Dis Colon Rectum 1976; 19:584–587.
43. Rutgeerts P, Hiele M, et al. Prevention of clinical recurrence after ileal resection for Crohn's disease with metronidazole: a placebo controlled study. Gastroenterology 1994; 106(4):764.
44. Simpson CJ, Smith IS, Young S, et al. Crohn's disease in the older patient. Gut 1986; 27:A595.
45. Prior P, Gyde S, Cooke WT, et al. Mortality in Crohn's disease. Gastroenterology 1981; 80:307–312.
46. Rhodes J, Rose J. Crohn's disease in the elderly. BMJ 1985; 291:1149.

COMMENTARY

Nadir Arber and Peter R. Holt   *St. Luke's–Roosevelt Hospital Center and Columbia University College of Physicians and Surgeons, New York, New York*

The reason to focus on a disease at a particular age is to emphasize possible differences in cause or in the interaction of age and the underlying cause in clinical presentation, differential diagnosis, therapy, or prognosis. Elderly subjects with Crohn's disease demonstrate a number of differences from younger patients, which results in changes in management of such patients as well as in the overall understanding of the disease.

Overall, inflammatory bowel disease in the elderly is more common than previously was recognized. Crohn's disease is becoming more important in the elderly population, in part, because of longer survival of patients with onset earlier in life and because there is a further peak of incidence in patients older than age 60 years. Newly diagnosed Crohn's disease in the elderly tends to be found in women, mainly with colonic involvement that especially affects the distal colon. This presentation can lead to a diagnostic dilemma because the clinical presentation may be difficult to distinguish from colon carcinoma, ischemic colitis, diverticulosis or diverticulitis.

Early epidemiological studies of a Johns' Hopkins group in Baltimore emphasized, perhaps for the first time, that Crohn's disease occurred commonly in older patients. That study clearly showed a bimodal age-specific incidence of Crohn's disease. In Baltimore, black women had a high prevalence of Crohn's disease affecting the distal colon. Subsequent observations in other parts of the world, including a carefully conducted epidemiological study from Cardiff, United Kingdom, also pointed out that this disease was not confined to the young. Some eminent authorities have argued that the manifestations and consequences of vascular disease of the bowel can so closely mimic the clinical features of Crohn's disease that the apparent high incidence in advanced age represents a disease of vascular origin. This hypothesis has been difficult to refute because many of the features of the two disorders unquestionably are similar. There is no specific diagnostic test for Crohn's disease because the histological presence of submucosal granulomas is too infrequent to use as a salient distinguishing feature.

Early descriptions of Crohn's disease in the elderly may have been slanted because the diagnosis was often made late in the course of the disease and only patients with classical small bowel disease were described initially. However, colonic involvement is common and the distal colon rather than proximal colon usually is involved in older patients. As a result, the differential diagnosis in the elderly patient has provided considerable clinical problems, particularly when diverticulosis is also present. In the elderly, chronic diverticulitis with possible chronic abscess formation, colon carcinoma and ischemic disease are the major issues in differential diagnosis. It is sometimes even difficult for the pathologist, with a specimen in hand after surgical resection, to provide a final answer.

The extensive cooperative studies headed by Tim deDombal from Leeds on inflammatory bowel disease in Europe originally described 244 patients older than age 60 years out of more than 2600 who were reported to the center. Colonic disease was present in more than 50% of patients, and the perforation rate was somewhat higher at 3.8% compared with 1.1% in younger patients. The authors concluded that recurrences of the disease were fewer and that surgery was performed less often in older patients.

Elderly patients who have had Crohn's disease for many years are at a significant risk of developing colorectal cancer. Whether the combination of age plus long-standing inflammatory bowel disease results in a much higher risk for the development of colorectal carcinoma is unknown. One recent study showed that colon cancer in Crohn's disease usually occurs in patients older than age 50 years but did not demonstrate a specific risk–effect of age. Furthermore, whether dysplasia occurs more or less frequently as a function of age has not been clarified. However, surveillance for malignancy is unjustified in patients older than age 70 years with a new diagnosis of Crohn's disease.

The original description of inflammatory bowel disease in the elderly emphasized a poor prognosis. This probably resulted in excessive delay in the performance of surgery, when surgery clearly was indicated because of the fear of increased complications. Since then, the overall risk of intestinal surgery in the elderly has been shown to be no greater than in younger patients as long as comorbid conditions are considered. One large mortality study indicates, however, that most postoperative deaths occurred in patients aged 74 to 84 years. The natural history of Crohn's disease in the elderly suggests that exacerbations and recurrences are muted when compared with those of younger patients. This might represent a relative reduced gut-associated immune response in older patients to the inciting agents.

Most elderly patients of Crohn's disease are treated medically rather than surgically. However, if obstructing strictures occur, these must be promptly treated. Medical treatment is similar in both the young and the elderly. Indeed, elderly patients with left-sided colonic involvement responded better to medical therapy than did young patients. 5-Amino-salicylic acid compounds are tolerated well. They have been reported to be especially effective in maintaining remission in patients older than age 30 years with ileal involvement of disease.

Corticosteroids should be used cautiously in all older patients and should be avoided when long-term therapy is needed. Acute psychosis has been reported more frequently in the elderly than in the young, dementia can be exacerbated, cataracts may be precipitated, and bone loss is greater. However, corticosteroids are not contraindicated and must be used to manage severe acute exacerbations that are not controlled by first line drugs. We believe that corticosteroids are far more dangerous than immunosuppressives when prolonged therapy is needed in older patients; thus, immunosuppressive agents are the treatment of choice when chronic suppressive therapy must be added to baseline 5-aminosalicylic acid compounds. Azathioprine and 6-mercaptopurine are well tolerated, and there is no report of secondary malignancy from the use of such immunosuppressives. The medical experience with methotrexate in this age group is limited, but the drug is widely used in elderly patients with rheumatic disorders, with few side effects. On the other hand, cyclosporin should be avoided if possible because older patients are susceptible to the common side effects of renal failure and hypertension. Drug-associated colitis, especially from non-steroidal anti-inflammatory drugs (NSAIDs), is increasingly being recognized; as the use of these drugs in this age group is extremely popular. Therefore, NSAID-induced nonspecific inflammatory Crohn's disease should be added to the differential diagnosis. In patients with known Crohn's disease, the use of NSAIDs should be avoided because they can activate quiescent disease.

Perhaps a better understanding of how the disease is modified in the older host may allow some further insight into cause and cellular responses.

20
Refractory Crohn's Disease

Stephen B. Hanauer   *University of Chicago Medical Center, Chicago, Illinois*

Crohn's disease is inherently refractory. The condition is medically incurable and recurs in a predictable pattern after surgical resection. Therefore, the concept of refractoriness must be considered in relative terms within the context of levels of treatment. Furthermore, in the absence of curability or a gold standard against which to measure disease activity defining response to refractory disease is also relative, depending on the circumstances of the disease state.

I. LIMITATIONS OF MEDICAL THERAPY

Previous chapters have delineated the positive responses to medical therapy and specific indications for surgery. Clinical trials have demonstrated the inadequacies of current approaches to Crohn's disease, although the confines of controlled trials should not be construed to define the ultimate value in clinical practice. Sulfasalazine has been ineffective in small bowel Crohn's disease and is of modest benefit in ileocolitis or colitis, although clinicians stand by its utility in mild to moderate disease (1–3). Nevertheless, according to the Crohn's Disease Activity Index (CDAI) as an endpoint, nearly half of patients treated fail to improve within 3 to 4 months, and, at doses of up to 3 g/day, no maintenance benefit has been observed (1,2). The newer salicylates have been shown to have modest benefits in mild to moderate Crohn's disease, but the remission rates are less than 50% (4,5). The long-term benefits of aminosalicylates are superior to placebo, but still only prevent less than one-half of predicted recurrences within one to 3 years after medical treatment or surgery (odds ratios of approximately 0.5) (6,7).

Corticosteroids also have limited benefits confined primarily to short-term therapy for active Crohn's disease, primarily to reduce the inflammatory sequelae; there has been no proven benefit for treatment of fistulas or the prevention of epiphenomena such as sclerosing cholangitis. The acute effects of steroids induce remission in approximately 70% to 80% of patients within 4 months, however, after 1 year, less than 45% of patients remain well and one-third become "steroid dependent" (1,2,8). The latter term must be distinguished from a "maintenance" therapy, which demonstrates a predictable dose-dependent benefit in reducing relapse. Steroids have not been demonstrated to have a maintenance role in Crohn's disease and "steroid dependency" is a primary reason why patients are considered refractory to standard interventions (5). Even the newer, nonsystemic steroids have failed to prevent relapses at doses that limit systemic side effects (9,10).

Finally, antibiotics, the common "underground" therapy for Crohn's disease, which have been least studied in clinical trials, have major limitations of usefulness. Metronidazole can only be considered as useful as sulfasalazine, although a small proportion of sulfasalazine failures respond to "crossover" therapy with metronidazole (11). In placebo-controlled trials, metronidazole at 10 to 20 mg/kg did reduce the CDAI more than did placebo but it was no more effective at inducing remission (CDAI < 150) (12). No other antibiotics have been systematically evaluated in controlled trials to compare their utility. However, antibiotics are commonly used in clinical practice, often on-top-of ongoing treatment to reduce perianal complications or as an adjunct for severe disease in hospitalized patients on intravenous steroids (3). Their efficacy in these situations has not been established.

II. LIMITATIONS OF SURGICAL THERAPY

Surgery is not curative in Crohn's disease. Recurrence after resection is inevitable, with endoscopic evidence of disease appearing in 80% of patients within 3 to 6 months (13). Symptomatic recurrences occur in half of patients within 3 years and reoperation is required in 50% of patients (14). Although surgery for perianal disease is palliative for suppurative complications, it does not halt recurrent fistulization or persistent drainage and may leave the patient partially incontinent after sphincterotomy. Only proctocolectomy for Crohn's disease confined to the colon can (sometimes) be curative, but the potential for recurrence in the small bowel persists. Thus, surgery is reserved for the treatment of medically refractory Crohn's disease, but it does not alter the eventual progression of disease.

III. REFRACTORY STATES

Treatment of refractory Crohn's disease is a relative concept usually applied to a specific scenario. The most common issues pertaining to steroid therapy are in patients who either do not respond to acute treatment ("steroid resistance") or are unable to taper steroids without relapsing ("steroid dependence") (8). Both are relative terms depending on the dose and duration of therapy. Although data are limited in these situations, both are frequently encountered in clinical practice and are the most common indications for immunomodulation or hyperalimentation and bowel rest (3). A third refractory setting is in cases of fistulizing disease (perianal, rectovaginal, enteroenteric, enterovesicular) when surgical therapy is undesirable because of postoperative sequelae (e.g., short-bowel, incontinence, need for ostomies, or established patterns or reoccurrence). Finally, postoperative recurrence, despite prophylaxis, is a novel challenge to clinicians.

A. Steroid Resistance

Approximately 25% of patients fail to respond to outpatient management with 1 mg/kg of prednisone therapy over 2 to 4 months (1,2). Predictors of poor response include colonic disease, perianal disease, malnutrition, and fistulization (5). To limit steroid therapy, many clinicians actually underdose patients. In a tertiary practice, I and my colleagues often find that patients are referred after having been tapered off therapy too quickly (before a complete response) or they have been treated with too small a dose (e.g., "beginning low" and "titrating up"). Our practice in using steroids is to begin effective doses (generally 40–60 mg of prednisone) and continue such dosing until patients achieve complete response (reach the chosen endpoint). Once-daily dosing in the morning is usually effective, but if patients are not responding, we divide the dose up to four times a day. Steroid tapering is never standardized outside of controlled trials but is individualized according to the time it takes for the patient to achieve the intended (complete) response. A patient who is tapered after a "partial" response is doomed to immediate relapse because the patient is already symptomatic at initiation of dose reduction.

An initial approach for patients who are failing or have failed outpatient therapy with adequate steroid dosing is hospitalization and initiation of intravenous steroids similar to the intensive intravenous regimen given for ulcerative colitis (15). Data are limited on the efficacy of this program, and the interpretation of results is obfuscated by elements of both increased dose and additional duration of therapy. Nevertheless, it is reasonable to hospitalize both severely ill patients as well as those who are failing to respond to an outpatient regimen (3). Patients with mild to moderate persisting symptoms receive intravenous steroids comparable to 1 mg/kg of prednisone—60 mg prednisolone, 40 to 60 mg methylprednisolone, or 300 to 400 mg/day hydrocortisone, in divided doses. (I and my colleagues prefer a continuous infusion based on our observations of patients who have failed divided dose therapy, and, we currently justify the continuous infusion on a cost basis to minimize "piggyback" setups). Some clinicians advocate intravenous adreno-corticotropin hormone (ACTH) infusions, but these data are even more limited in both acute and refractory situations (3).

In contrast to ulcerative colitis, Crohn's disease does respond to nutritional interventions. Therefore, similar to severely ill patients, sicker "steroid-resistant" patients benefit from either elemental feedings or bowel rest and total parenteral nutrition (TPN) (16,17). A single controlled trial failed to differentiate the benefits of TPN and bowel rest versus elemental feedings in conjunction with a standardized steroid regimen in hospitalized patients (18). The practicalities of both have been previously discussed and we still believe that bowel rest can be of benefit for patients who are unresponsive on oral regimens. However, in most cases, the benefits of nutritional intervention are transient and the long-term outcomes depend on the response to primary medical approaches (16).

Antibiotics may be effective for perianal complications but have not been evaluated for steroid-refractory Crohn's disease.

A primary indication for azathioprine or 6-mercaptopurine has been for steroid-resistant Crohn's disease (3,19). However, in most instances, the 3 to 6 month delay in response necessitates some temporizing or alternative short-term approach to modify disease activity (19). Up to 80% of patients can be expected to respond eventually, but, in a 1-year controlled crossover trail by Present et al., it was not possible to discern the response of steroid-resistant patients (19).

The potential for cyclosporin therapy to bridge the gap before long-acting immune modifiers take effect arises from the experience with both short-term trials of oral cyclosporin as well as the utility of intravenous cyclosporin for ulcerative colitis and Crohn's disease. In the first substantial controlled trial of oral cyclosporin for steroid-refractory Crohn's disease, Brynskov et al. reported a significantly higher improvement rate according to "individual goals" (59%) with cyclosporin, 5 to 7.5 mg/kg per day, compared with placebo treatment (32%)(20). Unfortunately, these results were not long lasting as other reports of oral cyclosporin have confirmed (21,22). The issues of dose and absorption are relevant because the bioavailability of cyclosporin is compromised by small bowel disease, length, and motility. In the Brynskov study, malabsorption was noted in 27% of patients, and there was a suggestion that response may correlate with tissue levels, although this premise has yet to be unequivocally demonstrated (20,21). Nevertheless, the response to intravenous cyclosporin is even more dramatic, suggesting that higher systemic availability may be critical for an initial response and that lower systemic levels may account for the failure of long-term cyclosporin treatment (23).

Methotrexate has recently been evaluated for refractory Crohn's disease but primarily as a "steroid-sparing" agent, although the initial, uncontrolled experience suggests that there may be a role for parenteral methotrexate in "steroid-refractory" disease (24).

Miscellaneous approaches have been evaluaed for steroid-refractory Crohn's disease, including alternative immunomodulators such as tacrolimus (FK 506), fusidic acid, chimeric anti-TNF monoclonal antibodies, anti-CD4 monoclonal antibodies, intravenous immunoglobulin, and razoxane, although controlled trials have not been performed to objectify expectations (25–30). In addition, lymphocytoplasmapheresis has been advocated for steroid-resistant disease (31). In one group's experience, 48 of 54 patients treated with lymphocytoplasmapheresis achieved long-lasting remissions. The method of Bicks et al. necessitates steroid withdrawal before initiating the pheresis to extract sufficient circulating lymphocytes (31). Often, these patients must be hospitalized and treated with TPN and bowel rest to control symptoms while they are receiving the pheresis. In controlled trials to maintain remission, however, lymphocytoplasmapheresis was not superior to placebo therapy (32).

B. Steroid-Dependent Crohn's Disease

The issue of how to get patients off of steroids once therapy has been initiated has been the major therapeutic controversy of the 1990s. The question arises based on two erroneous dogmas dating back to the National Cooperative Crohn's Disease Study (NCCDS) and the European Cooperative Crohn's Disease Study (ECCDS) (1,2). Both trials established the short-term efficacy of steroids but failed to demonstrate a maintenance role for low-dose prednisone (NCCDS) or a benefit from combined sulfasalazine and steroids (ECCDS). Hence, the standard practice has been to treat patients with short-term steroids then stop and wait for a relapse. Although these trials were innovative and large, they did not have sufficient numbers in all of the strata to avoid type II errors; hence, erroneous conclusions were based on small sample sizes in multiple strata. Subsequent clinical experience has demonstrated that the long-term response to a short-term course of steroids is not satisfactory in nearly 50% of patients who are either steroid dependent or unresponsive to therapy (8). In addition, using higher doses (4–6 g) of sulfasalazine, the response, over 4 months, can be boosted to the point of equivalence with prednisone (33). Finally, although there are minimal empirical data on the "steroid-sparing" benefits of amino-salicylates, a recent study from the Group d'Etudes Therapeutiques des Affections Inflammatoires Digestives (GETAID) suggests that, after a 3–7-week course of prednisolone (1 mg/kg), steroid tapering can be enhanced by the addition of 4 g of mesalamine daily (74%) compared with placebo (58%) (34). However, the study did not find any differences between continuation of mesalamine versus placebo after 1 year. These findings are in contrast to several trials that demonstrate a maintenance benefit from mesalamine therapy after medical or postoperative remissions (6,7).

Thus, data remain conflicting regarding a potential "steroid-sparing" role for sulfa-salazine and the newer aminosalicylates in Crohn's disease, and the lessons from the clinical trials can be summarized as follows: larger sample sizes for each clinical scenario (disease location, subtype, complication, treatment) and higher doses of aminosalicylates (i.e., 4–6 g sulfasalazine, greater than 4 g mesalamine) with appropriate release profiles for the disease location may be necessary to define a "steroid-sparing" role if one exists.

There are no data regarding "steroid-sparing" benefits of antibiotic therapy in Crohn's disease nor have studies evaluated elemental diets from this perspective. Certainly, elemental diets can provide equivalent benefits as steroid therapy, but the long-term results are no better or worse than after an adequate course of steroids.

Immunosuppressives, however, have demonstrated a "steroid-sparing" role in Crohn's disease in a number of clinical trials, and this has been the primary indication for use of azathioprine and 6-mercaptopurine (6-MP) in Crohn's disease. Early studies demonstrated a reduction in steroid use in patients treated with azathioprine (35–37). In a pivotal trial by Present et al., a 1-year crossover trial administering 6-MP, 1.5 mg/kg per day (adjusted to avoid leukopenia), 79% of patients improved compared with 29% receiving placebo. Subsequently, these findings were replicated by Ewe et al. who demonstrated that 76% of patients receiving a combination of tapering prednisone with 2.5 mg/kg of azathioprine achieved a remission at 4 months compared with 38% of patients on steroids plus placebo (38). Similarly, in a South African study published in abstract form, azathioprine in addition to a prednisone taper provided superior 1-year remission benefits (39).

The results with cyclosporin have not been as encouraging from a "steroid-sparing" perspective. Long-term maintenance benefits have not been demonstrated with oral cyclosporin despite the impressive short-term results (21,22). Hence, the therapeutic role of cyclosporin appears to be more of a "bridge" from short-term therapy for refractory or unresponsive patients to long-term therapy with azathioprine or 6-MP. Azathioprine does seem to give an additional benefit of maintaining the acute response to cyclosporin intervention (40,41).

The recently completed North American Methotrexate Study also demonstrated a "steroid-sparing" role for parenteral methotrexate in patients previously unable to wean off prednisone (42). In patients treated with a standardized steroid taper in addition to 25 mg of intramuscular or subcutaneous methotrexate, 39% of patients were tapered completely off steroids during the 16 weeks of the trial while remaining in remission compared with 19% of patients receiving placebo. The results were more impressive for patients requiring greater than 20 mg of prednisone before entering the trial. These results substantiate both the empirical observations by Kozarek et al. as well as smaller trials using oral methotrexate (24,43). More data regarding the dose response, need for parenteral versus oral methotrexate, duration of response, and toxicity are needed before final recommendations regarding the role of methotrexate can be asserted.

C. Fistulas

Fistulas can be a primary or complicating feature of Crohn's disease. When they are evaluated as a complicating feature, it is difficult to extract data from clinical trials regarding specific therapeutic efficacy related to fistula healing. Hence, there are, essentially, no data regarding any benefits from aminosalicylates or steroids related to fistula healing. Most experience dictates that fistula output improves when other inflammatory sequelae are subdued. However, some clinical investigators believe that steroids may actually increase the likelihood of fistulizing complications. Data specifically related to fistulizing complications are limited to case series and a few subgroups from controlled trials.

Original data regarding metronidazole come from observations on the role for this antibiotic in perianal Crohn's disease (44–46). Subsequently, it has become clear that withdrawal of metronidazole usually is associated with reopening of perianal disease, necessitating long-term (maintenance) therapy that requires careful monitoring for neurotoxicity (45). Ciprofloxacin also has been reported to be of benefit for perianal Crohn's disease, although no clinical trial data are available (47,48). Again, most clinicians recognize the need to maintain treatment to prevent relapse. Other antibiotics are used in practice but have not been studied in a controlled setting. Nevertheless, the extensive clinical experience and opinion is that antibiotic regimens can be useful to treat and maintian perianal fistulas in Crohn's disease. Similarly, without controlled data, many clinicians also use antibiotics for "internal" (e.g., enterovesicular, enterocolic) fistulas often associated with inflammatory masses, although there are even fewer data available to evaluate such circumstances (49).

This setting, again, is one in which immunosuppressives have a more clearly defined role. Both the original randomized crossover trial and subsequent observational series suggest that 6-MP (and presumably azathioprine) provide long-term benefits in fistulizing Crohn's disease (50). Controversy still remains as to the dose and long-term duration of therapy, and whether neutropenia should be "induced" or "averted" (51). The delay in onset of action for these agents has led to several reports on the use of cyclosporin to heal fistulas (52,53). Consistent with other experience in inflammatory bowel disease, the results of intravenous cyclosporin have been remarkable, with fistula healing occurring usually within 1 week. Again, the short-term benefits with cyclosporin cannot be maintained with this agent alone and probably require transition to a long-term regimen of alternative immunosuppressants (54).

Several other methods have been described to approach refractory perianal disease. These include local (depot) steroid injections or the use of hyperbaric oxygen (55,56). At all times, the principles of (surgical) drainage of pus and maintenance of the overall "quality of life" must be maintained; some patients do require diversion and eventual proctectomy to improve their short-and long-term well-being.

D. Postsurgical Considerations

Most patients do well after resection for Crohn's disease, but a number of factors increase the likelihood or rapidity of clinical relapse. Patients who require surgery within a short time after presentation, those with multifocal or phlegmaceous/fistulizing complications, and those who continue to smoke cigarettes have a worst postoperative prognosis (14,57,58). In addition, up to 80% of patients have endoscopic lesions noted around the anastomosis within 3 to 6 months after resection; the severity of these lesions can predict the likelihood of clinical relapse (13,59). Therefore, there is rationale to begin selecting subroups for potential therapy after surgical resection.

To date, however, there are limited prospective data regarding the benefits of postoperative maintenance for these "high-risk" subgroups. There are data that mesalamine can prevent both endoscopic and clinical relapse after surgery, although the benefits are still sublimated in the higher risk groups, especially in smokers (60–62). Likewise, there are some data that a 3-month course of high-dose metronidazole (20 mg/kg) can reduce the likelihood of endoscopic recurrences after resection, but clinical studies of prolonged metronidazole have not been completed (63). Combination antibiotic regimens targeted against atypical mycobacteria have not provided impressive results (64–66).

Finally, there are not controlled data regarding the role of immunosuppressive agents to prevent postoperative recurrence in surgically refractory patients. Case series do describe some patients who were treated to prevent recurrence according to "individual goals," although specific data are difficult to extract from these papers (67–70). Nevertheless, it is likely that continuation of azathioprine/6-MP will benefit patients with persisting Crohn's disease after resection similar to the benefits in chronically active disease. Controlled trials to evaluate the benefits of immunosuppressives to prevent postoperative relapse are underway.

IV. SUMMARY

Therapeutic alternatives for refractory Crohn's disease are the most difficult to interpret based on the diversity of patient subgroups, inadequate definitions, and the multiplicity of concurrent therapies. Nevertheless, the principles of treating patients with refractory disease are similar to treating Crohn's disease in general. Treatable complications (e.g., suppuration, concurrent enteric infections or infection with *Clostridium difficile*, administration of nonsteroidal anti-inflammatory drugs, or cigarette smoking) should be sought and remedied. Adequate "primary" therapeutic approaches, doses, and duration of therapy should be ascertained. Specifically, sulfasalazine should be prescribed at 4 to 6 g/day and mesalamine at 4 to 5 g/day before declaring therapeutic failures. Steroids should be administered at doses of 40 to 60 mg/day (or 1 mg/kg) until clinical remission is achieved. Failures should be treated with elemental diets or TPN and bowel rest but they do require long-term maintenance therapy. Alternatively, patients should be hospitalized for intravenous steroid "induction" therapy, and patients who fail this approach should be considered for cyclosporin treatment or surgery. Metronidazole (or alternative antibiotic) requires long-term treatment for perianal disease. Refractory Crohn's disease requires a long-term perspective on management, with prospective analysis of the chronic complications of persisting disease activity, toxicity of therapy, and surgical alternatives to maintain psychological well being, social functioning, and all aspects of "quality of life."

REFERENCES

1. Summers RW, Switz DM, Sessions Jr JT, et al. National Cooperative Crohn's Disease Study: results of drug treatment. Gastroenterology 1979; 77:847–869.
2. Anthonisen P, Barany F, Folkenborg O, et al. The clinical effect of salazosulphapyridine (Salazopyrin) in Crohn's disease. Scand J Gastroenterol 1974; 9:549–554.
3. Meyers S, Sachar DB. Medical therapy of Crohn's disease. In: Kirsner JB, Shorter RG, eds. Inflammatory Bowel Disease. 4th ed. Baltimore: Williams & Wilkins, 1995:695–714.
4. Singleton JW, Hanauer SB, Gitnick GL, et al. Mesalamine capsules for the treatment of active Crohn's disease: results of a 16-week trial. Gastroenterology 1993; 104:1293–1301.
5. Salomon P, Kornbluth A, Aisenberg J, Janowitz HD. How effective are current drugs for Crohn's disease? A meta-analysis. J Clin Gastroenterol 1992; 14:211–215.
6. Steinhart HA, Hemphill D, Greenberg R. Sulfasalazine and mesalazine for maintenance therapy of Crohn's disease: a meta-analysis. Am J Gastroenterol 1994; 89:2116–2124.
7. Messori A, Brignola C, Trallori G, et al. Effectiveness of 5-aminosalicylic acid for maintain-

ing remission in patients with Crohn's disease: a meta-analysis. Am J Gastroenterol 1994; 89:692–698.

8. Munkholm P, Langholz E, Davidsen M, Binder V. Frequency of glucocorticoid resistance and dependency in Crohn's disease. Gut 1994; 35:360–362.

9. Lofberg R, Rutgeerts P, Malchow H, Lamers C, Olaisson G, Jewell DP, Ostergaard Thomsen O, Lorenz-Meyer H, Goebell H, Hodgson H, Persson T, Seidegard C. Budesonide CIR for maintenance of remission in ileocecal Crohn's disease. A European multicenter placebo controlled trial for 12 months. Gastroenterology 1994; 106:A722.

10. Greenberg GR, Feagan BG, Martin F, Sutherland LR, Thomson ABR, Williams CN, Nilsson LG, Persson T, the Canadian Inflammatory Bowel Disease Study Group. Oral budesonide as maintenance treatment for Crohn's disease. Gastroenterology 1995; 108:A827.

11. Ursing B, Alm T, Barany F, et al. A comparative study of metronidazole and sulfasalazine for active Crohn's disease: the Cooperative Crohn's Disese Study in Sweden. II. Result. Gastroenterology 1982; 83:550–562.

12. Sutherland L, Singleton J, Sessions J, et al. Double-blind, placebo-controlled trial of metronidazole in Crohn's disease. Gut 1991; 32:1071–1075.

13. Rutgeerts P, Geboes K, Vantrappen G, Beyls J, Kerremans R, Hiele M. Predictability of the postoperative course of Crohn's disease. Gastroenterology 1990; 99:956–963.

14. Block GE, Hurst RD. Complications of the surgical treatment of ulcerative colitis and Crohn's disease. In: Kirsner JB, Shorter RG, eds. Inflammatory Bowel Disease. 4th Ed. Baltimore: Williams & Wilkins, 1995:898–922.

15. Shephard HA, Barr GD, Jewell DP. Use of an intravenous steroid regimen in the treatment of acute Crohn's disease. J Clin Gastroenterol 1986; 8:154–159.

16. Greenberg GR. Nutritional management of inflammatory bowel disease. Semin Gastroenterol Dis 1993; 4:69–86.

17. Ostro MJ, Greenberg GR, Jeejeebhoy KN. Total parenteral nutrition and complete bowel rest in the management of Crohn's disease. JPEN Parenter Enteral Nutr 1985; 9:280–287.

18. Greenberg GR, Fleming CR, Jeejeebhoy KN, et al. Controlled trial of bowel rest and nutritional support in the management of Crohn's disease. Gut 1988; 1309–1315.

19. Present DH, Korelitz BI, Wisch N, Glass JL, Sachar DB, Pasternack BS. Treatment of Crohn's disease with 6-mercaptopurine. A long-term randomized double blind study. N Engl J Med 1980; 302:981–987.

20. Brynskov J, Freund L, Rasmussen SN, et al. A placebo-controlled, double-blind, randomized, trial of cyclosporine therapy in active chronic Crohn's disease. N Engl J Med 1989; 321:845–850.

21. Brynskov J, Freund L, Rasmussen SN, et al. Final report on a placebo-controlled, double-blind, randomized, multicentre trial of cyclosporin treatment in active chronic Crohn's disease. Scand J Gastroenterol 1991; 26:689–695.

22. Feagan BG, McDonald JW, Rochon J, et al. Low-dose cyclosporin for the treatment of Crohn's disease. The Canadian Crohn's Relapse Prevention Trial Investigators. N Engl J Med 1994; 330:1846–1851.

23. Sandborn WJ. Clinical review: a critical review of cyclosporin therapy in inflammatory bowel disease. Inflammatory Bowel Diseases (J of CCFA) 1995; 1:48–63.

24. Kozarek RA, Patterson DJ, Gelfand MD, et al. Methotrexate induces clinical and histologic remission in patients with refractory inflammatory bowel disease. Ann Intern Med 1989; 110:353–356.

25. Reynolds JC, Trellis DR, Abu-Elmagd K, Fung J. The rationale for FK 506 in inflammatory bowel disease. Can J Gastroenterol 1993; 7:208–210.

26. Langholz E, Brynskov J, Bendtzen K, Vilien M, Binder V. Treatment of Crohn's disease with fusidic acid: an antibiotic with immunosuppressive properties similar to cyclosporin. Aliment Pharmacol Ther 1992; 6:495–502.

27. Derkx B, Taminiau J, Radema S, et al. Tumour necrosis factor antibody treatment in Crohn's disease. Lancet 1993; 342:173–174.

28. Emmrich J, Seyfarth M, Fleig WE, Emmrich F. Treatment of inflammatory bowel disease with anti-CD4 monoclonal antibody. Lancet 1991; 1:570–571.

29. Levine DS, Fischer SH, Haggitt RC, Christie DL, Ochs HD. Intravenous immunoglobulin therapy for active, extensive, and medically refractory idiopathic ulcerative or Crohn's colitis. Am J Gastroenterol 1992; 87:91–100.

30. Kingston RD, Hellman K. Razoxane for Crohn's colitis and non-specific proctitis. Br J Clin Pharmacol 1992; 46:252–255.

31. Bicks RO, Groshart KD. The current status of T-lymphocyte apheresis (TLA) treatment of Crohn's disease. J Clin Gastroenterol 1989; 11:136–138.

32. Lerebours E, Bussel A, Modigliani R, Bastit D, Florent C, Rabian C, Rene E, Soule JC, the Groupe d'Etudes Therapeutiques des Affections Inflammatoires Digestives. Treatment of Crohn's disease by lymphocyte apheresis: a randomized controlled trial. Gastroenterology 1994; 107:357–361.

33. Rijk MCM, Van Hogezand RA, Van Lier HJJ, Tongeren JHM. Sulphasalazine and prednisone compared with sulphasalazine for treating active Crohn's disease. Ann Intern Med 1991; 114:445–450.

34. Modigliani R, Colombel JF, Dupas JL, Dapoigny M, Bouhnik Y, Veyrac M, Cadiot G, Ducios B, Soule JC, Gendre JP, Danne O, Mary JY, on behalf of the GETAID, France. Mesalamine (M) in Crohn's disease (CD) patients with prednisolone-induced remission: effect on steroid weaning: a placebo-controlled, multicentre double-blind trial. Gastroenterology 1995; 108:A878.

35. Klein M, Binder HJ, Mitchell M, Aaronson R, Spiro H. Treatment of Crohn's disease with azathioprine: a controlled evaluation. Gastroenterology 1974; 66:916–922.

36. Rosenberg JL, Levin B, Wall AJ, Kirsner JB. A controlled trial of azathioprine in Crohn's disease. Am J Dig Dis 1975; 20:721–726.

37. Rhodes J, Bainton D, Beck P, et al. Controlled trial of azathioprine in Crohn's disease. Lancet 1971; 2:1273–1276.

38. Ewe K, Press AG, Singe CC, et al. Azathioprine combined with prednisolone or monotherapy with prednisolone in active Crohn's disease. Gastroenterology 1993; 105:367–372.

39. Wright JP, Candy S, Gerger M, Adams G, Gerig M, Goodman R. A double-blind controlled study of azathioprine in the treatment and maintenance of remission in Crohn's disease. Gastroenterology 1994; 106:A659.

40. Bertran X, Fernandez-Bariares F, Esteve M, Humbert P, Planas R, Gassull MA. Usefulness of azathioprine (AZA) to maintain cyclosporine (CyA)-induced remission in severe steroid-refractory inflammatory bowel disease (IBD). Gastroenterology 1995; 108:A782.

41. Actis GC, Pinna Pintor M, Salizzoni M, Verme G. Severe refractory ulcerative colitis (UC). Prolonged response after intravenous cyclosporin (IV-CYA) is told by the patient's previous history of steroid independence. Gastroenterlogy 1995; 108:A767.

42. Feagan BG, Rochon J, Fedorak RN, et al. Methotrexate for the treatment of Crohn's disease. N Engl J Med 1995; 332:292–297.

43. Baron TH, Truss CD, Elson CO. Low-dose oral methotrexate in refractory inflammatory bowel disease. Dig Dis Sci 1993; 38:1851–1856.

44. Bernstein LH, Frank MS, Brandt LJ, Boley SJ. Healing of perineal Crohn's disease with metronidazole. Gastroenterology 1980; 79:357–365.

45. Brandt LH, Bernstein LH, Boley SJ, Frank MS. Metronidazole therapy for perineal Crohn's disease: a follow-up study. Gastroenterology 1982; 83:383–387.

46. Jakobovits J, Schuster MM. Metronidazole therapy for Crohn's disease and associated fistulae. Am J Gastroenterol 1984; 79:533–540.

47. Turunen U, Farkkila M, Valtonen V, Seppala K. Long-term outcome of ciprofloxacin treatment in severe perianal or fistulous Crohn's disease. Gastroenterology 1993; 104:A793.

48. Solomon MJ, McLeod RS, O'Connor BI, Steinhart AH, Greenberg GR, Cohen Z. Combination ciprofloxacin and metronidazole in severe perianal Crohn's disease. Can J Gastroenterol 7:571–573.

49. Peppercorn MA. Is there a role for antibiotics as primary therapy in Crohn's ileitis? J Clin Gastroenterol 1993; 17:235–237.

50. Korelitz BI, Present DH. Favorable effect of 6-mercaptopurine on fistula of Crohn's disease. Dig Dis Sci 1985; 30:58–64.

51. Colonna T, Korelitz BI. The role of leukopenia in the 6-mercaptopurine–induced remission of refractory Crohn's disease. Am J Gastroenterol 1994; 879:362–366.

52. Hanauer SB, Smith MB. Rapid closure of Crohn's disease fistulas with continuous intravenous cyclosporin A. Am J Gastroenterol 1993; 88:646–649.

53. Present DH, Lichtiger S. Efficacy of cyclosporine in treatment of fistula of Crohn's disease. Dig Dis Sci 1994; 39:374–380.

54. Santos JV, Baudet JA, Casellas FJ, Guarner LA, Vilaseca JM, Malagelada JRB. Intravenous cyclosporine for steroid-refractory attacks of Crohn's disease: short- and long-term results. J Clin Gastroenterol 1995; 20:207–210.

55. Hughes LE, Donaldson DR, Williams JG, Taylor BA, Young HL. Local depot methylprednisolone injection for painful anal Crohn's disease. Gastroenterology 1988; 94:709–711.

56. Brady CE, Cooley BJ, Davis JC. Healing of severe perineal and cutaneous Crohn's disease with hyperbaric oxygen. Gastroenterology 1989; 97:756–760.

57. Griffiths AM, Wesson DE, Shandling B, Corey M, Sherman PM. Factors influencing postoperative recurrence of Crohn's disease in childhood. Gut 1991; 32:491–495.

58. Sutherland LR, Ramcharan S, Bryant H, Fick G. Effects of cigarette smoking on recurrence of Crohn's disease. Gastroenterology 1990; 98:1123–1128.

59. Caprilli R, Castro M, Cirillo LC, et al. Postoperative recurrence in Crohn's disease: definition, prediction and monitoring. Gastroenterol Int 1993; 6:145–148.

60. Brignola C, Cottone M, Pera A, et al. Mesalamine in the prevention of endoscopic recurrence after intestinal resection for Crohn's disease. Gastroenterology 1995; 108:345–349.

61. Caprilli R, Andreoli A, Capurso L, et al. 5-ASA in the prevention of Crohn's disease postoperative recurrence; an interim report of the Italian Study Group of the Colon (GISC). Ailment Tract Pharmacol 1994; 8:35–43.

62. Sutherland LR, Martin F, Bailey RJ, Fedorak R, Dallaire C, Rossman R, Poleski M, HarveyW, Lariviere L, for the Canadian Study of Pentasa for Remission of Crohn's Disease. 5-Aminosalicylic acid (Pentasa) in the maintenance of remission of Crohn's disease. Gastroenterology 1995; 108:A924.

63. Rutgeerts P, Peeters M, Hiele M, et al. A placebo controlled trial of metronidazole for recurrence prevention of Crohn's disease after resection of the terminal ileum. Gastroenterology 1992; 102:A688.

64. Rutgeerts P, Geboes K, Vantrappen G, et al. Rifabutin and ethambutol do not help recurrent Crohn's disease in the neoterminal ileum. J Clin Gastroenterol 1992; 15:24–28.

65. Swift GL, Srivastava ED, Stone R, et al. Controlled trial of anti-tuberculous chemotherapy for two years in Crohn's disease. Gut 1994; 35:363–368.

66. Prantera C, Kohn A, Mangiarotti R, Andreoli A, Luzi C. Antimycobacterial therapy in Crohn's disease: results of a controlled, double-blind trial with a multiple antibiotic regimen. Am J Gastroenterol 1994; 4:513–518.

67. Nyman M, Hansson I, Eriksson S. Long-term immunosuppressive treatment in Crohn's disease. Scand J Gastroenterol 1985; 20:1197–1203.

68. Markowitz J, Rosa J, Grancher K, Aiges H, Daum F. Long-term 6-mercaptopurine treatment in adolescents with Crohn's disease. Gastroenterology 1990; 99:1347–1351.

69. Verhave M, Winter HS, Grand RJ. Azathioprine in the treatment of children with inflammatory bowel disease. J Pediatr 1990; 117:809–114.

70. O'Brien JJ, Bayless TM, Bayless AJ. Use of azathioprine or 6-mercaptopurine in the treatment of Crohn's disease. Gastroenterology 1991; 101:39–46.

COMMENTARY

Theodore M. Bayless   *The Johns Hopkins University School of Medicine, Baltimore, Maryland*

Although gratifying strides have been made in the understanding and management of inflammatory bowel disease (IBD), a significant percentage of patients with Crohn's disease have symptoms or active disease that is refractory to the usual therapy. Fortunately, our awareness of this group of patients with "refractory" disease is continuing to expand. The cause of the refractoriness, or failure to respond to therapy, may reside with the disease, the patient, or the physician. Refractory disease refers to a disease process that does not improve (lessen) and allow the establishment of a complete endoscopic and histological remission despite adequate doses of 5-aminosalicylic acid products and prednisone, or it is a disease process for which daily doses of adrenocortical steroids cannot be discontinued or, at least, tapered to alternate-day administration. From the patient's perspective, refractory or recalcitrant means that some troublesome symptoms persist despite therapy. The symptoms may be due to drug side effects, such as hyperadrenocorticism, or to coexistent irritable bowel syndrome (1). The physician's definition of refractory may factor in his or her frustration with failure of his or her management to eliminate the patient's complaints or to correct endoscopic, radiographical or histological abnormalities.

An organized evaluation of the individual patient with "refractory" Crohn's disease, as proffered by Professor Hanauer, will often prove useful. My own outline follows.

I. UNRESPONSIVE DISTAL COLITIS

Approximately 5% of patients with resistant ulcerative proctitis are later found to have Crohn's disease. The true nature of the colitis usually results from review of additional biopsy material or from examination of the ileum. Management would then follow the outlined approaches for steroid-resistant disease, probably including long-term topical mesalamine therapy perhaps plus immunomodulator agents (2).

II. UNCOMPLICATED DISEASE ACTIVITY

Patients with Crohn's disease limited to 20 or 30 cm of ileum and, perhaps, the cecum are expected to respond to medical therapy. If there are no complications, such as fistulas or obstruction, a remission would be expected over the course of several weeks or a few months. In a series of prepubescent adolescents, disease activity could be suppressed adequately to allow a resumption of a normal growth velocity when the disease was limited to the terminal ileum. Those youngsters grew normally while on alternate-day steroids when all signs and symptoms of disease activity were suppressed (3). As outlined in this chapter, patients would be considered "refractory" if a symptomatic remission could not be achieved with prednisone, sulfasalazine, and metronidazole therapy or if daily prednisone therapy was needed for months to maintain a remission (4).

III. EXTENSIVE DISEASE

If extensive areas of the jejunum, ileum, or colon are involved with active Crohn's disease, the usual therapy outlined above may be inadequate to control symptoms. In the prepubescent adolescents, the disease activity could not be suppressed without using daily prednisone when there was extensive small bowel or colon disease activity (3).

A. Modification of the Lumenal Contents

Total parenteral nutrition (TPN) (with or without a limited oral intake) or an elemental diet can be expected to lead to a remission of uncomplicated small bowel disease in three-fourths of patients with active disease treated for 4 to 6 weeks. The studies are not restricted to patients with refractory disease, so the response data cannot be directly translated to all patients with refractory small bowel disease. If aggressive medical therapy, often including immunomodulators, is not started, patients with previously refractory disease are expected to relapse. The time on TPN provides an opportunity to start immunomodulators. I and my colleagues used prolonged TPN (at hospital and home) to achieve a remission in 14 of 16 patients with Crohn's colitis referred for a colectomy. Azathioprine was started in six of the patients (5).

The response rate to elemental diets in patients with colonic disease is less than 30%. Defunctioning ileostomy has been used in Oxford, England, for young patients with refractory colitis rather than using immunomodulators or before they were available. Approximately 50% of the procedures were successful and the patients could be reanasto-mosed (6). Most investigators would probably use prolonged TPN and immunomodulators in that setting today.

B. Immunomodulator Therapy

Azathioprine or 6-mercaptopurine (6-MP) (1 to 1.5 mg/kg) is expected to control extensive or refractory disease in 70% of adults and in the same percentage of teenagers. Steroid sparing would also be expected in 70% of patients in whom this was the objective of the therapy. Responses would be expected in 3 to 4 months. By 4 months, 80% of the responders had improved in our series of 72 patients who could tolerate azathioprine or 6-MP. In most published series, 5% to 8% of patients are allergic to these medications or have unacceptable side effects, such as pancreatitis (7).

Methotrexate (25 mg intramuscularly once per week for 12 weeks followed by 15 mg orally or parenterally once per week) can probably be expected to cause an improvement in 50% to 60% of adults with uncomplicated disease that is refractory to the usual therapy. Some of the responders had become or were refractory to azathioprine before methotrexate therapy (8).

Cyclosporine, usually given orally, has been of some effect as a rapidly acting immunosuppressant, allowing time to institute long-term immunomodulator therapy (9).

C. Surgery

In prepubescent adolescents who do not respond to immunomodulators, resection of a grossly involved colon may permit control of the remaining disease and allow a pre-pubescent growth spurt. Surgery done after the youngster has progressed in puberty (Tanner III or IV) does not usually permit any extra growth beyond that expected from puberty itself.

Patients with extensive and refractory colitis do well after colectomy. If the ileum was normal grossly by radiography or by endoscopy, recurrence in the ileostomy is not expected in 80% or 90% of the patients. With segmental Crohn's disease, ileo-left colon anastomoses are well tolerated if there is 20 or 30 cm of relatively uninvolved rectum and sigmoid and no perianal disease.

Because patients with refractory ileitis may have a 40% chance of not having recurrent disease in the next 5 to 10 years, some patients, physicians, and surgeons prefer ileal resection rather than bowel rest (TPN) and immunomodulators. This view may become more popular since oral mesalamine trials have suggested that perhaps they can lessen the rate and severity of recurrences postoperatively. These data may apply best to patients resected for obstruction, because only 50% will recur and it usually takes 8 to 10 years before another stricture requires surgery. Patients operated on for fistulizing or perforating disease have a poorer prognosis, and repeat surgery is needed in at least one-third of patients within the ensuing 3 or 4 years.

IV. OBSTRUCTION IN THE SMALL BOWEL

Obstruction in the small bowel is the most common cause of refractory symptoms in a patient with ileal disease who had been doing well for 8 to 10 years since the onset of disease or since a previous resection for obstruction. Patients can notice the difference in symptoms, and they describe pain 1 to 2 hours after eating as well as hearing borborygmi. This is the time to consider surgical resection or stricturoplasty for the patient with ileojejunitis and multiple short skip areas of disease. This is not the time to add high doses of anti-inflammatory drugs or immunomodulators. Obtaining a "road map" for the surgeon preoperatively is essential. This should usually include small bowel radiographs, colonoscopy, and perhaps computed tomography scanning.

V. FISTULIZING OR PERFORATING DISEASE

The fact that fistulization, perforation, or abscess formation has occurred may not be obvious on initial evaluation. The presence of one or more of these complications would usually prevent a complete response to the usual medical therapy for Crohn's disease. On the other hand, a number of patients form an entero-entero or entero-colic fistula during the course of otherwise clinically easily treated disease, and the fistula is only discovered at a later time. The presence of such a fistula without an abscess or co-existent obstruction is not in itself an indication for surgery.

VI. POSTILEECTOMY DIARRHEA

Watery diarrhea that starts immediately after surgery may be due to bile salt–induced colonic secretion and respond to cholestyramine and antidiarrheal medications. Steatorrhea as a result of an extensive resection and inadequate circulating bile salts for fat digestion respond to a low-fat diet. Diarrhea and left-sided abdominal pain immediately after ileocolonic resection may be due to large volumes of fluid and bile being rapidly delivered to a spastic left colon in a patient with coexistent irritable bowel syndrome (1). Diarrhea that begins a few months after resection could be due to an aggressive recurrence of disease in the neoterminal ileum or to unappreciated colonic disease that was not noted before surgery.

VII. PERIANAL DISEASE

The presence of perianal disease is one of the most common and most troublesome causes of patients being refractory to medical therapy. Several principles may be useful. Subclinical disease activity in the colon or ileum may need to be suppressed or resected before the perianal disease can be controlled. Pain in the perianal area usually indicates that there is purulent material under pressure and some type of drainage is needed. Recurrent abscesses may be prevented by use of a surgically placed drain (seton). Antibiotic therapy, usually metronidazole or ciprofloxacin can be helpful and may suppress drainage and recurrent abscesses. Immunomodulator therapy, azathioprine or 6-MP, can be helpful in decreasing drainage and extension of the fistulizing process. Some single fistulas will close and remain closed for long periods on continued azathioprine therapy. Most rectovaginal fistulas reopen at times of diarrhea but may be tolerable if there is no interference with intercourse.

VIII. CONCLUSIONS

The patient with refractory or recalcitrant inflammatory bowel disease needs to be considered as an individual based on disease location, type, extent, responsiveness to usual therapy, coexistent irritable bowel syndrome, presence of perianal disease, previous need for surgery, and tolerance of various medications. Recent studies with budesonide, a topically active corticosteroid that is rapidly metabolized in the liver, may eventually provide more rational and safer use of long-term corticosteroids in the patient with refractory disease (10,11).

REFERENCES

1. Bayless TM, Haris ML. Inflammatory bowel disease and irritable bowel syndrome. Med Clin North Am 1990; 74:21–28.
2. Connell WR, Kamm MA, Dickson M, et al. Long term neoplasia risk after azathioprine treatment in inflammatory bowel disease. Lancet 1994; 331:842.
3. Whittington PF, Barnes HV, Bayless TM. Medical management of Crohn's disease in adolescence. Gastroenterology 1977; 72:1338–1344.
4. Brignola C, DeSimone GD, Belloli C, et al. Steroid treatment in active Crohn's disease: a comparison between two regimens of different duration. Aliment Pharmacol Ther 1994; 8:465.
5. Sitzmann JV, Converse RL Jr, Bayless TM. Favorable response to parenteral nutrition and medical therapy in Crohn's colitis. A study of 38 patients comparing severe Crohn's disease and ulcerative colitis. Gastroenterology 1990; 99:1647–1652.
6. Jewell DP, Kettlewell MGW. Split ileostomy for Crohn's colitis. In: Current Management of Inflammatory Bowel Disease. Bayless TM, Ed. Toronto: BC Decker, 1989; 294–296.
7. O'Brien JJ, Bayless TM, Bayless JA. Use of azathioprine or 6-mercaptopurine in the treatment of Crohn's disease. Gastroenterology 1991; 101:39–46.
8. Kozarek RA. Immunosuppressive therapy for inflammatory bowel disease (review). Aliment Pharmacol Ther 1993; 7:117–123.
9. Present DH. Cyclosporine and other immunosuppressive agents: current and future role in the treatment of inflammatory bowel disease. Am J Gastroenterol 1993; 88:627–630.
10. Greenberg GR, Feagan BG, Martin F, et al. Oral budesonide for active Crohn's disease. N Engl J Med 1994; 331:836.
11. Rutgeerts P, Lofberg R, Malchow H, et al. A comparison of budesonide with prednisolone for active Crohn's disease. N Engl J Med 1994; 331:842.

21
The Role of Antibiotics
in Crohn's Disease

Peter S. Margolis and Walter R. Thayer, Jr.   *Rhode Island Hospital and*
Brown University, Providence, Rhode Island

The etiology and pathogenesis of Crohn's disease (CD) remains an enigma despite extensive worldwide research. Treatment for this disabling illness remains largely empirical based on well-designed clinical trials and physician experience. Several classes of pharmacological agents are the mainstay of medical therapy: sulfasalazine or its 5-aminosalicylate derivatives, corticosteroids, and immunosuppressive agents. Because an infectious cause of CD has long been postulated, antibiotics are prescribed in an attempt to improve clinical outcome. Broad-spectrum antibiotics held promise as evidenced by Ursing and Kamme's 1975 report of a positive response in CD patients treated with metronidazole (1). Although uncontrolled, the study stimulated interest in the therapeutic role of antimicrobial agents in the treatment of CD.

Bacterial infections complicate the course of CD patients in numerous settings such as small bowel bacterial overgrowth, toxic megacolon, abscess formation, fistulas and perianal disease. Infection plays a secondary role in CD, requiring antibiotic regimens for appropriate treatment. However, a small number of agents have been used as primary therapy for active CD. This chapter provides insight into what is known about the potential role for such therapy.

I. METRONIDAZOLE

Metronidazole, the most frequently studied antibiotic in inflammatory bowel disease (IBD), is a synthetic nitroimidazole effective against some parasites and most anaerobic bacteria (2). Metronidazole was first suggested as a salutary therapeutic agent in CD by Ursing and Kamme (1). Although uncontrolled, the trial benefited five patients with CD limited to the large bowel. Allan and Cooke noted metronidazole produced only a modest improvement in diarrheal symptoms of patients with colonic CD, but promoted healing of perianal lesions and erythema nodosum (3). Results of several control trials were disputed. In 1978, Blichfeldt et al. published the first double-blind, crossover study for drug assessment (4). Twenty-two patients received metronidazole (1000 mg/day) for two months compared with a placebo-administered group, with no significant difference found in the clinical outcome. However, an increase in hemoglobin concentration and a decrease in sedimentation rate were noted in the metronidazole group. A subgroup of patients with disease limited to the colon recorded a general sense of well-being with improvement in diarrhea and abdominal pain. Although the heterogeneity of the CD population was limited, some patients concurrently took sulfasalazine and/or corticosteroids, complicating the evaluation of the overall effect of the metronidazole.

The Swedish Cooperative Crohn's Disease Study compared the efficacy of metronidazole to sulfasalazine in a double-blind, crossover trial of active CD (5,6). Patient groups differed little with respect to treatment, severity of illness, and distribution of bowel involvement. Patients served as their own control for two separate study periods of 4 months each, using metronidazole, 400 mg twice a day and sulfasalazine, 1.5 g/day. No difference in efficacy between the two therapies was noted in Phase 1. Both metronidazole and sulfasalazine treatment resulted in a substantial decline in the Crohn's Disease Activity Index (CDAI) of 149 and 137 points, respectively. Additionally, the orosomucoid plasma level was reduced in both groups, with the decline being greater in the metronidazole group. During the crossover period, metronidazole was effective in patients who failed to favorably respond to sulfasalazine, but the reverse was not found. A subgroup of patients with disease limited to the small intestine demonstrated a poor response to both medications. The authors concluded that metronidazole was slightly more effective than sulfasalazine for the treatment of CD.

A double-blind multicenter control study recently compared two doses of metronidazole (10 mg/kg per day and 20 mg/kg per day) with placebo in CD; patients received no other medication (7,8). Significant improvement in disease activity as measured by the CDAI and decrease in orosomucoid plasma levels in the treated group compared with placebo were seen; a slightly greater, but not statistically significant, effect with higher doses was noted. Again, metronidazole was more effective in patients with colonic or ileocolonic CD than in patients with disease confined to the small intestine.

Metronidazole is useful in other manifestations of CD. Disabling perianal lesions occur in 60% to 80% of patients with large intestinal disease and in 25% of those with small bowel involvement (9). Early studies showed metronidazole improved perianal disease in small numbers of patients (5). Bernstein studied 21 patients in an unblinded and uncontrolled fashion with 20 mg/kg per day of metronidazole; 19 patients had failed one or more multiple forms of medical or surgical therapy (10). Improvement in lesions was seen in 20 of 21 patients with complete to near-complete resolution in 15 of 18. In long-term follow-up dose reduction was associated with exacerbation of disease activity; reinstitution of metronidazole at full strength showed healing to occur between 1 and 4 weeks (11). Only 20% of patients remained symptom free when therapy was discontinued. Long-term use of high-dose metronidazole showed an increased incidence of paresthesia, requiring cessation of treatment in only a few individuals (11).

Many potential mechanisms of action for metronidazole are proposed, and a chemical structure review is necessary to understand its varied effects. As a nitrogenated imidazole compound, metronidazole can function as both an antibiotic and an immunosuppressant (12). As an antimicrobial, it is active against most anaerobic bacteria and protozoans for which the nitro group attached to the imidazole ring is active against. Metronidazole is absorbed by bacteria and reduced by a nitroreductase enzyme, forming short-lived metabolites that are toxic to the bacteria and cause cell death (12). The nitro group may also interfere with DNA processing causing bacterial death. A beneficial response in CD occurs because metronidazole possibly alters the gut flora or sterilizes microabscesses. Krook evaluated stool cultures of CD patients and healthy control subjects before and after treatment with metronidazole (13). When compared with those of control patients, fecal bacteroides were markedly reduced, whereas streptococci increased (13,14). Interestingly, *Clostridium difficile* has been implicated in exacerbation of idiopathic colitis, although some studies are nonsupportive (15–18). Metronidazole is effective against most species of *C. difficile*.

As an immunosuppressant, metronidazole is an imidazole which, as a group of compounds, has immunomodulatory properties (19). The imidazole ring can interfere with the mammalian DNA process, causing the helical structure to unwind with subsequent strand breakage (12). Metronidazole interferes with various aspects of cell-mediated immunity in CD. Grove et al. showed suppression of cell-mediated granuloma formation after *Schistosoma mansoni* eggs were injected into mice (20). A dose-dependent response was seen, and granulomatous inflammation decreased as metronidazole was increased. The inability of the drug to suppress skin allograft rejection suggests a selective immuno-suppressive action (20). Other phenomena associated with metronidazole use may be immunomodulatory. An increased incidence of solid tumor and malignant lymphoma can result from an inhibitory response on tumor surveillance systems (21). A cytotoxic effect on hypoxic cells as well as a direct anti-inflammatory action have been reported (2,22). Through these varied mechanisms, metronidazole might affect CD, which is granulomatous and immunological in pathogenesis.

Generally, metronidazole is well tolerated, even at high doses used for CD therapy. More frequent side effects were encountered with the 20 mg/kg dose (nausea, headach, dry mouth, metallic taste, stomatitis, gastrointestinal distress), but few patients chose to discontinue the drug (11). Transient reversible neutropenia can occur at high doses and a well-documented disulfiram-like reaction is possible; strict avoidance of alcohol consumption is strongly advised (12). Neurotoxicity ranging from paresthesia, dizziness, and ataxia to a less frequent encephalopathy may occur; most worrisome is peripheral neuropathy. Studies of patients taking high-dosage (20 mg/kg per day for 4 to 6 months) metronidazole report a 50% to 85% instance of neuropathy (11,23). When using dosages of 0.8 to 1.0 mg per day, investigators report clinical effectiveness with infrequent neuropathy (5,8,24). Stahlberg et al., using sensitive electrophysiological methods, evaluated CD patients receiving metronidazole at dosages less than 0.8 mg/kg per day for 1 year (24). Motor and sensory nerve conduction studies, distal latency, and amplitude of sensory nerve action potential were determined. All patients taking metronidazole had normal sensory conduction velocities, and electric potentials that were unchanged and were comparable to those of untreated control subjects; some reported transient paresthesias not aggravated by continued treatment at the same doseage (24).

The potential mutagenic and carcinogenic effect of long-term metronidazole therapy is of concern. Prolonged feeding of the drug or of its metabolites has been carcinogenic to laboratory animals (21). No human cases directly linking metronidazole to cancer have been reported. A retrospective follow-up study of 771 women treated with metronidazole for gynecological infection showed no appreciable increase in cancer risk (25). However, the drug dose and length of treatment was much less than that recommended for CD, and longer surveillance is required for accurate assessment. The mutagenicity in a variety of bacteria including the Ames histidine auxotrophs of *Salmonella typhimurium* is recognized (2). One study reported increased chromosomal aberrations in a small number of CD patients treated with metronidazole when compared with an untreated group (26). This was not seen in a follow-up double-blind control trial (27). No data exist to support an increased risk in humans of either carcinogenesis or mutagenesis. Metronidazole has been prescribed through all stages of pregnancy without apparent teratogenic effects; however, its use during the first trimester is not recommended (12).

II. BROAD-SPECTRUM ANTIBIOTICS

Bacterial infections for which various broad-spectrum antibiotics are used, complicate the course of CD. The role of broad-spectrum antibiotics as a primary treatment of CD is limited. Forty-four CD patients were continuously given various broad-spectrum antibiotics (generally ampicillin and tetracycline) for more than 6 months (±5 years), resulting in 93% of patients showing symptomatic and 57% radiological improvement (28). Additionally, the pretreatment steroid dose was reduced in all responsive patients. The study was uncontrolled, with several different antibiotics and doses used, and the known beneficial effect of steroid therapy could not be dismissed. Although initially promising, data were too unreliable to justify antibiotic therapy as standard treatment for CD.

Individual broad-spectrum antibiotics have shown some beneficial effects with a positive response elicited in five ulcerative colitis (UC) and one CD patient treated with vancomycin (15). All patients were positive for *C. difficile* toxin and had unabated symptoms on standard IBD therapy. Even though a role for *C. difficile* in recurrent IBD was postulated, other studies were nonconfirmatory (15,16,18,29). Oral vancomycin as an adjunctive treatment in IBD was compared with placebo in a double-blind control trial (18). Forty patients (33 UC, 7 CD) were given either oral vancomycin (500 mg every 6 hours) or placebo for 7 days along with standard medical therapy; results showed no significant difference between the two groups. However, a trend was noted toward a reduction in surgical need for UC patients receiving vancomycin. *C. difficile*, which can complicate treatment, was not isolated from any patient studied.

Ciprofloxacin, a flouroquinalone, has possible usefulness in CD therapy (30,32). Active against gram-negative organisms, ciprofloxacin is only moderately active against anaerobic bacteria when compared with metronidazole. In a small uncontrolled series, five patients with perineal CD were given ciprofloxacin; four showed improvement of symptoms and some experienced complete healing of lesions (30). A high relapse rate occurred once treatment was discontinued. Peppercom reported resolution of symptoms in four patients with active CD after ciprofloxacin was given at a dosage of 500 mg twice a day for 1 week; remission was maintained for ±6 weeks of therapy (31). Ciprofloxacin may be a viable alternative to metronidazole, and further studies are needed.

III. NONABSORBABLE ANTIBIOTICS

A study of 37 moderately ill hospitalized CD patients compared prednisolone and a normal diet to an elemental diet plus nonabsorbable antibiotics (oral framycetin, colistin, nystatin) (33). Five patients withdrew due to elemental diet intolerance. Marked improvement in objective measures and a rapid decrease in disease activity occurred in both groups. The authors concluded that the combination of nonabsorbable antibiotics plus an elemental diet was as effective as prednisolone therapy. Elemental diets alone have been proposed as primary treatment in CD, but this separate study was not performed, resulting in uncertainty of the role of nonabsorbable antibiotics (34).

IV. ANTIMYCOBACTERIAL THERAPY

The earliest and most complete description of CD was made by Dalziel, a Scottish surgeon, who described a "non-tuberculous hyperplastic enteritis" similar to other mycobacterial disease (tuberculosis, Johne's disease) (35). Crohn, Ginzburg, and Oppenheimer later noted a disease bearing a pathological resemblance to tuberculous enteritis; they and subsequent investigators attempted to isolate mycobacteria from CD tissue (36).

Burnham et al. successfully isolated a strain of *Mycobacterium kansasii* from the lymph node of a CD patient in 1978 (37). Cultures from 22 of 27 other CD specimens grew pleomorphic organisms thought to be cell wall–deficient bacteria. Chiodini et al. isolated a previously unrecognized species from two CD patients, two additional specimens were isolated but a number of cultures again grew pleomorphic organisms (38,39). DNA-DNA hybridization studies, restriction polymorphism of the ribosomal 5s gene, and random gene sequencing proved the isolated species to be *Mycobacterium paratuberculosis* (39–43). Identical organisms have subsequently been isolated by other investigators, as have pleomorphic variable acid-fast organisms (44–46).

A chromosomal repetitive insertional element, IS-900, specific for *M. paratuberculosis* has been identified by several investigators, suggesting that some pleomorphic forms are *M. paratuberculosis* (47,48). Investigators examining pleomorphic cultures from Chiodini and others found one-third contained the IS-900 insertional element. Sanderson et al. identified the IS-900 element in CD tissue via polymerase chain reaction (PCR) technique, and alluded to the possible pathogenetic significance (49). Confirmation soon followed (50).

Howel-Jones and Lennard-Jones treated seven cases of CD with isoniazid, streptomycin (antituberculous therapy), and steroids. Although some improvement was noted, the small cohort made a firm conclusion difficult (51). French investigators studied rifampin alone and rifampin combined with antimycobacterial therapy (isoniazid, ethambutol, streptomycin); rapidity of response, improvement in overall health, disappearance of intestinal symptoms, and closure of fistulas were noted. Although not a cure, a positive response with antimycobacterial therapy was elicited (52,53).

The similar pathological process of CD to mycobacterial disease and the provocative work on CD tissue mycobacteria isolation led to solitary case reports on antimycobacterial efficacy (54–56). Wirostko et al. treated CD uveitis with rifampin and found coincidental improvement of intestinal disease (57). Rifampin withdrawal was associated with exacerbation of both conditions. Dapsone, an antileprosy drug, is effective in CD therapy (58,59).

Hampson et al. used multiple antibiotics (rifampin, ethambutol, isoniazid, pyrizinamide, clofazimine) in an uncontrolled study of 20 CD cases. Seventy-one percent of patients showed significant improvement in CDAI with 90% ultimately withdrawn from steroids (60). Kohn et al. showed definitive melioration with rifampin, ethambutol, dapsone, and clofazimine in a recent control trial (61).

Chiodini et al. performed antibiotic sensitivity tests on the *M. paratuberculosis* organism, resulting in significant in vitro antibacterial activity shown by rifabutin, kanamycin, ciprofloxacin, streptomycin, and amikacin (62). Also demonstrated was that monotherapy with rifabutin alone in *M. paratuberculosis*-infected mice did not eliminate the microbe unless administered in extremely high doses—in excess of recommended human allowance (63). Rifabutin combined with kanamycin in *M. paratuberculosis*-infected monkeys led to bacterial elimination (64). Thayer et al. studied rifabutin and streptomycin in 18 patients with prolonged steroid dependency or severe extra-

TABLE 1 Controlled Trials of Antimycobacterial Agents in Crohn's Disease

Author	Reference	Medication	Results
Shaffer et al.	55	Rifampin/ethambutol vs. placebo	No significant difference
Afdhal et al.	66	Clofazimine vs. placebo	No significant difference
Elliott et al.	67	Sulphadoxine/pyrimethamine vs. placebo	No significant difference
Rutgeerts et al.	68	Rifabutin/ethambutol vs. placebo	No significant improvement in endoscopic appearance of neoterminal ileum
Kohn et al.	61	Rifampin/ethambutol/ dapsone/clofazimine vs. placebo	Definite improvement in treatment group

colonic manifestations; seven successfully completed 1 year of therapy and required no further steroid medication (65). Five patients remain on rifabutin therapy and, after 6 years, are well.

Several controlled trials of antimycobacterial chemotherapy did not confirm any significant difference in the response of CD to chemotherapeutic agents (Table 1) (55,66–68). Evidence suggests that effective treatment of mycobacteria requires at least two drugs. Early tuberculosis studies with streptomycin and rifampin alone showed that highly effective bacteriocidal antimycobacterial drugs led to the emergence of resistant strains before a therapeutic end point was reached (69). *M. paratuberculosis* appears related to the *Mycobacterium avium* complex group of mycobacteria (70). Evidence strongly indicates that infection with *M. avium* often necessitates three or four antibiotics be given for up to 2 years (71,72). A recent in vivo study suggests that clarithromycin (macrolide antibiotic), when combined with ethambutol, is effective against *M. paratuberculosis*, including the agents isolated from CD patients (73).

V. ANTIBIOTICS IN THE MANAGEMENT OF OTHER DISEASE PROCESSES

A. Bacterial Overgrowth

An interruption of the orderly aborad flow of bowel contents can lead to bacterial colonization of the small intestine, resulting in small bowel dysfunction and diarrhea. Crohn's disease predisposes the patient to bacterial overgrowth by stricture of fistula formation (74). Antibiotic treatment may be beneficial as suggested by Rutgeerts et al., who evaluated the incidence of bacterial overgrowth in nonsurgical CD patients (74). Those with abnormal breath tests were given tetracycline; improvement was noted in both the C14 breath test and bacterial overgrowth symptoms. This valuable study allowed the correct diagnosis of concurrent ileal dysfunction and bile acid malabsorption. Metronidazole, aminoglycosides, and trimethoprim-sulfate reportedly induce remission of bacterial overgrowth symptoms (75). A pilot study by Pallone et al. suggested beneficial response with either broad-spectrum or nonabsorbable antibiotics (76). Further control trials are necessary before specific recommendations can be made regarding antibiotic use in bacterial overgrowth.

B. Fistulas

Fistula formation commonly complicates the medical course of CD. As previously described, evidence supports the role of antibiotics in the treatment of perianal fistulas (10,40,77–79). Metronidazole is possibly beneficial in the management of entero-enteric and enterocutaneous fistulas but, again, further studies with antibiotics are needed to accurately assess this parameter (78).

VI. PERIOPERATIVE ANTIBIOTICS

Postoperative infections often complicate surgery for inflammatory bowel disease, mostly in CD patients with fistula, abscess, or active disease (80,81). Varying rates of abdominal wound sepsis (18%–37%) are reported (80–83). Higgins et al. noted a 38% incidence of sepsis, that is, wound infections following small bowel resection for ileal disease (81). Risk for infection at the anastomotic site increased in those patients with histological evidence of residual disease despite macroscopically free resection margins (83).

Antibiotics and mechanical bowel decontamination in colorectal surgery have significantly reduced infectious complications (84). Data on preoperative and postoperative antibiotic use in IBD surgery is conflicting, running the gamut from beneficial to non-advantageous (80,81,84,84). Consequently, the ideal perioperative antibiotic regimen awaits further delineation. Metronidazole and gentamycin given perioperatively for 5 days significantly reduced the postoperative infection rate (80,85,86).

VII. SUMMARY

A possible link between an infectious agent and CD has intrigued investigators since 1913, and while the hypothesis remains unproven, various antibiotics have been employed in an attempt to improve clinical outcome. Both control trials and clinical experience support metronidazole use in certain manifestations of CD although the mechanism of its action is unknown; fluoroquinalone, particularly ciprofloxin, have shown a possible beneficial response. Evidence suggests an etiologic role for mycobacterium in a subset of CD, but the results with antimycobacterial therapy are unconclusive. Only through intensive research will the etiology of IBD be discovered, thereby allowing technologic and therapeutic breakthroughs to improve the quality of life.

REFERENCES

1. Ursing B, Kamme C. Metronidazole for Crohn's disease. Lancet 1975; 1:775–777.
2. Linn FV, Peppercorn MA. Drug therapy for inflammatory bowel disease: Part 1. Am J Surg 1992; 164:178–185.
3. Allan R, Cooke WT. Evaluation of metronidazole in the management of Crohn's disease. Gut 1977; 18:422a.
4. Blichfeldt P, Blomhoff JP, Myhre E, et al. Metronidazole in Crohn's disease: a double-blind cross-over clinical trial. Scand J Gastroenterol 1978; 13:123–127.
5. Ursing B, Alm T, Barany F, et al. A comparative study of metronidazole and sulfasalazine for

active Crohn's disease: the Cooperative Crohn's Disease Study in Sweden. Part II. Results. Gastroenterology 1982; 82:550–562.

6. Rosen A, Ursing B, Alm T, et al. A comparative study of metronidazole and sulfasalazine for active Crohn's disease: the Cooperative Crohn's Disease Study in Sweden. Part I. Design and methodologic considerations. Gastroenterology 1982; 83:541–549.

7. Singleton J. Metronidazole is more effective than placebo in treatment of active Crohn's disease. Gastroenterology 1989; 96:A477.

8. Sutherland L, Singleton J, Sessions J, et al. Double blind, placebo controlled trial of metronidazole in Crohn's disease. Gut 1991; 31:1071–1075.

9. Parks A, Morson B, Pegum J. Crohn's disease with cutaneous involvement. Proc R Soc Med 1965; 58:241.

10. Bernstein LH, Frank MS, Brandt LJ, et al. Healing of perianal Crohn's disease with metronidazole. Gastroenterology 1980; 79:357–365.

11. Brandt LJ, Bernstein LH, Boley SS, et al. Metronidazole therapy for perianal Crohn's disease: a follow-up study. Gastroenterology 1982; 83:383–387.

12. Goodman-Gillman A, Nies A. The Pharmacological Basis of Therapeutics. 7th ed. New York: Macmillan 1985; 22:1002–1005.

13. Krook A. Microbiological and clinical studies on Crohn's disease: effects of metronidazole and salazopyrine. Acta Univ Upp Abstr Diss Sci 1980; 20:378.

14. Gilat T. Metronidazole in Crohn's disease. Gastroenterology 1982; 83:702–704.

15. LaMont J, Trnka Y. Therapeutic implications of *Clostridium difficile* toxin during relapse of chronic inflammatory bowel disease. Lancet 1980; 1:381–383.

16. Trnka, LaMont J. Association of *Clostridium difficile* toxin with symptomatic relapse in chronic bowel disease. Gastroenterology 1981; 80:693–696.

17. Meyers S, Mayer L, Bottone E, et al. Occurrence of *Clostridium difficile* toxin during the course of inflammatory bowel disease. Gastroenterology 1981; 80:697–700.

18. Dickenson RJ, O'Connor HJ, Aner I, et al. Double-blind controlled trial of oral vancomycin as adjunctive treatment in acute exacerbation of idiopathic colitis. Gut 1985; 26:1380–1384.

19. Miller J. The imidazoles as immunosuppressive agents. Transplant Proc 1980; 2:300–303.

20. Grove DI, Mahmoud AAf, Warren KS. Suppression of cell-mediated immunity by metronidazole. Int Arch Allergy Appl Immunol 1977; 54:422–427.

21. Rustia M, Shubik P. Induction of lung tumors and malignant lymphomas in mice by metronidazole. J Natl Cancer Inst 1972; 48:721–729.

22. Tanga M, Antani J, Kabade S. Clinical evaluation of metronidazole as an anti-inflammatory agent. Int Surg 1975; 60:75–76.

23. Duffy L, Daum F, Fisher S, et al. Peripheral neuropathy in Crohn's disease patients treated with metronidazole. Gastroenterology 1985; 88:681–684.

24. Stahlberg D, Barany F, Einarsson K, et al. Neurophysiologic studies of patients with Crohn's disease on long-term treatment with metronidazole. Scand J Gastroenterol 1991; 26:219–224.

25. Beard C, Noller K, O'Fallon W, et al. Lack of evidence of cancer due to metronidazole use. N Engl J Med 1979; 301:519–522.

26. Mitelman F, Hartley-As B, Ursing B. Chromosome aberrations and metronidazole. Lancet 1976; 2:802.

27. Mitelman F, Strombeck B, Ursing B. No cytogenetic effect of metronidazole. Lancet 1980; 1:1249–1250.

28. Moss AA, Carbone JV, Kressel HY. Radiologic and clinical assessment of broad-spectrum antibiotic therapy in Crohn's disease. AJR Am J Roentgenol 1978; 1331:787–790.

29. Bolton R, Sherriff R, Read A. *Clostridium difficile* associated diarrhea: a role in inflammatory bowel disease? Lancet 1980; 1:383–384.

30. Wolf J. Ciprofloxacin may be useful in Crohn's disease. Gastroenterology 1990; 98:A212.

31. Peppercorn MA. Is there a role for antibiotics as primary therapy for Crohn's ileitis? J Clin Gastroenterol 1993; 17:235–237.

32. Spirt MJ. Antibiotics in inflammatory bowel disease: new choices for an old disease. Am J Gastroenterol 1994; 89:974–978.

33. Saverymuttu S, Hodgson HJF, Chadwick VS. Controlled trial comparing prednisolone with an elemental diet plus non-absorbable antibiotics in active Crohn's disease. Gut 1985; 26:994–998.

34. O'Morain L, Segal AW, Levi AJ. Elemental diet as primary treatment of acute Crohn's disease: a controlled trial. BMJ 1980; 181:1173–1175.

35. Dalziel TK. Chronic intestinal enteritis BMJ 1913; 2:1068–1070.

36. Crohn BB, Ginzburg L, Oppenheimer G. Regional ileitis: a pathologic and clinical entity. JAMA 1932; 99:1323–1329.

37. Burnham WR, Lennard-Jones JE, Stanford JL, et al. Mycobacteria as a possible cause of inflammatory bowel disease. Lancet 1978; 2:693–696.

38. Chiodini RJ, VanKruiningen HJ, Thayer WR, et al. Possible role of mycobacteria in inflammatory bowel disease. I. An unclassified *Mycobacterium* species isolated from patients with Crohn's disease. Dig Dis Sci 1984; 29:1073–1079.

39. Chiodini RJ, VanKruiningen HJ, Thayer WR, et al. Spheroplastic phase of mycobacteria isolated from patients wtih Crohn's disease. J Clin Microbiol 1986; 24:357–363.

40. Yoshimura HH, Graham DY, Estes MK, et al. Investigation of association of mycobacteria with inflammatory bowel disease by nucleic acid hybridization. J Clin Microbiol 1987; 25:45–51.

41. Chiodini RJ. Identification of mycobacteria from Crohn's disease by restriction polymorphism of the 5s ribosomal DNA genes. In: MacDermott RP, ed. Inflammatory Bowel Disease. Current Status and Future Approach. New York: Elsevier, 1988:509–514.

42. McFadden JJ, Butcher PD, Chiodini RJ, et al. Determination of genome size and DNA homology between an unclassified *Mycobacterium* species isolated from patients with Crohn's disease and other mycobacteria. J Gen Microbiol 1987; 133:211–214.

43. McFadden JJ, Butcher PD, Chiodini RJ, et al. Crohn's disease–isolated mycobacteria are identical to *Mycobacterium paratuberculosis* as determined by DNA probes that distinguish between mycobacterial species. J Clin Microbiol 1987; 25:796–801.

44. Tytgat GN, Mulder CJ. The aetiology of Crohn's disease. Int J Colonic Dis 1986; 1:188–192.

45. Coloe P, Wilke C, Lightfoot D, et al. Isolation of a *Mycobacterium* species resembling *M. paratuberculosis* from the bowel tissue of a patient with Crohn's disease. Aust J Microbiol 1986; 7:188.

46. Gitnick GL, Collins J, Beaman B. Prospective evaluation of mycobacterial infection in Crohn's disease: isolation and transmission studies. In: MacDermott RP, ed. Inflammatory Bowel Disease. Current Status and Future Approach. New York: Elsevier, 1988:527–534.

47. Green E, Tizard M, Moss M. Sequence and characteristics of IS-900, an insertional element identified in human Crohn's disease isolate of *Mycobacterium paratuberculosis*. Nucleic Acid Res 1989; 17:9063–9073.

48. Wall S, Kunze ZM, Saboor S, et al. Identificaiton of spheroplast-like agents isolated from tissues of patients with Crohn's disease and control tissues by polymerase chain reaction. J Clin Microbiol 1993; 31:1241–1245.

49. Sanderson J, Moss M, Tizard, et al. *Mycobacterium paratuberculosis* DNA in Crohn's disease tissue. Gut 1992; 33:890–896.

50. Dell'Isolo B, Poyart C, Goulet O, et al. Maladie de Crohn, maladie infectieuse? Detection de *Mycobacterium paratuberculosis* au cours de la maladie deCrohn par amplification genique (PCR). Resultats preliminaire. Rev Med Interne 1992; 13:S401.

51. Howel-Jones J, Lennard-Jones J. Corticosteroids and corticotrophin in the treatment of Crohn's disease. Gut 1966; 7:181–187.

52. Paris J, Paris JC Simon V. Etude critique des effets de la medication antituberculeuse dans une serie de 18 cas de formes severes de maladie de Crohn. Lille Med 1975; 20:333–338.

53. Paris J, Paris JC, Claerbout JF, et al. Resultats a distance du traitement de la maladie de Crohn par medication antituberculeuse. Lille Med 1978; 23:494–496.

54. Picciotto A, Gesu GP, Schito GC, et al. Antimycobacterial chemotherapy in two cases of inflammatory bowel disease. Lancet 1988; 1:536–537.

55. Shaffer J, Hughes S, Linaker B, et al. Controlled trial of rifampicin and ethambutol in Crohn's disease. Gut 1984; 25:203–205.

56. Warren J, Rees H, Cox T. Remission of Crohn's disease with tuberculosis chemotherapy. N Engl J Med 1986; 314:182.

57. Wirostko E, Johnson L, Wirostko B. Crohn's disease. Rifampin treatment of the ocular and gut disease. Hepatogastroenterologica 1987; 34:90–93.

58. Prantera C, Argentieri R, Mangiarotti R, et al. Dapsone and remission of Crohn's disease. Lancet 1988; 1:536.

59. Ward M, McManus JPA. Dapsone in Crohn's disease. Lancet 1975; 1:1236–1237.

60. Hampson S, Parker M, Saverymuttu S, et al. Quadruple antimycobacterial chemotherapy in Crohn's disease: results at nine months of a pilot study in 20 patients. Aliment Pharmacol Ther 1989; 3:343–352.

61. Kohn A, Prantera C, Mangiaroth F. Antimycobacterial therapy and Crohn's disease: a randomized placebo controlled trial. Gastroenterology 1992; 102:A657.

62. Chiodini R, VanKruiningen HJ, Thayer WR. In vitro antimicrobial susceptibility of a *Mycobacterium sp.* isolated from patients with Crohn's disease. Antimicrob Agents Chemother 1984; 26:930–932.

63. Chiodini R, Kreeger J, Thayer WR. Use of rifabutin in treatment of systemic *Mycobacterium paratuberculosis* infection in mice. Antimicrob Agents Chemother 1993; 37:1645–1648.

64. McClure H, Chiodini R, Anderson D, et al. *Mycobacterium paratuberculosis* infection in a colony of stumptail Macaques (*Macaca arctoides*). J Infect Dis 1987; 155:1011–1019.

65. Thayer WR, Coutu JA, Chiodini RJ. Use of rifabutin and streptomycin in the therapy of Crohn's disease. In: MacDermott RP, ed. Inflammatory Bowel disease. Current Status and Future Approach. New York: Elsevier, 1988; 565–568.

66. Afdhal N, Long A, Lennon J, et al. Controlled trial of antimycobacterial therapy in Crohn's disease. Clofazimine versus placebo. Dig Dis Sci 1991; 36:449–453.

67. Elliott PR, Burnham WR, Berghouse LM, et al. Sulphadoxine-pyrimethamine therapy in Crohn's disease. Digestion 1982; 23:132–134.

68. Rutgeerts P, Geboes M, VanTrappen G, et al. Treatment of severe recurrence of Crohn's disease in the neoterminal ileum with rifabutin and ethambutol. J Clin Gastroenterol 1992; 15:24–28.

69. Raleigh J. Chemotherapy of tuberculosis. In: Kubica GP, Wayne LG, eds. The Mycobacteria: A Source Book. Vol. 15. New York: Dekker, 1984:1007–1020.

70. Chiodini RJ. Characterization of *Mycobacterium paratuberculosis* and organisms of the *Mycobacterium avium* complex by restriction polymorphism of the DNA gene region. *J Clin Microbiol* 1990; 28:489–494.

71. Yeager H, Raleigh J. Pulmonary disease due to *Mycobacterium intracellulare*. Am Rev Respir Dis 1973; 108:547–552.

72. Izeman M, Carpe R, O'Brien R, et al. Disease due to *Mycobacterium avium intracellulare*. Chest 1987; 87:129S–149S.

73. Rastogi N, Goh K, Labrousse V. Activities of clarithromycin compared with those of other drugs against *Mycobacterium paratuberculosis* and further enhancement of its extracellular and intracellular activities by ethambutol. Antimicrob Agents Chemother 1992; 36:2843–2846.

74. Rutgeerts P, Ghoos Y, VanTrappen G, et al. Ileal dysfunction and bacterial overgrowth in patients with Crohn's disease. Eur J Clin Invest 1981; 11:199–206.

75. Sherman PM. Bacterial overgrowth. In: Yamada T, ed. Textbook of Gastroenterology. New York: JB Lippincott, 1991:1530–1539.

76. Pallone F, Boirivant M, Fais S, et al. Antibacterial drugs in Crohn's disease. Ital J Gastroenterol 1992; 24(suppl 2):17–18.

77. Allan A, Keighley M. Management of perianal Crohn's disease. World J Surg 1988; 12:198–202.

78. Jakobovitis J, Schuster M. Metronidazole therapy for Crohn's disease and associated fistulae. Am J Gastroenterol 1984; 79:533–540.

79. Turanen U, Farkkile M, Valtonen V, et al. Longterm outcome of ciprofloxacin treatment in severe perianal or fistulous Crohn's disease. Gastroenterology 1993; 104:A793.

80. Ambrose NS, Alexander-Williams J, Keighley MRB. Audit of sepsis in operations for inflammatory bowel disease. Dis Colon Rectum 1984; 27:602–604.

81. Higgins C, Allan R, Keighley M, et al. Sepsis following operation for inflammatory intestinal disease. Dis Colon Rectum 1980; 23:102–105.

82. Becker J, Alexander D. Colectomy, mucosal proctectomy, and ileal pouch anal anastomosis. Ann Surg 1991; 213:242–247.

83. Simi M, Leardi S, Minervini S, et al. Early complications after surgery for Crohn's disease. Neth J Surg 1990; 42:105–109.

84. Alexander D, Becker J. Cefoxitin disposition in colorectal surgery. Ann Surg 1988; 208:162–168.

85. Hares M, Bentley S, Allan R, et al. Clinical trials on the efficacy and duration of antibacterial cover for elective resection in inflammatory bowel disease. Br J Surg 1982; 69:215–217.

86. Keighley M. Infection and the use of antibiotics in Crohn's disease. Can J Surg 1984; 27:438–441.

Commentary

Cosimo Prantera   *Ospedale Nuovo Regina Magherita, Rome, Italy*

Antibiotics are used worldwide in the treatment of Crohn's disease; there is no doubt that their use is helpful and, in some patients, decisive for improving symptoms and inducing remission of active phases.

Unfortunately, we do not know exactly how or why they are successful. One first explanation is that bacteria play a secondary role in perpetuating the inflammatory process after the primary agents of Crohn's disease have broken through the epithelial barrier, thus inducing the initial lesion. In this context, the antibacterial action of the antibiotics could influence symptoms and the secondary pathologic condition. A second hypothesis is that one or different bacterial species are the primary cause of Crohn's disease and that their eradication could, therefore, induce not only the remission of symptoms but also the healing of the disease itself.

So far, no drug has definitely been shown to have therapeutic efficacy on the lesions of Crohn's disease; such efficacy would be a clue indicating that the cause of Crohn's disease is in some way being affected. Similarly, no bacterium has unequivocally been shown to be a causative agent of Crohn's disease.

The search for a single causative agent has been hindered by the fact that Crohn's disease is probably a melting pot of different pathologic conditions and of various etiological agents acting via different pathological routes. Some Crohn's disease patients experience a complete regression of their lesions—either without any apparent reason or following treatment; but this happens so rarely that when there is permanent complete regression of all the lesions there is a strong suspicion of wrong diagnosis. Permanent healing can sometimes be seen in cases of initial and mild disease, but when it occurs after antibiotic therapy in chronic, refractory forms, then it would appear that the antibiotic has acted on a bacterium that is the primary cause of lesion.

From the results of clinical practice in which antibiotics are used, it can be deduced that any bacterium considered to be a putative cause of Crohn's disease should have certain characteristics. First, this hypothetical bacterium should be resistant to several different antibiotics, and it is therefore unlikely that it could be combatted by one antibiotic alone. Second, the bacterium should show little response to short- or medium-term treatment. And, third, it could easily develop resistance to the antibiotic during treatment, and relapses could therefore occur after its suspension.

Unfortunately, no controlled trial has ever been carried out taking these bacterial characteristics into consideration. Certain chemotherapeutic drugs such as ciprofloxacin, metronidazole, some antimycobacterials, and other antibiotics with high fecal concentration should be experimented with in multiple combinations and for long periods of time. But, inasmuch as treatment with multiple antibiotics for long periods can give rise to a large number of side effects, these can only be accepted if the therapy leads to complete regression of all anatomical lesions, thus probably confirming the action of the drugs on the primary cause of disease. Finally, in the selection of patients for such research, the clinicopathological and immunological characteristics leading to suspect those of bacterial origin of Crohn's disease should be considered.

22
Pregnancy and Fertility in Crohn's Disease

Daniel H. Present   *Mount Sinai School of Medicine, New York, New York*

Crohn's disease is a chronic inflammatory disorder that can affect the entire gastrointestinal tract. It occurs predominantly in young adults with peak occurrences in the second to third decade of life. Because these are the main childbearing ages, data regarding pregnancy in Crohn's disease patients are vital in terms of future quality of life issues and medical management. Unfortunately, there are few case-controlled trials and no prospective therapeutic trials of pregnancy in patients with Crohn's disease.

The ability to distinguish ulcerative colitis from Crohn's disease has improved over the years; however, these entities may have been confused and 10% of patients with only colonic involvement of disease are still classified as "indeterminate." This potential error as well as lack of information regarding smoking, physician advice regarding conception, and variability in medical management leaves much uncertainty regarding physician recommendations. This chapter reviews current data regarding genetics and inheritance, fertility, influence of inflammatory bowel disease on pregnancy, influence of pregnancy on inflammatory bowel disease, current medical therapy before and during pregnancy, advice on delivery, and the influence of surgical management on pregnancy in Crohn's disease. Controlled trials that will provide more accurate answers to this often difficult management problem are needed.

I. GENETICS AND INHERITANCE

Extensive data indicate that a major risk of developing Crohn's disease is to have a family history of inflammatory bowel disease. The frequency of occurrence in such patients ranges from 6% to 33% (1). First degree relatives appear to have a ten-fold increased risk of developing Crohn's disease. The disease is more common among Jews, especially those whose ancestry is in middle Europe. Recent studies have provided some data that may be useful in genetic counseling. The lifetime risk of developing Crohn's disease in a first degree relative of non-Jewish probands is 5.2% (risk to siblings of 7.0%, to parents of 4.8%, to offspring of 0%) (2). The lifetime risk is increased in Jewish probands to 7.8% overall (risk to siblings of 16.8%, to parents of 3.8% to offspring of 7.4%).

In ulcerative colitis, the risks are lower in both Jews and non-Jews; however, some studies disagree with this finding and show a similar risk for ulcerative colitis. Identical twin studies have shown increased monozygotic twin concordance rates in ulcerative colitis but more so in twins with Crohn's disease. Another study reporting on 19 husbands and wives with inflammatory bowel disease showed an incidence of inflammatory bowel disease in 36% of the children, with an increased proclivity toward Crohn's disease, especially when the parents were concordant for Crohn's disease (3). Although it is a unique situation when both parents have inflammatory bowel disease, in future marriages, couples with inflammatory bowel disease should be alerted to the marked potential increased risk to their children of developing inflammatory bowel disease.

Recently developed animal mouse models should provide an important resource for genetic studies. Thus far, there is no evidence for a single mendelian model for Crohn's disease. Other hypothetical possibilities are that two or more major genes act together to predispose the person to inflammatory bowel disease and that ulcerative colitis and Crohn's disease are a genetically heterogeneous group of disorders that share a common clinical end point of gastrointestinal inflammation. Gene mapping studies may determine the genetic origin of Crohn's disease.

When couples request advice on the risk to their children of developing inflammatory bowel disease, they should also be informed that, in addition to the genetic pattern, there are also significant environmental factors to be considered. These include smoking, geographic variations, seasonality of conception, and infectious agents (4). Much remains to be learned before accurate extensive advice can be dispensed to propective parents.

II. FERTILITY IN CROHN'S DISEASE PATIENTS

Crohn's disease patients often ask whether they are able to conceive and whether their offspring will be normal.

Initial descriptive reports were flawed in that they lacked important data and failed to adjust for factors such as whether women were attempting to conceive, what were the methods of birth control, and whether their physicians advised against having children. Other neglected factors related to the duration of observations, severity of bowel disease, and fertility of the husband. Any of these factors might result in a voluntary decrease in fertility rather than a disease-related impairment.

There have been several reviews of the early descriptive reports noting clearly that the prior data was conflicting. Crohn et al. suggested that fertility was not impaired, whereas Fielding and Cooke in 1970 reported that one-third of married women with Crohn's disease were infertile (5,6). DeDombal et al. in 1972 described fertility problems in more than 50% of married women (7). The authors noted that there was greater infertility in Crohn's colitis compared with infertility in patients with ileitis or ileocolitis, but they failed to exclude patients who were taking contraceptives. However, it was noted that, after surgery, the ability to conceive increased and, therefore, many of these patients were not truly infertile. The authors used the term "subfertile" in patients who had active disease.

Homan and Thorbjarnarson's study in 1976 also showed a decrease in the frequency of pregnancy compared with that of control subjects, but only in women with small intestinal disease and not in patients with ileocolitis and colitis (8). Vender and Spiro's recalculation of these data confirmed statistical significance. It was not noted whether patients with small bowel disease were malabsorbing and nutritional factors may have played an important role.

In a series by Khosla et al. 112 married women younger than age 45 years were evaluated; the infertility rate was lower (12%) than in prior studies and was similar to that observed in the general population (10). Infertility also seemed to be related to colonic involvement. A larger case-controlled trial by Mayberry and Weterman in 1986 matched 275 Crohn's disease patients with women of the same age (11). More data were provided in terms of marital status and obstetrical history. This study noted that there was a significant reduction in both fertility and pregnancy in women between the ages of 18 and 45 years in whom Crohn's disease developed. The number of children born after diagnosis was 0.4 in Crohn's disease patients compared with 0.7 in control subjects. The authors could find no correlation with site of disease, nor was it related to the rate of miscarriage. The authors also noted that although medical advice against conception may play a role, Crohn's disease patients practiced less contraception than control subjects and there was still a decreased ability to conceive (42%) compared with controls (28%). The conclusion of this European survey was that Crohn's disease in women results in "subfertility."

In another controlled study by Baird et al. 177 Crohn's disease patients were compared with 84 women with ulcerative colitis and 216 control subjects (12). Patients with inflammatory bowel disease whose first pregnancy occurred after onset of disease symptoms had fewer total pregnancies than control subjects, whereas women whose first pregnancies occurred before the onset of symptoms had the same total number of pregnancies as control subjects. There was, therefore, reduced fertility but it was suggested that it was the patient's choice and not due to disease impairment. Many patients voluntarily limited their conception because of fear of exacerbation of symptoms and because of medication difficulties or because they had been told not to become pregnant by their physician. An increased use of oral contraceptives or intrauterine devices (IUDs) was observed in women diagnosed with Crohn's disease compared with control subjects, confirming once again that some patients avoid pregnancy after disease onset. Other factors may diminish the desire for pregnancy, such as the occurrence of perianal disease with abscesses and fistula, especially with fistula to the vagina and labia as well as the rectum. This may result in dyspareunia, difficulty with hygiene, and an overall decrease in interest in or fear of sexual relations. Other factors leading to subfertility may include fallopian tube obstruction and nutritional deficiency. In conclusion, fertility is reduced in women with Crohn's disease for multiple reasons.

There have been few studies of infertility in men with Crohn's disease. Sulfasalazine decreases spermatozoa count and alters their motility, with an increased number of abnormal spermatozoa forms. However, in a fertility study by Burnell, of 70 men with Crohn's disease who were compared with age-matched control subjects, there was a significant decrease in family size regardless of whether the patients took sulfasalazine or steroids (12a). Control patients had 2.3 children compared with male Crohn's disease patients who produced 1.6 children. Once again, this may be related to other factors, such as an increased use of contraception or a desire not to increase family size because of fear of future disability. The authors concluded that further studies are needed to prospectively compare quality of spermatozoa, independent of medications and correlating with and without perineal fistulization. A more recent study in 106 men with Crohn's disease who were contrasted with colitis patients and normal patients showed that the overall reproductive capacity of men with inflammatory bowel disease was not markedly diminished (13).

III.   INFLUENCE OF CROHN'S DISEASE ON PREGNANCY

Multiple reviews have attempted to determine the effect of Crohn's disease on pregnancy outcome. Initial case reports were pessimistic as to pregnancy outcome; however, in the first series by Crohn et al. 84 patients with only small bowel involvement had a pregnancy survival rate of almost 90% (5). This rate was similar to that seen in normal populations, and Crohn's disease was noted to be deleterious only for pregnancies in which the disease developed during the gestation period. The latter data were confirmed in a report by Martinbeau in which there was a mortality in over 55% of 11 infants in which the disease developed in the mother during pregnancy (14). Almost 15 years later, the next studies appeared as summarized in 1982 both by Vender and Spiro and by Jarnerot and Into-Malmberg (9, 15). The latter review included data from six studies, including 388 pregnancies in Crohn's disease patients. This information was contrasted with that of 1155 pregnancies in ulcerative colitis patients. There were normal births in 83% in Crohn's disease patients (83% in ulcerative colitis), congenital abnormalities in 1.2% (1.1% in ulcerative colitis), spontaneous abortions in 11% (9.1% in ulcerative colitis), and stillbirths in 2% in both groups. Outcomes are similar as those for a normal population, except when the disease appears for the first time during pregnancy. A further update on 746 pregnancies in nine studies in Crohn's disease patients by Miller showed similar results (16). Normal babies were observed in 83% of pregnancies, directly comparable with the normal population. Miller noted that the coexistence of severe disease may increase the risk of spontaneous abortions (twice as likely), stillbirths, and premature deliveries.

Most recent case-controlled studies have revealed similar results with some minor differences. In a case-controlled retrospective analysis of 82 pregnancies in ulcerative colitis and Crohn's disease patients, Porter and Stirrat suggested that neither disease had a major effect on pregnancy outcome (17). Birth weight was statistically less in babies born to women with Crohn's disease, but there was no effect on pregnancy duration or mode of delivery. Low birth weight was not affected by the state of disease at onset of pregnancy, the need for medication, or whether Crohn's disease deteriorated during gestation. The number of premature deliveries was increased in women with Crohn's disease, but not significantly. Other studies have also found an increase in premature deliveries, noting the danger in pregnancy if there is a marked deterioration in the inflammatory bowel disease, especially if surgery is required (18). However, the authors also noted that deterioration occurred no more frequently than in women with Crohn's disease who were not pregnant and that symptoms in approximately 30% of all patients exacerbate during a 9 to 12 month period. Another retrospective controlled trial by Fedorkow et al. in 98 patients also showed a statistically higher preterm delivery rate than in control subjects (19). Exacerbations, especially in the first trimester, increased the risk of preterm delivery.

In a final matched controlled trial in 177 women with Crohn's disease, the data showed no risk of loss of pregnancy except in those patients with the subset of severe active disease (12). There was a statistically significant increased risk of preterm births, not always correlated with active disease. The authors note that preterm delivery occurs in Crohn's disease before the onset of symptoms, which may represent a nutritional or immunological factor affecting pregnancy. Smoking protected against preterm birth in patients with ulcerative colitis but not in women with Crohn's disease.

In conclusion, the treating physician can be sanguine about the outcome of pregnancy in Crohn's disease patients. Congenital abnormalities, spontaneous abortions, and still-births occur in a similar percentage as in the general population, except when there is increased inflammatory activity of the disease. Obstetrical management should be the same as for patient's without inflammatory bowel disease, except cesarean section may be preferred when there is severe perianal disease.

IV. INFLUENCE OF PREGNANCY ON INFLAMMATORY BOWEL DISEASE

Many studies looking into the effect of pregnancy on inflammatory bowel disease have used Abramson's four-group classification (20). Group 1 is made up of patients with known Crohn's disease that is quiescent at the time of conception. In Group 2, disease is active at conception. Group 3 patients are those in whom Crohn's disease develops for the first time during pregnancy, and Group 4 patients develop Crohn's disease for the first time in the puerperium. Using these criteria, the initial report by Crohn et al. on women with small bowel disease reveals that 62% in Group 1 complete a pregnancy without relapse and a greater number of women improved rather than worsened in Group 2 pregnancies (5). They concluded that pregnancy in Crohn's ileitis was not as much of a problem as it was in ulcerative colitis. The subsequent literature varied between unfavorable and favorable reports (the latter in most cases). Fielding and Cooke reported easy control of Crohn's disease during pregnancy, and deDombal et al. noted a relapse rate of only 10% (6,7). Khosla et al. using Abramson's criteria, reported that 44 of 52 (85%) patients in Group 1 stayed in remission during pregnancy and seven out of eight relapses occurred in the first trimester. In Miller's 1986 review, of 186 inactive patients who became pregnant, 73% (61%–91%) remained in remission (16). These relapse rates are statistically similar to those seen in nonpregnant women with Crohn's disease. When relapse occurs, it is primarily in the first trimester, with some reports noting a higher relapse rate in the puerperium.

In Group 2 patients, the outcome is not as good. In the series by Khosla et al., disease in 13 of 20 (65%) patients either stayed active or worsened during the course of the pregnancy (10). In Miller's review of three large series of 93 pregnancies, approximately one-third worsened, one-third continued with active disease, and one-third improved (16).

The overall conclusion is that in two-thirds of patients with active Crohn's disease who become pregnant, the disease stays persistently active during the pregnancy. This may not be the recent experience of many gastroenterologists who are treating these patients more aggressively with 5-aminosalicylic acid agents (5-ASA), antibiotics, steroids, and immunosuppressives. There is great need for a prospective trial of outcome that stratifies current therapeutic modalities. There are limited data with regard to Group 3 patients whose onset occurs during pregnancy. There appears to be a poor prognosis, especially for the fetus. Postpartum exacerbations appear to follow a similar course as the usual Crohn's disease exacerbation. As regards the prognosis for subsequent pregnancies, Vender and Spiro state that, although there are limited data in ulcerative colitis, there are no studies in Crohn's disease patients to provide a recommendation (9). However, Korelitz reports that there is no evidence that the course of the inflammatory bowel disease will be the same in subsequent pregnancies (21). My personal experience agrees with the latter opinion, so that, although a patient may have had difficulties during a prior pregnancy, there is no reason to discourage future pregnancies, especially when conception is being attempted during a clinical remission. Although there are several reports studying pregnancies associated with severe ulcerative colitis, there are little data on fulminant Crohn's disease in pregnancy, and, therefore, no conclusions can be made regarding clinical outcome (22).

In conclusion, conception occurring at the time a patient is in remission is usually successful and results in a small percentage of exacerbations. Conception at the time of disease activity results in persistent activity or worsening in two-thirds of cases. In this situation, the Crohn's disease should be treated aggressively. Therapeutic abortions are rarely required. Therefore, in long-term planning for women with Crohn's disease, they should be encouraged to conceive only when the disease is quiescent.

V. MEDICATIONS IN PREGNANCY

There are several general considerations regarding the administration of medications to pregnant Crohn's disease patients. Most drugs do cross the placenta, and although pregnant women usually want to avoid all drugs during pregnancy, they sometimes take medications for several weeks before they are aware of the gestation. The basic concept in medicating is to give Crohn's disease patients as little medication as possible while maintaining control of the disease. However, higher doses may be required to induce and maintain remission. Recommendations as to drug usage and dosage are often theoretical and lack controlled clinical experience. Animal studies demonstrating teratogenesis may not apply to humans. Alteration in maternal physiology (delayed gastric emptying, decreased gastric acidity, enhanced hepatic metabolism) may alter the effect of medication (23). Furthermore, toxicity may not be evident early after administration of medication and may require long-term observation to be identified.

Few studies have been done on the effect of pregnancy when the male partner is receiving medications. There has been a clear decline in the semen volume and spermatozoa count in studies performed in semen over the last 50 years (24). This may be due to environmental factors, especially the ingestion of drugs. Despite the scarcity of data, it has been shown that many drugs are excreted into semen and may play a role in fertility and teratogenesis.

A. Nonspecific Symptomatic Medications

Prior reports on aspirin ingestion show conflicting data regarding teratogenesis and, although high doses are associated with prolonged pregnancy and labor and increased blood loss, low doses may be of value in coagulation disorders, such as deep vein thrombosis. In the latter situation, the benefits may outweigh the risks later in pregnancy. Although there are no definite data to restrict the use of aspirin for potential teratogenesis or the risk of stillbirth in premature labor, there is the risk of intracranial bleeding and the possibility of pulmonary hypertension. The latter requires caution and an appropriate indication for the use of aspirin. Approximately 20% of the maternal dose of salicylate passes into breast milk.

On the other hand, neither paracetamol nor aspirin, which can be given for pain control, has been associated with congenital malformations (23). There is no contra-indication to the ingestion of these drugs during breast-feeding. Prostaglandins play a significant role in the development of the fetus, and nonsteroidal anti-inflammatory drugs (NSAIDs) are contraindicated, especially during the third trimester, for fear of their effects on fetal blood vessels, which may result in pulmonary hypertension. Likewise, the safety of NSAIDs in nursing mothers is in doubt; therefore, they should not be ingested during nursing. Many other widely used drugs have all been investigated in a large series of more than 6500 infants and have not been shown to be associated with congenital disorders (25).

B. Sulfasalazine and 5-Aminosalicylic Acid Agents

Sulfasalazine (Azulfidine) consists of sulfapyridine linked to 5-ASA (mesalamine) by an azo bond that is cleaved by colonic bacteria. The active agent (5-ASA) is released predominantly in the colon. As discussed, sulfasalazine can cause reversible male infertility (oligospermia, decreased motility, and increased abnormal forms of spermatozoa) (26). Discontinuation of sulfasalazine or switching to an oral or rectal 5-ASA preparation reverses the abnormalities within 3 months and is often followed by pregnancies. Multiple studies have demonstrated no harmful effect on pregnancy with the use of sulfasalazine, whether the patient is treated for active disease or prophylaxis. There has been no statistically significant increase in spontaneous abortions or congenital malformations. A national survey in inflammatory bowel disease patients comparing the use of sulfasalazine and steroids showed no difference in outcome compared with outcome of untreated women (27). In fact, there was a decreased incidence of prematurity, spontaneous abortions, and developmental birth defects compared with that of the general population. Serum concentrations of sulfasalazine and sulfapyridine are similar in both mothers and children at delivery. There is no significant transfer of sulfasalazine in breast milk, but the concentration of sulfapyridine in breast milk is approximately 45% of maternal serum. The bilirubin displacing capacity is negligible, and there is no increased risk of kernicterus in the child (28). Therefore, the drug can be safely used during nursing.

There is no contraindication to the use of sulfasalazine during pregnancy. Conversely, the drug should be maintained as prophylaxis throughout the pregnancy and postpartum period. A major error in management of Crohn's disease is to discontinue this drug in the last trimester because such action may result in postpartum exacerbation of disease.

The newer 5-ASA (mesalamine) agents contain the same ingredient as sulfasalazine without the sulfapyridine. They are coated and released in various areas of the small and large bowel. Clinical data show that they are effective agents in the treatment of active Crohn's disease (29, 30). Furthermore, there is statistically significant evidence from meta-analysis that the 5-ASA drugs are effective in maintaining remission in patients with Crohn's disease (31). All patients with Crohn's disease, then should be continuously taking these agents at all phases of activity. Thus far, animal reproductive studies have not demonstrated a fetal risk, but there are no prospective controlled studies in pregnant women. Several uncontrolled studies have reported on more than 100 pregnancies in both ulcerative colitis and Crohn's disease patients taking 5-ASA drugs (32–34). These limited data suggest that oral 5-ASA is safe in the management of active inflammatory bowel disease during pregnancy and can protect against recurrences without damaging the fetus. There have been no reports of increased fetal abnormalities associated with 5-ASA delivered topically by enema or suppository. Studies showed 5-ASA concentration to be lower in fetal than maternal plasma, although acetyl-5-ASA had similar levels of concentration (35). Calculations of the total dose of 5-ASA received by the newborn indicate that, in conventionally used doses, 5-ASA preparations are without risk to the fetus and newborn. There have been scattered rare allergic diarrheal reactions in infants who received 5-ASA transferred through nursing. Further extensive studies are awaited, but, in view of the prophylactic nature of these agents, they should not be discontinued during pregnancy and can be used in the postpartum nursing period.

C. Steroids

Based on animal data, there has been some concern regarding the use of steroids during pregnancy. Mice have a significant increase in the incidence of cleft palate, especially after high doses of steroids are administered early in pregnancy. Increased abortion rates and decreased litter size in other animals have also been noted. In humans, steroids readily cross the placenta, but cortisol is rapidly converted to the more inactive cortisone, with fetal circulation concentration being only 10% of that of the mother's circulation. Prednisone and prednisolone poorly cross into the fetal circulation, and it is rare to observe pituitary–adrenal axis suppression. The literature varies in looking at outcomes of pregnancy when steroids are used in patients with inflammatory bowel disease (9). ACTH has been used successfully in a small series with no negative effects on pregnancy or the fetus (36). Other studies have reported a reduction in birth weight and an increased number of stillbirths, but much clinical information was not made available. Most publications, whether they are reporting on patients with inflammatory bowel disease or other disorders requiring steroids (systemic lupus erythematosus, rheumatoid arthritis, asthma) are more positive. As was noted in a survey of 531 pregnancies in patients with inflammatory bowel disease, the complication rate was increased with severe Crohn's disease, although this was thought to be due to disease-related activity and not medication. The incidence of underweight infants, spontaneous abortions, prematurity, and congenital defects was not increased. Only one child was born with a cleft palate. In general, patients taking corticosteroids should be given increased doses during labor and delivery. As regards nursing, the amount of steroids received by the infant is minimal. However, there are no reports of use of more than 30 mg per day, and caution should be used when higher dosages are given.

In summary, use of steroids appears to be safe during pregnancy, and the risk of continued active disease in the mother is considered to be greater than any risk to the fetus.

D. Antibiotics

There is frequent need during pregnancy for the use of antibiotics for intercurrent infections. Although there is wide variation in types and dosages of antibiotics given in different stages of gestation, due to dosage differences and stage of gestation, almost all antibiotics pass through the placenta to the fetus. There have been few rigorous controlled trials of antibiotics in pregnancy. Ampicillin, the cephalosporins and erythromycin are generally considered safe in pregnancy (37). Several antibiotics carry a potentially toxic risk to the fetus or neonate. These include sulfonamides, which increase the risk of kernicterus in neonates and, therefore, should not be given late in pregnancy. Tetracyclines bind to developing fetal teeth and are containdicated. Nitrofurantoin may cause hemolysis, and trimethoprim-sulfamethoxazole may increase the teratogenic risk.

Although broad-spectrum antibiotics are anecdotally used for treatment of Crohn's disease, metronidazole has been shown to be effective in controlled trials in the treatment of active Crohn's disease. Efficacy is especially seen in the colon as well as in perianal fistula. Metronidazole crosses the placenta and enters the fetal circulation rapidly. It is a known carcinogen in rodents, causing pulmonary, hepatic, and mammary tumors. Consequently, its use during human pregnancy has been questioned. Reproductive studies in animals have shown no impairment in fertility. There are no well-controlled trials in human pregnancies, but there has been no pattern of congenital defects, and, in several reports, there has been no apparent deleterious effect to the fetus. A small number of studies have suggested an increased abortion rate and malformations if metronidazole is used in the first trimester of pregnancy. Long-term follow-up studies of pregnant women treated with metronidazole for trichomonal vaginitis have shown no increase in complications compared with matched control subjects (38). The drug appears in high concentrations in breast milk, and discontinuation of nursing is advised. The conclusion of most studies is that metronidazole is safe in the second and third trimesters of pregnancy, but data are inconclusive for the first trimester. There are no data regarding patients with Crohn's disease in whom higher dosages are used for more prolonged periods.

Ciprofloxacin HCl has recently been used either alone or in combination with metronidazole in the treatment of active Crohn's disease or perianal fistula. Data from the manufacturing pharmaceutical company and investigators are limited (39). Although I know of no conclusive implication of ciprofloxacin in fetal death, increased abortion rates, or congenital abnormalities, more information is required before chronic use can be advised for Crohn's disease patients. Ciprofloxacin is excreted in breast milk and is not recommended for postpartum use because its effect in nursing infants is uncertain.

E. Immunosuppressives

Six-mercaptopurine and azathioprine have shown efficacy in controlled and uncontrolled trials in the therapy of active Crohn's disease with steroid-sparing effects as well as the healing of perianal and internal fistula (40). Similar efficacy has been demonstrated in the maintenance of remission after there has been a therapeutic response to either drug. Azathioprine and 6-mercaptopurine have shown teratogenicity in rats, whereas azathioprine alone has shown no teratogenicity in rats but has shown this effect in rabbits and some mice. Chromosomal abnormalities have occasionally been observed in adults and in two children; these abnormalities disappeared after 20 and 32 months, respectively. Although the drugs cross the placenta in humans, there has been no teratogenicity observed. Azathioprine is also transmitted through breast milk.

Pregnancy has been successful in women with chronic renal disease who take azathioprine as well as in women receiving immunosuppressive therapy for systemic lupus erythematosus. There does not appear to be any impairment of fertility with use of these agents. A summary of the literature showed no increased incidence of congenital anomalies among offspring of patients with systemic lupus erythematosus receiving prednisone or azathioprine (41). These data are similar to those in women with renal transplants who were taking these drugs (42).

In a small series of 14 pregnancies, azathioprine was maintained throughout the pregnancy in seven of the patients, and there was no evidence of increased premature deliveries, perinatal problems, or congenital abnormalities. Further close observation showed no increase in childhood infections or neoplasia (43). A case-controlled study in 74 patients showed no increased number of premature deliveries, miscarriages, or congenital abnormalities (44).

In summary, clinical experience suggests that azathioprine and 6-mercaptopurine are safe at the time of conception and when the drug is maintained throughout the pregnancy. There are no data on their effect during nursing.

Methotrexate has recently been shown to be effective in chronic Crohn's disease, with significant steroid-sparing effect when high doses are administered. Oligospermia is observed during treatment with methotrexate in men, and the drug is contraindicated during pregnancy because there is a high incidence of chromosomal abnormalities and teratogenicity (45). Patients are advised to discontinue methotrexate at least 3 to 4 months before attempting conception. The drug is also contraindicated during nursing.

F. Cyclosporin

Cyclosporin has shown efficacy in both controlled and uncontrolled trials in active Crohn's disease. Closure of fistulas has been dramatic in several uncontrolled reports. Long-term maintenance of remission has been unsuccessful using oral cyclosporin.

There has been limited experience with use of cyclosporin in pregnancy in auto immune disorders. However, in registries of transplant patients, although the incidence of prematurity is high (58%) and the birth weight is low (38%), survival of the infant was greater than 90% (46). The outcome in male transplant patients who are taking cyclosporin and who impregnate women is similar to that of the general population. There are no data that suggest specific congenital malformations or induction of birth defects with use of cyclosporin. The increased incidence of complications seen in these patients is thought to be likely due to the organ transplantation. The active ingredient in cyclosporin is expressed in breast milk, and breast-feeding is not advised. A recent report has suggested that the presence of cyclosporin throughout pregnancy has only a minimal effect on fetal immune development and concludes that children exposed to cyclosporin in utero are not likely to be at risk for immune deficiency or long-term autoimmunity (47). There are no data available regarding pregnancy in patients with inflammatory bowel disease.

VI. DELIVERY

Plans for delivery of patients with Crohn's disease should be the same as for the normal population, except when there is perianal disease (perineal or rectovaginal fistula). In this situation, delivery by cesarean sections should be strongly considered, and episiotomy, in particular should be avoided.

VII. DIAGNOSTIC STUDIES

There is no contraindication to a limited endoscopic evaluation (flexible sigmoidoscopy) of the colon during pregnancy. Colonoscopy may occasionally be performed but should generally be avoided. Upper endoscopy is safe during pregnancy, and almost all endoscopic procedures can be performed with no sequelae.

Radiographic examinations are potentially harmful to the fetus, but the amount of exposure required for diagnosis in a patient with inflammatory bowel disease is usually not significant. Limited radiographic studies can be performed when there is an appropriate clinical indication. Barium enemas should be avoided because of their excessive radiation.

VIII. SURGERY

Patients who have undergone surgery for Crohn's disease are capable of delivering normal children. In the study by Nielson et al., patients who underwent bowel resection had a slightly increased risk of delivering a premature baby compared with nonresected women (18). Other series have shown no difference in live births compared with the general population after patients had undergone a resection for Crohn's disease. After total colectomy and ileostomy, pregnancy is possible, but fertility may be reduced. When conception occurred in patients who underwent a total colectomy, the pregnancy proceeded without incidence, and approximately one-third of patients required delivery by cesarean section.

IX. SUMMARY

Despite their subfertility, most women with Crohn's disease can expect to have normal pregnancies and deliveries, and the gastroenterologist can treat the disease in a normal manner. For the most part, medications can be used in a similar manner as to when there is no pregnancy. Most drugs used for the treatment of Crohn's disease are safe during pregnancy; however, data on the effects on nursing are limited.

REFERENCES

1. Orholm M, Munkholm P, Langholz E et al. Familial occurrence of inflammatory bowel disease. N Engl J Med 1991; 324:84–88.
2. Yang H, McElree C, Roth MP, et al. Familial empirical risks for inflammatory bowel disease: differences between Jews and non Jews. Gut 1993;34:517–524.
3. Bennett RA, Rubin PH, Present DH. Frequency of inflammatory bowel disease in offspring of couples both presenting with inflammatory bowel disease. Gastroenterology 1991; 100:1638–1643.
4. Sonnenberg A, McCarty DJ, Jacobsen SJ. Geographic variation of inflammatory bowel disease within the United States. Gastroenterology 1991; 100:143–149.
5. Crohn BB, Yarnis H, Korelitz BI. Regional ileitis complicating pregnancy. Gastroenterology 1956; 31:615–628.
6. Fielding JF, Cooke WT. Pregnancy and Crohn's disease. BMJ 1970; 2:76–77.
7. DeDombal FT, Burton IL, Goligher JC. Crohn's disease and pregnancy. BMJ 1972; 3:550–553
8. Homan WP, Thorbjarnarson NB. Crohn's disease and pregnancy. Arch Surg 1976; 111:545–547.
9. Vender RJ, Spiro HM. Inflammatory bowel disease in pregnancy. J Clin Gastroenterol 1982; 4:231–249.
10. Khosla P, Willoughby CP, Jewell DP. Crohn's disease and pregnancy. Gut 1984; 25:52–56.
11. Mayberry JF, Weterman IT. European survey of fertility and pregnancy in women with Crohn's disease: a case control study by European collaborative group. Gut 1986; 27:821–825.
12. Baird DD, Narendranathan M, Sandler RS. Increased risk of preterm birth for women with inflammatory bowel disease. Gastroenterology 1990; 99:987–994.
12a. Burnell D, Mayberry J, Calcraft BJ, et al. Postgraduate Med. Journal 1986: 62:269–272.
13. Narendranathan M, Sandler RS, Suchindran M. Male infertility in inflammatory bowel disease. J Clin Gastroenterol 1989; 11:403–406.
14. Martinbeau PN, Welch JS, Weiland LH. Crohn's disease and pregnancy. Am J Obstet Gynecol 1975; 122:746–749.
15. Jarnerot G, Into-Malmberg MD. Review fertility, sterility and pregnancy in chronic inflammatory bowel disease. Scand J Gastroenterol 1982; 17:1–4.
16. Miller JP. Inflammatory bowel disease in pregnancy—a review. J Soc Med 1986; 79:221–225.
17. Porter RJ, Stirrat GM. The effects of inflammatory bowel disease on pregnancy: a case-controlled retrospective analysis. Br J Obstet Gynecol 1986; 93:1124–1131.
18. Nielson OH, Andreasson B, Bondesen S, et al. Pregnancy in Crohn's disease. Scand J Gastroenterol 1984; 19:724–732.
19. Fedorkow DM, Persaud D, Nimrod MB. Inflammatory bowel disease: a controlled study of late pregnancy outcome. Am J Obstet Gynecol 1989; 160:998–1001.

20. Abramson D, Jankelson IR, Milner LR. Pregnancy in idiopathic ulcerative colitis. Am J Obstet Gynecol 1951; 61:121–129.
21. Korelitz BI. Pregnancy—seminars in colon and rectal surgery. 1993; 4:48–54.
22. Boulton R, Hamilton M, Lewis A, et al. Fulminant ulcerative colitis in pregnancy. Am J Gastroenterol 1994; 89:931–933.
23. Brooks PM, Needs CJ. Antirheumatic drugs in pregnancy and lactation. Bailliers Clin Rheumatol 1990; 4:157–171.
24. Pichini S, Zuccaro P, Pacifici R. Drugs in semen. Clin Pharmacokinet 1994; 26:356–373.
25. Aselton P, Jick H, Milunsky A, et al. First trimester drug use and congenital disorders. Obstet Gynecol 1985; 65:451–455.
26. O'Morain C, Smethurst P, Dore CJ, et al. Reversible male infertility due to sulfasalazine. Studies in man and rat. Gut 1984; 25:1078–1084.
27. Mogadam M, Dobbins WO, Korelitz BI, et al. Pregnancy in inflammatory bowel disease effects of sulfasalazine and corticosteroids on fetal outcome. Gastroenterology 1981; 80:72–76.
28. Esbjorner E, Jamerot G, Wranne L. Sulfasalazine and sulfapyridine serum levels in children to mothers treated with sufasalazine during pregnancy and lactation. Acta Pediatr Scand 1987; 76:137–142.
29. Singleton JW, Hanauer SB, Gitnick GL, et al. Mesalamine capsules for the treatment of active Crohn's disease. Gastroenterology 1993; 104:1293–1300.
30. Tremaine WJ, Schroeder JW, Harrison JN. A randomized double blind placebo controlled trial of oral mesalamine (Asacol) in the treatment of symptomatic Crohn's colitis and ileocolitis. J Clin Gastroenterol 1994; 19:278–282.
31. Messori D, Brignola C, Trallori G, et al. 5-Aminosalicylic acid in maintaining remission in patients with Crohn's disease: a meta-analysis. Am J Gastroenterol 1994; 89:692–698.
32. Trallori G, D'Albasio G, Bardazzi G, et al. 5-Aminosalicylic acid in pregnancy: clinical report. Ital J Gastroenterol 1994; 26:75–78.
33. Habal FM, Hui G, Greenberg GR. Oral 5-ASA for inflammatory bowel disease in pregnancy. Safety and clinical course. Gastroenterology 1993; 105:1057–1060.
34. Marteau PH, Grand J, Devaux CB. Mesalazine in pregnancy: fetal outcome in 76 IBD patients treated with Pentasa (abstr). Gastroenterology 1995; 108:871.
35. Christensen LA, Rasmussen SN, Hansen SH. Disposition of 5-aminosalicylic acid and N-acetal 5-aminosalicylic acid in fetal and maternal body fluids during treatment with different 5-aminosalicylic acid preparations. Acta Obstet Gynecol Scand 1994; 73:399–402.
36. Margulis RR, Hodgkinson CP. Evaluation of the safety of ACTH and cortisone in pregnancy. Obstet Gynecol 1953; 1:276–281.
37. Landers DV, Green JR, Sweet RL. Antibiotic use during pregnancy and the postpartum period. Clin Obstet Gynecol 1983; 26:391–406.
38. Rosa RW, Baum C, Shaw M. Pregnancy outcomes after first trimester vaginitis drug therapy. Obstet Gynecol 1987; 69:751–755.
39. Bomford JAL, Ledger JC, O'Keefe BJ, et al. Ciprofloxacin used during pregnancy. Drugs 1993; 45:461–462.
40. Present DH. 6-Mercaptopurine and other immunosuppressive agents in the treatment of Crohn's disease and ulcerative colitis. Gastroenterol Clin North Am 1989; 18:57–72.
41. Meehan RT, Dorsey JK. Pregnancy among patients with systemic lupus erythematosus receiving immunosuppressive therapy. J Rheumatol 1987; 14:252–258.
42. Hou S. Pregnancy in women with chronic renal disease. N Engl J Med 1985; 312:836–839.
43. Alstead EM, Ritchie JK, Lennard-Jones JE, et al. Saftey of azathioprine in pregnancy in inflammatory bowel disease. Gastroenterology 1990; 99:443–446.
44. Dayan A, Present DH, Rubin P, et al. 6-Mercaptopurine in inflammatory bowel disease patients of childbearing age: no increase in congenital anomalies. A case controlled study (abstr). Gastroenterology 1991; 100:A824.
45. Weinstein GD. Methotrexate. Ann Intern Med 1977; 86:199–204.

46. Armenti VT. The National Transplantation Pregnancy Registry: An analysis of 504 pregnancies. Presented at the 18th annual meeting of the American Society of Transplant Sugeons 1992.
47. Pilarski LM, Yacyshyn BR, Lazarobits AI. Analysis of peripheral blood lymphocyte populations and immune function from children exposed to cyclosporin and to azathioprine in utero. Transplantation 1994; 57:133–144.

COMMENTARY

Robert Burakoff   *Winthrop–University Hospital, Mineola, and State University of New York at Stony Brook, Stony Brook, New York*

As stated by Dr. Present, there are no controlled randomized prospective studies regarding the various issues involving the pregnancy with Crohn's disease. Despite the paucity of studies, however, I would like to summarize some important observations and my own clinical observations.

I. FERTILITY

Fertility is not decreased in Crohn's disease patients, but rather decreased fecundity (the biological ability to conceive) is a result of the presence of disease activity.

II. EFFECT OF CROHN'S DISEASE ON PREGNANCY

Active Crohn's disease during pregnancy or at conception may predispose the patient to abnormal pregnancy outcome, that is, developmental defects, stillbirth, or spontaneous abortion. Active Crohn's disease occurring either at conception or during pregnancy significantly increases abnormal outcomes indpendent of the use of medication or requirement for surgery (1). Furthermore, there are credible epidemiological data that do bear out the fact that patients with Crohn's disease, even if it is inactive, have a higher rate of preterm delivery (less than 37 weeks).

III. EFFECT OF PREGNANCY ON CROHN'S DISEASE

I echo Dr. Present's observations and literature analysis that exacerbations of Crohn's disease are no more frequent during the pregnancy than during any other 9-month period and that there is approximately a 25% relapse rate during the pregnancy and puerperium (2). Furthermore, analysis of the literature indicating that disease activity at conception may worsen or remain the same during the pregnancy is based on literature written prior to the era of aggressive medical therapy for Crohn's disease. It is clear that maintaining a patient with Crohn's disease in remission prior to the conception and during pregnancy is paramount for a normal pregnancy and results in a healthy newborn. Additionally, there is significant need for prospective studies to stratify outcomes with current therapeutic regimens during pregnancy.

IV. DRUG THERAPY IN CROHN'S DISEASE DURING PREGNANCY

The use of prednisone, sulfasalazine, and the new 5-aminosalicylic acid (5-ASA) drugs can be safely used during pregnancy and nursing and the use of these drugs to maintain a clinical remission is the most important factor for a normal pregnancy and delivery of a healthy newborn. But because sulfasalazine can inhibit absorption of folate, it is essential that daily folate supplements be taken, especially because during pregnancy there is a heightened requirement for folate. Recent studies have shown that there is a decrease in fetal neural tube defects with folate supplementation (3,4).

The use of metronidazole for Crohn's colitis and perirectal disease during pregnancy is a problematic issue. Because metronidazole crosses the placenta and passes into breast milk and because it has been shown to cause cranial–facial defects when taken in the first trimester, physicians must currently recommend the avoidance of metronidazole during pregnancy (5).

Regarding the use of immunosuppressive therapy with 6-mercaptopurine and azathioprine, there are accumulating data from Drs. Present and Korelitz et al. and Alstead supporting the safety of 6-mercaptopurine and azathroprine during pregnancy, although the numbers of patients studied are still small. However, these drugs cross the placenta in humans and have been associated with teratogenicity. Their routine use during pregnancy cannot be recommended at this time. My own observations support that of Present and Korelitz, that a patient becoming pregnant while on 6-mp and in remission, discontinuation of the 6-mp, does not have an increased risk of exacerbation during the course of pregnancy. Therefore, I advise my patients who are on 6-MP therapy at the time of conception to stop 6-MP therapy and attempt to maintain their remission during pregnancy with 5-ASA therapy. In the more difficult scenario of a patient who can only maintain disease remission with 6-MP and who becomes pregnant, the patient must decide whether to continue the pregnancy. Finally, despite the data on the relative safety of cyclosporin in transplantations and pregnancy extrapolated from the transplantation literature, there are no data regarding patients with Crohn's disease. Because of the risk of hypertension, nephrotoxicity, and the theoretical long-term risk of neoplasm, cyclosporin cannot be recommended before conception or during pregnancy.

V. ALTERNATIVES

Alternative medical therapies for Crohn's disease should be considered during pregnancy. Maternal malnutrition has adverse effects on the fetus, and scrupulous attention to appropriate nutritional supplementation should be maintained for any patient with active Crohn's disease during pregnancy. Furthermore, although the literature is limited, pregnancies have been completed successfully using total parental nutritional for patients with active Crohn's disease during pregnancy (6). Furthermore, patients who have active Crohn's disease during pregnancy can also be nutritionally supported with the use of elemental diet. In one small study by Teahon et al. of four patients with active Crohn's disease, elemental diet resulted in the induction of clinical remission (7).

VI. CONCLUSION

Women who are contemplating pregnancy and have Crohn's disease that is well controlled by medical therapy can look forward to a normal pregnancy with the only risk being the possibility of having a preterm delivery. Women should be counseled that the risk of a flare-up of Crohn's disease during pregnancy is no greater than at any other time unrelated to the pregnancy. Additionally, pregnancy does not cause exacerbation of inactive Crohn's disease and exacerbation of Crohn's disease during pregnancy can usually be treated effectively with aggressive medical management with the use of 5-ASA drugs and corticosteroids, if necssary. Furthermore, enteral and parenteral nutrition can be used safely and efficiently during pregnancy. Finally, women who are contemplating pregnancy should be further informed that the course of Crohn's disease during one pregnancy has no relation to subsequent pregnancies.

REFERENCES

1. Woolfson K, Cohen Z, McLeod, RS. Crohn's disease and pregnancy. Dis Colon Rectum 1990; 33:869–873.
2. Nielson OH, Andreasson B, Bondersen S, et al. Pregnancy in ulcerative colitis. Scand J Gastroenterol 1983; 18:735–742.
3. Czeizel EA, Dudas I. Prevention of the first occurrence of neural tube defects with folic acid supplementation. N Engl J Med 1992; 327:1832–1835.
4. Rush D. Periconceptional folate and neural tube defects. Am J Clin Nutr 1994; 59(suppl):511s–516s.
5. Cantu JM, Garcia-Cruz D. Midline facial defects as a teratogenic effect of metronidazole. Birth Defects 1982; 18:85–88.
6. Jacobson LB, Clapp DH. Total parenteral nutrition in pregnancy complicated by Crohn's disease. JPEN J Parenter Enteral Nutr 1987; 11:93–96.
7. Teahon K, Pearson M, Levi J, et al. Elemental diet in the management of Crohn's disease during pregnancy. Gut 1991; 32:1079–1081.

23
Psychosocial Issues in Crohn's Disease

Susan Levenstein   *Ospedale Nuovo Regina Margherita, Rome, Italy*

My heart is like wax; it is melted in the midst of my bowels. —Psalms 22:14

I. HISTORY AND OVERVIEW

From the golden days of star billing for ulcerative colitis among official "psychosomatic" disorders to a recent major review of inflammatory bowel disease that never mentions psychology, the hypothesis that psychosocial factors can influence the development and course of inflammatory diseases of the intestine has undergone remarkable vicissitudes (1–3). Such swings are not new, although perhaps the pace of the 20th century has sent them by at a dizzying rate; medical thinking has always oscillated between periods when first the psychosocial, then the biophysical has the upper hand.

The history of the psychosomatic hypothesis for inflammatory bowel disease begins in the 1930s with the nascent psychosomatics movement, when these chronic diarrheal conditions (especially ulcerative colitis, which was better described) rapidly acquired a full set of "psychosomatic" baggage (4). Physicians were still somewhat vague as to the difference between ulcerative colitis and irritable bowel syndrome, undoubtedly increasing their openness to psychosomatic explanations for disease onset, the appearance of exacerbations, and symptom fluctuations within periods of activity (3). Even the presence of amebas in a patient's loose stools didn't stop enthusiasts from offering psychodynamic interpretations (5).

The pioneer psychosomatic theorists did try to keep their feet on the ground regarding psychophysiological mechanisms, favoring the autonomic nervous system as a mediator and tending to exclude the kind of symbolic interpretations that they considered appropriate for conversion symptoms (6,7). An inflammatory bowel disease–prone personality was only one of several types of predisposition, and disease would develop when the individual encountered precipitating factors that could be physical (probably infectious), psychosocial, or both. Successive theorists stripped the subtleties from this complex model and, in the place of plausible psychophysiological mechanisms, often substituted symbolic ones; the Crohn's disease patient might develop diarrhea, for example, when confronted with a problem that indicated "trying to get rid of it" (8).

The psychosomatic baggage accrued steadily until the early 1960s, only to be discarded in a flurry of spring cleaning that heralded the biologizing phase that dominated the 2 subsequent decades of medical thinking. Although this phase often merely substituted biophysical for psychological reductionism, common sense also gained coin: physicians and researchers could begin to notice that living with the specter of fecal incontinence could lead one to be obsessed with toilets, or to admit that chronic illness can be depressing.

Biological reductionism has again passed its peak. The biopsychosocial model for medical disease has made inroads into the popular imagination, while advances in psychoneuroimmunology have suggested plausible etiological mechanisms (9–11). In tune with the "mind–body" theme song, interest in possible psychological influences on inflammatory bowel disease has been reappearing (12–16).

The current state of the psychosomatic hypothesis within the medical profession is that American gastroenterologists think that psychological factors have little to do with the origins of inflammatory bowel disease (rated at an importance of 2.2 on a scale of 0–10 for ulcerative colitis and 1.7 for Crohn's disease) (17). Their opinions have, in part, been molded by the shabby state of the scientific literature: a major review of 138 published studies of the association between personality or psychopathology and ulcerative colitis found only seven of them to have represented solid investigation; only one of the seven found positive results (18). The profession as a whole remains convinced, on the other hand, that psychological influences have considerable impact on the ups and downs of disease (rated at 5.3 for ulcerative colitis and 4.3 for Crohn's disease, again on a scale of 0–10), such that a consensus document could write that psychological stress "has been positively correlated with exacerbation (17,19)."

Outside the scientific community, ordinary folk continue to think diseases ought to make sense, whether the cause be a chill, stress, or divine punishment. All physicians must parry the perennial and unanswerable question, "Why did this happen to me?" asked by patients with everything from earache to cancer. This yearning after explanations is nurtured by the waxing and waning course of inflammatory bowel disease: each episode offers a new opportunity to search for causes. Furthermore, we all know we get diarrhea if we're nervous, so "common sense" links a chronic diarrheal disease to nervousness. The upshot is that a surprisingly high percentage (53% to 59%) of patients with inflammatory bowel disease are convinced that stress or their own personality was the main, or a principal, cause of their disease, and more than 90% think it influences their disease course (20,21).

However, even the stress-exacerbation thesis rests on a feeble scientific basis. Support thus far has been largely retrospective or anecdotal, and even retrospective studies have given mixed results (22–25). One careful review concluded that the concept is "unfortunately backed by very little data" (26). Recent attempts to show a relation between stress and disease activity using methodologies free of recall bias have thus far been unable to reach definitive conclusions (15,16). Since the question remains open, this chapter emphasizes critical presentation of the scientific evidence. Studies of ulcerative colitis as well as of Crohn's disease are examined; patients with the two diseases are often inextricably mixed in study populations, results for one disease may to some extent be generalizeable to the other, and many series of ulcerative colitis patients, especially the earlier ones, are likely to have included many misdiagnosed cases of Crohn's colitis.

II. PERSON VARIABLES

A. Personality

1. General

The notion that people who share a common diagnosis also share a common set of personality characteristics and that the latter contribute to creating the former was a cornerstone of the psychosomatic thinking of the 1940s and 1950s, reaching its full expression in Alexander's so-called "specificity hypothesis" (1). After many years out of favor, the specificity hypothesis has been undergoing selective resurrection recently, for example, in the possibility that a hostile personality may presage coronary artery disease (2). In broad terms, there seems to be little to resurrect regarding inflammatory bowel disease because most studies have found patients to have similar personality profiles to controls (24,28). But a few doubts remain.

2. Obsessiveness

Many clinicians have found patients with inflammatory bowel disease to be fussy, overcontrolled, and preoccupied with filth (29–31). Some empirical studies agree. One found both ulcerative colitis and Crohn's disease patients to be slightly more obsessive than control subjects with other chronic medical conditions (23,32). Another group found ulcerative colitis patients to be less flexible and more punctual than duodenal ulcer patients, and to be more concerned about their own rigidity (33).

But do these mild obsessive traits have any etiological significance? Currently, most workers think that they rather result from the onerous task of coexisting, often since adolescence, with an embarrassing diarrheal condition (34). Patients with severe inflammatory bowel disease are spurred by potential loss of bowel control to develop a mental map of their habitual stomping grounds, studded with imaginary gold stars to mark available toilets; even the most slapdash turn meticulous when haunted by an unpredictable colon.

3. Alexithymia

Psychological processes capable of producing organ damage may not always be mediated by such subjective distress states as anxiety and depression. On the contrary, some theorists have suggested a particular vulnerability to psychosomatic phenomena in the "alexithymic" individual who is unable to verbalize or be fully in touch with his or her own emotions (35). Such an individual is held to be especially prone to develop organic disease as an outlet for stress or inner conflict. This mechanism has long been hypothesized as a cause for ulcerative colitis, and it has found some support in controlled studies of both ulcerative colitis and Crohn's disease (4,36,37).

But, the familiar refrain returns: might these traits merely develop in reaction to the illness experience? The reports of alexithymia in an array of long-standing diseases suggests that one method of coping with chronic illness may be to turn away from (potentially overwhelming) emotional reactions.

4. Miscellaneous Personality Traits

Inflammatory bowel disease patients have been found to be less self-confident and less aggressive than patients with other chronic diseases, and to score higher on the hysteria and hypochondriasis scales of the Minnesota Multiphasic Personality Inventory (MMPI) than their siblings and than general-population volunteers (38,40). Disease effects can obviously not be excluded in any of these instances.

B. Psychopathology

1. Mood Disorders

A number of workers have reported high rates of anxiety and depression in both ulcerative colitis and Crohn's disease (21,32,38,40–43). One study found high lifetime rates of depression before disease onset in patients with Crohn's disease, but this study must be considered with the usual reservations accorded to retrospective interviews.

On the other hand, one study found no increased anxiety or depression in a mixed group of patients with inflammatory bowel disease on the Profile of Mood States when patients' siblings were used as an astute comparison group (39). Patients with ulcerative colitis, not Crohn's disease, have not only been reported to be not depressed but to be models of good cheer as compared with patients having other medical conditions (24,44).

These contradictory results reflect, in part, the natural history of inflammatory bowel disease. During first attacks or symptom flares, patients are more distressed than in quiescent phases, suggesting that anxiety and depression occur as reactions to acute illness or to the shock of the recent diagnosis of a potentially grave disease (16,21,42,45). The passage of time seems to soften the impact of a major diagnosis and to allow the individual to rise above it. Many patients with serious, chronic diseases reportedly achieve a "philosophical" attitude that goes beyond resignation to their fate to a heightened appreciation of life and even to spiritual fulfillment (46–48).

2. Other Psychiatric Disorders

During the 1940s and 1950s, inflammatory bowel disease patients were claimed to have a high rate of severe psychopathological impairments. Alexander thought ulcerative colitis sufferers even had "a tendency toward . . . psychotic episodes," a concept supported by at least one well-known case series (49). But the samples examined by these observers were lopsided; they included only patients who were being seen by psychiatrists. When unselected ulcerative colitis patients have been studied through use of interviews or standardized testing, they have usually been found to harbor no more psychiatric disorders than control subjects, although one study did report strikingly elevated scores on virtually every subscale of the Hopkins Symptom Checklist (SCL-90) (23,24,36,41,43). Results using the Eysenck Personality Inventory have been conflicting. One study found patients with ulcerative colitis to be less neurotic and introverted than other medical patients, whereas another found them to score higher on both scales than control patients with diabetes but lower than patients with Crohn's disease (21,44).

Controlled studies of persons with Crohn's disease, on the other hand, have usually found patients to have a variety of psychiatric syndromes. One group using the National Institutes of Mental Health (NIMH) Diagnostic Interview Schedule found an excess of panic disorder among patients with Crohn's disease over normal control subjects, and another found trends toward high rates of obsessive–compulsive neurosis and hysteria (32,43). Studies using the Eysenck Personality Inventory have consistently reported higher neuroticism and introversion among patients with Crohn's disease over those in control patients with or without other medical disorders, although, in one such study, these characteristics were present only among men (21,28,32).

C. Ulcerative Colitis Versus Crohn's Disease

Patients with ulcerative colitis, although distressed during acute episodes, otherwise enjoy remarkable psychological health as a group. Crohn's disease patients, on the other hand, are somewhat more likely to have persistent, yet minor, psychopathological impairment.

The difference in the clinical patterns of the two diseases provides some basis for explaining why it may be more difficult for a person living with Crohn's disease to keep on an even psychic keel. In ulcerative colitis, symptomatic episodes are more often interspersed with periods of complete well-being. Crohn's disease is more likely to give chronic pain or unrelenting symptoms (fewer disease-free spaces for contemplation and distancing) and to require medications with central nervous system side effects or repeated surgical operations. One study reporting more psychological distress in Crohn's disease than in ulcerative colitis found the difference to disappear when the amount of distress was adjusted for disease severity (50). Furthermore, there is no cure for Crohn's disease, whereas ulcerative colitis patients know they can be cured by surgery.

III. SOCIAL VARIABLES

Early psychosomaticists theorized that a pattern of dependency in interpersonal relationships predisposed the patient to ulcerative colitis. Male patients were described as "passive, pathologically attached to their mothers, frequently unmarried" (51). But, although it may be true that some patients with inflammatory bowel disease lack self-reliance, their tendency to lean on others may well be a product of the disease, especially when illness begins in adolescence and hampers the normal process of maturation and separation.

Epidemiologists have unearthed occupational patterns of disease that might suggest influences of the broader social context: both ulcerative colitis and Crohn's disease are usually reported to be more common in higher socioeconomic classes (52,53). But, psychological mechanisms seem less likely to account for occupational differences than do physiological ones such as specific toxic exposures (e.g., yeast antigens in bakers or the protective effect of physical exertion or work in the open air)(54,55).

Inflammatory bowel disease is also sometimes considered one of the "diseases of civilization," more common in the north of the world than in the south, more common in the city than in the country (56). Whereas some of the other diseases on the list probably are induced, in part, by the stressors of urban life—blood pressure, for instance, can be raised by acoustic pollution—few researchers have dared make such a suggestion for inflammatory bowel disease (57). Misreporting (e.g., in the tropics, all diarrhea is dysentery) and variation in infectious exposures are more likely explanations.

IV. STRESS, STRESSORS, AND
INFLAMMATORY BOWEL DISEASE

A. Onset Setting

Few researchers believe that the first attack of inflammatory bowel disease is set off by stress, despite uncontrolled case series reporting recent major loss of a loved one or other severely stressful life events in an overwhelming majority of cases of both Crohn's disease and ulcerative colitis (45). The introduction of appropriate comparison groups causes the apparent excess of potential psychosocial precipitants to decline precipitously

(23,58). There are few exceptions, and at least one of them, which found a high rate of undesirable life events in the 6 months before the onset of ulcerative colitis, used interviews that were unblinded and performed after a considerable lag time (22,59). Even a prompt, blinded comparison of cases with healthy individuals would not eliminate a bias in favor of an association, because sick individuals typically remember more life events than healthy ones as part of their effort to make sense out of their illness ("effort after meaning") (60).

B.   Stress and Fluctuations in Disease Activity

Patients with inflammatory bowel disease and their physicians share the belief that there is a connection between stress and relapse. The evidence, however, is surprisingly weak.

Not only case series but also cross-sectional controlled studies have suggested that major negative life events often precede exacerbations in Crohn's disease (25,29,61,62). For ulcerative colitis, the retrospective literature includes some reports of stressful life events before exacerbations, but there are also several reports to the contrary (16,23–25).

Recall bias can never be eliminated in a cross-sectional/retrospective study, even when every effort is made to tally up only the most objective of life events. The suspicion that associations between events and symptoms are due to artifacts or to bias can be definitively resolved only by using a study design in which psychosocial stressors are observed first and symptoms later.

One possible research design, attentive prospective observation of individuals, has been characterized by anecdotal reports in which psychoanalysts and gastroenterologists who follow patients with inflammatory bowel disease have claimed to observe exacerbations to follow close on the heels of major life stressors (8,63). Even though such observers are in a privileged position to detect relapse precipitants in real time, their recognition and elaboration of the temporal relations is, in practice, retrospective, compromising this privileged vantage point and allowing bias by the observer's own and often quite powerful preconceptions of what the connections between the psyche and the some "ought" to be. And, observations can be unconsiously selective. In a relapsing–remitting disease, some exacerbations are bound to fall in stressful periods by chance alone.

Several groups have, therefore, attempted to evaluate the relation between inflammatory bowel disease activity and stress by obtaining serial assessments of both (12–15).

Two of these studies performed only period-by-period cross-sectional analyses and thus were retrospective in practice, though prospective in form. They were, therefore, likely to be biased in favor of a stress–activity relationship. However, one study was completely negative, finding no increase in life events, anxiety, or depression before exacerbations of ulcerative colitis, and the other yielded unclear results—Crohn's disease and ulcerative colitis patients in relapse recalled more perceived stress than inactive controls, but reported no more life events (13,14).

Two other studies used a true prospective design, examining the lag time relation between monthly assessments of stress and subsequent relapse. One study found no association of major life events or depression with subsequent disease activity in either Crohn's disease or ulcerative colitis; some question may be raised as to whether these two measures of stress are sufficiently sensitive for this purpose (15,16). The second study concluded that there was a causative relation between major life events and disease activity in a mixed ulcerative colitis/Crohn's disease population, with a risk ratio of 2.9 (12). Unfortunately, symptomatic episodes occurred only in the same month as life events, raising the question of direction of causality. Further analysis of this group's data revealed that many of these same-month stress events were rated as "health-related," casting further doubt on the authors' conclusion that it was the stress that caused the relapse (64).

The literature thus leaves open the question of whether stress precipitates relapses, though tending to answer "no." Because ulcerative colitis activity may be detected through the proctoscope regardless of symptoms. I and my colleagues established a model for investigating the relation of life stress to the activity of this disease. The psychological state of patients in clinical remission, some of whom have mild colonic inflammation without realizing it, could be compared, free of confounding by the effect of symptoms, with the simultaneous state of the rectal mucosa. The resulting model, though it was cross-sectional in form, was double-blind and free from the usual biases of the retrospective approach. We found that asymptomatic patients who had endoscopic abnormalities reported substantially higher levels of perceived stress than similarly asymptomatic patients with normal proctoscopic results (16).

Stress can also influence the microfluctuations of inflammatory bowel disease. In a patient whose intestine is already inflamed, psychological distress might precipitate or worsen symptoms on a daily, hourly, or even minute-to-minute basis (65). One recent study did find the daily symptoms of Crohn's disease to vary with stress levels, but, unfortunately, the direction of causality was indeterminate (66).

Whatever the overall relation between stress and inflammatory bowel disease, patients are heterogeneous and able to escape from statistical associations. Among migraine patients, for example, only a subgroup say their headaches are set off by stress (67,68). Some patients with Crohn's disease may similarly be particularly susceptible to stress effects, either because their psychological makeup is ill-equipped to buffer life's slings and arrows or because their immunological and gastrointestinal systems possess a specific form of reactivity (69).

V.   POSSIBLE PATHOPHYSIOLOGICAL MECHANISMS

A.   Autonomic Nervous System Activation

The direct effect of autonomic discharge has been proposed as the cause of hourly and daily symptom activation by psychological stressors as well as to account for longer term influences on disease evolution (1,65). It has recently been suggested that phenomena usually considered typical of the irritable bowel syndrome may explain some of the clinical picture in inflammatory bowel disease (70). The empirical evidence is greater for ulcerative colitis. Not only do patients with inactive disease have a high rate of "irritable bowel" symptoms, but manometry studies have also found that low-amplitude, postprandial propagating contractions occur more frequently in ulcerative colitis than in healthy subjects (71–73). Furthermore, in an old study, anger or fear induced by stress interviews caused a prompt increase in bowel motility in ulcerative colitis patients (74). Adrenergic blockade in the form of lidocaine enemas seems to have a salutary effect (75). Given the well-known sensitivity of the irritable bowel syndrome to psychological distress, the stress–symptom relation might, therefore, involve a genuine cause and effect relation as a result of autonomic discharge, without implying any impact of psychological factors on mucosal inflammation (76).

B. Psychoneuroimmunology

The recent revelation of complex interaction pathways between the psychological and immunological systems has opened new vistas on the understanding of psychosomatic phenomena (11). Deregulation of the immune system—possibly through the mediation of autonomic nerves that innervate lymphoid tissue—seems to be a frequent consequence of stress (77).

Most psychoneuroimmunology research has focused on the psychogenic depression of immunological defenses (78). However, the dysregulatory effect of stress on the immune system is more complex and can result in stimulation as well as suppression (79). There is some evidence that acute and chronic stress may have contrasting effects (80). These findings may help give a basis for the often-postulated theory that stress triggers chronic idiopathic inflammatory diseases with an autoimmune component, such as rheumatoid arthritis and inflammatory bowel disease (81,82).

Recent advances in unscrambling the cascade of events in inflammatory bowel disease relapses have shown that immune mechanisms play a major role in the instigation and maintenance of mucosal inflammation. Immune dysregulation, with altered response of the immune system to normal intraluminal substances, has been proposed to be the root defect in these disorders (83). Levels of local and circulating cytokines are correlated with clinical activity in both ulcerative colitis and Crohn's disease, and sulfasalazine (not 5-aminosalicylate) has been found to inhibit cell-mediated cytotoxicity (84,85). The ability of stressors to disrupt immune regulation, possibly via autonomic nervous pathways, might therefore be a mediating mechanism for effects on disease activity.

C. Behavioral Changes

Patients' behavior may often be responsible for "psychological" effects on organic pathologic conditions. This concept may be less exciting in terms of etiological trailblazing than are psychoneuroimmunological interweavings, but it must be kept in mind. Self-neglect is a major contributor to the excess mortality rate among the recently bereaved, hostile people may develop coronary artery disease partly because they smoke more cigarettes, and a "fighting spirit" may improve cancer prognosis partly by increasing compliance with chemotherapy (86–88).

There are several ways this mechanism might come into play in Crohn's disease. Many patients avoid specific foods that precipitate their symptoms, and they might tend to throw dietary caution to the winds during difficult periods. Other stressed individuals may increase their risk of a relapse by neglecting their maintenance therapy or by smoking more cigarettes (89–92).

VI. RESEARCH ISSUES

This chapter has emphasized the flaws in studies that purport to demonstrate a relation between psychological factors and inflammatory bowel disease. Psychosomatics is a methodological bag of worms, and the researcher must be tediously scrupulous to sort out the variety of biases and confounding factors that cause spuriously positive findings, even when functional disorders are the object of study (93). But the reverse can occasionally be the case, especially when there is an organic pathologic condition: researchers may fail to detect subtle but genuine associations because of inappropriate measures of disease or insensitive measures of stress. A case in point is the difficulties encountered in demonstrating the relation between stressful life events and duodenal ulcer (94–97). The case of inflammatory bowel disease presents one peculiar negative confound, that is, cigarette smoking, an activity that is often indulged in under stress and that can actually improve ulcerative colitis (16,91,98,99). Smoking could, therefore, artifactually lower the association between stress and colitis activity.

It is not likely to be verified or disproved that obsessiveness or any other "person variable" may predispose a person to Crohn's disease. Because of the profound effects of the disease, studies of patients who are already ill, however carefully conducted, cannot be trusted for evaluation of premorbid psychological conditions. Convincing evidence must, therefore, be prospective, which presents daunting methodological barriers.

The theoretical ideal is to examine the psychological traits of a large number of healthy individuals and to determine in which of them Crohn's disease develops over the years. Unfortunately, this condition is too rare, at an incidence rate of perhaps 5/100,000 per year, to justify a dedicated project (100,101). A good-sized longitudinal study, enrolling 8000 subjects and achieving an unheard-of 100% follow-up, would see only four new cases within 10 years.

Another possible approach, secondary analysis of existing longitudinal data sources, involves its own problems. Not only must a very large number of subjects be enrolled and Crohn's disease specifically enquired after at follow-up, but it is also crucial that subjects be specifically screened for disease at enrollment. This is because Crohn's disease typically goes undiagnosed for several years, and a patient with the appropriate personality features may learn later that he or she has the disorder, after having the effects of its symptoms, without the benefit of a diagnosis, at the time of initial testing (102).

Another source, which must be handled cautiously, is the observations of physicians and psychotherapists in whose patients Crohn's disease subsequently develops. At least one authoritative observer of current research suggests such a return to scrupulous use of anecdotal evidence (103).

The prospective evaluation of the relation between stress and exacerbations, on the other hand, is feasible because remission zeros out the score for a substantial group of patients, and the high relapse rate ensures that enough adverse events will occur within a practicable time frame to permit statistical analysis. Ideally, such studies should take into account behavioral mediators and confounders (e.g., smoking and compliance with therapy).

VII. IMPLICATIONS FOR THERAPY

Both patients and physicians have generally taken eagerly to the idea that psychological factors influence Crohn's disease. This belief has repercussions on both sides of the coin (Table 1).

Says one physician-patient cited by Spiro, "When I dared expose myself to close friends and relate distress over worsening symptoms, I felt vulnerable to statements like, 'Well, it does sound like your job has been stressful lately' " (104). Probably many patients are told by their physicians, or decide on their own accord, to slow down and take it easy.

Throughout the course of disease, patients need an open ear, sensitivity to the impact of the disease on their daily lives, and a license to bring up their emotional state without being dismissed as "psychosomatic." Some require additional psychological support, generally best given by their treating physician. A joint session with the spouse or the family may occasionally be useful to demystify the disease, allow ventilation of frustra-

TABLE 1 Pros and Cons of Psychological Factors Influencing Crohn's Disease

Pros	Cons
The doctor–patient relationship may be humanized if the physician talks with the patient about something other than blood and guts.	The doctor–patient relationship may be dehumanized if the physician stigmatizes the patient as "psychosomatic." A patient may be afraid to voice any distress for fear it will be interpreted as "tainted anxiety" (104).
Undertanding of the complexity of mind–body interactions may be enriched by serious scrutiny of the quirks of a patient's saga.	Understanding of the complexity of mind–body interactions may be diminished by simplistic attribution of all disease swings to "stress."
Patients' lives may be enhanced by the consideration of autonomy-building, nontoxic, nonpharmacological therapeutic approaches such as relaxation techniques or job changes.	Patients' lives may be interfered with by unnecessary fiddling, restrictions, or therapies— a life devoted to relaxation techniques can be the modern equivalent of taking to one's bed.
Interpersonal relatinships may be deepened if psychological as well as physical needs are met, and they may be improved by efforts to create a calmer, less conflict-ridden atmosphere.	Interpersonal relationships may be damaged if the severity and impact of the disease are belittled. The conviction that personality and stress can predispose a patient to the disease or its swings carries a serious danger of blaming the victim.

tions, clear up sexual questions, defuse conflicts over control issues, and assess dependency levels. Sometimes, a patient may welcome referral to a psychiatrist or psychologist for counseling around these issues, but the clinician must be familiar enough with local resources to decide whether referral to a patient support group might be more appropriate. If possible, any therapist chosen should have specific interest and experience in treating patients with Crohn's disease.

The indications for formal psychotherapy and for psychopharmacological treatment are generally thought to be the same for patients with inflammatory bowel disease as for anyone else, because optimism regarding the potential for psychotherapeutic interventions to affect the long-term course of the disease has long since faded (105). Although prolonged psychotherapy did seem to improve the course of one group of patients with ulcerative colitis, these patients were atypical in having major psychopathological conditions (35% were diagnosed as schizophrenic), and control groups were inadequate. More recent studies have found no beneficial physiological effect on either Crohn's disease or ulcerative colitis from either psychotherapeutic or behavioral medicine techniques (23,106,107).

Psychotherapy can certainly, however, increase the patient's sense of control (29,106). Furthermore, if disease induces vulnerability and dependency, these may in turn decrease the individual's ability to withstand stressors that might otherwise not induce exacerbations; helplessness and hopelessness may be psychological precipitants of attacks (29). When it seems that this kind of cycle has been established, individual or family therapy might help the patient to emerge from it. Therapy can also improve the individual's coping strategies, which may condition physiological vulnerability in the face of stress (69). However, coping style per se seemed to have no relation to the success of therapy in one study of ulcerative colitis (108). Most patients with Crohn's disease use adaptive ways of coping (50). The minority who display such maladaptive styles as escapism or self-blame might be selective targets for formal psychotherapy.

REFERENCES

1. Alexander F. Psychosomatic Medicine: Its Principles and Applications. New York: WW Norton, 1950.
2. Podolsky DK. Inflammatory bowel disease (Part 1). N Engl J Med 1991; 325(13):928–937.
3. Aronowitz R, Spiro HM. The rise and fall of the psychosomatic hypothesis in ulcerative colitis. J Clin Gastroenterol 1988; 10(3):298–305.
4. Daniels GE. Nonspecific ulcerative colitis as a psychosomatic disease. Med Clin North Am 1944; 28:593–602.
5. Murray CD. Psychogenic factors in the etiology of ulcerative colitis and bloody diarrhea. Am J Med Sci 1930; 180:239–248
6. Alexander F, French TM. Studies in Psychosomatic Medicine. New York: The Ronald Press Company, 1948.
7. Alexander F. Fundamental concepts of psychosomatic research: psychogenesis, conversion, specificity. Psychosom Med 1943; 5:205–210.
8. Grace WJ. Life stress and regional enteritis. Gastroenterology 1953; 23:542–553.
9. Engel GL. The need for a new medical model: a challenge for biomedicine. Science 1977; 196(4286):129–136.
10. Moyers B. Wounded healers. In: Public Affairs Television, 1993.
11. Ader R, Felten DL, Cohen N. Psychoneuroimmunology. 2d ed. San Diego: Academic Press, 1991.
12. Duffy LC, Zielezny MA, Marshall JR, et al. Lag time between stress events and risk of recurrent episodes of inflammatory bowel disease. Epidemiology 1991; 2(2):141–145.
13. Riley SA, Masni V, Goodman MJ, Lucas S. Why do patients with ulcerative colitis relapse? Gut 1990; 31:179–183.
14. Weitersheim JV, Köhler T, Feiereis H. Relapse-precipitating life events and feelings in patients with inflammatory bowel disease. Psychother Psychosom 1992; 58:103–112.
15. North CS, Alpers DH, Helzer JE, Spitznagel EL, Clouse RE. Do life events or depression exacerbate inflammatory bowel disease? A prospective study. Ann Intern Med 1991; 114:381–386.
16. Levenstein S, Prantera C, Varvo V, et al. Psychological stress and disease activity in ulcerative colitis: a multidimensional cross-sectional study. Am J Gastroenterol 1994; 89:1219–1225.
17. Mitchel CM, Drossman DA. Survey of the AGA membership relating to patients with functional gastrointestinal disorders. Gastroenterology 1987; 92:1282–1284.
18. North CS, Clouse RE, Spitznagel EL, Alpers DH. The relation of ulcerative colitis to psychiatric factors: a review of findings and methods. Am J Psychiatry 1990; 147:974–981.
19. National Foundation for Ileitis and Colitis. Challenges in IBD Research: Agenda for the '90's. Washington, D.C., 1990.
20. Lewis MC. Attributions and inflammatory bowel disease: patients' perceptions of illness causes and the effects of these perceptions on relationships. AARN Newsletter 1988; May:16–17.
21. Robertson DAF, Ray J, Diamond I, Edwards JG. Personality profile and affective state of patients with inflammatory bowel disease. Gut 1989; 30:623–626.
22. Fava GA, Pavan L. Large bowel disorders I, illness configuration and life events. Psychother Psychosom 1976; 77;27:93–99.
23. Feldman F, Cantor D, Soll S, Bachrach W. Psychiatric study of a consecutive series of 34 patients with ulcerative colitis. BMJ 1967; 3(July1):14–19.
24. Helzer JE, Stillings WA, Chammas S, Norland CC, Alpers DH. A controlled study of

the association between ulcerative colitis and psychiatric diagnosis. Dig Dis Sci 1982; 27(6):513–518.

25. Paar GH, Bezzenberger U, Lorenz-Meyer H. Über den Zusammenhang von psychosozialem Streb und Krankheitsactivität bei Patienten mit Morbus Crohn and Colitis ulcerosa. Z Gastroenterol 1988; 26:648–657.

26. Schwarz SP, Blanchard EB. Inflammatory bowel disease: a review of the psychological assessment and treatment literature. Ann Behav Med 1990; 12(3):95–105.

27. Hearn MD, Murray DM, Luepker RV. Hostility, coronary heart disease, and total mortality: a 33-year old follow-up study of university students. J Behav Med 1989; 12(2):105–121.

28. Gazzard BG, Price HL, Libby GW, Dawson AM. The social toll of Crohn's disease. BMJ 1978; 2:1117–1119.

29. Engel G. Studies of ulcerative colitis. V. Psychological aspects and their implications for treatment. Am J Dig Dis 1958; 3(4):315–337.

30. Sundby H, Austed A. Ulcerative colitis in children: a follow-up study with special reference to psychosomatic aspects. Acta Psychiatr Scand 1967; 43:410–423.

31. Karush A, Daniels GE, O'Connor JF, Stern LO. The response to psychotherapy in chronic ulcerative colitis. I. Pretreatment factors. Psychosom Med 1968; 30(3):225–276.

32. Helzer JE, Chammas S, Norland CC, Stillings WA, Alpers DH. A study of the association between Crohn's disease and psychiatric illness. Gastroenterology 1984; 86:324–330.

33. Bellini M, Tansella M. Obsessional scores and subjective general psychiatric complaints of patients with duodenal ulcer or ulcerative colitis. Psych Med 1976; 6:461–467.

34. Drossman DA. Psychosocial aspects of ulcerative colitis and Crohn's disease. In: Kirsner JB, Shorter RG, eds. Inflammatory Bowel Disease 3rd ed. Philadelphia: Lea & Febiger, 1988: 209–226.

35. Nemiah JC. Denial revisited: reflections on psychosomatic theory. Psychother Psychosom 1975; 26:140–147.

36. Fava GA, Pavan L. Large bowel disorders. II. Psychopathology and alexithymia. Psychother Psychosom 1976-77;27:100–105.

37. Taylor G, Doody K, Newman A. Alexithymic characteristics in patients with inflammatory bowel disease. Can J Psychiatr 1981; 26(7):470–474.

38. Arapakis G, Lyketsos CG, Gerolymatos K, Richardson SC, Lyketsos GC. Low dominance and high intropunitiveness in ulcerative colitis and irritable bowel syndrome. Psychother Psychosom 1986; 46:171–176.

39. McMahon AW, Schmitt P, Patterson JF, Rothman E. Personality differences between inflammatory bowel disease patients and their healthy siblings. Psychosom Med 1973; 35(2):91–103.

40. Schwarz SP, Blanchard EB, Berreman CF, et al. Psychological aspects of irritable bowel syndrome: comparisons with inflammatory bowel disease and nonpatient controls. Behav Res Ther 1993; 31(3):297–304.

41. Magni G, Bernasconi G, Mauro P, et al. Psychiatric diagnoses in ulcerative colitis: a controlled study. Br J Psychiatr 1991; 158:413–415.

42. Andrews H, Barczak P, Allan RN. Psychiatric illness in patients with inflammatory bowel disease. Gut 1987; 28:1600–1604.

43. Tarter RE, Switala J, Carra J, Edwards KL, Thiel DHV. Inflammatory bowel disease: psychiatric status of patients before and after disease onset. Int J Psychiatr Med 1987; 17(2)173–181.

44. Esler MD, Goulston KJ. Levels of anxiety in colonic disorders. N Engl J Med 1973; 228(1):16–20.

45. McKegney FP, Gordon RO, Levine SM. A psychosomatic comparison of patients with ulcerative colitis and Crohn's disease. Psychosom Med 1970; 32(2):153–166.

46. Beard BH, Sampson TF. Denial and objectivity in hemodialysis patients. In: Levy NB, ed.

Psychonephrology 1: Psychological Factors in Hemodialysis and Transplantation. New York: Plenum, 1983.

47. House A. Psychosocial problems of patients on the renal unit and their relation to treatment outcome. J Psychosom Res 1987; 31(4):441–452.

48. Kübler-Ross E. On Death and Dying: What the Dying Have to Teach Doctors, Nurses, Clergy and Their Own Families. New York: Macmillan, 1969.

49. O'Connor JF, Daniels G, Flood C, Karush A, Moses L, Stern LO. An evaluation of the effectiveness of psychotherapy in the treatment of ulcerative colitis. Ann Intern Med 1964; 60(4):587–602.

50. Drossman DA, Thompson WG. The irritable bowel syndrome: review and a graduated multicomponent treatment approach. Ann Intern Med 1992; 116(12 pt. 1):1009–1016.

51. Weiss E, English OS. Psychosomatic Medicine: The Clinical Application of Psychopathology to General Medical Problems. 2d ed. Philadelphia: WB Saunders, 1949.

52. Keighley A, Miller DS, Hughes AO, Langman MJS. The demographic and social characteristics of patients with Crohn's disease in the Nottingham area. Scand J Gastroenterol 1976; 11:293–296.

53. Bonnevie O. A socio-economic study of patients with ulcerative colitis. Scand J Gastroenterol 1967; 2:129–136.

54. Young CA, Sonnenberg A, Burns EA. Lymphocyte proliferation response to baker's yeast in Crohn's disease. Digestion 1994; 55:40–43.

55. Sonnenberg A. Occupational distribution of inflammatory bowel disease among German employees. Gut 1990; 31:1037–1040.

56. Trowell HC, Burkitt DP, eds. Western Diseases: Their Emergence and Prevention. Cambridge, MA: Harvard University Press, 1981.

57. Ortiz GA, Arguelles AE, Crespin HA, Sposari G, Villafane CT. Modifications of epinephrine, norepinephrine, blood lipid fractions and the cardiovascular system produced by noise in an industrial medium. Horm Res 1974; 5:57–64.

58. Monk M, Mendeloff AI, Siegel CI, Lilienfeld A. An epidemiological study of ulcerative colitis and regional enteritis among adults in Baltimore: III. Psychological and possible stress-precipitating factors. J Chronic Dis 1970; 22:564–578.

59. Hislop IG. Onset setting in inflammatory bowel disease. Med J Aust 1974; 1:981–984.

60. Brown GW, Harris TO. Social Origins of Depression: A study of Psychiatric Disorder in Women. London: Tavistock, 1978.

61. Lindemann E. Modifications in the course of ulcerative colitis in relation to changes in life situations and reaction patterns. Res Pub Assoc Res Nerv Ment Dis 1949; 29:706–723.

62. Kiss A, Nemeskeri N, Maritesch F, et al. Stressful life events and acute relapse of Crohn's disease. Psychosom Med 1991; 53:215–227.

63. Spiro HM. Can a colon burst from grief? J Clin Gastroenterol 1987; 9(3):251–252.

64. Duffy LC, Zielezny MA, Marshall JR, et al. Relevance of major stress events as an indicator of disease activity prevalence in inflammatory bowel disease. Behav Med 1991; (Fall):101–109.

65. Prugh DG. The influence of emotional factors on the clinical course of ulcerative colitis in children. Gastroenterology 1951; 18(3):339–354.

66. Garrett VD, Brantley PJ, Jones GN, McKnight GT. The relation between daily stress and Crohn's disease. J Behav Med 1991; 14(1):87–96.

67. Vandenbergh V, Amery WK, Waelkens J. Trigger factors in migraine: a study conducted by the Belgian Migraine Society. Headache 1987; 27(April):191–196.

68. Amery WK, Vandenbergh V. What can precipitating factors teach us about the pathogenesis of migraine? Headache 1987; 27(March):146–150.

69. Gentry WD, Kobasa SCO. Social and psychological resources mediating stress–illness relationships in humans. In: Gentry WD, ed. Handbook of Behavioral Medicine. New York: Guilford Press, 1984.

70. Bayless TM, Harris ML. Inflammatory bowel disease and irritable bowel syndrome. Med Clin North Am 1990; 74(1):21–29.

71. Isgar B, Harman M, Kaye MD, Whorwell PJ. Symptoms of irritable bowel syndrome in ulcerative colitis in remission. Gut 1983; 24:190–192.

72. Snape WJ. The role of a colonic motility disturbance in ulcerative colitis. Keio J Med 1991; 40(1):6–8.

73. Reddy SN, Bazzocchi G, Chan S, et al. Colonic motility and transit in health and ulcerative colitis. Gastroenterology 1991; 101:1289–1297.

74. Karush A, Hiatt RB, Daniels GE. Psychophysiological correlations in ulcerative colitis. Psychosom Med 1955; 17(1):36–56.

75. Bjorck S, Dahlstrom A, Ahlman H. Topical treatment of ulcerative proctitis with lidocaine. Scand J Gastroenterol 1989; 24:1061–1072.

76. Whitehead WE, Crowell MD, Robinson JC, Heller BR, Schuster MM. Effects of stressful life events on bowel symptoms: subjects with irritable bowel syndrome compared with subjects without bowel dysfunction. Gut 1992; 33:825–830.

77. Daruna JH, Morgan JE. Psychosocial effects on immune function: neuroendocrine pathways. Psychosomatics 1990; 31(1):4–12.

78. Stein M, Schleifer SJ. Frontiers of stress research: stress and immunity. In: Zales M, ed. Stress in Health and Disease. New York: Brunner/Mazel, 1985.

79. Baker GHB. Psychological factors and immunity. J Psychosom Res 1987; 31(1):1–10.

80. Ader R, Cohen N. Behavior and the immune system. In: Gentry WD, ed. Handbook of Behavioral Medicine. New York: Guilford Press, 1984.

81. Baker GHB, Brewerton DA. Rheumatoid arthritis: a psychiatric assessment. BMJ 1981; 282(20 June):2014.

82. Rekola JK. Rheumatoid arthritis and the family. Scand J Rheumatol 1973; 2(suppl 3):1–117.

83. MacDermott RP, Stenson WF. Alterations of the immune system in ulcerative colitis and Crohn's disease. Adv Immunol 1988; 42:285–328.

84. Ligumsky M, Simon PL, Karmeli F, Rachmilewitz D. Role of interleukin 1 in inflammatory bowel disease—enhanced production during active disease. Gut 1990; 31:686–689.

85. MacDermott RP, Kane MG, Steele LL, Stenson WF. Immunopharmacology 1986; 11:101–109.

86. Jacobs S, Ostfield A. An epidemiological review of the mortality of bereavement. Psychosom Med 1977; 39(5):244–357.

87. Siegler IC, Peterson BL, Barefoot JC, Williams RB. Hostility during late adolescence predicts coronary risk factors at mid-life. Am J Epi 1992; 136(2):146–154.

88. Ayres A, Hoon PW, Franzoni JB, Matheny KB, Cotanch PH, Takayanagi S. Influence of mood and adjustment to cancer on compliance with chemotherapy among breast cancer patients. J Psychosom Res 1994; 38(5):393–402.

89. Ginsberg AL, Albert MB. Treatment of patient with severe steroid-dependent Crohn's disease with nonelemental formula diet: identification of possible etiologic dietary factor. Dig Dis Sci 1989; 34(10):1624–1628.

90. Levenstein S, Prantera C, Luzi C, D'Ubaldi A. Low residue or normal diet in Crohn's disease: a prospective controlled study in Italian patients. Gut 1985; 26:989–993.

91. Calkins BM. A meta-analysis of the role of smoking in inflammatory bowel disease. Dig Dis Sci 1989; 34(12):1841–1854.

92. Vessey M, Jewell K, Smith A, Yeates D, McPherson K. Chronic inflammatory bowel disease, cigarette smoking, and use of oral contraceptives: findings in a large cohort of women of childbearing age. BMJ 1986; 292(26 April):1101–1103.

93. Drossman D, McKee DC, Sandler RS, et al. Psychosocial factors in the irritable bowel syndrome: a multivariate study of patients and nonpatients with irritable bowel syndrome. Gastroenterology 1988; 95(3):701–708.

94. Piper DW, McIntosh JH, Ariotti DE, Calogiuri JV, Brown RW, Shy CM. Life events and chronic duodenal ulcer: a case control study. Gut 1981; 22:1011–1017.

95. Adami HO, Bergström R, Nyren O, et al. Is duodenal ulcer really a psychosomatic disease? A population-based case-control study. Scand J Gastroenterol 1987; 22:889–896.

96. Ellard K, Beaurepaire J, Jones M, Piper D, Tennant C. Acute and chronic stress in duodenal ulcer disease. Gastroenterology 1990; 99:1628–1632.

97. Feldman M, Walker P, Green JI, Weingarden K. Life events, stress and psychosocial factors in men with peptic ulcer disease: a multidimensional case-controlled study. Gastreonterology 1986; 91(December):1370–1379.

98. Levenstein S, Prantera C, Varvo C, Spinella S, Arcà M, Bassi O. Life events, personality, and physical risk factors in recent-onset duodenal ulcers: a preliminary study. J Clin Gastroenterol 1992; 14(3):203–210.

99. Pullan RD, Rhodes J, Ganesh S, et al. Transdermal nicotine for active ulcerative colitis. N Engl J Med 1994; 330(March 24):811–815.

100. Garland CF, Lilienfeld AM, Mendeloff AI, Markowitz JA, Terrell KB, Garland FC. Incidence rates of ulcerative colitis and Crohn's disease in fifteen areas of the United States. Gastroenterology 1981; 81:1115–1124.

101. Ekbom A, Helmick C, Zack M, Adami H. The epidemiology of inflammatory bowel disease: a large, population-based study in Sweden. Gastroenterology 1991; 100:350–358.

102. Summers RW, Switz DM, Sessions JT Jr, et al. National Cooperative Crohn's Disease Study. Gastroenterology 1979; 77:827–944.

103. Fava GA, Wise TN. Recommendations for clinical studies in psychosomatic medicine. Psychosomatics 1988; 29(4):424–427.

104. Spiro HM. Six physicians with inflammatory bowel disease. J Clin Gastroenterol 1990; 12(6):636–642.

105. Weinstock H. Successful treatment of ulcerative colitis by psychoanalysts: a survey of 28 cases, with follow-up. J Psychosom Res 1962; 6:243–249.

106. Schwarz SP, Blanchard EB. Evaluation of a psychological treatment for inflammatory bowel disease. Behav Res Ther 1991; 29(2):167–177.

107. Whitehead WE. Behavioral medicine approaches to gastrointestinal disorders. J Consult Clin Psychol 1992; 60(4):605–612.

108. Alberts MS, Lyons JS, Anderson RH. Relations of coping style and illness variables in ulcerative colitis. Psychol Rep 1988; 62:71–79.

24
Quality of Life Issues in Crohn's Disease

Douglas A. Drossman   *University of North Carolina at Chapel Hill, Chapel Hill, North Carolina*

I. CONCEPTS AND DEFINITIONS

In the preceding chapter, the putative effects of psychosocial factors on the cause or exacerbation of Crohn's disease as well as the psychosocial concomitant factors of the disorder are discussed. In this chapter, the psychosocial impact of Crohn's disease and its measurements are reviewed. The distinction relating to cause and effect, however, is made for convenience; from a systems or biopsychosocial perspective, these factors mutually interact.

For the most part, clinicians and investigators have learned that the physical examination, laboratory studies, pathology reports, and endoscopic and radiological findings do not adequately explain the patient's experience and behavior in the face of illness. Two patients with ileitis may have the same degree of inflammation and the same size stricture of the ileum, yet they respond quite differently. One person may be disabled with chronic pain, and the other may only note an occasional ache, not worthy of further consideration. One may be paralyzed with fears, and the other may ignore them. One may feel helpless and victimized, and the other may seem in full control and able to get on with life. Although symptoms are frequently attributed directly to the degree of pathological change or disease activity, this concept is somewhat simplistic and does not explain the wide range of responses among persons to other medical diseases such as cancer, arthritis, or acquired immunodeficiency syndrome (AIDS). The combination of attributes and behaviors related to illness is unique for every individual and results from several psychosocial factors (a) sociocultural influences that shape attitudes beginning early in life, (b) predisposing psychiatric or personality traits, (c) previous experiences with medical illness, (d) current psychological state (e.g., anxious or sad), and (e) the social network and coping strategies that can "buffer" adverse experiences (1). These factors are particularly important for chronic disorders such as Crohn's disease (2).

Recent investigations also show that measures of disease activity for Crohn's disease are insensitive and discrepant with patient perceptions of their health status (3–5). These psychosocial factors are independent predictors of various outcomes. Among patients with inflammatory bowel disease, quality of life measures such as functional status and

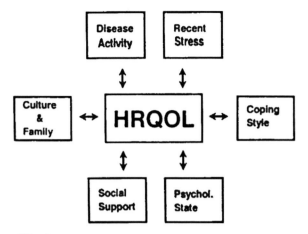

FIG. 1 The association of disease activity and psychosocial factors with health-related quality of life (HRQOL). There is a reciprocating relationship between HRQOL and its determinants. (From Ref. 6.)

disease-related concerns correlate better with scores of well-being and health care utilization than do the physician's rating of disease activity (4).

Health-related quality of life (HRQOL), also called health status, is a global concept that incorporates the patient's perceptions, attributions, and daily level of function in response to an illness (3,6). Taken from this perspective, the biological nature of the disease contributes only a part of the person's HRQOL, which is also strongly influenced by social, cultural, and psychological factors (Fig. 1). Therefore, the evaluate of HRQOL differs from disease measurement in two important ways: (a) it must include psychosocial parameters as well as disease-related factors, and (b) the validation standard rests with the patient, not with the physician, and they are not based on biological tests or other externally measurable factors (3). In effect, HRQOL evaluation quantifies the experience of the illness, much like laboratory or disease activity measures *disease* (i.e., the type and extent of inflammation or pathological condition).

Whereas clinicians readily obtain this information in clinical practice (with simple questions like "How are you doing?"), the capability to obtain HRQOL data for research has evolved only in the last several years. Reliable and valid questionnaires have recently been developed to quantitate the subjective experience of ill health.

II. METHODOLOGICAL ISSUES IN
HEALTH-RELATED QUALITY OF LIFE RESEARCH

The choice of an HRQOL scale usually depends on the interests and needs of the clinician and investigator. The scales possess certain qualities that are helpful to investigors (7). An instrument that can differentiate between persons or groups in terms of a better and worse HRQOL is said to be discriminative. When it measures how much HRQOL has changed in a given patient or group of patients, it has evaluative capability. For a discriminative instrument, *reliability*, that is, the condition when the variability between patients is greater than variability within patients, is most important. For an evaluative measure, *responsiveness*, that is, the ability to detect change, is most important. Several types of research instruments meet these needs.

A. Global Measures

The simplest approach to assess quality of life is to use a single question in which the patient intuitively integrates all the domains of HRQOL into a single global response. One example, "How would you rate your general well-being?" (or "How would you rate the quality of your life?") is usually scored on a 5-point scale (excellent, very good, good, fair, poor). The response can give a clinically relevant global measure of health status, and it is a strong predictor of physician visits for patients with inflammatory bowel disease (5). Global measures, however, yield no information about the factors leading to the patient's response.

B. Generic Measures

Generic measures evaluate HRQOL independent of the specific features of the disease. Therefore, the values can either characterize a range of responses for a patient group or compare HRQOL across patient groups, even with different diseases. There are two types of generic measures—health profiles and utility measures (7,8).

Multi-item health profiles incorporate several domains of experience and behavior, such as physical or psychosocial functioning, or perceptions of disease impact. For example, the Sickness Impact Profile (SIP), a commonly used health profile, encompasses 12 areas of daily function: an "overall" score, a "physical" domain containing three subscales (ambulation, mobility, body care and movement), a "psychosocial" domain with four subscales (social interaction, communication, alertness behavior, and emotional behavior), and five "independent" domains (sleep and rest, eating, work, home management, and recreation and pastimes) (9). As a generic scale, the SIP can be used in health policy planning to compare the functional status of patients having different diseases. For Crohn's disease, values on the overall scale show patients with Crohn's disease to have poorer HRQOL than a random sample or than patients with obesity, but better HRQOL than patients with rheumatoid arthritis, chronic obstructive pulmonary disease, or chronic back pain (6).

Single-item utility measures relate self-perception to a reference point. For example, the "Time Trade-Off Technique (TTOT)" evaluates the patient's perception of existing health compared with death (10). The score ranges from 0.0 (equal to death) to 1.0 (full health). The patient chooses between living in the present state of health with all its physical and psychosocial limitations and living a shorter life span but in perfect health. For two patients with Crohn's disease having a life expectancy of 75 years, the one with good HRQOL may feel well enough to only trade 5 years of life (and live until age 70) in full health. This person would have a utility score of $70/75 = 0.93$. In comparison, the other patient in poorer health might be willing to trade more years (e.g., 30) (and live until age 45) to be in perfect health. So the utility score would be $45/75 = 0.60$. This technique has been used to evaluate HRQOL in response to colectomy for patients with ulcerative colitis, and it can be used to factor patient preferences in ulcerative colitis relating to surveillance versus prophylactic colectomy (11,12). Similar to global measures, a utility measure is more useful as an evaluative rather than a discriminative measure because the determinants leading to the score are not known (7).

C. Specific Measures

Disease-specific measures evaluate the special states and concerns of patients having a particular disease. A scale developed for Crohn's disease would likely have questions relating to bowel habit, abdominal pain, and sexual functioning, whereas one for rheumatoid arthritis might ask about hand strength and mobility. Disease-specific measures are more responsive to clinical changes that occur over time, and the questions relate closely to areas routinely evaluated by physicians (13). Therefore, they are considered useful for clinical trials. However, they cannot discriminate between patients with different diseases and they may not be generalizable to different clinical populations even with the same disease. For example, a quality of life scale developed for hospitalized patients with inflammatory bowel disease (containing items related to fever, abdominal mass, and anemia, among others) may not adequately assess changes in HRQOL among ambulatory patients with milder illness, the so-called "ceiling" effect (7). Table 1 lists the features of the HRQOL instruments developed for inflammatory bowel disease.

TABLE 1 Specific Health Status Instruments for Inflammatory Bowel Disease

Name	Scales	Comments
Inflammatory Bowel Disease Questionnaire (IBDQ) (14)	Bowel symptoms	Well standardized
	Systemic symptoms	Designed for clinical trials
32-Item Likert Scale, interiew format	Social function	Developed on "sick" patients—
	Emotional function	gastrointestinal referrals and inpatients
Modified IBDQ (16)	Bowel symptoms	Derived from IBDQ
36-Item Likert Scale, self-administered	Systemic symptoms	Developed on "well" patients—
	Social function	Local chapter of NFIC
	Emotional function	
	Functional impairment	
Cleveland Clinic IBD Questionnaire (17)	Functional/economic	Correlates with SIP
	Social/recreational	Developed on ulcerative colitis/
47-Item Likert Scale, interview format	Affect/life in general	Crohn's disease surgery and
	Medical/symptoms	nonsurgery groups
		Quality of life index distinguishes groups
Rating Form of IBD Patient Concerns (RFIPC) (18)	Impact of disease	Correlates with Sickness Impact Profile and SCL-90
	Sexual intimacy	
25-Item Visual Analog Scale, self-administered	Complications	Developed on "well" patients—
	Body stigma	CCFA national sample
UC/CD Health Status Scales (19)	Ulcerative colitis	Standardized to health care
9 or 10-item Likert Scale, physician/patient scoring	Crohn's disease	use, function, psychological distress in CCFA
		Designed to discriminate mild/ severe illness and predict outcome
		Better predictor than Crohn's Disease Activity Index

Source: Ref. 6.

There are certain features that are unique to each scale. The Inflammatory Bowel Disease Questionnaire (IBDQ) was developed to evaluate bowel and systemic symptoms and emotional and social function in treatment trials (14). The questionnaire is psychometrically sound and has been shown to be reproducible, stable, and responsive to change in an IBD population (15). The Modified IBDQ was tested in a sample of patients with milder disease (16). Although it is not fully standardized (the IBD data was only compared with those of normal control group), the modified IBDQ used many of the same questions as the IBDQ, providing concurrent validity with the more standard IBDQ. The Cleveland Clinic questionnaire evaluated activities of daily living rather than medical symptoms, and the items successfully discriminated patients with ulcerative colitis and Crohn's disease as well as those with milder (i.e., no surgery history) and more severe disease (17). The Rating Form of IBD Patient Concerns (RFIPC) rates the 25 most important worries and concerns of patients with inflammatory bowel disease (18). It can help clinicians easily obtain this type of information and could be used as a responsive measure of counceling or educational interventions. The scores on the RFIPC correlate well with self-reports of well-being, psychological distress (SCL-90), and daily function (SIP). Finally, the *UC/CD Health Status Scales* were designed to discriminate mild from severe illness and to predict a composite outcome measure that incorporates health care use, daily function, and psychologic distress (19). The symptom items in the scale were stronger predictors of these outcomes than the Crohn's Disease Activity Index (20).

III. RESULTS FROM CLINICAL STUDIES OF HEALTH-RELATED QUALITY OF LIFE IN INFLAMMATORY BOWEL DISEASE

Most reports of quality of life in inflammatory bowel disease are based on physician assessment or nonstandardized questionnaires. This section reviews the HRQOL studies using standardized measures of assessment.

A. National Studies of Nonclinical Populations with Inflammatory Bowel Disease

In an American study, 997 members belonging to the Crohn's and Colitis Foundation of America (CCFA) were surveyed with regard to demographic factors, symptoms, and clinical data including HRQOL (5). The key findings were (a) the health status of this population based on global measures, psychological distress scores (SCL-90) and daily function (SIP) was generally good, (b) impairment in daily functioning occurred more in the psychological and social realms than the physical realm, (c) when compared with patients with ulcerative colitis, those with Crohn's disease had greater psychosocial difficulties and health care use; however, the Crohn's disease group had more psychosocial difficulties because of greater disease severity, (d) the members effectively coped with disease-related distress through social support and problem-based coping strategies, and (e) psychosocial and quality of life measures (e.g., general well-being, psychologic distress, and functional status) were strong predictors of physician visits (21). Disease activity measures did not have a significant influence on physician visits, but were strong predictors of hospitalization and surgery.

The RFIPC was tested and standardized on this population (18). The most intense concerns related to the uncertain future of the disease, the effects of medication, energy level, surgery (and having an ostomy bag), being a burden on others, loss of bowel control, and development of cancer. It was also found that those with Crohn's disease were more concerned with their energy level, being a burden on others, achieving their full potential, experiencing pain or suffering, financial costs, and passing on the disease to others. In comparison, those with ulcerative colitis were more concerned with development of cancer. The authors suggested that identifying and addressing patient concerns through education or counseling may improve their health status.

B. Clinical and Referral Patient Data

The SIP was also used in a sample of outpatients and hospitalized patients with inflammatory disease, and most of the national data findings were supported in this clinical patient sample (4). Also, as expected, much higher scores were obtained for hospitalized patients (SIP overall score 28) than outpatients (SIP overall score 8), thereby confirming usefulness of this scale as an evaluative measure. In using the Cleveland Clinic questionnaire for referred patients, Farmer et al. also found that patients with Crohn's disease have poorer HRQOL than those with ulcerative colitis and patients with surgical histories reported poorer HRQOL than those with no history (17).

C. Ulcerative Colitis Postsurgical Data

Two issues relevant to ulcerative colitis are whether colectomy leads to improvement in HRQOL and whether there is a differential effect among the three surgical procedures: conventional ileostomy, Kock pouch, and ileal pouch–anal anastomosis. McLeod et al. used two utility measures, the TTOT and the Direct Questioning of Objectives (DQO) to answer these questions (11). In the first study, the authors studied 20 patients before colectomy and again 1 year postoperatively. The mean utility scores for the TTOT increased from 0.58 ± 0.34 to 0.98 ± 0.07 after surgery, and, similarly, the DQO increased from 0.38 ± 0.27 to 0.88 ± 0.19 ($p < 0.05$). In the second study, the authors compared the utility scores for patients who had colectomy and these three surgeries at least 1 year previously. The TTOT and DQO scores for the three groups were not significantly different (ranging from 0.95–0.97 for TTOT and 0.86–0.89 for DQO), suggesting that the choice of surgery is irrelevant at least 1 year later.

In another study, more than 1000 ulcerative colitis patients who had colectomy and the three types of operations beginning in 1981 were surveyed retrospectively to assess the degree of restriction related to social activity, recreation interpersonal relationships, sexual activity, and travel (22). The authors found that patients with ileal pouch–anal anastomoses had fewer restrictions in sports and sexual activities than those with Kock pouches ($p < 0.05$), whereas those with Kock pouches had fewer restrictions in these activities, but more restrictions in travel than those with Brooke ileostomies ($p < 0.05$). All others categories were similar among groups.

When the RFIPC was used to compare patient's concerns between CCFA patients with ostomies to those without ostomies, it was found that those with ostomies had fewer disease-related concerns about cancer, surgery, and having an ostomy. Furthermore, they did not report more body-image concerns (sexuality, intimacy, attractiveness) (23). These three studies suggest that quality of life is improved in response to colectomy for ulcerative colitis and that the presence of an ostomy diminishes or at least does not worsen disease-related concerns.

IV. CONCLUSION

Clinicians and investigators have come to realize that disease-related measures such as laboratory data, histopathology, and endoscopic/radiological findings do not adequately explain the health status of patients with inflammatory bowel disease. The evaluation of health-related quality of life broadens our understanding of the impact of these disorders in a manner that cannot be accomplished through these traditional methods.

The recent interest in HRQOL research has led to the development of several standardized instruments for inflammatory bowel disease. Although there are only limited data from studies using standardized instruments, a few conclusions derived from these studies can be made: (a) for most ambulatory patients, HRQOL is generally good, (b) functional impairment is greater in the psychological and social dimensions than in physical dimensions, (c) patients with Crohn's disease have greater impairment of HRQOL than those with ulcerative colitis, (d) there is a strong relationship between disease severity and HRQOL impairment, which accounts for the greater impairment in HRQOL with Crohn's disease, (e) disease-related worries and concerns are associated with psychological distress and poor function, so reduction in these concerns through education/counseling may improve HRQOL, (f) impaired HRQOL appears to be successfully mediated through problem-based coping strategies, (g) HRQOL measures, such as daily functional status and disease-related concerns, correlate better with general well-being than with the physician's rating of disease activity, and they are stronger predictors of health care visits than disease activity, and (h) for ulcerative colitis, colectomy, regardless of surgical repair, is associated with improved HRQOL, reduced worries about disease, and no worsening of body image concerns (4,5,16,17,18,24–26).

REFERENCES

1. Drossman DA. Psychosocial considerations in gastroenterology. In: Sleisenger MH, Fordtran JS, Scharschmidt BF, Feldman M, eds. Gastrointestinal disease: Pathophysiology, Diagnosis, Management. 5th ed. Philadelphia: WB Saunders, 1993:3–17.

2. Drossman DA. Psychosocial factors in ulcerative colitis and Crohn's disease. In: Kirsner JB, Shorter RG, eds. Inflammatory Bowel Disease. 4th ed. Philadelphia: Lea & Febiger, 1994.

3. Garrett JW, Drossman DA. Health status in inflammatory bowel disease: biological and behavioral considerations. Gastroenterology 1990; 99:90–96.

4. Drossman DA, Patrick DL, Mitchell CM, Zagami EA, Appelbaum MI. Health related quality of life in inflammatory bowel disease: functional status and patient worries and concerns. Dig Dis Sci 1989; 34:1379–1386.

5. Drossman DA, Leserman J, Mitchell CM, Li Z, Zagami EA, Patrick DL. Health status and health care use in persons with inflammatory bowel disease: a national sample. Dig Dis Sci 1991; 36:1746–1755.

6. Drossman DA. Quality of life in IBD: methods and findings. In: Rachmilewitz D, ed. Falk Symposium #72; Inflammatory Bowel Disease—1994. Dordrecht: Kluwer Academic Publishers, 1994:105–116.

7. Guyatt GH, Feeny DH, Patrick DL. Measuring health-related quality of life. Ann Intern Med 1993; 118:662–629.

8. Patrick DL, Deyo RA. Generic and disease-specific measures in assessing health status and quality of life. Med Care 1989; 27:S217–S232.

9. Bergner M, Bobbitt RA, Carter WB. The Sickness Impact Profile: development and final revision of a health status measure. Med Care 1981; 19:787–805.

10. Torrance GW, Thomas WH, Sackett DL. A utility maximization model for evaluation of health care program. Health Serv Res 1972; 7:118–133.

11. McLeod RS, Churchill DN, Lock AM, Vanderburgh S, Cohen Z. Quality of life of patients with ulcerative colitis preoperatively and postoperatively. Gastroenterology 1991; 101:1307–1313.

12. Provenzale D, Shearin M, Tillinger B, et al. The effect of patient preferences on policy recommendations for prophylactic colectomy or surveillance in patients with ulcerative colitis (abstr). Gastroenterology 1994; 4:A22.

13. Guyatt GH, Walter S, Norman G. Measuring change over time: assessing the usefulness of evaluative instruments. J Chron Dis 1987; 40:171–178.

14. Guyatt G, Mitchell A, Irvine EJ, et al. A new measure of health status for clinical trials in inflammatory bowel disease. Gastroenterology 1989; 96:804–10.

15. Irvine EJ, Feagan B, Rochon J, et al. Quality of life: a valid and reliable measure of therapeutic efficacy in the treatment of inflammatory bowel disease. Gastroenterology 1994; 106:287–296.

16. Love JR, Irvine EJ, Fedorak RN. Quality of life in inflammatory bowel disease. J Clin Gastroenterol 1992; 14:15–19.

17. Farmer RG, Easley KA, Farmer JM. Quality of life assessment by patients with inflammatory bowel disease. Cleve Clin J Med 1992; 59:35–42.

18. Drossman DA, Leserman J, Li Z, Mitchell CM, Zagami EA, Patrick DL. The rating form of IBD patient concerns: a new measure of health status. Psychosom Med 1991; 53:701–712.

19. Drossman DA, Li Z, Leserman J, Patrick DL. Ulcerative colitis and Crohn's disease health status scales for research and clinical practice. J Clin Gastroenterol 1992; 15:104–112.

20. Best WR, Becktel JM, Singleton JW, Kern FJ. Development of a Crohn's disease activity index. National Cooperative Crohn's Disease Study. Gastroenterology 1976; 70:439–444.

21. Lazarus RS, Folkman S. Stress, appraisal and coping. New York: Springer, 1984:1–445.

22. Kohler LW, Pemberton JH, Zinsmeister AR, Kelly KA. Quality of life after proctocolectomy. A comparison of Brooke ileostomy, Kock pouch, and ileal pouch–anal anastomosis. Gastroenterology 1991, 101:679–684.

23. Drossman DA, Mitchell CM, Appelbaum MI, Patrick DL, Zagami EA. Do IBD ostomates do better? a study of symptoms and health-related quality of life (abstr). Gastroenterology 1989, 96:A130.

24. Mitchell A, Guyatt G, Singer J, et al. Quality of life in patients with inflammatory bowel disease. J Clin Gastroenterol 1988, 10:306–310.

25. Whitehead WE, Engel BT, Schuster MM. Irritable bowel syndrome: physiological and psychological differences between diarrhea-predominant and constipation-predominant patients. Dig Dis Sci 1980; 25:6:404–413.

26. Tjandra JJ, Fazio VW, Church JM, Oakley JR, Milsom JW, Lavery IC. Similar functional results after restorative proctocolectomy in patients with familial adenomatous polyposis and mucosal ulcerative colitis life quality and psychological morbidity with an ileostomy. Am J Surg 1993; 165:322–325.

COMMENTARY

Barbara S. Kirschner   *Wyler Children's Hospital, The University of Chicago, Chicago, Illinois*

One of the more interesting aspects of the history of Crohn's disease and ulcerative colitis is the change in thought from psychological issues as being causative to their being a consequence of the recurrent intestinal (and extraintestinal) symptoms. The background for much of this progression in thought is reviewed in the accompanying chapters. Unfortunately, outdated stereotypical characterizations of the personalities of patients with inflammatory bowel disease are still heard in the lay public and are spoken by therapists, some of whom are entrusted with counseling these patients.

As a pediatric gastroenterologist caring for a large population of children and adolescents with inflammatory bowel disease, it is apparent to me that the psychological impact of these conditions is often vastly different between periods of disease activity and remission. In the acute situation, recurring episodes of severe pain induce fear of hospitalization and the need for diagnostic studies and procedures, possible surgery, and even death. Illness prompts constant attention from family members (especially parents) into what would otherwise be private matters (e.g., stool frequency and consistency, weight changes). With chronic disease, the effect of repeated unanticipated school (or work) absenteeism, having to leave a classroom early (to the obvious gaze of peers), or showing the cosmetic effects of corticosteroid therapy can produce significant emotional reactions. Under these circumstances, the two emotional states (anxiety and depression) observed to be greater in pediatric patients with inflammatory bowel disease than control subjects are understandable.

The recommendation that patients need a sensitive member of the medical team ("an open ear") to prepare them to cope with the changing course of their Crohn's disease is important. One has to identify the specific concerns of the individual patient so that they can be addressed constructively. Based on my experience, the list of factors that contribute to anxiety and depression is extensive including anger at a parent for having "given" the patient the disease, anger at a physician who cannot cure the disease, thoughts that the patient is being punished by God, frustration over the lack of control of symptoms, recognition that having Crohn's disease makes the patient "different" from peers, and guilt for the cost of therapy incurred by the family.

Dr. Drossman describes his studies with objective measures of health-related quality of life (HRQOL) and suggests that this can be improved in patients with Crohn's disease by "education or counseling using problem-based coping strategies." He noted that psychosocial and quality of life measures correlated with physician visits, and disease activity scores more closely predicted hospitalization.

Fortunately, despite the physical and psychosocial problems described above, a recent study from Scotland of 70 adult patients with inflammatory bowel disease (50 juvenile-onset Crohn's disease and 20 ulcerative colitis) was generally encouraging regarding the eventual outcome of patients with Crohn's disease. Although Crohn's disease had an adverse effect on school attendance, the percent of patients with Crohn's disease entering college was higher than for high school graduates as a whole. In addition, the rate of "involuntary unemployment" was low (6 of 70) in young adults with Crohn's disease. These authors concluded that "most patients were successful in gaining and retaining a satisfactory job."

25

The Psychiatric Treatment of Patients with Crohn's Disease

Marvin Kaplan   *Lenox Hill Hospital, New York, New York*

In comparison with ulcerative colitis, Crohn's disease occurs earlier in life, can be more widespread throughout the gastrointestinal tract, is generally more painful, and has no cure. Crohn's disease has an unpredictable course, and it can create numerous psychiatric problems such as depression, anxiety, and drug dependence for patients, putting considerable stress on their families. In a subset of patients, certain psychiatric problems seem to exacerbate Crohn's disease. When these situations arise, psychiatric consultation and treatment can be beneficial.

The psychiatric consultant's job is to correctly assess (a) the nature of the current psychological problems and their relationship to Crohn's disease, (b) the patient's personality structure, including its strengths and weaknesses, and (c) the role that the patient's family may be playing in mitigating or exacerbating the problems. After this information is collected, the psychiatrist should create a therapeutic plan that is consistent with the ongoing medical or surgical treatment. Because this can take a considerable amount of time, the sooner the consultant is involved with the patient, the better.

I. RELATIONSHIP BETWEEN PSYCHIATRIC ILLNESS AND CROHN'S DISEASE: A REVIEW OF THE ENGLISH LITERATURE

Because ulcerative colitis was conceptualized as strictly a psychosomatic illness, there is a considerable amount of literature about its psychiatric aspects (1,2). By comparison, the literature concerning psychiatric problems in Crohn's disease is relatively sparse. As with ulcerative colitis, over the past several decades, there has been a shift in focus from etiological psychiatric factors to the psychological effect of Crohn's disease on the patient and family.

Despite this change in outlook, a number of studies repeatedly show that a variety of stressful events coincide with the onset or exacerbation of Crohn's disease (3–7). Although these reports suffer from the not inconsiderable problem of being retrospective, they are consistent with similar research in other illnesses, including ulcerative colitis (6). There is evidence that the illness is influenced by psychological stressors in some Crohn's disease patients, and the idea should not be discarded.

A large number of studies show that patients with Crohn's disease have significant concurrent psychiatric morbidity when compared with patients with ulcerative colitis, patients with other chronic medical illnesses and normal control subjects (1,2,4,8–10). These studies are fairly uniform in finding that most of the increased psychiatric morbidity is due to a higher incidence of depression in patients with Crohn's disease.

Surprisingly, this latter literature reports little correlation between the severity of Crohn's disease and the development of psychiatric symptoms. (McKegney et al. report an exception (6).) This implies that, most likely, there are biochemical personality or social factors that mediate how well a patient adapts to this illness, and some reports attempt to elucidate these variables (11–14). Some such factors that have been identified are an accurate knowledge of Crohn's disease, having a sense of control over the illness, and strong social supports, These may be indicators of more basic underlying psychiatric issues such as the structure of the patient's psychic defenses or the neurochemical vulnerability of the patient to depression. Further research is needed to more specifically identify these factors, which seem crucial in determining a successful adaptation to Crohn's disease.

II. CLINICAL ISSUES

All chronic painful illnesses with unpredictable courses put obvious burdens on a patient's emotional life (with unpredictability often being the psychologically most difficult hardship). Admixtures of anger, depression, denial, and anxiety are all common and normal reactions to living with Crohn's disease. Psychiatric intervention is needed when one or more specific clinical syndromes develop.

A. Major Depressive Disorder

The most common psychiatric problem in patients with Crohn's disease is the development of a major depressive disorder; almost 50% of patients with Crohn's disease were so diagnosed in one study (8). A patient with Crohn's disease and major depression has two serious illnesses. Major depression itself can cause severe fatigue, anorexia, weight loss, insomnia, impaired concentration, and poor memory; major depressive disorder also carries a 15% lifetime chance of suicide. In addition, major depression significantly affects the ability to cope with Crohn's disease. For example, it creates increased abdominal pain by decreasing pain thresholds, and patients often stop taking their medications or keeping their doctor's appointments because they feel hopeless. This can easily initiate a downward spiral, with Crohn's disease and a major depression negatively reinforcing each other.

Because the severity of bowel symptoms does not seem to correlate with the severity of psychiatric symptoms, a careful history is needed to determine why a particular patient has become depressed. It is often puzzling why a major depression develops in someone with relatively mild Crohn's disease. First, the specific precipitating circumstances (e.g., pain, "living from bathroom to bathroom," fatigue, or the uncertainty of the course of the illness) must be determined. Second, it must be discovered what these issues mean to the patients beyond the obvious interference with their lives and sense of well-being. For example, for a younger patient, chronic diarrhea may mean "I'm smelly, who would want me? I'll never marry," whereas for an older patient, fatigue can be guiltily experienced as "I'm a terrible burden to my family." There are also patients with a probable biochemical vulnerability to major depression (assessed by a history of prior major depressions, manic episodes or a family history of affective illness) regardless of Crohn's disease.

The other key area to assess is the use of depresogenic substances, which can cause or exacerbate the picture of a major depression. Corticosteroids and narcotics are common offenders, but alcohol, tranquilizers, sedatives, and other drugs of abuse may also be involved; at times, a drug screen of both blood and urine is helpful.

The treatment of a major depressive disorder usually involves starting antidepressant medication and psychotherapy. Psychotherapy is short term and is aimed at strengthening the patient's defenses to better cope with the precipitating problems and their underlying meaning to the patient (supportive psychotherapy). A selective serotonin reuptake inhibitor (SSRI) such as fluoxetine or sertraline is usually the drug of choice, although, if diarrhea is a major problem, a constipating antidepressant (e.g., a tertiary tricyclic such as triimipramine) is often better tolerated. Specific psychopharmacological issues in patients with Crohn's disease include, at times, poor absorption of antidepressants requiring the use of high oral doses and frequent monitoring of serum drug levels; on rare occasions, parenteral administration is necessary. If corticosteroids, narcotics, or other drugs are causing or exacerbating a major depression, they should be reduced or stopped if possible. When not possible, substituting adrenocorticotropic hormone (ACTH) for oral or intravenous corticosteroids often preserves the therapeutic effect without being depresogenic.

Psychotherapeutically, much has been made of patients with certain medical illnesses having difficulty expressing their feelings, fantasies, and the psychological connection between events. The term "alexithymia" has been coined to describe this condition (15,16). In my experience, this certainly does occur in patients with Crohn's disease but not particularly more so than in other patients seeking psychiatric treatment (17). The therapist should recognize that the patient is concrete or regressed and the psychotherapeutic technique should be adapted accordingly.

If the patient is well understood and the issues that are depressing the patient are correctly identified, the aggressive use of both antidepressants and psychotherapy is usually successful in improving or curing a major depressive episode. Outpatients need to be seen at least once per week, although those at risk for suicide or with complicated personality structures may need to be seen more often until the depressive episode resolves. If patients are in the hospital (for either medical or psychiatric reasons), they are seen daily until their condition is significantly improved. In selected cases, spouses or families are included in the treatment if they are part of the problem or if additional emotional support is necessary. If a patient's condition has not improved after several months (which allows adequate trials of two different antidepressants and a reasonable period of psychotherapy), the case should be reconceptualized and a different approach tried.

B. Psychogenic Precipitation and Exacerbation

1. Psychogenicity

Clinical experience supports the literature in identifying a subgroup of patients with Crohn's disease whose illness is psychologically precipitated or exacerbated, that is, specific feelings or emotional conflicts play some role in activating Crohn's disease. In many of these patients, a full remission is difficult to achieve without psychiatric treatment. A general rule is that patients who are unable to obtain a remission or have frequent relapses despite good compliance with a medical regimen should have a psychiatric evaluation to determine whether there is evidence for psychogenicity.

A detailed history is the key to determining whether a patient's Crohn's disease is psychogenically precipitated or exacerbated. Setting the tone of the initial consultation is crucial because some patients are puzzled by or hostile to a psychiatric evaluation. Most helpful is an early acknowledgement that the consultant has no bias and believes that some cases of Crohn's disease are psychologically influenced and others are not. The patient is then asked to engage with the interviewer to examine the facts and find out the truth of the situation. This approach is also useful with a patient who is refusing a psychiatric consultation.

Once there is a working relationship with the patient, a standard psychiatric history is obtained. The essential issues to review (in detail) are the emotional events surrounding the current exacerbation as well those events that preceded the initial onset of Crohn's disease and prior exacerbations. Other issues to assess are the prodromal activation of psychodynamic conflicts (which usually involve dependency or aggression and may be outside the patient's awareness), anniversary reactions of significant losses, and the family's response to patient's illness. At least one to two hours spread over several days are needed for this type of evaluation.

With this approach, it generally becomes clear whether emotional factors are playing a role; if they are, most patients are aware of the fact. Usually, anxiety is a factor, but, at times, depression or guilt is the problem. Sexual conflicts, even if attended with overt anxiety or guilt, are rarely factors. Also most patients with Crohn's disease who are in this subgroup seem to stay in it. That is, if the initial onset of disease has evidence of being psychogenically precipitated, so will subsequent exacerbations. Occasionally, this is not the case, and evidence can be found for one relapse but not for another.

If a case of psychogenic precipitation of disease is questionable, the patient is instructed to keep a diary for at least two weeks, charting bowel symptoms with concurrent events and feelings. This is especially useful for patients who have trouble remembering their feelings, and a review of the diary usually clarifies the issue.

2. Restoration of Responsiveness to Medical Treatment

Once psychogenicity of disease is established, vigorous psychiatric treatment is generally needed. The most dramatic example of this is when such a patient is unresponsive to medical treatment and needs surgery. Because these patients are invariably in the hospital, aggressive treatment of anxiety and depression is possible, necessary, and frequently effective in establishing responsiveness to medical treatment. If anxiety is exacerbating a patient's Crohn's disease, the patient is heavily tranquilized (almost sedated) for several days with a benzodiazepine such as clonazepam. If the patient cannot take anything orally, lorazepam, clonazepam, and traizolam are all effective sublingually at their usual oral doses; other benzodiazepines may also work sublingually but experience with them is lacking. Lorazepam can also be administered intravenously or, if necessary, intramuscularly. In selected cases, the medication schedule is adjusted so that patients are alert enough to be seen daily in psychotherapy. Psychotherapy is aimed at concretely solving current problems and reducing anxiety. Similarly, with a nonagitated depression, psychostimulants are preferred because of their more rapid onset, and a similar type of intensive psychotherapy is started. If the patient's medical condition allows the necessary two to five days for these measures to start to work, clinical experience is that many patients begin responding to medical treatment and immediate surgery can be avoided.

More common are patients whose Crohn's disease is partially improved but who do not achieve a full remission or are having frequent relapses. If psychogenic factors are determined to be affecting their illness, many of these patients can be helped to achieve a full and stable remission. Again, the cornerstones of treatment are the accurate identification of the psychogenic precipitants, appropriate psychopharmacological treatment of anxiety or depression, and a focused psychotherapy aimed at minimizing the intensity of the aggravating emotion. Customarily, this is done on an outpatient basis, and the patient is seen at least weekly until the Crohn's disease remits; this is concurrent with active medical treatment. It is crucial to understand (and to explain to the patient) that some of these patients are experiencing a low level of anxiety or depression that would not warrant any treatment except that there is evidence that these emotions are worsening their illness.

C. Pathological Denial of Illness

1. Nature of the Problem

In clinical practice, pathological denial of Crohn's disease is a relatively common and serious problem, particularly among younger patients. Denial is the emotional inability to accept a painful reality, and it exists on a continuum. Too much (pathological) denial results in the feeling that "I'm not sick," leading to a refusal to take medications or see physicians; too little denial leads to hypochondriasis and high levels of anxiety. Optimally, patients achieve a moderate state of denial in which they are fully compliant with treatment yet are not preoccupied with their disease.

Most patients with significant denial are not seen by physicians unless they are quite ill, their lives are seriously disrupted by their symptoms, or they are coerced by their families. In Crohn's disease, pathological denial is seen in all age groups but seems most common in adolescents and young adults. These younger people are in the midst of developing a stable self-image as well as a vision of their future and, for some, the reality of having a lifelong incurable illness is psychologically intolerable. Of note is that patients who have had Crohn's disease since childhood do not seem to have this problem in adolescence or adulthood.

Once it is clear that pathological denial is the reason that a patient has neglected the illness, psychiatric consultation is indicated. Otherwise, the patient will "disappear" once the acute exacerbation is treated or family pressure abates. Emphasizing the medical risks of continued noncompliance is counterproductive: at best, the patient agrees intellectually but emotionally the patient is made more anxious, which often strengthens the use of denial as a defense. Having patients agree to a psychiatric consultation is generally best done by emphasizing how intolerable having Crohn's disease seems to be for them and that perhaps a better way of coping can be found. Initial refusals of psychiatric care are expected, but, with perseverance and a conviction that there can be no good treatment of the illness with pathological denial present, some patients can be persuaded to become engaged with a psychiatrist.

2. Treatment

The psychiatric treatment of pathological denial is psychotherapy. The specific techniques depend on the patient's overall personality structure and underlying anxieties. Common anxieties that feed pathological denial are fear of death, fear of pain, fear of being sexually unattractive and alone the rest of one's life, fear of not being able to control and plan the future, and, in narcissistic individuals, fear of "not being perfect." Many patients have histories of using significant denial since childhood, with early histories of counterphobic behavior being not uncommon.

Psychotherapy is conducted on an outpatient basis usually once or twice per week. It is exploratory in nature, aiming at gradually uncovering the specific fears that generate such severe denial and developing other sets of defenses to cope with them. At the forefront of this type of treatment is how patients currently cope with their Crohn's disease, with noncompliance taking priority over other issues. There needs to be ongoing communication between the psychiatrist and gastroenterologist, with the patient being apprised of what has been discussed. The main psychotherapeutic issue is keeping the patient in treatment. Pathological denial often extends to the need for psychiatric treatment, and such patients are, as a rule, tenuously engaged in psychotherapy for extended periods. The therapist needs to carefully gauge how much anxiety the patient is able to tolerate, particularly early in treatment, when the basic defense is still to deny that there is any problem. Such patients stop psychotherapy suddenly if too much anxiety is generated too soon.

D. Drug Dependence

1. Scope of the Problem

Drug dependence is defined as repeated intoxication or inability to decrease drug use persisting for at least one month, impairment in social or occupational functioning, and evidence of physiological tolerance or withdrawal symptoms (18). There is controversy about the incidence of drug dependence among medically ill patients, with the current consensus being that it is rare among patients with no prior history of substance abuse (19–23). These reports overlook certain practical clinical problems. First, because drug dependence is relatively common, a percentage of medically ill patients have a prior or current history of it. The incidence of drug dependence in the general population is estimated to be 1% to 5%, excluding alcohol dependence, and 7% to 14% when alcohol dependence is included (24). There is no basis in thinking that medically ill patients would have a lower incidence. Secondly, the diagnosis of drug dependence is difficult to make until it is far advanced. Third, clear distinction should be made concerning the use of narcotics (and other dependence-producing medications) in acute versus chronic situations and, most importantly, between inpatient and outpatient settings. The literature focuses almost exclusively on inpatients, and the problem in Crohn's disease probably mainly occurs in outpatients (25).

In one study that specifically looked at drug dependence in inflammatory bowel disease, it was conservatively estimated that 5% of all inflammatory bowel disease patients may be drug dependent (25). Although the sample studied was not random, most patients developed drug dependence without a prior history of it, most developed it on an outpatient basis, and patients with Crohn's disease seemed at higher risk than patients with ulcerative colitis. Until there is further research, it seems prudent to consider drug dependence to be a complication of Crohn's disease.

2. Diagnosis

Making the diagnosis of drug dependence is difficult because the patient does not report it and frequently denies it when questioned. There are usually few clues until the problem has escalated. On occasion, difficult to explain bowel symptoms (narcotic bowel syndrome) may arouse suspicion as may a patient's preoccupation with the amounts and doses of narcotics, sedatives, or other drugs. Signs of intoxication or withdrawal observed by the prescribing physician are late signs of drug dependence; usually, patients try to protect the supply of drugs by not misusing them on the day of an appointment.

If there is any suspicion of drug dependence, the key to making the diagnosis lies in interviewing the patient's family or friends. In contrast to the patient's efforts to hide the problem, family and friends are generally forthright and concerned. They may report the use of medication in the absence of pain, the presence of multiple prescriptions from multiple physicians, signs of repeated intoxication, and impairment in functioning. This is so consistent that it is suggested that drug dependence not be ruled out until after interviewing a family member or friend of the patient.

3. Treatment

Prevention is the key to drug dependence in Crohn's disease because the dependencies is usually iatrogenic. The source of pain should be sought and treated with a specific medical or surgical program rather than masking the pain with narcotics or other drugs. If narcotics are prescribed, only one of the patient's physicians should be designated to prescribe them. This physician should rule out prior or concurrent substance abuse, which are relative contraindications to chronic narcotic prescription. The first approach in treatment (other than treating the underlying Crohn's disease) is to increase the patient's pain tolerance. Both depression and anxiety can dramatically lower pain tolerance, and, if either is present, it should be treated with appropriate psychotropic medication or psychotherapy. At times, hypnosis or relaxation training is helpful. Chronic narcotic use can lead to lower pain thresholds, and narcotics should be prescribed on a scheduled rather than an as needed basis (26–28). Development of the early signs of drug dependence (e.g., increasing doses, "lost" prescriptions, a focus on pain medications, or family concerns) should not be ignored.

If patients develop iatrogenic drug dependence on a single medication (usually an oral narcotic), they can often be treated without psychiatric intervention. They need firm confrontation of their drug dependence and gradual detoxification. If a patient is obtaining the drug from multiple physicians, the various physicians should coordinate a therapeutic plan, and only one will prescribe drugs. Generally, drug-dependent patients have a good prognosis as long as their access to the drug abuse is eliminated or well controlled.

Patients with iatrogenic multiple drug dependence or noniatrogenic dependence almost always need specialized psychiatric treatment. Usually, psychiatric hospitalization in a drug rehabilitation unit is necessary in the beginning of therapy. The prognosis of such patients is much poorer.

E. Coping with the Illness

1. Burden of Crohn's Disease

Most reports say that patients with Crohn's disease cope well, and more than 90% say that such patients have a fair to good long-term quality of life (29,30). As expected, patients did better when they had more localized illness, did not need surgery, or, if they did need surgery, had a resection rather than an ileostomy. However, there is still a psychological burden of living with Crohn's disease and a subgroup of patients who do not cope well and often request psychiatric treatment.

The issues that patients with Crohn's disease must face are numerous: pain or the fear of pain, diarrhea, incontinence, chronic fatigue, fear of medication side effects, worries about self-appearance and sexual life, fear of surgery, unpredictability of the illness, and fear of disability and financial hardship. If patients have had surgery, then coping with an ileostomy, colostomy, or short bowel syndrome poses other special issues (31). Not all patients are concerned with every issue, but the psychological burden can be substantial.

The severity of the underlying illness, personality strengths, problems unrelated to Crohn's disease, and quality of social supports are crucial variables in determining psychiatric well-being (32).

The subgroup of patients who do not cope well show varying combinations of maladaptive symptoms such as chronic anxiety, depression, social withdrawal, the adoption of a dependent "sick" role, pathological denial, and drug dependence. Many of these patients have little support from family or friends and pose a challenge in helping them cope better with their illness.

2. Treatment

The psychiatric treatment of poor adaptation to Crohn's disease is varied and is based on an accurate assessment of the patient's personality and social strengths as well as the severity of the illness. The psychiatrist must often be creative in using a variety of psychotherapeutic, behavioral, environmental, and psychopharmacological interventions. Whatever modalities are used, there are two general phases of treatment. The first is to stabilize the patient's psychological state. This involves the development of a therapeutic alliance with the patient and the treatment of depression, anxiety, and/or drug dependence. Additionally, education, additional social supports, and participation in a support group can be helpful. This first stage may be accomplished quickly, or it may take many months, but further treatment should not proceed until the patient's psychological state seems to be stabilized.

The second phase is to help patients mourn their previous state of health; maladaptive patterns of coping result from the avoidance of doing so (33). Ideally, patients gradually face and emotionally accept the limitations that Crohn's disease has placed on their lives while emphasizing and enlarging what they can still do. For example, patients are helped to accept that they may have to live with severe fatigue. Whatever sense of themselves as a healthy person as well as whatever dreams they have that are no longer possible need to be grieved in a process analogous to what happens after someone dies. Patients are helped to realize that their chronic anxiety and social withdrawal are ways of avoiding mourning these losses. This is a painful process accompanied by much resentment and sadness; patients go through periods of feeling worse before they get better.

To buffer this, patients are encouraged to expand their life if it has been unrealistically constrained by their illness. For example, fears about needing a bathroom or being unattractive, which cause social isolation, are often exaggerated. Patients respond to clarification and encouragement to begin to take some risks in these areas. Regressed patients who have identified themselves as "sick" beyond the actual severity of their illness are a particular challenge because they have often built a life revolving around this identity. In these cases, there is usually secondary gain operating; that is, the patients are either being emotionally rewarded by family for being ill (sometime in subtle ways) or they are financially rewarded by disability insurance. These reinforcements must be interrupted, although strong resistance to changing them is the norm.

In practice, this approach of stabilizing the patients psychological state, undoing maladaptive patterns so that the patients can mourn, and encouraging the patients to try things they had previously feared does work for most patients. However, for some, the inherent unpredictability of Crohn's disease does not allow a normal mourning process; these patients have a strong need for feeling in control and insist on knowing with certainty what their future will be. For such people, it is easier to adapt to more severe illness with a clear-cut prognosis than a milder illness with chronic unpredictability, as long as a reasonably normal life is feasible. In these situations, when mourning one's old reality so as to accept a new one is not possible, patients are encouraged to learn to tolerate uncertainty and adopt a "1 month at a time" attitude. If the patient remains psychologically stable, then this attitude can gradually be increased to "2 months at a time," and so on.

For the psychiatrist, realistic goals coupled with flexibility and perseverance are necessary in this maladaptive group. For those patients who are able to mourn, psychiatric treatment can usually be completed within 1 to 2 years. For those who cannot, treatment is interminable. Its frequency should be lessened when the patient is doing well, but the psychiatrist should expect patients to return on a maintenance basis and during periods when they are not coping well.

III. CONCLUSION

This chapter is a summary of the psychiatric problems that affect certain patients with Crohn's disease. The issues of depression, psychogenic activation, pathological denial, drug dependence, and maladaptation have been presented separately; in practice, they often occur together in varying combinations, leading to complicated clinical problems. This chapter is intended to help gastroenterologist identify those patients with Crohn's disease who need psychiatric treatment and to stimulate more psychiatrists to become knowledgeable about this illness, so they can enhance their therapeutic skills. In terms of future research, issues abound; especially necessary is a physiological understanding of how psychiatric illnesses and Crohn's disease mutually affect each other.

REFERENCES

1. Andrews H, Barczak P, Allan RN. Psychiatric illness in patients with inflammatory bowel disease. Gut 1987; 28:1600–1604.
2. Tarter RE, Switala J, Carra J, et al. Inflammatory bowel disease: psychiatric status before and after disease onset. Int J Psychiatr Med 1987; 17:173–181.
3. Feldman F, Cantor D, Soll S, Bachrach W. Psychiatric study of a consecutive series of 19 patients with regional ilietis. BMJ 1967; 4:711.
4. Whybrow PC, Kane TJ, Lipton MA. Regional ileitis and psychiatric disorders. Psychosom Med 1968; 30:209.
5. Ford CV, Glober GA, Castelnuovo-Tedesco P. A psychiatric study of patients with regional enteritis. JAMA 1969; 208:311.
6. McKegney FP, Gordon RO, Levine SM. A psychosomatic comparison of patients with ulcerative colitis and Crohn's disease. Psychosom Med 1970; 32:153.
7. Cohn EM, Lederman II, Shore E. Regional enteritis and its relation to emotional disorders. Am J Gastroenterol 1970; 54:378.
8. Helter JE, Channas S, Norland CC, et al. A study of the association between Crohn's disease and psychiatric illness. Gastroenterology 1984; 86:324–330.
9. Heltzer JE, Stillings WA, Chammas S, et al. A controlled study of the association between ulcerative colitis and psychiatric diagnoses. Dig Dis Sci 1982; 27:513–518.
10. Latimer PR. Crohns' disease: a review of the psychological and social outcome. Psychol Med 1978; 8:469–482.
11. Sadler HH, Gransz H. A clinical challenge. West J Med 1976; 125:393–396.
12. Gazzard, BG, Price H, Libby GW, Dawson AM. The social toll of Crohn's disease. BMJ 1978; 2:1117–1126.
13. Olbrisch ME, Ziegler SW. Psychological adjustment to inflammatory bowel disease: informational control and private self-consciousness. J Chron Dis 1982; 35:573.

14. Schneider AP. Coping with Crohn's disease: some factors contributing to the appraisal of a chronic stressor. Dissertation, Department of Psychology, New York University, New York, NY, 1985.

15. Sifneos PE. The prevalence of "alexithymic" characteristics in psychosomatic patients. Psychother Psychosom 1973; 22:255–261.

16. Lesser IM, Lesser BZ. Alexithymia: examining the development of a psychological concept. Am J Psychiatry 1983; 140:1305–1312.

17. Giovaccini PL. The concrete and difficult patient. In: Giovaccini PL, ed. Tactics and Techniques in Psychoanalytic Therapy. New York: Science House, 1972:351–363.

18. Diagnostic and Statistical Manual of Mental Disorders. 3rd ed. Washington DC: American Psychiatric Association, 1980.

19. Pescor M. The Kolb Classification of Drug Addicts. Public Health Report Supplement 155. Washington DC: United States Public Health Service, Divison of Sanitary Reports and Statistics, 1931.

20. Rayport M. Experience in the management of patients medically addicted to narcotics. JAMA 1954; 156:684–691.

21. Porter J, Jick H. Addiction rare in patients treated with narcotics. N Engl J Med 1980; 302:123.

22. Portenoy RK. Chronic opioid therapy in non-malignant pain. J Pain Symptom Manage 1990; 5:S46–S62.

23. Portenoy RK. Chronic pain management. In: Stoudemire A, Fogel B, eds. Psychiatric Care of the Medical Patient. New York: Oxford University Press, 1993: 341–363.

24. Millman R. The opiates. In: Wyngarden S, Smith L, eds. Textbook of Medicine. Philadelphia: WB Saunders, 1982:2006–2010.

25. Kaplan MA, Korelitz BI. Narcotic dependence in inflammatory bowel disease. J Clin Gastro-enterol 1988; 10(3):275–278.

26. Wolff BB, Kantor TG, Jarvik ME, Laska E. Response of experimental pain to analgesic drugs (I). Morphine, aspirin and placebo. Clin Pharmacol Ther 1966; 7:224–238.

27. Wolff BB, Kantor TG, Jarvik ME, Laska E. Response of experimental pain to analgesic drugs (III). Codeine, aspirin, secobarbital and placebo. Clin Pharmacol Ther 1969; 10:217–228.

28. Fordyce W, Fowler R, Lehmann, JF, et al. Operant conditioning in the treatment of chronic pain. Arhc Phys Rehab Med 1973; 54:399–408.

29. Farmer RG, Whelan G, Fazio VW. Long-term follow-up of patients with Crohn's disease. Relationship between the clinical pattern and prognosis. Gastroenterology 1985; 88:1818–1823.

30. Meyers S, et al. Quality of life after surgery for Crohn's disease: a psychosocial survey. Gastroenterology 1980; 78:1–13.

31. Drossman D. Psychosocial aspects of ulcerative colitis and Crohn's disease. In: Kirsner J, Shorter R, eds. Inflammatory Bowel Disease. Philadelphia: Lea & Febiger, 1988:209–226.

32. Gazzard BG, Price HL, Libby GW, Dawson AM. The social toll of Crohn's disease. BMJ 1978; 2:1117–1121.

33. Green SA. Principles of medical psychotherapy. In: Stoudemire A, Fogel BS, eds. Psychiatric Care of the Medical Patient. New York: Oxford University Press, 1993:3–18.

COMMENTARY

Barbara S. Kirschner   *Wyler Children's Hospital, University of Chicago, Chicago, Illinois*

The chapter by Kaplan addresses the recognition and treatment of psychiatric conditions, which, in some patients with Crohn's disease, may precipitate or prolong their symptoms. As discussed in previous chapters by Levenstein and Drossman, most attention is directed toward the alleviation of anxiety and depression. The author clearly points out that the intensity of psychiatric symptoms is not well correlated with disease severity. For gastroenterologist, the notion that "unpredictability . . . is psychologically the most difficult hardship" emphasizes the need for addressing this topic with patients with Crohn's disease.

An interesting but controversial idea is that patients with refractory disease (unable to achieve remission or suffer frequent relapses despite medical therapy) should undergo psychiatric evaluation for "psychogenicity." According to the author, the most common contributing feelings are anxiety, depression, and guilt. The concept that such a patient should be "heavily tranquilized" is probably not widely practiced. Certainly, I and my colleagues have managed occasional patients for whom intensive psychotherapy and medication have been indicated. Most of these instances have been in patients who demonstrated emotional lability, including depression, prior to the diagnosis of Crohn's disease and whose psychiatric symptoms were exacerbated by corticosteroid therapy. I have found that the author's observation that patients are more likely to agree to psychiatric consultation if it is presented as providing "a better way of coping" is the most effective approach in this situation.

For most patients, especially teenagers, the goal of achieving "a moderate state of denial," which fosters compliance with medical therapy while avoiding preoccupation with Crohn's disease, is the one I use most consistently in this population. At times, this means being an advocate for the patient, contrary to the thoughts of the family, so that Crohn's disease does not become the focus of the patient's life. It is my impression that the risk of pathological denial leading to cessation of medical therapy is lessened by regular follow-up visits, which provide opportunities to adjust medications based on history, physical examination, and laboratory tests. For some patients in whom anxiety or irritable bowel symptoms play a role, relaxation techniques can be helpful.

The role of social support systems in helping patients cope with the recurrent symptoms of Crohn's disease is critically important. These include not only parents, friends, and organized support groups but also teachers who may need to be sensitized to the effects of Crohn's disease, especially when patients "look well." Brochures from organizations such as the Crohn's and Colitis Foundation specifically address these points and can be helpful to pediatric patients.

It is my impression that trying to convince patients "to tolerate uncertainty" (or fluctuations in the course of disease) while reconsidering and adjusting combinations of medications to reduce disease symptoms is a useful approach. Whether it is necessary to encourage patients to "mourn their previous state of health" is not clear to me.

26
Extraintestinal Manifestations

Andrew S. Warner and Richard P. MacDermott   *Lahey Hitchcock Clinic,*
Burlington, Massachusetts

Crohn's disease is often associated with manifestations at sites separate and distinct from the gastrointestinal tract (1–3). The presence of these "extraintestinal" manifestations suggests that Crohn's disease may be a systemic disorder in which the gastrointestinal tract is the predominant but not the only organ involved. The extraintestinal manifestations that are associated with Crohn's disease can occasionally overshadow and may sometimes be more devastating to the patient's quality of life than the underlying bowel disease. This chapter reviews the extraintestinal manifestations of Crohn's disease, describes their relationship to the location and activity of intestinal inflammation, discusses therapy, and differentiates between extraintestinal manifestations of Crohn's disease and those that are direct complications of the underlying bowel disease. Most of the extraintestinal manifestations reviewed in this chapter can also be seen in association with ulcerative colitis. Therefore, issues that are relevant to extraintestinal manifestations in ulcerative colitis are also reviewed.

I. SKIN AND MUCOUS MEMBRANES

A. Aseptic Neutrophilic Dermatosis

The mucocutaneous abnormalities that accompany inflammatory bowel disease (IBD) can be viewed as a spectrum of changes resulting from leukocyte migration to different sites in the skin and mucous membranes (4,5). Pyostomatitis vegetans, psoriasis, vesiculo-pustular eruptions, epidermolysis bullosa acquisita, Sweet's syndrome, erythema nodosum, and pyoderma gangrenosum can all be considered various forms of an aseptic neutrophilic dermatosis. These same mucocutaneous changes can also be seen in other intestinal/multisystem disorders, such as Behçet's disease, Reiter's syndrome, infectious entero-colitis, bowel-associated dermatosis-arthritis syndrome, and collagen vascular disorders (rheumatoid arthritis and systemic lupus erythematosus, in particular).

1. Erythema Nodosum

Erythema nodosum is the most common cutaneous lesion in Crohn's disease, with a reported incidence of up to 15% (6). It is also seen in diseases other than IBD, such as streptococcal infections, sarcoidosis, and as a reaction to various drugs. Erythema nodosum classically occurs with the sudden appearance of one or more red, warm, nonulcerating, tender nodules approximately 1 to 1.5 cm in diameter on the anterior tibial surfaces of one or both legs, but can be found at many other sites as well. Erythema nodosum lesions can be accompanied by fever, chills, and leukocytosis, but these nonspecific findings can also be due to the underlying active Crohn's disease. Classified as a septal panniculitis, erythema nodosum is a subcutaneous process that leaves relative sparing of the overlying dermis. Erythema nodosum is characterized by an initial dense neutrophilic infiltrate that subsequently progresses to a predominance of both mononuclear and histiocytic giant cells. Neither leukocytoclastic vasculitis nor fat necrosis is seen. Direct immunofluorescent studies have not revealed a consistent pattern of immunoglobulin deposition.

Within a few days of onset, the raised nodules usually evolve into red-brown to purple macules. Healing with medical therapy occurs in 3 to 6 weeks, with desquamation and hyperpigmentation. New lesions may arise as others resolve. Erythema nodosum closely parallels the activity of the underlying bowel disease. Many patients can sometimes predict a flare of Crohn's disease by the antecedent finding of erythema nodosum lesions. Therapy aimed at the underlying bowel disease using steroids, 5-aminosalicylic acid (5-ASA) compounds or Cyclosporin A in resistant or severe cases, almost always leads to resolution of the skin lesions.

2. Pyoderma Gangrenosum

Pyoderma gangrenosum is one of the most serious extraintestinal manifestations of IBD, occurring in 1% to 2% of Crohn's disease patients and slightly less often in ulcerative colitis patients (7,8). Pyoderma gangrenosum is also associated with many other diseases such as systemic bacterial infections, vasculitis, chronic hepatitis, arthritis, and myelo-proliferative disorders. Pyoderma gangrenosum can often resemble squamous cell carcinoma and may require biopsies for diagnosis. Pyoderma gangrenosum is a chronic, persistent skin disorder that, when it is extensive, is often resistant to therapy. Pyoderma gangrenosum begins as a tender papulopustule that gradually ulcerates as the lesion expands, forming a necrotic center surrounded by a dusky, purple-blue border that is raised and undermined. The healed lesion leaves a hyperpigmented area or cribriform scar. Lesions may be solitary or multiple and, when multiple, can be in different stages of development. In some patients, the ulcers arise as discrete lesions; in others, the primary pustules occur in crops and coalesce to involve large areas of skin. Pyoderma gangrenosum can occur anywhere on the body, although, like erythema nodosum, it tends to initially form on the lower extremities. These lesions often erupt at a site of trauma (pathergy phenomena) (9,10).

The histologic findings of pyoderma gangrenosum are nonspecific (11,12). Either neutrophilic or mononuclear cell infiltrates can be seen, depending on the biopsy site and the stage of the lesion. No clear-cut pattern of immunoglobulin deposition has been demonstrated. Pyoderma gangrenosum tends to be seen more often in the setting of active disease involving the colon and occurs less often in inactive disease or Crohn's disease isolated to the small bowel (13). The onset of pyoderma gangrenosum can precede the onset of bowel symptoms, but can also develop after diseased bowel has been removed. Initial treatment of pyoderma gangrenosum is aimed at controlling intestinal inflammation (7). Nontraumatic local care of the skin ulcer should also be used. Various topical regimens can be used initially, including topical corticosteroids, cromolyn sodium, benzoyl peroxide, and polysporin and silver sulfadine to protect the ulcer from secondary infection.

Intralesional corticosteroids may also be helpful, particularly in early, small lesions. Pyoderma gangrenosum ulcers resistant to local therapy usually require aggressive systemic therapy with intravenous corticosteroids. Many other drugs have been tried with varying success including sulfasalazine, clofazimine, dapsone, azathioprine, and recently, cyclosporin A. Administration of hyperbaric oxygen has resulted in only limited benefit. Surgical debridement of pyoderma gangrenosum only promotes further ulceration due to pathergy response and should be absolutely avoided.

3. Sweet's Syndrome

Sweet's Syndrome, or acute febrile neutrophilic dermatosis, is characterized by the sudden eruption of multiple, 1 to 2-cm erythematous plaques accompanies by fever, arthralgias, and leukocytosis (14). Histologically, a dense, diffuse neutrophilic infiltrate with dermal edema is seen. Some dermatopathologists speculate that Sweet's syndrome is a variant of pyoderma gangrenosum (15,16). The relationship of Sweet's syndrome to the activity and extent of Crohn's disease is unknown. Sweet's syndrome–like lesions can also be seen in systemic lupus erythematosus, rheumatoid arthritis, blind loop syndrome, Behçet's disease, and hematologic malignancies, especially acute nonlymphocytic leukemia (17). Systemic corticosteroids are usually effective. Other therapies that can be tried include dapsone, colchicine, potassium iodide, indomethacin, and isotretinoin.

4. Epidermolysis Bullosa Acquisita

Epidermolysis bullosa acquisita is an autoimmune subepidermal blistering disease that has occasionally been seen with Crohn's colitis (18,19). Epidermolysis bullosa acquisita has also been described in patients with rheumatoid arthritis and diabetes mellitus as well as malignancies and systemic infections. Patients with epidermolysis bullosa acquisita develop generalized blisters with an intact blister roof, usually over bony prominences. After healing, residual hyperpigmentation and scarring are seen. Histologically, a characteristic neutrophilic infiltrate is seen between the dermal–epidermal junction. Treatment with immunosuppressive therapy is often required.

5. Other Mucocutaneous Abnormalities

There have been scattered case reports of dermatomyositis/myositis occurring in Crohn's colitis (20,21). In approximately half of the patients reported, a distinct correlation between the dermatomyositis/myositis and severity of Crohn's disease can be found. Corticosteroids are usually rapidly effective.

The vesiculopustular eruptions described in ulcerative colitis have not been found in Crohn's disease (22,23). Psoriasis is seen more frequently in patients with IBD than in the general population (24). The appearance and response to therapy of psoriasis is the same in IBD as in non-IBD patients.

B. Oral Lesions

1. Aphthous Stomatitis

Aphthous stomatitis is a common occurrence in IBD, with an incidence of 10% to 20%. Although found primarily in Crohn's disease, idiopathic aphthous stomatitis can occasionally be observed in ulcerative colitis patients and in patients without IBD. In patients with IBD, the lesions are often painless, whereas in patients without IBD, the aphthous ulcers are usually painful. Most lesions occur in the setting of active Crohn's disease. It should be reiterated that aphthous stomatitis is not pathognomonic for Crohn's disease; it is also seen in other disorders, such as ulcerative colitis, Behçet's disease, and cyclic neutropenia.

2. Cobblestone-Like Lesions

Cobblestone-like lesions, usually of the buccal mucosa, can also be seen in the oral cavity of patients with Crohn's disease (25,26). As in intestinal Crohn's disease, the histologic appearance shows chronic inflammation and granuloma formation. These cobblestone-like lesions are often asymptomatic, and there is no apparent relationship to the activity or location of intestinal inflammation. Whether cobblestone-like lesions of the mouth are either proximal components of small or large bowel Crohn's disease or are true extraintestinal manifestations of Crohn's disease is unclear. In older patients with Crohn's disease, the finding of cobblestone mucosa in the oral cavity must be differentiated from denture granulomata, which has a similar appearance.

3. Pyostomatitis Vegetans

Pyostomatitis vegetans is a rare oral manifestation of Crohn's disease (25,26). Some dermatologists consider it to be an oral presentation of pyoderma gangrenosum. Patients present with multiple 2 to 3 mm pustules in the oral cavity that eventually ulcerate and form abscesses. Histologic examination shows a dense neutrophilic and eosinophilic infiltrate. Most patients with pyostomatitis vegetans have quiescent bowel disease. Improvement has been noted after treatment with either sulfasalazine or dapsone, in conjunction with topical therapy. In patients with active Crohn's disease, initial therapy is aimed at control of the intestinal inflammation, and systemic corticosteroids are usually required.

4. Other Oral Lesions

Other oral lesions reported in Crohn's disease include stomatitis and glossitis. These lesions are usually due to malnutrition and subsequent vitamin deficiency. Granulomatous tonsillitis has also been described (27).

C. "Metastatic" Crohn's Disease

"Metastatic" Crohn's disease refers to the presence of nodular, ulcerating skin lesions containing noncaseating granulomas found at sites distant from the gastrointestinal tract (28,29). "Metastatic" Crohn's disease can be found in any location and may take the form of a papule, nodule, or plaque that may or may not ulcerate. These lesions can be solitary or multiple and are usually painful and tender to the touch. Diagnosis is made by skin biopsy. The activity of these lesions seems to be independent from the activity of the intestinal disease. Therapy can include both topical and systemic medications. Granulomas are commonly found in a multitude of dermatologic conditions. Hidradenitis suppurativa, in particular, must be differentiated from metastatic Crohn's disease (30). Similar in histologic appearance, hidradenitis suppurativa is more likely to have foreign body type granulomas, whereas Crohn's disease is characterized by discrete epithelioid granulomas.

II. JOINTS

Joint involvement is the most common extraintestinal manifestation of Crohn's disease, with a reported incidence of up to 25% (31–33). There are four general patterns of joint involvement in IBD: (a) peripheral joint involvement, (b) central or axial joint involvement, principally ankylosing spondylitis and sacroileitis, (c) hypertrophic osteoarthropathy (clubbing), and (d) direct complications of Crohn's disease and complications of therapy.

A. Peripheral Arthralgias/Arthritis

Many patients with Crohn's disease have episodes of peripheral joint arthralgias. Clinical presentation with low grade, intermittent, asymmetric, pauciarticular (less than 6 joints) arthralgias is characteristic. The joints most commonly affected are the knees, hips, ankles, elbows, and wrists. An effusion can sometime be demonstrated on palpation of the joint. These findings most commonly do not represent frank destructive arthritis. Nevertheless, in 15% of Crohn's disease patients with joint symptoms, overt arthritis can develop, mimicking rheumatoid arthritis. A subset of IBD patients with peripheral arthralgias have frank arthritis and test positive for rheumatoid factor. However, unlike rheumatoid arthritis, the arthritis of IBD lacks bony destruction or joint deformity. Patients with IBD also have normal serum uric acid levels and test negative for antinuclear antibodies. Analysis of synovial fluid is nondescript, with turbid fluid containing 10,000 to 50,000 cells per milliliter. Joint fluid contains polymorphonuclear leukocytes, but no bacteria, normal glucose, normal protein, and no rheumatoid factor. The use of arthrocentesis in IBD patients should be reserved for specific situations to exclude other potential causes for joint inflammation, such as septic arthritis. Synovial biopsy, when used experimentally, usually shows a nonspecific, mononuclear cell infiltrate without destruction.

Arthralgias are observed more commonly in patients with colonic or ileocolonic disease and less often in IBD patients with disease isolated to the small bowel. The activity of the arthralgias usually parallels the activity and extent of the underlying intestinal inflammation. However, in some patients, arthralgias may appear before onset of bowel symptoms, and many of these patients often have recurrence of their arthralgias before relapses of their Crohn's disease. Unusual cases in patients with Crohn's disease have been reported in which true arthritis can present as a monoarticular process with erosive lesions and a granulomatous synovitis that can lead to joint destruction (31,34,35). Peripheral arthralgias are seen more often in patients who also have other extraintestinal manifestations, especially skin and eye involvement (3). This has led to the subclassification of skin, joint, mucous membrane, and eye manifestations as the "itis" or inflammation-related extraintestinal complications of IBD. Other diseases that can have a similar appearance with arthralgias include reactive arthritis secondary to intestinal infections, bowel-associated dermatosis-arthritis syndrome, gluten-sensitive enteropathy, Whipple's disease, Poncet's disease (tuberculous rheumatism), and psoriatic arthritis.

Treatment for arthralgias in IBD is aimed at the underlying bowel disease. A major problem that should be avoided is the use of aspirin or nonsteroidal anti-inflammatory drugs (NSAIDs), which may exacerbate the Crohn's disease. Therefore, the pain medication of choice is acetaminophen. Systemic corticosteroids usually work well, but should only be reserved for the most severe cases. In addition, interarticular steroid injection and physiotherapy have been found to be beneficial.

B. Ankylosing Spondylitis

Ankylosing spondylitis is a chronic inflammatory process of the lower back. It occurs insidiously as low back pain and morning stiffness that improves with exercise and becomes worse again with rest. In later stages, destructive changes from the arthritis can lead to stooped posturing. Fortunately, ankylosing spondylitis often runs a mild course with destructive disease usually confined to the distal spine. The radiological findings include a spectrum of changes from squaring of the vertebral bodies to ankylosed joints and a "bamboo spine." Twenty percent of patient with ankylosing spondylitis can also have peripheral joint involvement, particularly of the larger joints, such as the hips and shoulders.

Ankylosing spondylitis occurs less frequently in Crohn's disease than in ulcerative colitis. Ankylosing spondylitis in IBD is associated with the HLA B27 phenotype in up to 70% of patients, which is less than an idiopathic ankylosing spondylitis in which the HLA B27 phenotype is found in 90% of patients (36). Some patients with what was previously thought to be idiopathic ankylosing spondylitis have subsequently been found to have underlying IBD that was asymptomatic (37). Conversely, patients with IBD may have asymptomatic ankylosing spondylitis. An increased incidence of aortic valve disease and cardiac conduction defects have been reported in patients with ankylosing spondylitis associated with IBD.

Sacroileitis is a more common central arthritis in IBD than is ankylosing spondylitis. Whereas sacroileitis was originally believed to occur in approximately 15% of patients, most of whom were symptomatic, the incidence has been reported in up to 70% of IBD patients when more sensitive imaging techniques (bone scans) are used (38). Most of these patients are asymptomatic.

In contrast to symptoms of peripheral joint involvement, symptoms due to either sacroileitis or ankylosing spondylitis are usually independent of the activity of the underlying inflammatory bowel disease (31). Furthermore, there is usually no improvement with medical or surgical therapy aimed at the underlying IBD. Treatment is, therefore, primarily supportive in nature, with physiotherapy often providing the best symptomatic relief. NSAIDs can be used to help with morning stiffness, but, because they can also exacerbate the underlying IBD, acetaminophen is preferred.

C. Hypertrophic Osteoarthropathy

Clubbing is the most common form of hypertrophic osteoarthropathy; other forms are synovitis and periostosis (39). Clubbing is more common in Crohn's disease than in ulcerative colitis. Although in some series there is a 40% to 60% incidence, most clinicians find clubbing to be uncommon in IBD (40,41). Osteoarthropathy is thought to be related to both the activity and proximal extent of small bowel Crohn's disease.

D. Direct Complications

Pelvic osteomyelitis is a direct septic complication of Crohn's disease (39). It is associated with psoas abscess and further extension into the hip joint. Fistulas may be present in patients with pelvic osteomyelitis.

III. EYE

Ophthalmologic conditions are among the more common and serious extraintestinal manifestations of Crohn's disease. Although eye manifestations occur more frequently in ulcerative colitis, 2% to 4% of Crohn's disease patients experience ocular inflammation (3,40,43,44). Patients with colonic involvement are more likely to experience ocular disorders than patients with isolated small bowel Crohn's disease. Although the ocular manifestations often parallel bowel disease activity, they can also run an independent course. Inflammatory bowel disease patients with eye manifestations are also more likely to have joint and skin involvement as well (3).

A. Iritis and Uveitis

Iritis and uveitis occur as the result of inflammation in the anterior chamber of the eye and have an incidence of 0.5% to 3.5%. Their onset can be before, during, or after the diagnosis of IBD. Unilateral conjunctival injection, blurred vision, eye pain, photophobia, and headache are clinical manifestations of uveitis. When it recurs, it is often in the contralateral eye. A split lamp examination is required for accurate diagnosis and reveals inflammatory cells or "flares" in the anterior chamber. When left untreated, uveitis/iritis can progress to scarring and blindness. For mild cases, treatment with mydriatic agents such as atropine can provide symptomatic relief. For more severe cases, topical and systemic corticosteroids are often needed. Cyclosporin A has been used for refractory disease (45). Uveitis/iritis usually improves after bowel surgery, although there has been recurrence after total colectomy. Asymptomatic uveitis with spontaneous resolution has been reported in children (46).

B. Episcleritis

Episcleritis is the most common of the ocular abnormalities and does not lead to scarring or blindness. Clinical presentation can range from the patient being asymptomatic to the patients noticing the gradual development of redness and burning of the eye, or, in occasional cases, the patient may present with loss of vision. As with uveitis/iritis, patients with episcleritis are more likely to have colitis or ileocolitis than small bowel disease alone. Unlike uveitis/iritis, the presence and severity of episcleritis is associated with ongoing, active intestinal disease. Therapy with topical corticosteroids usually achieves rapid relief. Systemic therapy aimed at controlling the intestinal inflammation is often equally effective.

C. Retinal Vascular Disease and Retrobulbar Neuritis

Retinal vascular disease and retrobulbar neuritis have only occasionally been reported in Crohn's disease (47). Other potential ophthalmologic complications that may arise include cataracts or candidiasis of the eye secondary to corticosteroid therapy.

IV. GENITOURINARY

Most genitourinary disorders associated with Crohn's disease are complications secondary to the bowel disease itself and not true extraintestinal manifestations. In general, insults to the kidneys, ureters, and bladder in Crohn's disease result from excessive diarrhea with water and electrolyte losses, malabsorption, or direct complications from the disease process, such as obstruction and fistulization.

A. Renal Stones

Renal stones are the most common urologic complication in Crohn's disease with an incidence ranging from 2% to 40% (48). Renal calculi should be suspected when a patient with IBD presents with severe flank or abdominal pain but is otherwise in remission. This complication occurs more frequently in Crohn's disease than in ulcerative colitis, with oxalate stones the predominant type in Crohn's disease and urate stones being most common in ulcerative colitis. The pathophysiology of oxalate stone formation has been well described (49,50). Normally, calcium binds to oxalate in the intestinal lumen to form an insoluble, nonabsorbable complex. However, in the presence of significant ileal disease or extensive ileal resection, the enterohepatic circulation of bile acids is interrupted, leading to fat malabsorption. This allows the malabsorbed free fatty acids to bind the free calcium and, therefore, leaves less calcium available to bind with oxalate. The excess free oxalate is then absorbed within the colon and excreted in the urine. Hence, calcium oxalate renal stones do not develop in patients who have undergone colectomy because the absorption site for the free oxalate is removed along with the colon. Conversely, in patients who have an ileostomy, urate stones predominate (51,52). This is because excessive ileostomy output can lead to chronic dehydration and metabolic acidosis from loss of bicarbonate. These two factors result in supersaturation of uric acid in the urine. In addition to fluid and alkaline losses, sodium, magnesium and citric acid can also be lost through the ileostomy, which can increase the insolubility of the calcium. This can, therefore, lead to both calcium urate as well as calcium pyrophosphate precipitation with subsequent stone formation. Treatment of renal calculi includes hydration, analgesia, and alkalinization of the urine as well as reduction of the ileostomy output.

B. Obstructive Hydronephrosis

Obstructive hydronephrosis is usually right-sided and a direct result of active ileal Crohn's disease (53). Rarely, the hydronephrosis can be left-sided or bilateral, which, when seen, is usually due to Crohn's disease involving the colon. Hydronephrosis can be diagnosed using either ultrasonography or an intravenous pyelogram. Treatment of the underlying inflammatory process medically is sometimes effective in relieving the obstruction, but usually surgery is necessary. Ureteral stents may also be needed in severe cases.

C. Bladder Involvement

Bladder involvement is another complication that can occur in Crohn's disease. Characteristically, an enterovesical fistula presents with pneumaturia and recurrent urinary tract infections, often with multiple types of enteric bacteria (54). Fecaluria is rarely seen. Although medical therapy of both the infection and intestinal inflammation is often effective, these patients frequently require surgery. At times, patients with active Crohn's disease describe urinary tract infection–like symptoms but have sterile pyuria or a completely normal urinanalysis and urine culture and no demonstrable fistula. This type of presentation is characteristic of irritation of the bladder or ureter by an external inflammatory process. Treatment of the underlying bowel disease is usually effective. Kaliopenic nephropathy is an infrequent disorder in which chronic potassium losses can lead to renal dysfunction (55). Glomerulonephritis is a rare genitourinary disorder in IBD patients (56). It occurs in either Crohn's disease or ulcerative colitis and usually responds to treatment with corticosteroids. The pathogenesis of this entity is unclear, but could be due to immune complex disease.

V. AMYLOIDOSIS

Secondary or reactive amyloidosis (AA-type) has been frequently associated with Crohn's disease but only rarely observed in ulcerative colitis (57). The incidence of amyloidosis varies from 1%, if the diagnosis is made premortem, to 29%, if the diagnosis is made postmortem (2,58). Crohn's disease–associated amyloidosis has been described involving the intestines, heart, liver, spleen, and thyroid, but amyloid infiltration of the kidney is the most frequent site of AA deposition. Amyloid nephropathy is a potential cause of serious illness or even death for Crohn's disease patients. Patients may present with only mild proteinuria or full blown nephrotic syndrome. The diagnosis can be made by abdominal subcutaneous fat pad biopsy or rectal biopsy. The kidney itself can also be sampled for biopsy, less invasive approaches are preferred. Intestinal amyloidosis may present as malabsorption out of proportion to the extent of bowel disease. Amyloidosis has not been related to the extent or severity of Crohn's disease. Although colchicine has often been used for amyloidosis, there is no proven effective treatment. Most authors have also found no improvement in amyloidosis following resection of active Crohn's disease.

VI. ANEMIA

A. Iron Deficiency Anemia

Hematologic abnormalities are commonly seen in many IBD patients and they are often multifactorial. Chronic occult gastrointestinal blood loss can result in iron deficiency anemia (59). The degree of iron deficiency can be used as a marker for disease activity and is one of the parameters in the Crohn's Disease Activity Index. Even though many patients are treated with iron supplementation, anemia is more often corrected in conjunction with treatment of intestinal inflammation. Crohn's disease patients may also exhibit anemia of chronic disease, which sometimes makes the diagnosis of iron deficiency anemia difficult, because both types of anemia occur with low serum iron. Ferritin is not a good marker because it is an acute phase reactant and can be elevated in the setting of active Crohn's disease. The ratios of serum iron to TIBS (percent of saturation) is the most helpful index. A low value (less than 10%) is seen in iron deficiency anemia and high values (greater than 15%) are seen in anemia of chronic disease. However, even this index can be unreliable because a patient with active Crohn's disease can exhibit a low TIBC due to enteric protein loss.

B. Vitamin B$_{12}$ and Folate Deficiency

Vitamin B$_{12}$ and folate deficiency can lead to a macrocytic anemia (60). These nutritional anemias are usually due to malabsorption of ingested nutrients but occasionally can occur from inadequate intake. Vitamin B$_{12}$ is absorbed in the ileum and is often deficient in patients with significant ileal disease or extensive ileal resection. Bacterial overgrowth can also lead to vitamin B$_{12}$ deficiency due to bacterial degradation. Parenteral vitamin B$_{12}$ injections (usually 1000 μg per month) rapidly reverses this deficiency. In the case of bacterial overgrowth, antimicrobial therapy with tetracycline, metronidazole, or trimethoprim-sulfamethoxazole is usually effective. Folate deficiency occurs less frequently and can be seen in patients with severe proximal disease involving the duodenum and jejunum, the site of folate absorption. Folate deficiency can also be seen associated with sulfasalazine therapy. It is readily treated with supplemental oral folate.

C. Autoimmune Hemolytic Anemia

Autoimmune hemolytic anemia has been described in association with ulcerative colitis, but has not been seen in Crohn's disease (61). It is often confused with hemolysis secondary to sulfasalazine therapy in patients with G6PD deficiency (62).

VII. THROMBOEMBOLIC EVENTS

Patients with IBD are at risk for serious thromboembolic disease. Potential life-threatening complications include deep venous thrombosis, stroke, and pulmonary emboli (63,64). Clots usually form in the lower extremities and pelvic veins, although clots from most other locations have also been seen. Arterial thrombosis is rare. Coagulation abnormalities have been noted in some patients and include thrombocytosis; increase in the levels of factors V, VIII, and fibrinogen; protein S deficiency; and decreased levels of antithrombin III (65–67). Many of these laboratory abnormalities return to normal with resolution of disease activity. Patients with Crohn's disease have an activated coagulation cascade, with increased levels of fibrinopeptide and monocyte tissue factor that correlate with disease activity (65). There does not appear to be any relationship between the location of Crohn's disease and the development of thromboembolism. However, patients with active IBD can be confined to bed, can be septic, may have just undergone surgery, may have central venous catheters in place, all of which may be contributing risk factors to thromboembolism.

Therapy includes prophylactic subcutaneous heparin therapy in patients who are at bed rest or who are immediately postoperative and chronic anticoagulation in patients on home total parenteral nutrition. Treatment of thromboembolic complications using anti-coagulation, antiplatelet drugs, and thrombolysis needs to be performed cautiously.

VIII. VASCULITIS

Vascular changes are commonly found in patients with Crohn's disease, but rarely in patients with ulcerative colitis (63,68). These changes include minor, nonspecific alterations in the arteries that supply the intestine and adjacent mesentery as well as major alterations such as giant vessel arteritis, similar to that of Takayasu's disease. Polyarteritis nodosa has also been noted in small and medium-sized vessels. Other findings have included a leukocytoclastic vasculitis involving small vessels in muscle, cutaneous vasculitis with subsequent peripheral gangrene, and pulmonary vasculitis. Cryoglobulins and cryofibrinogens in the serum have also been documented. There has been no correlation found between the presence of vasculitis and the activity or location of the Crohn's disease. Most patients respond quickly to corticosteroid therapy.

IX. HEART

Cardiovascular disorders are rarely associated with IBD. As in idiopathic ankylosing spondylitis, valvular lesions, especially aortic insufficiency, and cardiac conduction defects have also been seen in IBD patients, both with and without spondyloarthritis (69). Pericarditis and pleuropericarditis have also been observed and treated either with non-steroidals or corticosteroids (70,71). An increased incidence of infectious endocarditis has also been reported in patients with Crohn's disease (72).

X. LUNG

Bronchopulmonary abnormalities are only rarely seen in Crohn's disease, with impaired pulmonary function, alveolar lymphocytosis, and radiological abnormalities occasionally being noted (73,74). Granulomatous lung disease has been seen in patients with Crohn's disease (75). In this setting, Crohn's disease must be differentiated from sarcoidosis. This can occasionally be difficult because sarcoidosis is characterized by noncaseating epithelioid granulomas associated with "extrapulmonic manifestations," such as erythema nodosum, uveitis, and arthritis. Furthermore, sarcoidosis can, on occasion, involve the intestinal tract as well. Sarcoidosis and Crohn's disease have been reported to coexist in the same family, suggesting the possibility of shared underlying genetic risk factors (76). The pulmonary abnormalities in Crohn's disease appear to run a course independent from the underlying bowel disease. Crohn's disease with lung involvement can be treated with aerosolized or systemic corticosteroids.

XI. PANCREAS

Acute pancreatitis has been reported in Crohn's disease (77–80). The pathophysiology is unknown. Some authors have hypothesized that, in duodenal Crohn's disease, pancreatitis may develop from papillary obstruction or, alternatively, from papillary incompetence leading to reflux of duodenal contents into the pancreatic duct (81–83). Other causes of pancreatitis in Crohn's disease patients include medications (Imuran or 6-mercaptopurine [6-MP]), and gallstones, which are increased in frequency due to decreased bile salt recirculation and cholesterol supersaturated bile.

XII. GROWTH RETARDATION

Growth retardation in adolescents is found more often in Crohn's disease than in ulcerative colitis (84). Delayed onset of puberty, short stature, and being below expected weight are often the predominant findings, with improvement in growth parameters being a marker of effective therapy. Growth retardation may precede the clinical recognition of bowel symptoms by years (85). No specific endocrine or metabolic abnormality has been defined as yet. The cause of growth retardation is multifactorial and includes malnutrition due to inadequate caloric intake and malabsorption of fats, vitamins, and minerals. Patients with active disease may also have increased intestinal losses of proteins and minerals along with increased nutritional requirements. In the past, medical therapy of children and adolescents with Crohn's disease has been almost identical to that of adults. Recently, however, studies have demonstrated that nutritional therapy with elemental or polymeric diet is as effective in inducing remission and reversing growth failure as are corticosteroids, which also can cause growth retardation (86–88). Whether used as primary or adjuvant therapy, ensuring adequate caloric intake should be the cornerstone of treatment of Crohn's disease in children and adolescents to prevent or reverse growth retardation.

XIII. NEUROLOGIC SYMPTOMS

Various nonspecific neurological disturbances have been found in Crohn's disease (90–92). The cause of these neurological changes in unknown, although cerebral vasculitis and cerebral thrombosis are possible mechanisms. Whether the neurological disturbances are related to the activity and extent of Crohn's disease is unclear.

XIV. THERAPY-RELATED EXTRAINTESTINAL MANIFESTATIONS

A. Sulfasalazine

Side effects due to sulfasalazine can occur in patients who are slow acetylaters or who are receiving high doses of sulfasalazine (93). Cutaneous effects can include urticaria, exfoliative dermatitis, and toxic epidermal necrolysis. "Sulfasalazine lung" classically occurs as scattered pulmonary infiltrates with peripheral eosinophilia. Interstitial pulmonary fibrosis has also been reported. Hepatotoxicity is rare and, when present, is usually associated with rash and eosinophilia. Granulomatous hepatitis has also been described in patients taking sulfasalazine (94,95). Agranulocytosis, leukopenia, and hemolytic anemia have also been seen. Sulfasalazine can induce a decrease in spermatozoa count that is usually reversible upon cessation of sulfasalazine or changing the patient's therapy to a mesalamine (5-aminosalicylic acid) preparation.

B. Corticosteroids

Long-term use of corticosteroids may aggravate growth retardation in adolescents (89). Corticosteroids can also promote renal calculi formation by increasing calcium secretion in urine. Cataracts, diabetes, osteoporosis, and avascular necrosis are other well-known side effects of long-term steroid use (96).

C. Immunomodulator Therapy

6-Mercaptopurine and azathioprine can lead to bone marrow suppression, pancreatitis, and hepatotoxicity (97–99). These side effects almost always reverse upon withdrawal of the drug. Cyclosporin A can cause a wide variety of side effects, including nephrotoxicity, hepatotoxicity, and neurotoxicity. Methotrexate can result in both hepatic and pulmonary fibrosis.

Total parenteral nutrition can cause nonspecific changes in liver chemistries (100). These changes are often reversible by infusing the diet over a twelve-hour cycle. Actigall (ursodeoxycholic acid) has also been shown to improve liver chemistries.

XV. THE ROLE OF THE IMMUNE SYSTEM IN EXTRAINTESTINAL MANIFESTATIONS OF CROHN'S DISEASE

The stimulatory molecules present within the intestinal lumen that activate and induce the acute and chronic mucosal immunological and inflammatory events appear to be bacterial cell wall products (101–103). These potent activating molecules include peptidoglycans, lipopolysaccharides, and other chemotactic bacterial products that are produced by the many different types of bacteria within the gastrointestinal tract. Bacterial cell wall products activate macrophages and T lymphocytes to release a group of potent proinflammatory cytokines, including interleukin-1, interleukin-6, and tumor necrosis factor (TNF)-α (101–103). These proinflammatory cytokines normally serve to heighten host protective mucosal immune processes. Interleukin-1, interleukin-6, and TNF-α, as well as interferon-γ, increase human leukocyte antigen (HLA) class II antigen-presenting molecules on the surfaces of epithelial cells, endothelial cells, macrophages, and B cells. This increases the ability of a variety of cell types to present lumenal antigens and bacterial products in order to stimulate an immune response.

The proinflammatory cytokines interleukin-1 and TNF-α also increase secretion of potent chemotactic cytokines, such as interleukin-8, and macrophage chemotactic and activating factors by epithelial cells, endothelial cells, macrophages, and fibroblasts (101–103). The chemokines along with other chemotactic molecules (e.g., leukotriene B$_4$), complement components, and bacterial products (e.g., N-formyl-methionine-leucine-phenylalanine) markedly increase the attraction of macrophages and granulocytes so that they move from the circulation into the inflamed mucosa (101–103). The stimulatory and activation processes also lead to heightened antibody (immunoglobulin G) synthesis and secretion with resultant complement activation and increased T-cell activation.

Due to the continuous lumenal exposure to potent, nonspecific stimulatory bacterial products, the state of activation of the intestinal immune system and mucosal inflammatory pathways is markedly up-regulated. In contrast to the mucosal immune response to a self-limited infection, in IBD, there appears to be a deficiency in effective down-regulation through decreased production of suppressive cytokines such as interleukin-10, transforming growth factor-β, interleukin-4, and interleukin-1 receptor antagonist. Normally, active immunological and inflammatory events should turn off after the effective resolution of a bacterial or viral infection (101–103). In IBD, however, the down-regulatory events and processes that should turn off immunological and inflammatory protective processes appear to be deficient, resulting in a continuously up-regulated and highly activated mucosal immune system which, in turn, leads to continuous damage to the intestine (101–103).

Chronic inflammation leads to a rapid increase in the number of high endothelial venules (identified morphologically by their typical cuboidal, plump appearance). Increase in the number of high endothelial venules is due to both enhanced differentiation as well as stimulation of proliferation by cytokines (104–106). Cytokines, including interleukin-1, interferon-γ, and TNF, increase lymphoblast adherence to endothelial cells and both trigger the development of endothelial cell differentiation markers and enhance the expression of endothelial adhesion molecules. Increased expression of adhesion molecules on endothelial cells allows an increase in the influx of antigen-specific, sensitized lymphocytes as well as monocytes and granulocytes into areas of chronic inflammation (104–106). High endothelial venules increase in number in areas that are in close proximity to developing granulomas. The presence of high endothelial venules is thus closely associated with dense, lymphocytic infiltrates, particularly when mononuclear cell–mediated processes are persistent. Although most studies have focused on the maturation and homing events related to lymphocytes, the migration of granulocytes and macrophages into both mucosal and extraintestinal sites is also regulated by interactions with similar endothelial cell adhesion molecules [104–107].

Mucosal lymphoblasts from the intestine can circulate to a number of other mucosal secretory sites that comprise the common mucosal immune system, including the breast, lung, and eye (108,109). Recent work implicates synovial tissue as a similar site. Thus, for example, homing of stimulated lymphoblasts to diverse mucosal secretory sites allows the secretion into lung, breast, and eye fluids of protective IgA antibodies directed against antigens within the gastrointestinal lumen (108,109). Once lymphoblasts have "homed" to the gastrointestinal mucosa and have matured into effector cells, they provide protective immunity within the lamina propria. The appearance of activated T cells in the peripheral blood of patients with IBD as well as enhanced IgA secretion by peripheral blood B cells during active disease may represent activated lymphoblasts migrating from involved intestine and participation in the homing process in active IBD (101–103). Recent studies have demonstrated that activated lymphoblasts from the intestine also adhere to human synovial tissue (110–113). This raises the possibility that altered cell homing to the synovium could lead to the joint manifestations (arthralgias) observed in active IBD (110–113).

Selective migration of lymphocytes is directed by organ-specific binding of lymphocytes to high endothelial venules. Separate but related lymphocyte–endothelial cell recognition systems exist in the mucosa-associated lymphatic tissues, peripheral lymph node, synovium, and skin (114–116). Lymphocyte–endothelial cell interaction involves many lymphocyte adhesion receptors and their endothelial ligands, which act in concert to establish appropriate contacts between appropriately activated lymphocytes and endothelial cells. The integrins direct lymphocyte binding to mucosal sites (117,118). Selectins mediate lymphocyte homing to peripheral lymph nodes (107,119). The endothelial adhesion molecule E-selectin is involved in the binding of lymphocytes (120).

Intestinal immunoblasts from normal and inflamed gut bind differently to vascular endothelium. Immunoblasts from the normal gut bind extremely well to mucosal high endothelial venules but not at all to peripheral lymph node high endothelial venules, whereas blasts from patients with IBD interact efficiently with peripheral lymph node high endothelial venules (110–113). Therefore, it appears that immunoblasts from the inflamed gut lose their selectivity of HEV binding. Differences in the selectivity of homing from the inflamed gut may be caused by the inflammation-related alterations in the adhesion molecule patterns expressed on the immunoblasts (110–113). Mucosal immunoblasts can bind almost equally well to both mucosal and synovial high endothelial venules and use distinct sets of homing receptors for binding to mucosal and synovial high endothelial venules. The well-described homing-associated molecules of mucosal lymphocytes do not fully account for the synovial adherence (110–113). Unique homing molecules that mediate binding of mucosal lymphoblasts to synovial high endothelial venules remain to be discovered (113). Lymphoblast cells from human intestine, therefore, have a strong ability to interact efficiently with synovial high endothelial venules, raising the possibility that homing of lymphoblasts from the intestine to joint synovium may contribute to arthralgias and arthritis in patients with active IBD (110–113).

After intestinal antigenic stimulation, activated immunoblasts return to the blood circulation (108,109). Subsequently, blast cells home either back to mucosal sites or alternately to synovium (108,109). Accumulation of antigen-specific, highly activated immunoblasts in joints could lead to aggravation of synovitis, with arthralgias or arthritis (110–113). The pathophysiology of the arthralgias and arthritis could be related to cytokine and chemokine secretion from the activated lymphocytes or stimulated synovial cells, which might then lead to increased influx of granulocytes and macrophages (110–113).

Other endothelial cell adhesion molecule regulated sites may be found to be points of accumulation of activated intestinal immunoblasts and thereby be involved in the pathogenesis of other extraintestinal manifestations of IBD (110–113).

REFERENCES

1. Kirsner JB. The local and systemic complications of inflammatory bowel disease. JAMA 1979; 242:1177–1183.
2. Greenstein AJ, Janowitz HD, Sachar DB. The extraintestinal complications of Crohn's disease and ulcerative colitis: a study of 700 patients. Medicine 1976; 55:401–412.
3. Rankin GB, Watts DH, Melnyk CS, Kelley ML. National Cooperative Crohn's Disease Study: extraintestinal manifestations and perianal complications. Gastroenterology 1979; 77:914–920.

4. Moschella SL. Review of so-called aseptic neutrophilic dermatoses. Aust J Dermatol 1983; 24(2):55–62.

5. McCord ML, Hall RP. Cutaneous manifestations of inflammatory bowel disease. In: Targan SR, Shanahan F, eds. Inflammatory Bowel Disease. Baltimore: Williams & Wilkins, 1994:682–694.

6. Jorizzo JL. Blood vessel–based inflammatory disorders. In: Moschella SL, Hurley HJ, eds. Dermatology. 3d ed. Philadelphia: WB Saunders, 1992:584–586.

7. Jorizzo JL. Blood vessel–based inflammatory disorders. In: Moschella SL, Hurley HJ, eds. Dermatology. 3d ed. Philadelphia: WB Saunders, 1992:589–590.

8. Schoetz DJ Jr, Coller JA, Veidenheimer MG. Pyoderma gangrenosum and Crohn's disease. Eight cases and a review of the literature. Dis Colon Rectum 1983; 26:155.

9. Hickman JG. Pyoderma gangrenosum. Clin Dermatol 1983; 1:102–113.

10. Schwaegerle SM, Bergfeld WF, Senitzer D, Tidrick TR. Pyoderma gangrenosum: a review. J Am Acad Dermatol 1988; 18:559–568.

11. Holt PJA, Davies MG, Saunders KC, Nuki G. Pyoderma gangrenosum. Medicine 1980; 59:114–133.

12. Su WPD, Schroeter AL, Perry HO, Powell FC. Histopathologic and immunopathologic study of pyoderma gangrenosum. J Cutan Pathol 1986; 13:223–230.

13. Powell FC, Schroeter AL, Su WPD, Perry HO. Pyoderma gangrenosum: a review of 86 patients. Q J Med 1985; 217:173–186.

14. Fetto DL, Gibson LE, Su WPD. Sweet's syndrome: systemic signs and symptoms and associated disorders. Mayo Clinic Proc 1995; 70:234–240.

15. Jackson RM, Duvic M. Pyoderma gangrenosum/Sweet's syndrome. In: Jordon RE, ed. Immunologic Disease of the Skin. Norwalk, CT: Appleton & Lange, 1991:477–485.

16. Callen JP. Pyoderma gangrenosum and related disorders. Med Clin North Am 1989; 73:1247–1261.

17. Jorizzo JL. Blood vessel–based inflammatory disorders. In: Moschella SC, Hurley HJ, eds. Dermatology. 3d ed. Philadelphia: WB Saunders, 1992:586–587.

18. Fine J. Bullous disease. In: Moschella SL, Hurley HJ, eds. Dermatology. 3d ed. Philadelphia: WB Saunders, 1992:

19. Ray TL, Leivne JB, Weiss W, Ward PA. Epidermolysis bullosa acquisita and inflammatory bowel disease. J Am Acad Dermatol 1982; 6:242–252.

20. Leibowitz G, Eliakim R, Amir G, Rachmilewitz D. Dermatomyositis associated with Crohn's disease. J Clin Gastroenterol 1994; 18(1):48–52.

21. Drabble EM, Gani S. Acute gastrochemius myositis. Med J Australia 1992; 157:318–319.

22. O'Loughlin S, Perry HO. A diffuse pustular eruption associated with ulcerative colitis. Arch Dermatol 1978; 114:1061–1064.

23. Fenske NA, Gern JE, Pierce D, Vasey FB. Vesiculopustular eruption of ulcerative colitis. Arch Dermatol 1983; 199:664–669.

24. Lee FI, Bellary SV, Francis C. Increased occurrence of psoriasis in patients with Crohn's disease and their relatives. Am J Gastroenterol 1990; 85:962–963.

25. Plauth M, Jensu H, Meyle J. Oral manifestations of Crohn's disease: an analysis of 79 cases. J Clin Gastro 1991; 13(1):29–37.

26. Frankel DH, Mostofi RS, Lorincz AL. Oral Crohn's disease: report of two cases in brothers with metallic dysgeusia and a review of the literature. J Am Acad Dermatol 1985; 12:260–268.

27. Bozkurt T, Langer M, Fendel K, Lux G. Granulomatous tonsillitis: a rare extraintestinal manifestation of Crohn's disease. DDS 1992; 37(7):1127–1130.

28. Kafity AA, Pellegrini AE, Fromkes JJ. Metastatic Crohn's disease: a rare cutaneous manifestation. J Clin Gastroenterol 1993; 17(4):300–303.

29. Mooney EE, Sweeney E, Barnes L. Granulomatous leg ulcers: an unusual presentation of Crohn's in a young man. J Am Acad Dermatol 1993; 28(1):115–117.

30. Attanoos RL, Appleton MAC, Hughes LE, Ansell ID, Douglas-Jones AG, Williams GT.

Granulomatous hidradenitis suppurativa and cutaneous Crohn's disease. Histopathology 1993; 23:111–115.

31. Gravallese EM, Kantrowitz FG. Arthritic manifestations of inflammatory bowel disease. Am J Gastroenterol 1988; 83:703–709.

32. Wollheim FA. Enteropathic arthritis. In: Kelly W, Harris E Jr, Ruddy S, Sledge CB, eds. Textbook of Rheumatology. 3d ed. Philadelphia: WB Saunders, 1989.

33. Levine JB. Arthropathies and ocular complications of inflammatory bowel disease. In: Targan SR, Shanahan F, eds. Inflammatory Bowel Disease. Baltimore: Williams & Wilkins, 1994:668–680.

34. Norton KI, Eichenfield AH, Rosh JR, Stern MT, Hermann G. Atypical arthropathy associated with Crohn's disease. Am J Gastroenterol 1993; 88(6):948–952.

35. Hermans PJ, Fievez ML, Descamps L, Aupaix MA. Granulomatous synovitis and Crohn's disease. J Rheumatol 1984; 11:710–712.

36. Purrmann J, Zeidler H, Bertrams J, Juli E, Cleveland S, Berges W, Gemsa R, Specker C, Reis HE. HLA antigens in ankylosing spondylitis associated with Crohn's disease. Increased frequency of the HLA phenotype B27,B44. J Rheumatol 1988; 15:1658–1661.

37. De Vos M, Cuvelier C, Mielants H, Veys E, Barbier F, Elewaut A. Ileo-colonoscopy in seronegative spondyloarthropathy. Gastroenterology 1989; 96:339–344.

38. Davis P, Thomson A, Lentle B. Quantitative sacroiliac scintigraphy in patients with Crohn's disease. Arthritis Rheum 1978; 21:234–237.

39. Mayer L, Janowitz H. Extraintestinal manifestations of inflammatory bowel disease. In: Kirsner JB, Shorter RG, eds. Inflammatory bowel disease, ed ed. Philadelphia: Lea & Febiger, 1988: .

40. Fielding JF, Cooke WT. Finger clubbing and regional enteritis. Gut 1971; 12:442.

41. Perry PM, Evans GA, Davies JD. Regional ileitis, ulcerative colitis and clubbed fingers. Dis Colon Rectum 1972; 15:278.

42. Billson FA, De Dombal FT, Watkinson G, Goligher JG, Ocular complications of ulcerative colitis. Gut 1967; 8:102–106.

43. Knox DL, Schachat AP, Mustonen E. Primary, secondary and coincidental ocular complications of Crohn's disease. Ophthalmology 1984; 91:163–173.

44. Salmon JF, Wright JP, Murray AD. Ocular inflammation in Crohn's disease. Ophthalmology 1991; 98:480–484.

45. Soukiasian SH, Foster CS, Raizman MB. Treatment strategies for scleritis and uveitis associates with inflammatory bowel disease. Am J Opthalmol 1994; 118:601–611.

46. Hofley P, Roerty J, McGinnity G, Griffiths AM, Marcon M, Kraft S, Sherman P. Asymptomatic uveitis in children with chronic inflammatory bowel disease. J Pediatr Gastroenterol Nutr 1993; 17(4):397–400.

47. Ruby AJ, Jampol LM. Crohn's disease and retinal vascular disease. Am J Ophthalmol 1990; 110:349–353.

48. Gelzayd EA, Breuer RI, Kirsner JB. Nephrolithiasis in inflammatory bowel disease. Am J Dig Dis 1986; 13:1027–1034.

49. Hylander E, Jarnum S, Frandsen J. Urolithiasis and hyperoxaluria in chronic inflammatory bowel disease. Scand J Gastroenterol 1979; 14:475.

50. Chadwick VS, Modka K, Dowling RH. Mechanism for hyperoxaluria in patients with ileal dysfunction. N Engl J Med 1973; 289:172–176.

51. Grossman MS, Nugent FW. Urolithiasis as a complication of chronic diarrheal disease. Am J Dig Dis 1967; 12:491.

52. Maratka Z, Nedbal J. Urolithiasis as a complication of the surgical treatment of ulcerative colitis. Gut 1964; 5:214.

53. Present D, et al. Obstructive hydronephrosis—a frequent but seldom recognized complication of granulomatous disease of the bowel. N Engl J Med 1969; 280:523.

54. Banner MP. Genitourinary complications of inflammatory bowel disease. Radiol Clin North Am 1987; 25:199–209.

55. Lichtman SN, Sartor B. Extraintestinal manifestations of inflammatory bowel disease: clinical aspects and natural history. In: Targan SR, Shanahan F, eds. Inflammatory bowel disease. Baltimore: Williams & Wilkins, 1994:317–333.

56. Wilcox GM, Aretz HT, Roy MA, Roche JK. Glomerulonephritis associated with inflammatory bowel disease. Gastroenterology 1990; 98:786–791.

57. Greenstein AJ, Sachar D, et al. Amyloidosis and inflammatory bowel disease: a 50-year experience with 25 patients. Medicine 1992; 71(5):261–270.

58. Meyers S, Janowitz HD. Complications of Crohn's disease. In: Berk JE, Haubrich WS, Kalser MH, Roth JLA, Schaffner F, eds. Bockus gastroenterology. Phildelphia: WB Saunders, 1985:2294–2305.

59. Dyer NH, Child JA, Mollin DL, et al. Anemia in Crohn's disease. Q J Med (New Series) 1972; 41:419.

60. Elsborg L, Larsen L. Folate deficiency in chronic inflammatory bowel disease. Scand J Gastroenterol 1979; 14:1019.

61. Altman AR, Matlz CR, Janowitz HD. Auto immune hemolytic anemia in ulcerative colitis. Dig Dis Sci 1979; 24:282–285.

62. Das KM, Eastwood MA, McManus JP, Sircus W. Adverse reactions during salicylazo-sulfapyridine therapy. N Engl J Med 1973; 289:491.

63. Talbot RW, Heppel J, Dozois RR, Beart RW. Vascular complications of inflammatory bowel disease. May Clin Proc 1986; 61:140–145.

64. Koenigs KP, McPhedran P, Sprio H. Thrombosis in inflammatory bowel disease. J Clin Gastroenterol 1987; 9(6):627–631.

65. Edwards RL, Levine JB, Green R, Duffy M, Mathews E, Brande W, Ricles FR. Activation of blood coagulation in Crohn's disease. Gastroenterology 1987; 92:329–337.

66. Conlan MG, Haire WD, Burnett DA. Prothrombotic abnormalities in inflammatory bowel disease. Dig Dis Sci 1989; 34:1089–1093.

67. Wyshock E, Caldwell M, Crowley JP. Deep venous thrombosis, inflammatory bowel disease, and protein S deficiency. Am J Clin Pathol 1988; 90:633–635.

68. Yassinger S, et al. Association of inflammatory bowel disease and large vascular lesions. Gastroenterology 1976; 71:844.

69. Burdick S, Tresch DD, Komokowski RA. Cardiac valvular dysfunction associated with Crohn's disease in the absence of ankylosing spondylitis. Am Heart J 1989; 118:174–176.

70. Abid MA, Gitlin N. Pericarditis—an extraintestinal complication of inflammatory bowel disease. West J Med 1990; 153:314–315.

71. Patwardhan RV, Heilpern J, Brewster AC, Darrah JJ. Pleuropericarditis: an extraintestinal complication of inflammatory bowel disease. Arch Intern Med 1983; 143:94–96.

72. Wong JSK. Infective endocarditis in Crohn's disease. Br Heart J 1989; 62:163–164.

73. Heatley RV, Thomas P, Prokipchuk EJ, Gauldie J, Sieniewicz DJ, Bienenstock J. Pulmonary function abnormalities in patients with inflammatory bowel disease. Q J Med 1982; 203:241–250.

74. Bonniere P, Wallaert B, Cortot A, Marchandise X, Riou Y, Tonnel AB, Colombel JF, Voisin C, Paris JC. Latent pulmonary involvement in Crohn's disease: biological, functional, bronchoalveolar lavage and scintigraphic studies. Gut 1986; 27:919–925.

75. Calder CJ, Lacy D, Raafat F, Weller PH, Booth IW. Crohn's disease with pulmonary involvement in a 3 year old boy. Gut 1993; 34:1636–1638.

76. Willoughby JMT, Mitchell DN, Wilson JD. Sarcoidosis and Crohn's disease in siblings. Am Rev Respir Dis 1971; 104:249–254.

77. Niemela S, Lehtola J, Lähde S. Pancreatitis in patients with chronic inflammatory bowel disease. Hepatogastroenterology 1989; 36:175–177.

78. Seyrig J, Jian R, et al. Idiopathic pancreatitis associated with inflammatory bowel disease. Dig Dis Sci 1985; 30(12):1121–1126.

79. Meyers S, Greenspan J, et al. Pancreatitis coincident with Crohn's ileocolitis: report of a case and review of the literature. Dis Colon Rectum 1987; 30:119–122.

80. Matsumoto T, Matsoi T, Iida M, Nunoi K, Fujishima M. Acute pancreatitis as a complication of Crohn's disease. Am J Gastroenterol 1989; 84(7):804–807.

81. Newman LH, Wellinger JR, Present DH, Aufses AH. Crohn's disease of the duodenum associated with pancreatitis: a case report and review of the literature. Mt Sinai J Med 1987; 54(5):429–432.

82. Altman HS, Phillips G, Bank S, Klotz H. Pancreatitis associated with duodenal Crohn's disease. Am J Gastroenterol 1983; 78(3):174–177.

83. Meltzer SJ, Korelitz BI. Pancreatitis and duodenopancreatic reflux in Crohn's disease: case report and review of the literature. J Clin Gastroenterol 1988; 10(5):555–558.

84. Korschner BS. Inflammatory bowel disease in children. Pediatr Clin North Am 1988; 35:189–208.

85. Kanof ME, Lake AM, Bayless TM. Decreased height velocity in children and adolescents before the diagnosis of Crohn's disease. Gastroenterology 1988; 95:1523–1527.

86. Kirschner BS, Klich JR, Kalman SS, DeFavaro MV, Rosenberg IH. Reversal of growth retardation in Crohn's disease with therapy emphasizing oral nutritional restitution. Gastroenterology 1981; 80:10–15.

87. Aiges H, Markowitz J, Rosa J, Daum F. Home nocturnal supplemental nasogastric feedings in growth-retarded adolescents with Crohn's disease. Gastroenterology 1989; 97:905–910.

88. Seidman E. Nutritional management of inflammatory bowel disease. Gastroenterol Clin North Am 1989; 17:129–155.

89. Hyams JS, Carey DE. Corticosteroids and growth. J Pediatr 1988; 113:249-254.

90. Gendelman S, present D, Janowitz HD. Neurological complications of inflammatory bowel disease. Gastroenterology 1982; 82:1065.

91. Schneiderman JH, Sharpe JA, Sutton DMC. Cerebral and retinal vascular complications of inflammatory bowel disease. Ann Neurol 1979; 5:331–337.

92. Adamek RJ, Wegener M, Wedmann B, Buttner T, Ricken D. Cerebral vasculitis in Crohn's disease. Leber Magen Darm 1993; 23(2):91–93.

93. Fich A, et al. Sulfasalazine hepatotoxicity. Am J Gastroenterol 1984; 79:401.

94. Janner RS, Tedesco FJ, Kalser MH. Azulfidine (sulfasalazine)-induced hepatic injury. Am J Dig Dis 1974; 19:465.

95. Losek JD, Werlin SL. Sulfasalazine hepatotoxicity. Am J Dig Dis Child 1981; 135:1071.

96. Compston JE, Judd D, Crawley ED, Evans WD, Evans C, Church HA, Reid EM, Rhodes J. Osteoprosis in patients with inflammatory bowel disease. Gut 1987; 28:410–415.

97. Klein M, et al. Treatment of Crohn's disease with azathioprine: a controlled evaulation. Gastronenterology 1974; 66:916.

98. Present DH, et al. Treatment of Crohn's disease with 6-mercaptopurine. A long-term randomized, double blind study. N Engl J Med 1980; 301:981.

99. Nogueria JR, Freedman MA. Acute pancreatitis as a complication of Imuran therapy in regional enteritis. Gastroenterology 1972; 62:1040.

100. Benogoa JM, et al. Pattern and prognosis of liver function test abnormalities during parenteral nutrition in inflammatory bowel disease. Hepatology 1985; 5:79.

101. Schreiber S, Raedler A, Stenson WF, MacDermott RP. The role of the mucosal immune system in inflammatory bowel disease [Review]. In: MacDermott RP, Elson CO, eds. Mucosal immunology II: clinical applications. Gastroenterology Clinics North Am 1992; 21(2):451–502.

102. Reinecker HC, Schreiber S, Stenson WF, MacDermott RP. The role of the mucosal immune system in ulcerative colitis and Crohn's disease. In: Orga P, et al, eds. Handbook of Mucosal Immunology. San Diego: Academic Press, 1994:439–456.

103. MacDermott RP. Alterations in the mucosal immune system in ulcerative colitis and

Crohn's disease. In: Katz J, ed. Inflammatory bowel disease. Med Clin North Am 1994; 78(6):1207–31.

104. Hamann A, Jablonski-Westrich D, Scholz KU, Duijvestijn A, Butcher EC, Thiele HG. Regulation of lymphocte homing I. Alterations in homing receptor expression and organ-specific high endothelial venule binding of lymphocytes upon activation. J Immunol 1988; 140:737–743.

105. Jalkanen S, Reichert RA, Gallatin WM, Bargatze RF, Weissman IL, Butcher EC. Homing receptors and the control of lymphocyte migration. Immunol Rev 1986; 91:39–60.

106. Jalkanen S, Streeter P, Lakey E, Bargatze R, Butcher EC. Lymphocytic and endothelial cell recognition elements that control lymphocyte traffic to mucosa-associated lymphatic tissues. Monogr Allergy 1988; 24:144–149.

107. Streeter PR, Berg EL, Rouse BT, Bargatze RF, Butcher EC. A tissue-specific endothelial cell molecule involved in lymphocyte homing. Nature 1988; 331:441–446.

108. Mestecky J. The common mucosal immune system and current strategies for induction of immune responses in external secretions. J Clin Immunol 1987; 7:265–276.

109. Mestecky J, McGhee JR. Immunoglobulin A (IgA): Molecular and cellular interactions involved in IgA biosynthesis and immune repsonse. Adv. Immunol. 1987; 40:153–245.

110. Jalkanen S, Nash GS, de los Toyos J, MacDermott RP, Butcher EC. Human lamina propria lymphocytes bear homing receptors and bind selectively to mucosal lymphoid high endo-therlium. Eur J Immunol 1989; 19:63–68.

111. Salmi M, Granfors K, Leirisalo-Repo M, Hämäläinen M, MacDermott RP, Leino R, Havia T, Jalkanen S. Selective endothelial binding of interleukin-2 dependent human T-cell lines derived from different tissues. Proc Natl Acad Sci U S A 1992; 89:11436–11440.

112. Salmi M, Granfors K, MacDermott RP, Jalkanen S. Aberrant binding of lamina propria lymphocytes to vascular endothelium in inflammatory bowel disease. Gastroenterology 1994; 106:596–605.

113. Salmi M, Andrew DP, Butcher EC, Jalkanen S. Dual binding capacity of mucosal im-munoblasts to mucosal and synovial endothelium in humans: dissection of the molecular mechanisms. J Exp Med 1995; 181(1):137–149.

114. Butcher EC, Scollary RG, Weissman IL. Organ specificity of lymphocyte homing: mediation by highly selective lymphocyte interaction with organ-specific determinants on high endo-thelial venule. Eur J Immunol 1980; 10:556–561.

115. Jalkanen S, Steere AC, Fox RI, Butcher EC. A distinct endothelial recognition system that controls lymphocyte traffic into inflamed synovium. Science 1986; 233:556–560.

116. Picker LJ, Koshimoto TK, Smith XW, Warnock RA, Butcher EC. ELAM-1 is an adhesion molecule for skin-homing T cells. Nature 1991; 349:796–799.

117. Holzmann B, Weissman IL. Integrin molecules involved in lymphocyte homing to Peyer's patches. Immunol Rev 1989; 108:45–61.

118. Hu MC-T, Crowe DT, Weissman IL, Holzmann B. Cloning and expression of mouse integrin beta P (beta 7): a functional role in Peyer's patch-specific lymphocyte homing. Proc Natl Acad Sci U S A 1992; 89:8254–8258.

119. Gallatin WM, Butcher EC, Weismann IL. A cell surface molecule involved in organ-specific homing of lymphocytes. Nature 1983; 304:30–34.

120. Stoolman LM. Adhesion molecules controlling lymphocyte migration. Cell 1989; 56:907–910.

COMMENTARY: THE SYSTEMIC NATURE OF INFLAMMATORY BOWEL DISEASE

Lloyd Mayer   *Mount Sinai Medical Center, New York, New York*

There is a growing awareness that organ-specific inflammatory disorders are not truly organ specific but rather spill over to the rest of the body. This is not to say that there is not a primary event or predisposing factor that is organ specific in a given disease, but that many inflammatory events may be more generalizable. This appears to be true for inflammatory bowel disease (IBD). Once thought of as a localized disorder, IBD is now viewed as a systemic disease. This is due to the increasing recognition of manifestations that occur outside the bowel and, as noted in the preceding chapter, may even overshadow the bowel disease itself. The incidence of extraintestinal manifestations is staggering with more than 60% of all patients with IBD experiencing one or more such manifestations during the course of their disease.

The unique feature in IBD is that extraintestinal manifestations can be broken down into several subdivisions. The common subclassification relates to those manifestations that are disease activity–related versus those that have an independent course. Even further subdivisions have been described. Some extraintestinal manifestations occur more commonly in Crohn's disease than ulcerative colitis and vice versa; others occur in patients with predominantly colonic disease versus those with isolated small intestinal disease. Some extraintestinal manifestations occur in groups; others are isolated. Some extraintestinal manifestations occur in all forms of intestinal inflammation (non-IBD and IBD) and others are IBD selective. Lastly, there are those manifestations that are common to many inflammatory diseases (e.g., sarcoid, infectious disease), reflecting a more uniform type of abnormality. Some extraintestinal manifestations are a direct consequence of the disease process and do not fit into the concept of systemic diseases. These various subdivisions underscore potential differences in the pathogenetic mechanisms involved in extraintestinal manifestations and may be helpful when evaluating IBD patients with these problems.

Knowing the potential complications, is there anything that the physician can do to intervene?

To screen for all extraintestinal manifestations would be inefficient given the low incidence of each manifestation and the generally benign course of many of these disorders. However, intervention is warranted in those patients in whom the extraintestinal manifestations are a direct consequence of the disease process (e.g., nephrolithiasis due to increased oxalate absorption or excessive water and alkali loss from ostomies, anemia from iron loss). Prudent fluid and electrolyte management as well as acidification of the urine could help prevent such complications. However, most extraintestinal manifestations do not allow for prior intervention.

If early intervention is limited, what important concepts can be learned from studying the subdivisions described? Because these manifestations represent components of a systemic process, there may be clues to the pathogenesis of IBD itself. As detailed in the accompanying chapter, mucosal lymphocytes and macrophages are activated in IBD by interaction with luminal contents, bacterial products, or some other as yet undefined factors. The activated cells spill over into the systemic circulation and can migrate to other tissues and promote inflammation. The degree of activation of cells in the mucosa correlates well with the activity of disease. Therefore, the concept that some extraintestinal manifestations correlate with disease activity supports the concept of cell migration. The key issue is specificity. Why do patients manifest specific extraintestinal manifestations? Part of the answer may relate to the types of homing receptors expressed on immunologically activated cells. There is strong evidence for "homing" of intestinally primed lymphocytes to other mucosal sites. Migration here is directed by a series of homing molecules and their receptors. This phenomenon has evolved into the concept of a common mucosal immune system, disseminating protection from the gut to the lungs, mammary glands (and breast milk), and genitourinary tract. However, few extraintestinal manifestations occur in these mucosal organs, so mucosa-specific homing is not likely to be relevant to the origin of extraintestinal manifestations. Several groups have identified specific homing receptors for the skin, lymph nodes, and intestinal mucosa. To invoke specific homing of mucosally activated lymphocytes, it would have to be postulated that lymphocyte activation in IBD changes the homing receptor expression on these cells, making them localize to the skin, anterior chamber to the eye, bile duct, and so on. There is little evidence for this. Specificity would more likely be due to recognition of some cross-reactive antigen by immunocompetent cells. In this scenario, mucosal cells would migrate to all sites but only be induced to cause local inflammation in the setting of specific antigenic stimulation. This is the case for general lymphocyte recirculation in lymph nodes. Here naive cells exit the circulation after binding to high endothelial venules and, if Ag is present (to which they have been primed), then cells are trapped, induced to proliferate, and eventually lose the expression of their homing receptors. This subsequently allows them to leave the lymph node and distribute themselves throughout the host. Recent data from Das suggest a similar scenario may exist at sites of extraintestinal inflammation. This group has identified in patients with ulcerative colitis an IgG antibody against a 40-kd protein expressed on normal intestinal epithelial cells. Although the killing of epithelial cells by this antibody is not prominent, complement activation and deposition occur at the antibody–antigen binding site. Activated complement components may attract and activate neutrophils and mast cells causing nonspecific tissue injury. More recently, Das and coworkers detected the expression of the 40-kd protein in bile duct and corneal epithelium. Thus, one scenario is that 40-kd Ag–reactive lymphocytes may circulate and get trapped at extraintestinal sites where this Ag is expressed, setting up a similar scenario of complement activation and inflammation at these sites. Similar Ags have not been identified in Crohn's disease, suggesting that other pathways may be involved or other unique Ags are recognized by lymphocytes in these patients.

This latter issue may be important with regard to the understanding of extraintestinal manifestations that are different in ulcerative colitis versus Crohn's disease as well as to those that have a commonality in the two diseases. For example, the presence of anti–40-kd Ab in ulcerative colitis and not Crohn's disease may help to explain the clear association of sclerosing cholangitis with ulcerative colitis and not Crohn's disease (the 40-kd Ag is expressed on bile duct epithelium). These similarities and dichotomies should be used to gain insight into IBD mechanisms. Unfortunately, there are little available data. Recent studies have supported the concept that Crohn's disease reflects a local cell-mediated immune response. This is true not only from the histologic features (granuloma formation, macrophage activation) but also from the profile of cytokines produced in the lamina propria. In contrast, ulcerative colitis appears to resemble more of an immune complex–mediated injury process with complement activation, neutrophil infiltration, and autoantibody production. Even though there is overlap, it would be interesting to view the specific extraintestinal manifestations in the context of T-cell versus B-cell pathogenesis. For example, erythema nodosum is seen in a number of other diseases in which T-cell and macrophage activation is evident (e.g., *Mycobacterium leprae* infections, sarcoidosis). Thus it would make sense that this extraintestinal manifestation is more common in Crohn's disease. Pyoderma gangrenosum has more of the gross appearance of a vasculitic lesion (generally immune complex mediated) and is more common in ulcerative colitis. However, on immunohistochemical analysis, these lesions do not have true vasculitic features. Furthermore, ankylosing spondylitis (idiopathic) is thought to be T cell mediated (cytolytic T-cell attack on an altered HLA-B27 molecule) but occurs more commonly in ulcerative colitis than Crohn's disease. Thus, correlating pathogenetic mechanisms of the bowel disease with extraintestinal manifestations is still a concept that remains to be tested with more well-defined tools.

All is not lost however. There is the repeated observation that extraintestinal manifestations are much more common in patients with colonic rather than ileal disease. Given the differences in flora between the two sites, this might support a role for bacterial products. As alluded to earlier, bacterial products might activate mucosal lymphocytes, macrophages, and neutrophils, nonspecifically allowing them to circulate throughout the body, alter their homing patterns, and cause nonspecific tissue injury at sites where they deposit. Alternatively, they might also activate normally suppressed autoreactive cross-reactive lymphocytes. A similar scenario has been proposed for the formation of anti-DNA antibodies in systemic lupus erythematosus since cross-reactivity of anti-DNA Abs with phosphorylated bacterial products has been noted. However, even here, a direct relationship has not been substantiated. There are several extraintestinal manifestations that are common to many forms of intestinal inflammation (celiac sprue, blind loop syndrome, diverticulitis, infectious colitis). More typically, these manifest as polyarticular arthritis. In some of these disorders, the arthritis appears to correlate with the level of circulating immune complexes (e.g., blind loop or the arthropathy of intestinal bypass), which can deposit in joints as part of a serum sickness reaction. However, in ulcerative colitis and Crohn's disease joints do not appear to be the site for immune complex deposition because complement levels are normal and cellular infiltration is limited.

What is left is an assessment of extraintestinal manifestations that cluster versus those that occur individually. The classic triad of colitic arthritis, iritis, and erythema nodosum (with and without aphthous stomatitis) suggests that there is some common pathogenetic mechanism for these extraintestinal manifestations. Again, given the diseases that this group of manifestations is seen with, it is suggested that this might be a T-cell–mediated process. It is much more difficult to identify antigens that stimulate T cells because these are processed peptides presented in the context of an MHC molecule. Such antigens are not freshly expressed on cell surfaces or in tissues. T-cell clones from locally affected areas would have to be generated to demonstrate that these recognize tissue antigens at other sites. Given the recent advances in technology, this is not impossible, but it would be a major undertaking.

The extraintestinal manifestations open a window to the understanding of IBD. Specific attention should be paid to patients with these types of presentations, and it should be determined what is truly IBD specific versus what is specific to Crohn's disease or ulcerative colitis. These should be analyzed accordingly. Careful attention is required to identify those extraintestinal manifestations that are related to therapy rather than to IBD and those that are consequences of the disease process as opposed to its pathogenesis. The potential for such analyses is great as general knowledge of immunological defects in IBD expands.

27
Liver Complications

Harvey M. Lieberman   *Lenox Hill Hospital and New York University School of Medicine, New York, New York*

Liver disease complicating Crohn's disease, specifically pyelphlebitis and hepatic abscess, was first reported by Snavely in 1946 (1). Since then, our appreciation for the occurrence of liver and biliary disease in individuals with Crohn's disease has increased dramatically. Most liver disease was initially believed to be associated with ulcerative colitis, but, in the majority of cases, the incidence and types of liver disease in patients with Crohn's disease are similar to that of ulcerative colitis. Particularly because there is an increasing incidence of Crohn's disease, it is of paramount importance that the clinician be aware of the types of diseases of the liver and biliary tract that may affect such patients.

The reported incidence of hepatic disorders in individuals with inflammatory bowel disease varies from 5% to more than 90% (2–8). This incidence varies according to the means by which patients are selected and the criteria used for determining the presence of liver disease. For example, studies that use wedge liver biopsies at the time of laparotomy for inflammatory bowel disease tend to have the highest percentages of occurrence of hepatobiliary disease (2,3). If these biopsies are reviewed and individuals having only minor histological changes of the liver are excluded or only those individuals undergoing needle biopsy of the liver are considered, the incidence of such disease is significantly less (4–6). These observations may be attributed to, at least in part, the patchy histological distribution of some disorders of the liver. Furthermore, if the diagnosis of liver disease is based solely on clinical and laboratory information, the incidence of liver disease is only approximately 2% to 6% (7–9). Individuals having wedge biopsies at the time of bowel surgery are likely to be the most ill and are likely to suffer from the greatest extent of malnutrition, which may also affect the liver biopsies. An important observation of several studies of patients with significant liver disease documented by liver biopsy is that many of these patients had either lacked biochemical evidence of liver disease or had developed normal values of biochemical liver function tests subsequent to the performance of liver biopsy (3,5,6). This observation is supported by the fact that those individuals screened for liver disease solely by clinical and laboratory information represent the smallest group of patients with Crohn's disease also having liver disease. Therefore, if only clinical and laboratory screening methods are used to detect liver disease, then the presence of significant liver disease in some patients with Crohn's disease will be missed.

In considering hepatic complications of Crohn's disease, an etiological relation-ship between the liver disease and bowel disease must also be considered. In general, little is known about such a relationship. In most diseases of the liver discussed here, there is a poor correlation between the presence of liver disease and the activity of the inflammatory bowel disease (5,6). Such hepatic disorders have been described as variably occurring before or at the time of diagnosis of inflammatory bowel disease, during the course of the bowel disease, even when relatively quiescent, and, in some cases, after surgical removal of affected bowel. Therefore, in many instances of liver disease compli-cating inflammatory bowel disease, a simple cause-and-effect relationship between these processes cannot be established.

Finally, although the main emphasis of this chapter is on diseases of the liver that complicate Crohn's disease, certain disorders of the biliary tree have an increased inci-dence or association with inflammatory bowel disease (10–12). In certain circumstances, these may be considered to be extraintestinal manifestations of such inflammatory bowel disease (12). Therefore, disorders of the biliary tree that complicate Crohn's disease are also considered.

I. HEPATIC DISORDERS

A. Fatty Liver or Steatosis

Fatty liver or hepatic steatosis is one the most common disorders of the liver that complicate Crohn's disease; in some series, it is the most common hepatic disorder (6,13,14). This is particularly true of the earlier reports and series based on autopsy studies. Depending on the indication for liver biopsy, the incidence of steatosis of the liver in inflammatory bowel disease varies from 20% to 45% (15).

Fatty infiltration of the liver, or hepatic steatosis, is characterized by large droplets of fat within the cytoplasm of the hepatocyte, with minimal inflammation, if any, present within the hepatic lobule (15). A typical microscopic picture of hepatic steatosis is seen in Figure 1. The histological lesion is variable, usually of the macrovesicular type, although all distributions have been described (13). In one series, based on liver biopsies of patients with Crohn's disease in which fatty changes were the most common disorder observed, biopsies showed a distinct vacuolization of the hepatocytes (5). Of 22 specimens in this series, two showed complete fatty metamorphosis or fatty liver, five showed fatty changes in more than half of the parenchymal cells (severe fatty changes), and 11 showed fatty changes of one-fourth to one-half of the parenchymal cells (moderate fatty change), whereas four specimens contained only scattered small groups of fat-laden cells (focal fatty change). Grossly, the fatty infiltration may diffusely involve the liver, but may also be localized, mimicking hepatic abscess or tumor, when visualized by computed tomography (CT) scan, as seen in Figure 2 (16).

The relationship of fatty infiltration to inflammatory bowel disease is complex, but does not appear to be related to any specific localization of Crohn's disease or disease activity. This entity is found most frequently in series using liver biopsies performed either at autopsy or on patients undergoing laparotomy for bowel resection, suggesting an increased incidence when bowel disease has been most severe. However, these observa-tions have led to the general conclusion that fatty infiltration of the liver, rather than being a specific complication related to the inflammatory bowel disease activity per se, is more closely related to chronic debilitating disease and consequent malnutrition, itself often the

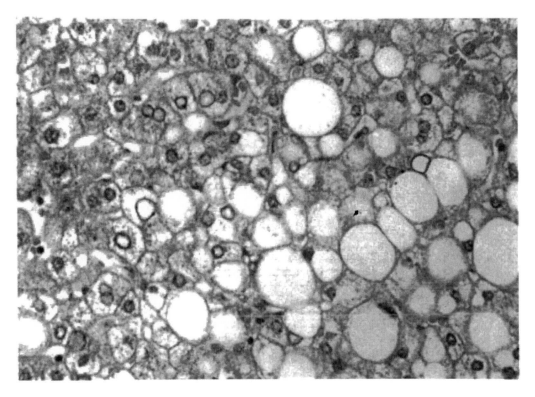

FIG. 1 Fatty liver. Many liver cells are distended with fat droplets and the nuclei are vacuo-lated. The fatty change is most marked around the portal zones. Hematoxylin-eosin stain ×100. (From Sherlock S, Summerfield JA, eds. Color Atlas of Liver Disease. 1st ed. Chicago: Year Book, 1979, with permission.)

result of active intestinal disease (13,15,17,18). Therefore, therapy is generally directed at improving nutrition and controlling the inflammatory process. Often, the hepatic disorder is asymptomatic, although hepatomegaly may be found in such individuals and is generally regarded as not likely to progress to more serious liver disease (13,15,17).

B. Pericholangitis

Studies have demonstrated the presence of inflammatory lesions of the portal tract in many individuals with hepatic disease who also have inflammatory bowel disease. Pericholan-gitis is a histological diagnosis that, in most antemortem studies, is the most common hepatic disease occurring in the presence of Crohn's disease, ranging in incidence from 20% to 80% (3–5,13,15,17,19). Because the term pericholangitis refers to a nonspecific inflammation of the portal tract, other terms such as interlobular hepatitis, intrahepatic or intralobular cholangitic hepatitis, and portal triaditis have also been used to describe the same lesion, resulting in some confusion.

The histological course of this disease has been well studied, with acute, subacute, and chronic lesions being described (20–22). The acute phase is characterized by marked edema of the bile ductules, dilation of portal venules and lymphatics, and an acute cellular infiltrate of the periductular and hepatic parenchyma that is associated with pericentral

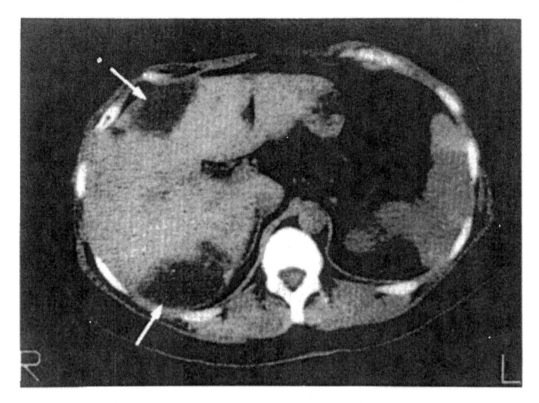

FIG. 2 Focal fat. Fatty infiltration of the liver reduces the density of liver parenchyma in computed tomography scans so that the fatty liver appears darker. Two low-attenuation filling defects (arrows) are present anteriorly and posteriorly in the right lobe of the liver. The appearance of fatty infiltration of the liver, when occurring as focal fat, may be confused with malignant infiltration of the liver. (From Sherlock S, Summerfield JA, eds. Color Atlas of the liver. 2nd ed. Chicago: Mosby-Year Book, 1991, with permission.)

hepatic cholestasis. The disease is, at this stage, reversible (20). The subacute phase, no longer reversible, is characterized by hyaline changes in the walls of the bile ductules and a fibroblastic proliferation; there is increased fibrous tissue. The chronic phase, characterized by established circumductal fibrosis, lacks an acute cellular infiltrate. It is additionally characterized by periportal fibrosis, phlebosclerosis, lymphangiectasia, and piecemeal hepatic necrosis. This phase is irreversible and may progress to cirrhosis and portal hypertension (20,21). A typical microscopic picture of pericholangitis is seen in Figure 3.

The clinical course of this disease has also been elucidated; it may either be asymptomatic or have features of cholestasis or cholangitis (21). In asymptomatic disease, the most common manifestation is a variably elevated serum alkaline phosphatase; portal hypertension and esophageal varices may still develop (21). The most common course of symptomatic patients is one of intermittent episodes of cholestasis, frequently of sudden onset and characterized by icterus and pruritis. A second, less common type of symptomatic course is characterized by recurrent episodes of cholangitis (21).

Some investigators believe that pericholangitis is part of a spectrum of liver disease, including primary sclerosing cholangitis, but only having involvement of the intrahepatic ducts (15,23,24). This view is supported by the study of Wee and Ludwig in which six of

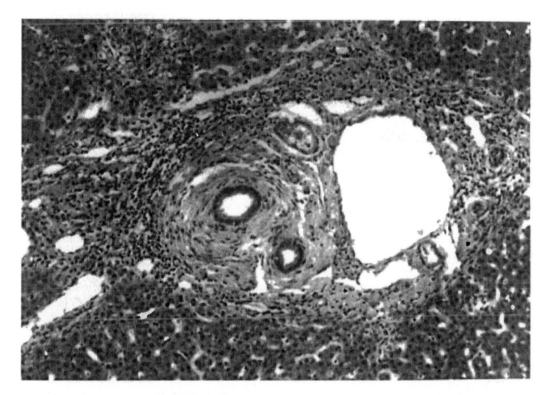

FIG. 3 Pericholangitis. Progressive fibrosis and inflammation of the portal triads. Rings of fibrosis tissue enclose the small bile duct in the portal tracts and there is chronic inflammatory cell infiltration. Aematoxylin-eosin stain ×40. (From Sherlock S, Summerfield JA, eds. Color Atlas of Liver Disease. 1st ed. Chicago: Year Book, 1979, with permission.)

18 patients with primary sclerosing cholangitis had evidence from a prior liver biopsy of pericholangitis (which the authors call small duct primary sclerosing cholangitis), with an earlier normal cholangiogram. The hepatic microscopic findings of both small duct primary sclerosing cholangitis and primary sclerosing cholangitis are identical and include hepatic portal edema with bile duct proliferation, fibrous cholangitis, pleomorphic cholangitis, and fibro-obliterative cholangitis (15,24). Periportal hepatitis with piecemeal necrosis may also be seen histologically. In addition, this same study demonstrated that five of 37 patients with small duct sclerosing cholangitis progressed to primary sclerosing cholangitis and four of 37 patients progressed to secondary biliary cirrhosis (24). Twenty-seven of 37 patients with small duct primary sclerosing cholangitis had stable liver function for a mean period of 13 years, and, of those 18 patients with primary sclerosing cholangitis, 11 individuals progressed to secondary biliary cirrhosis and biliary cholangiocarcinomas developed in three patients (25). The evidence that some cases of small duct sclerosing cholangitis, or pericholangitis, develop into primary sclerosing cholangitis and that both lesions are associated with the development of cholangiocarcinoma, therefore, support the view that these two pathological entities are related and represent different parts of a spectrum of the same disease.

Liver biopsy and cholangiography of both the extrahepatic and intrahepatic biliary systems are required to adequately diagnose small duct primary sclerosing cholangitis (i.e., pericholangitis) or primary sclerosing cholangitis of the extrahepatic biliary system. In addition, because the histological picture may resemble chronic active hepatitis or primary biliary cirrhosis, serological testing for antimitochondrial, anti-smooth muscle, and antinuclear antibodies are indicated in this setting (15).

C. Cirrhosis

The incidence of cirrhosis of the liver associated with inflammatory bowel disease varies from 1% to 5% in most studies (2,3,5,13,15,17). The histological features of the cirrhosis varies with different studies. Some studies report the cirrhosis to be mainly of the postnecrotic type, and others report the majority of cases to be portal-biliary cirrhosis (2,3,5,17). In most studies, at least some of the cases of cirrhosis do not fall into either of these two categories.

In attempting to determine the cause of the cirrhosis, most series do report a number of these patients having received blood transfusions; however, when these cases are subjected to serological study, hepatitis B is unable to be implicated as a causative agent. Whether some of these cases are due to hepatitis C is unknown, because this serological test was unavailable at the time of these studies. Many instances of hepatitis C lack identifiable risk factors, and the incidence of infection with hepatitis C virus, of development of persistent infection, and of cirrhosis is substantial. Therefore, it is important to test subjects having cirrhosis and inflammatory bowel disease for hepatitis C antibody in future studies. Determination of progression to postnecrotic cirrhosis by prior liver biopsies that demonstrate chronic active hepatitis, especially hepatitis C, would also be supportive for such a role of this virus.

In contrast, some of the cases of histologically documented cirrhosis are likely to represent the end stage of primary sclerosing cholangitis, or pericholangitis, which is known to progress to cirrhosis (20–23). In some instances, previous cholangiograms or liver biopsy demonstrating preexisting sclerosing cholangitis, or pericholangitis, are available. In other series, such diagnostic studies are either unavailable or have failed to demonstrate these underlying conditions, again suggesting the variable nature of cirrhosis when associated with inflammatory bowel disease.

D. Amyloidosis

Of the numerous liver disease discussed in this chapter, amyloidosis is one of the few that is associated primarily with Crohn's disease (8,13). The incidence in several large series is approximately 1% but this is probably an underestimation of the actual occurrence of this entity in Crohn's disease, suggesting that patient selection may play an important role in determining the presence of this entity (3,4,5,8,12,26). Although involvement of the ileum is thought to be of crucial importance in the development of amyloidosis in Crohn's disease, amyloidosis has also been found in patients with Crohn's disease of only the colon (4,26,27). Amyloidosis has been historically found in patients with long-standing Crohn's disease, usually described as having preceded the development of amyloidosis by a period of between 4 and 21 years; however, in at least one study, this period was less than five years, and, in two cases, amyloidosis was present at the time of initial diagnosis of inflammatory bowel disease (26). This suggests that the presence of amyloidosis is underestimated and that aggressive diagnostic approaches will find this entity more frequently and earlier in the course of Crohn's disease than previously supposed. This disease should be considered in any patient with hepatomegaly and Crohn's disease of significant duration.

The clinical course of amyloidosis, when associated with Crohn's disease, is variable, and no relationship has been found between steroid treatment or the duration or extent of Crohn's disease and the development of amyloidosis (8,12,26). Although one study has described regression of hepatic amyloidosis after surgical removal of the involved bowel, in general, no correlation between therapy of the Crohn's disease and regression of hepatic amyloidosis has been found (28).

Amyloidosis, when associated with inflammatory bowel disease, is found in the kidneys as well as the liver, resulting in nephrotic syndrome and renal failure (29). Kidney transplantation may temporize this process, if renal amyloidosis is believed to play a significant role in the clinical course of such patients, but the long-term impact of such a procedure is questionable in view of the multiple organs that are often involved with amyloidosis.

E. Granulomatous Hepatitis and Granulomas

Granulomatous hepatitis is a well-described entity associated with Crohn's disease, occurring in approximately 1% of such individuals (30). The granulomas found in the liver are histologically similar to those found in the bowel wall and lymph nodes of patients with Crohn's disease (3). The hallmark of this disease, hepatic granulomas, occur within the liver lobule and are not necessarily found in the portal triad (15,30). Typical hepatic granulomas are seen in Figure 4. The patients may be asymptomatic and show minimal hepatic dysfunction by laboratory testing; most characteristically, an elevation in serum alkaline phosphatase is seen in approximately one-half of the individuals (12). Other patients may be symptomatic and have hepatomegaly or fever. The prognosis of these patients is generally good, and the disease rarely progresses to cirrhosis or portal hypertension (12). Treatment is nonspecific and is directed toward treating the underlying inflammatory bowel disease; hepatic granulomas have been reported to regress after surgical removal of the inflamed portion of the bowel (30). The finding of granulomatous hepatitis or hepatic granulomas may occur alone or in the presence of other hepatic disorders such as pericholangitis or cirrhosis, making the interpretation of this entity somewhat difficult in some cases (17,20). Significantly, other diseases causing granulomatous hepatitis, such as sarcoidosis and fungal and tuberculous infections, may mimic this picture (30). Drugs, including sulfasalazine, have been implicated as a cause of granulomatous hepatitis (31). The diagnosis of granulomatous hepatitis is made by liver biopsy and fastidious exclusion of other causes of granulomatous hepatitis, including those noted above. Treatment of specific underlying causes of granulomatous hepatitis, when indicated, is of paramount importance.

F. Chronic Active Hepatitis

Although usually associated with ulcerative colitis, chronic active hepatitis has rarely been associated with Crohn's disease, the overall incidence being approximately 1% or less (3,17). Piecemeal necrosis, the main diagnostic feature of chronic active hepatitis histologically, is found in many cases of pericholangitis, and changes in bile ductules are also found in some case of chronic active hepatitis, as well as pericholangitis, complicating the histological distinction in certain instances (12,20). Even in the presence of a normal cholangiogram, the diagnosis of chronic active hepatitis is therefore uncertain in many

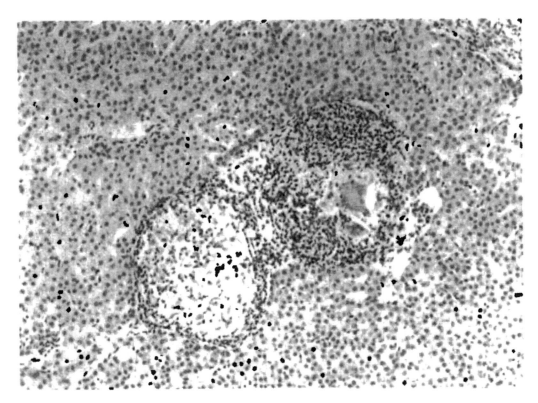

FIG. 4 Granulomas as found in the liver in both ulcerative colitis and Crohn's disease. These may be well developed with a cuff of lymphocytes enclosing epithelioid cells and giant cells. Caseation does not occur. Hematoxylin-eosin stain ×40. (From Sherlock S, Summerfield JA, eds. Color Atlas of Liver Disease. 1st ed. Chicago: Year Book, 1979, with permission.)

cases of inflammatory bowel disease, but it has, nonetheless, been diagnosed in several series of patients with pericholangitis using the aforementioned histological criteria.

In a review of 1911 patients with ulcerative colitis at the Mayo Clinic, Wee and Ludwig found a 13% incidence of chronic active hepatitis, including the histological features of periportal hepatitis but excluding the finding of periportal edema or bile duct changes (24). It is unclear why this study, so frequently cited, has such an inordinately high incidence of chronic active hepatitis and, in general, significant liver disease; this issue was not addressed by those authors (24). The cause of chronic active hepatitis in association with inflammatory bowel disease does not appear to have any relationship to prior infection with the hepatitis B virus, because no evidence of hepatitis B infection was noted in any patient in the aforementioned study who was found to have chronic active hepatitis (24). Furthermore, 11 of 18 such patients, followed up for a mean period of 12 years, progressed to postnecrotic cirrhosis (15). In an early report of a few patients having chronic active hepatitis and either ulcerative colitis or Crohn's disease, the patients also had concomitant diseases such as acquired hemolytic anemia or Hashimoto's thyroiditis (32). Although it is tempting to attribute an autoimmune origin to chronic active hepatitis associated with inflammatory bowel disease, especially in view of the recent emphasis on immune phenomenon in Crohn's disease, the limited number of such patients is this study and the lack of subsequent descriptions of such associations of any consistency make it difficult to make such a conclusion. As to the relationship of chronic active hepatitis to inflammatory bowel disease itself, the activity of chronic active hepatitis has not been consistently related to the activity or severity of the inflammatory bowel disease, and hepatic function has improved in only some patients after colectomy for ulcerative colitis, which has been better studied than Crohn's disease in this respect (17,18,33).

G. Primary Biliary Cirrhosis

Although primary biliary cirrhosis and ulcerative colitis have been described, I am not aware of any reports of primary biliary cirrhosis and Crohn's disease (22,34,35). Secondary biliary cirrhosis occurs as a complication of primary sclerosing cholangitis, and this relationship is likely to account for the observation of the portal–biliary type of cirrhosis described in inflammatory bowel disease (5,14). Primary biliary cirrhosis may be distinguished from secondary biliary cirrhosis by the presence of IgM antibody, normal cholangiogram, absence of gallstones, and the distinctive clinical occurrence in young women (36). Although primary biliary cirrhosis may histologically overlap pericholangitis because of the presence of granulomas, bile duct changes, and fibrosis in both diseases, the two entities are distinguished from each other by the criteria already described (20,22,36). Despite the reported occurrence of primary biliary cirrhosis and inflammatory bowel disease, the increasing incidence of inflammatory bowel disease and increasing detection of primary biliary cirrhosis occurring separately and the lack of reports of concomitant occurrence in patients with Crohn's disease make it difficult to ascribe an association between these two entities.

H. Drugs

Patients having inflammatory bowel disease frequently take a variety of medications. Drugs that are used in the treatment of inflammatory bowel disease are known to cause a large spectrum of hepatic disorders, ranging from mild abnormalities in serum liver function tests to acute and chronic inflammatory and cholestatic liver disease. One of the most commonly used drugs, sulfasalazine, is also one of the most studied in this regard. Liver injury from this agent is well documented and may result in a spectrum of hepatotoxicity including acute hepatitis, cholestasis, granulomatous hepatitis, and a syndrome comprised of abnormal serum liver chemistries that reflect both parenchymal inflammation and cholestasis (22,31,37–41).

However, despite the known hepatotoxicity of sulfasalazine and other drugs, most large series that have considered drugs as a possible cause of liver disease have not found them to be a cause of significant or frequent liver disease in inflammatory bowel disease. These conclusions have been based on the lack of occurrence of drug-associated liver disease, the lack of a relationship between liver disease and the time of drug ingestion, or an equal incidence of liver disease and severity in subjects either taking or not taking these medications during specific studies (3–6,8). Although such drugs can cause liver disease in any one patient, the incidence of drug-related liver disease in inflammatory bowel disease has not been regarded as of great significance in a number of studies, some involving large numbers of patients with inflammatory bowel disease (3–6,8).

I. Hepatic Abscess

Hepatic abscess is rare in Crohn's disease. Occasional case reports have been reviewed by Sparberg et al. (42). With antibiotic therapy, the incidence of pyogenic liver abscess is rare (43). More recent reviews have supported the increasing rarity of this entity with the widespread use of antibiotics (44). Only one case in a study of 700 patients with inflammatory bowel disease was reported by Greenstein (8). Crass reviewed 10 cases and found that the occurrence of hepatic abscess was associated with additional extrahepatic inflammatory conditions, such as fistulas, multiple mesenteric abscesses, and pylephlebitis (45). Using CT scan or abdominal ultrasonography, such a lesion is suggested when a focal liver lesion is detected in the presence of other abdominal inflammatory processes, such as those already discussed. The use of nuclear scans may be of benefit in the differentiation of such a process from other entities such as malignancy (44).

J. Thrombosis of the Portal Vein

Thrombosis of the portal vein has been described in patients with inflammatory bowel disease (17,22,46). In these reports, four patients had Crohn's disease and one had ulcerative colitis. One patient had associated pancreatitis, which may have been the causative factor, and hepatic infarct was described in two of the patients with Crohn's colitis.

K. Parenteral Nutrition–Related Liver Disease

Total parenteral nutrition (TPN) is frequently used in the therapy of inflammatory bowel disease (47). However, TPN is associated with abnormalities of liver function tests and a variety of hepatic disorders including fatty infiltration of the liver and cholestatsis (48–51). A study by Bengoa et al. considered the effects of TPN on the liver in patients with inflammatory bowel disease, including ulcerative colitis and Crohn's disease (47). Abnormal serum liver function tests frequently occurred in patients with Crohn's disease receiving total parenteral nutrition, but, in none of the 69 such patients did symptoms of liver disease develop, and liver biopsies of those patients with severe liver chemical abnormalities failed to demonstrate severe or progressive liver disease, demonstrating abnormalities "indistinguishable from mild abnormalities reported in patients with Crohn's disease of ulcerative colitis not on TPN" (47). When the TPN was discontinued, liver chemistry levels returned to normal, suggesting no permanent adverse effects of this therapy on the liver (47). Because patients without inflammatory bowel disease were not included in this study, no direct comment can be made as to whether patients with Crohn's disease have an increased incidence of hepatic disorders due to parenteral nutrition compared with individuals without inflammatory bowel disease. However, they do develop the types of liver disease typically associated with parenteral hyperalimentation in the absence of inflammatory bowel disease (48–51). It appears that when the course of TPN is short, the liver disease is typically reversible and not progressive. Under such circumstances, that is, short courses of TPN, it seems unnecessary to discontinue TPN despite the development of sometimes severely abnormal liver function tests in patients with inflammatory bowel disease (47).

L. Miscellaneous Hepatic Lesions

A variety of liver lesions have been described in patients with inflammatory bowel disease including Crohn's disease. These include hepatoma and sarcoidosis (52,53). It is unlikely that a true association exists between these liver disease, and inflammatory bowel disease.

Undoubtedly, there will be reports of additional diseases of the liver in such patients, despite any logical evidence of an etiological association with Crohn's disease.

II. DISEASES OF THE BILIARY TRACT

A. Gallstones

The incidence of cholelithiasis is increased in Crohn's disease (8,10,12,13,15–18). The reported incidence of gallstones in these patients ranges from 13% to 34% compared with a 10% to 15% incidence in the general population (8,10,18,19). The gallstones occur in patients with Crohn's ileitis, ileal resection, or intestinal bypass (10,18,19). The incidence of cholelithiasis is significantly increased in patients with regional enteritis, specifically distal ileitis, compared with either ulcerative colitis or Crohn's colitis (8,10). The most sensitive test for cholelithiasis is abdominal ultrasonography (18). Because many patients with gallstones are asymptomatic, the studies with the highest incidences of gallstones in such patients were those in which this entity was specifically sought by sonography regardless of the presence of symptoms (18,54).

The origin of this increased incidence of cholelithiasis in patients with Crohn's disease of the ileum has been well studied (8,10,54,55). The development of gallstones appears to be related to the extent of ileal disease or dysfunction, including length of diseased ileum, and duration of the ileal disease (10,17,19). Inflammation or absence of the terminal ileum has been demonstrated to result in malabsorption of bile salts, ultimately leading to a contraction or depletion of the bile salt pool (55–57). Cholesterol is normally rendered soluble by incorporation into lecithin liquid crystals, which are broken down into soluble aggregates known as mixed micelles (58–62). In states of relative deficiencies of bile salts, that is, lithogenic bile, cholesterol may precipitate and gallstone calculi may form. This theory is usually invoked to account for the increased incidence of gallstones in patients with either ileal dysfunction or resection as related to Crohn's disease (8,19). However, this theory may not be the sole reason for the formation of gallstones in such patients. Additional mechanisms may be present and may account for the observation that increased cholesterol saturation of bile is found more commonly than stone formation in patients after ileal resection (18). Furthermore, most gallstones in such patients are not purely cholesterol but contain enough pigment to be radiopaque (18). Several additional mechanisms have been suggested that may contribute to the role of secretion of lithogenic bile in the formation of gallstones (56–59). Thus the exact role of ileal dysfunction in the formation of gallstones in patients with Crohn's ileitis remains to be fully elucidated.

Because cholelithiasis occurs more frequently in patients with Crohn's disease, the presence of this disease should be considered in any patient having abdominal pain or signs and symptoms of biliary tract disease. Although ultrasonography is the most sensitive diagnostic test for the detection of gallstones, a careful review should be made of any other radiological procedures previously performed, including abdominal flat plate and CT scan of the abdomen, that may also reveal the presence of cholelithiasis.

B. Primary Sclerosing Cholangitis

Primary sclerosing cholangitis was first described by Delbet in 1924 (63). Until recently, it was regarded as a rare disease, with fewer than 100 cases reported in the English language literature by 1980 (12). However, with more frequent monitoring of liver enzyme tests and the use of endoscopic retrograde or percutaneous transhepatic cholangiography, the syndrome is being recognized with increasing frequency (11,18). Primary sclerosing cholangitis is a slowly progressive disease characterized by inflammatory, obliterative changes and fibrosis of the extrahepatic bile ducts, often associated with the same involvement of the intrahepatic bile ducts (11). The term "primary" is used to distinguish this process from cholangitis, which may occur secondary to choledocholithiasis, prior biliary surgery, or congenital anomalies of the biliary tree (18), because up to 70% of all patients with primary sclerosing cholangitis have inflammatory bowel diseases at some time in their life (11). Conversely, up to 4% of all patients with inflammatory bowel disease develop primary sclerosing cholangitis (12). Although previously believed to be associated only with ulcerative colitis, primary sclerosing cholangitis may also develop in up to approximately 10% of patients with Crohn's disease; this figure may represent an unusually strong association of the two entities (11,12,64). In one study, all three cases of primary sclerosing cholangitis occurred in individuals with Crohn's disease, usually with extensive colitis (64). In general, however, symptoms of bowel disease are modest, and the inflammatory bowel disease is usually present at the time of diagnosis of cholangitis, that is, preceding the development of biliary disease. However, primary sclerosing cholangitis can occur before the bowel disease becomes clinically evident, when it is quiescent, or, in some cases, after the affected bowel has been removed surgically, sometimes years later (12,18).

Sclerosing cholangitis is usually a disease of young men, occurring in the third to fifth decade of life (11,23). The clinical presentation is usually insidious, with gradual development of fatigue, jaundice, and pruritus, associated with intermittent episodes of abdominal pain and fever (11,18). The experience from the Mayo Clinic is that ascending bacterial cholangitis is rare unless previous biliary reconstructive surgery was performed or unless the biliary tract has been manipulated to obtain a cholangiogram or to introduce a stent into a strictured area (11,23). Liver function tests demonstrate a cholestatic profile, with the serum alkaline phosphatase, despite fluctuations, being always abnormal and serological tests for viral hepatitis being negative (11,23). Abnormalities in liver function tests ultimately lead to evaluation by cholangiography, which is essential for the diagnosis. The cholangiogram characteristically reveals a beaded contour of the extrahepatic, and sometimes intrahepatic bile ducts, representing areas of stricture and dilation of the biliary tree. A typical cholangiogram is shown in Figure 5. The course of the disease is variable and slowly progressive, ultimately developing into biliary cirrhosis and death from complications of liver failure and portal hypertension in some individuals. In addition, development of bile duct carcinoma is a rare complication of this entity (12,18,25,65,66).

The cause of primary sclerosing cholangitis is unknown. The erratic relationship to the time of active bowel disease makes a directly causal relationship unlikely. However, because of some reports, increased associations with certain human leukocyte antigen (HLA) types such as HLA-B8 and HLA-DR3, an underlying immune cause has been considered (12). In addition, an association of primary sclerosing cholangitis with "autoimmune" diseases such as thyroiditis, hypothyroidism, and chronic active hepatitis has also been described, although autoantibodies, such as antimitochondrial antibody or antinuclear antibody have been either negative or only minimally elevated (12,23). Because histopathological findings of chronic active hepatitis may be seen with primary sclerosing cholangitis, it is probably wise not to attribute these two diagnoses to the same patient when both are identified (12). Another abnormality that has received attention is the elevations in serum copper levels seen in primary sclerosing cholangitis. However, because copper is mainly excreted in the bile, these elevations have also been identified in other cholestatic diseases such as primary biliary cirrhosis and Wilson's disease, and it is likely that the

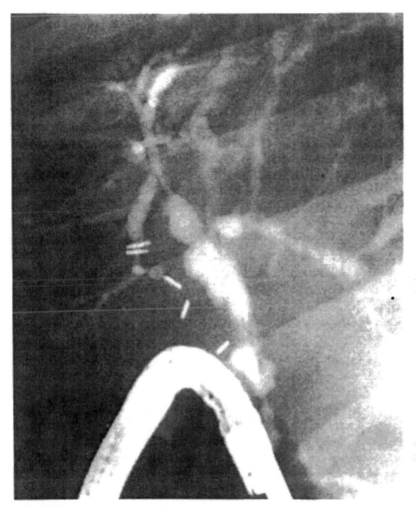

FIG. 5 Diffuse extrahepatic and intrahepatic disease consistent with sclerosing cholangitis as demonstrated by endoscopic cholangiography. (From Siegel JH. Endoscopic Retrograde Cholangiopancreatography. Technique, Diagnosis and Therapy. New York: Raven Press, 1991, with permission.)

elevations of serum copper reported in primary sclerosing cholangitis represent a secondary phenomenon rather than a cause of this disease (23).

The relationship between primary sclerosing cholangitis and pericholangitis is controversial. Some researchers prefer to regard these diseases as separate entities, whereas others have attempted to consider, as discussed previously, both primary sclerosing cholangitis and pericholangitis as parts of a spectrum of cholestatic liver disease (12,23,24). In such a scheme, pericholangitis represents the small bile duct manifestations of primary sclerosing cholangitis and is called by these authors "small bile duct sclerosing cholangitis" with specific stages leading to biliary cirrhosis (23,24). Most patients with pericholangitis do show primary sclerosing cholangitis (12). However, the reverse is often not true; whereas liver biopsies of patients with primary sclerosing cholangitis frequently show nonspecific changes, only 25% of such individuals demonstrate histopathological changes consistent with pericholangitis by liver biopsy. In addition, some of these liver biopsies also contain the characteristics of chronic active hepatitis. Despite the finding of biliary cirrhosis in liver biopsies of another 30% of such patients with primary sclerosing cholangitis, this relationship between primary sclerosing cholangitis and pericholangitis is not universally accepted (12,18).

Treatment of primary sclerosing cholangitis is controversial. As discussed, although there are some reports of improvement with surgical removal of disease bowel, most series report no definitive improvement after such surgery and sometimes report the development of primary sclerosing cholangitis even years after such surgery has been performed (11,12,18,23). A variety of drugs such as corticosteroids, penicillamine, and cyclosporine have been used for therapy, and mechanical relief of obstructed areas have been undertaken by surgical, radiological, or endoscopic means, without significant success, and, in some cases, with increased occurrence of ascending bacterial cholangitis (11,12,23). Therefore, there is no proven curative treatment for primary sclerosing cholangitis, and treatment is generally reserved for patients in whom symptomatic complications of the disease develop (11,23). This conservative approach is particularly important because many of these patients are young and may be candidates for liver transplantation, which would be made more difficult by previous biliary or abdominal surgery.

C. Cholangiocarcinoma

The association between biliary tract carcinoma and ulcerative colitis was first described by Parker and Kendall in 1954 (67). Since then, the incidence of this tumor in such patients has been estimated between 0.4% and 1.4% (18). They occur at least 10-fold more frequently, usually in the absence of cholelithiasis, and, on average, 20 to 30 years earlier than in patients without inflammatory bowel disease (15). They also usually occur in the presence of primary sclerosing cholangitis, which often precedes the development of this tumor by years (12,18). Initially, cholangiocarcinomas were thought to be associated only with ulcerative colitis, but the occurrence of such tumors in individuals with Crohn's disease has been well described (9,13,66).

The most common clinical presentation is general malaise, pain in the right upper quadrant of the abdomen, fever, and progressive jaundice, although the onset may be insidious, with symptoms only referable to the bowel (13,17,18). As with primary sclerosing cholangitis, development of tumor may precede the development of inflammatory bowel disease, or occur in absence of active disease, even after bowel resection; it also occurs predominantly in men (13,18). The tumor is usually an adenocarcinoma and is often multicentric in origin. Most tumors involve the larger extrahepatic ducts or bifurcation of the intrahepatic ducts (18). The diagnosis is usually made by cholangiography, although this is sometimes difficult to interpret because of the irregular contours of underlying sclerosing cholangitis. Use of biliary brush cytology or demonstration of a mass by abdominal CT scan can aid in the diagnostic accuracy (12,18). Use of endoscopic stenting may prolong life, but the overall prognosis is poor to dismal (13,17).

III. EVALUATION OF HEPATOBILIARY DISEASE IN CROHN'S DISEASE

As discussed earlier, the finding of liver disease in Crohn's disease varies widely with the method used to screen such patients. In general, all patients with Crohn's disease should have periodic monitoring of serum liver function tests, even in the absence of signs or symptoms referable to the hepatobiliary system, such as pain in the right upper quadrant of the abdomen or abdominal tenderness in this area, nausea, vomiting, or jaundice. The persistence of such biochemical abnormalities requires further investigation with liver biopsy, radiological visualization of the liver and biliary tree and cholangiography, which is commonly performed endoscopically. Ultrasonography and abdominal CT scan are the most widely used techniques for radiological visualization. In general, ultrasonography is the most cost-efficient of the two tests and has the advantage of greater sensitivity for detection of cholesterol gallstones and, perhaps, diffusely abnormal parenchymal liver disease, which is reflected by abnormalities in echogenicity of the liver. Abdominal CT scan may be more sensitive in the detection of focal lesions of the liver, particularly vascular lesions. An ultrasound determination of "fatty liver" is actually a statement about abnormal hepatic echogenicity and may not necessarily be reflected histologically by hepatic steatosis but by other diffusely infiltrative abnormalities of the hepatic parenchyma. Thus, when abnormalities in liver function tests or radiological testing are noted, other diseases of the liver must be excluded, especially because they may coexist with Crohn's disease. When hepatic steatosis is demonstrated by hepatic imaging, the presence of other hepatic diseases that may be associated with this process, such as hepatitis C, or, in any young person, Wilson's disease, as well as other nonsteatotic diseases of the liver, must be considered. Even in the absence of hepatic steatosis, patients must be evaluated for specific diseases of the liver, including those not commonly associated with Crohn's disease, which may require specific treatment.

IV.   THERAPY OF THE PATIENT
WITH LIVER DISEASE IN CROHN'S DISEASE

Therapy of the patient with hepatobiliary disease having Crohn's disease depends on the specific hepatic process present. In some instances, no specific therapy has been found to be beneficial. In addition, therapy of the underlying inflammatory bowel disease does not have any consistent effect on the concomitant liver disease. Hepatobiliary disorders occur before, during, and after the occurrence of clinically active inflammatory bowel disease, and, in many cases, there is no correlation between the severity of the two processes. In some cases, such hepatobiliary disease has occurred even after involved bowel has been surgically removed. Because of these observations, the importance of excluding other diseases of the hepatobiliary system, including those not commonly associated with Crohn's disease, some of which may respond to specific medical therapy, cannot be overstated. The role of liver transplantation in individuals with severe liver disease and inflammatory bowel disease is intriguing, and the decision to have such patients undergo hepatic transplantation must be made individually. Many of the immunomodulatory agents used in the patient with liver transplantation, most notably cyclosporin, are being applied in therapy of inflammatory bowel disease.

V.   SUMMARY

With few exceptions, disorders of the hepatobiliary system complicating Crohn's disease appear to be similar in nature and incidence to those previously described in patients with ulcerative colitis. The actual incidence of such disorders varies widely with the method used for screening such patients for potential liver disease and indications used for liver biopsy. When routine screening with serum liver function tests is used, the incidence of significant liver disease in most series is approximately 5%. In general, the presence of hepatobiliary disorders in individuals with Crohn's disease does not correlate with the severity or timing of activity of the Crohn's disease. Therefore, therapy of underlying bowel disease has an inconsistent effect on activity of the liver disease. This further emphasizes the need to fully elucidate the nature of the hepatic disorder and to exclude the presence of other types of liver diseases not commonly associated with Crohn's disease, which may respond to specific therapies. In addition, patients with persistently abnormal liver function tests should undergo further evaluation with radiological visualization of the liver and biliary tract as well as with liver biopsy.

REFERENCES

1. Snavely JR. Diarrhea and abdominal tenderness. Bull Tulane Med Fac 1946; 6:22–25.
2. Eade MN. Liver disease in ulcerative colitis. I. Analysis of operative liver biopsy in 138 consecutive patients having colectomy. Ann Intern Med 1970; 72:475–487.
3. Eade MN, Cooke WT, Williams JA. Liver disease in Crohn's disease. A study of 100 consecutive patients. Scand J Gastroenterol 1971; 6:199–204.
4. Eade MN, Cooke WT, Brooke BN, Thompson H. Liver disease in Crohn's colitis. A study of 21 consecutive patients having colectomy. Ann Intern Med 1971; 74:518–521.
5. Dordal E, Glagov S, Kirsner JB. Hepatic lesions in chronic inflammatory bowel disease. I. Clinical correlations with liver biopsy diagnosis in 103 patients. Gastroenterology 1967; 52:239–253.
6. Perrett AD, Higgins G, Johnston HH, Massarella GR, Truelove SC, Wright R. The liver in Crohn's disease. Q J Med 1971; 158:187–209.
7. Rankin GB, Watts H, Melnyk CS, Kelley ML Jr. National Cooperative Crohn's Disease Study: extraintestinal manifestations and perianal complications. Gastroenterology 1979; 77:914–920.
8. Greenstein AJ, Janowitz HD, Sachar DB. The extra-intestinal complications of Crohn's disease and ulcerative colitis: a study of 700 patients. Medicine 1976; 55:401–412.
9. Present DH. Extraintestinal manifestations. Mt Sinai J Med 1983; 50:126–132.
10. Baker AL, Kaplan MM, Norton RA, Patterson JF. Gallstones in inflammatory bowel disease. Dig Dis 1974; 19:109–112.
11. Wiesner RH, LaRusso NF. Clinicopathologic features of the syndrome of primary sclerosing cholangitis. Gastroeneterology 1980; 79:200–206.
12. Schrumpf E, Fausa O, Elgjo K, Kolmannskog F. Hepatobiliary complications of inflammatory bowel disease. Semin Liver Dis 1988; 8:201–209.
13. Rankin GB. Extraintestinal and systemic manifestations of inflammatory bowel disease. Med Clin North Am 1990; 74:39–50.
14. Kleckner MS Jr. The liver in regional enteritis. Gastroenterology 1956; 30:415–420.
15. Danzi JT. Extraintestinal manifestations of idiopathic inflammatory bowel disease. Arch Intern Med 1988; 148:297–302.
16. Halvorsen RA. CT appearance of focal fatty infiltration of the liver. Am J Radiol 1982; 139:277–281.
17. Christophi C, Hughes ER. Hepatobiliary disorders in inflammatory bowel disease. Surg Gynecol Obstet 1985; 160:187–193.
18. Williams SM, Harned RK. Hepatobiliary complications of inflammatory bowel disease. Radiol Clin North Am 1987; 25:175–188.
19. Cohen S, Kaplan M, Gottlieb L, Patterson J. Liver disease and gallstones in regional enteritis. Gastroenterol 1971; 60:237–245.

20. Mistilis SP. Pericholangitis and ulcerative colitis. I. Pathology, etiology and pathogenesis. Ann Int Med 1965; 63:1–16.
21. Mistilis SP, Skyring AP, Gouston SJM. Pericholangitis and ulcerative colitis. II. Clinical aspects. Ann Intern Med 1965; 63:17–26.
22. Stauffer MH, Sauer WG, Dearing WH, Baggenstoss AH. The spectrum of cholestatic liver disease. JAMA 1965; 191:829–837.
23. LaRusso NF, Wiesner RH, Ludwig J, MacCarty RL. Primary sclerosing cholangitis. N Engl J Med 1984; 310:899–903.
24. Wee A, Ludwig, J. Pericholangitis in chronic ulcerative colitis: primary sclerosing cholangitis of the small bile ducts. Ann Intern Med 1985; 102:581–587.
25. Wee A, Ludwig J, Coffrey RJ Jr, LaRusso NF, Wiesner RH. Hepatobiliary carcinoma associated with primary sclerosing cholangitis and chronic ulcerative colitis. Hum Pathol 1985; 16:719–726.
26. Fausa O, Nygaard K, Elgjo K. Amyloidosis and Crohn's disease. Scand J Gastroeneterol 1977; 12:657–662.
27. Mir-Madjlessi SH, Brown CH, Hawk WA. Amyloidosis associated with Crohn's disease. Am J Gastroenterol 1977; 58:563–577.
28. Fitchen JH. Amyloidosis and granulomatous ileocolitis. Regression after surgical removal of the involved bowel. N Engl J Med 1975; 292:352–353.
29. Mayer L, Janowitz HD. Extra-intestianl manifestations of ulcerative colitis including reference to Crohn's disease. In: Allan RN, Keighley, MRB, Alexander-Williams J, eds. Inflammatory Bowel Disease. London, Churchill Livingstone, 1983.
30. Maurer LH, Hughes RW Jr, Folley JH, Mosenthal WT. Granulomatous hepatitis associated with regional enteritis. Gastroenterology 1967; 53:301–305.
31. Peppercorn MA. Sulfasalazine. Pharmacology, clinical use, toxicity and related new drug development. Ann Intern Med 1984; 3:377–386.
32. Soloway RD, Summerskill WHJ, Baggenstoss AH. Clinical, biochemical, and histological remission of severe chronic active liver disease: a controlled study of treatment and early prognosis. Gastroenterology 1972; 63:820–833.
33. Holdsworth CD, Hall EW, Dawson AM, Sherlock S. Ulcerative colitis in chronic liver disease. Q J Med 1965; 34:211–216.
34. Kato Y, Morimoto H, Unoura M. Primary biliary cirrhosis and chronic pancreatitis in a patient with ulcerative colitis. J Clin Gastroenterol 1985; 7:425–427.
35. Bush A, Mitchison H, Walt R, Baron JH, Boylston AW, Summerfield JA. Primary biliary cirrhosis and ulcerative colitis. Gastroenterology 1987; 92:2009–2013.
36. Sherlock S, Dooley J. Diseases of the Liver and Biliary System. 9th ed. Oxford: Blackwell Scientific, 1993.
37. Callen JP, Soderstrom RM. Granulomatous hepatitis associated with salicylazosulfapyridine therapy. South Med J 1978; 71:1159–1160.
38. Kanner RS, Tedesco FJ, Kalser MH. Azulfidine (sulfasalazine)-induced hepatic injury. Am J Dig Dis 1978; 23:956–9581.
39. Jacobs E, Paulet P, Rahier J. Hypersensitivity reaction to sulfasalazine—another case (letter). Gastroenterology 1978; 75:1193.
40. Namias A, Bhalotra R, Donowitz M. Reversible sulfasalazine-induced granulomatous hepatitis. J Clin Gastroenterol 1981; 3:191–195.
41. Gulley RM, Mirza A, Kelly CE. Hepatotoxicity of salicylazosulfapyridine and review of the literature. Am J Gastroenterol 1979; 72:561–564.
42. Sparberg M, Gottschalk A, Kirsner JB. Gastroenterology 1965; 49:548–551.
43. Schiff L. Diseases of the Liver. 2d ed. Philadelphia: JB Lippincott, 1963.
44. Saverymutta SH, Keshavarzian A, Gibson R, Chadwick VS, Hodgson HJF. Hepatic abscess associated with Crohn's disease detected by [111]Indium leukocyte scanning. J Clin Gastroenterol 1985; 7:273–276.

45. Crass JR. Liver abscesses as a complication of regional enteritis: interventional considerations. Am J Gastroenterol 1983; 78:747–749.

46. Chapin LE, Scudmore HH, Baggeenstoss AH, Bargen JA. Regional enteritis associated with visceral changes. Gastroenterology 1956; 30:404–415.

47. Bengoa JM, Hanauer SB, Sitrin MD, Baker AL, Rosenberg IH. Pattern and prognosis of liver function test abnormalities during parenteral nutrition in inflammatory bowel disease. Hepatology 1985; 5:79–84.

48. Grant JP, Cox CE, Kleinman LM, Maher MM, Pittman MA. Serum hepatic enzyme and bilirubin elevations during parenteral nutrition. Surg Gynecol Obstet 1977; 145:573–580.

49. Lindor KD, Fleming CR, Abrams A, Hirschkorn MA. Liver function values in adults receiving total parenteral nutrition. JAMA 1979; 241:2398–2400.

50. Rodgers BM, Hollenbeck JI, Donnelly WH, Talbert JL. Intrahepatic cholestasis with parenteral nutrition. Am J Surg 1976; 131:149–154.

51. Postuma R, Trevenen CL. Liver disease in infants receiving total parenteral nutrition. Pediatrics 1979; 63:110–115.

52. Smith PM. Hepatoma associated with ulcerative colitis. Dis Colon Rectum 1974; 17:554–556.

53. Dew MJ, Thompson H, Allan, RN. The spectrum of hepatic dysfunction in inflammatory bowel disease. Q J Med 1979; 48:113–121.

54. Whorwell PJ, Hawkins R, Dewbury K, Wright R. Ultrasound survey of gallstones and other hepatobiliary disorders in patients with Crohn's disease. Dig Dis Sci 1984; 29:930–933.

55. Abaurre R, Gordon SG, Mann JG, Kern F Jr. Fasting bile salt pool size and composition after ileal resection. Gastroenterology 1969; 57:679–688.

56. Heaton KW, Read AE. Gallstones in patients with disorders of the terminal ileum and disturbed bile salt metabolism. BMJ 1969; 3:494–496.

57. Pitt HA, Lewinski MA, Muller EL, Porter-Fink V, DenBesten L. Ileal resection induced gallstones. Surgery 1984; 96:154–160.

58. Small DM. Current concepts: gallstones. N Engl J Med 1968; 279:588–593.

59. Admirand WH, Small DM. The physicochemical basis of cholesterol gallstone formation in man. J Clin Invest 1968; 47:1043–1052.

60. Dowling RH, Bell GD, White J. Lithogenic bile in patients with ileal dysfunction. Gut 1972; 13:415–420.

61. Hill GL, Mair WSJ, Goligher JC. Gallstones after ileostomy and ileal resection. Gut 1975; 16:932–936.

62. Vlahcevic ZR, Bell CC, Buhac I, Farrar JT, Swell L. Diminished bile acid and pool size in patients with gallstones. Gastroenterology 1970; 59:165–173.

63. Delbet P. Retrecissement du choedoque cholecystoduodenostomie. Bull Mem Soc Chir Paris 1924; 50:1144–1146.

64. Aadland E, Schrumppf E, Fausa O, Elgjo K, Heilo A, Aakhus T, Gjone E. Primary sclerosing cholangitis: a long-term follow-up study. Scand J Gastroenterol 1987; 22:655–664.

65. Akwari OE, Van Heerden JA, Foulk WT, Baggenstoss AH. Cancer of the bile ducts associated with ulcerative colitis. Ann Surg 1975; 181:303–309.

66. Berman MD, Falchuck KR, Trey C. Carcinoma of the biliary tree complicating Crohn's disease. Dig Dis Sci 1980; 25:795–797.

67. Parker RJF, Kendall EJC. The liver in ulcerative colitis. BMJ 1954; 2:1030–1032.

COMMENTARY

Nicholas F. LaRusso   *Mayo Clinic, Rochester, Minnesota*

Lieberman has written a thorough and comprehensive, well-referenced chapter on the association of liver and inflammatory bowel disease (IBD) with a particular emphasis on Crohn's disease. To complement this excellent review, I submit several points based heavily on the huge experience at the Mayo Clinic with both inflammatory bowel disease and chronic liver disease. First, a few general concepts are necessary to initiate this commentary: (a) hepatobiliary abnormalities are more frequent in patients with IBD than in the general population, (b) the frequency of association of hepatobiliary abnormalities with chronic ulcerative colitis and Crohn's disease is variable; however, in our experience, hepatobiliary abnormalities are much more common in association with chronic ulcerative colitis than with Crohn's disease, and (c) associated "hepatobiliary abnormalities" are not synonymous with clinical hepatobiliary disease. As is pointed out by Lieberman, the list of abnormalities found on liver biopsy in patients with IBD is long; frequently, these abnormalities are unassociated with symptoms or signs of liver disease. Nevertheless, there are at least four clinically significant hepatobiliary diseases associated with IBD; these include, in order of importance, primary sclerosing cholangitis (PSC), which is unquestionably the most frequent and clinically important hepatobiliary disease associated with IBD, adenocarcinoma of the bile ducts, idiopathic or autoimmune chronic active hepatitis, and cholelithiasis. The term "pericholangitis" is a descriptive morphological term and is not, in itself, a disease entity. This morphological abnormality on liver biopsy can be found in association with IBD, PSC (with or without associated IBD), primary biliary cirrhosis, extrahepatic obstruction, and graft versus host disease. In the judgement of the Mayo Clinic group, when the morphological lesion of pericholangitis is found in association with IBD, it represents the hepatic histological manifestation of PSC.

Although the issue is controversial, it is reasonable to address the relationship of hepatobiliary disease and IBD by asking the question, "Does the inflammatory bowel disease cause the underlying hepatobiliary disease?" Reasons for answering this question "yes" include historical perspectives in which hepatobiliary abnormalities were considered "extracolonic manifestations" of IBD, experimental data in which animal models of colitis may have associated hepatobiliary tract lesions, and clinical data of two types: (a) most patients with selective types of hepatobiliary diseases (e.g., PSC) have IBD and (b) data from our institution support the conclusion that IBD is an independent risk factor for survival of patients with PSC. Evidence for a "no" answer falls under two general categories: clinical and theoretical. Clinical evidence against the relationship includes the fact that not all patients with the most common form of liver disease seen in association with IBD (i.e., PSC) have associated IBD. As was pointed out by Lieberman and originally suggested by work from the Mayo Clinic, patients can develop hepatobiliary disorders including PSC, after proctocolectomy for chronic ulcerative colitis. Furthermore, proctocolectomy, at least in a relatively large retrospective study from our institution, did not affect the progression of the underlying hepatobiliary disease. In addition, cholangiograms and liver biopsies do not appear to be different in patients with PSC with or without associated IBD. At a theoretical level, hypotheses account for association without causation. The question could reasonably be reversed as "Is inflammatory bowel disease an extrahepatic manifestation of primary sclerosing cholangitis?" Although the answer to this question, despite the preceding analysis, remains uncertain, the opinion of my group is that, even though the two diseases are related and the relationship remains obscure, the clarification of this relationship will almost certainly have pathogenic relevance for both entities. Nevertheless, the two diseases appear to progress independently and thus should be dealt with, in most circumstances, as independent entities. The IBD, as seen in association with a variety of hepatobiliary disorders, most importantly PSC, is usually mild, although recent data have raised the possibility that the existence of PSC may be an independent risk factor for the development of adenocarcinoma of the colon in patients with chronic ulcerative colitis.

With regard to the other clinically significant entities (cholelithiasis, adenocarcinoma of the bile duct, and chronic active hepatitis) seen in association with inflammatory bowel disease, I agree with Lieberman that cholelithiasis is particularly frequent in Crohn's disease for the reasons outlined in his chapter. These gallstones are usually cholesterol in nature and their treatment should generally be no different from the treatment of this condition in patients without IBD. Both chronic persistent and chronic active hepatitis are seen in association with IBD. Idiopathic or autoimmune varieties of chronic hepatitis can be seen in association with chronic ulcerative colitis and, perhaps most importantly, may represent an overlap syndrome between chronic active hepatitis and PSC. In my practice, patients who have biochemical evidence of chronic hepatitis in association with IBD usually have a cholangiogram, particularly if they are being considered for liver transplantation (when it is critically important to know whether or not the extrahepatic duct may be involved as a manifestation of sclerosing cholangitis). I agree with Lieberman that adenocarcinoma of the bile duct is a devastating and generally fatal disorder. However, the development of adenocarcinoma in association with IBD is virtually always a manifestation of underlying PSC. I do not believe that IBD unaccompanied by PSC predisposes the patient to the development of adenocarcinoma of the bile duct.

In conclusion, liver test abnormalities, which are commonly found in association with both types of IBD, in my experience tend to occur more commonly in chronic ulcerative colitis and are not always a manifestation of clinically important, hepatobiliary disorders. PSC is the most common and clinically important hepatobiliary disorder found in association with IBD, especially chronic ulcerative colitis. I consider these disorders associated and not causally related, although common pathogenetic mechanisms are likely involved.

28
Malignancy in Crohn's Disease

Paul M. Choi   *UCLA School of Medicine, Los Angeles, California*

Since the initial description of Crohn's disease in 1932, much has been learned about the natural history of this complex disease (1). In 1948, Warren and Sommers reported the first case of colorectal carcinoma associated with Crohn's disease (2). Since that time, the risk of developing cancer in Crohn's disease has become better appreciated. In particular, recent studies suggest that the risk of developing colorectal cancer in patients with Crohn's disease may be significantly elevated (3–8). In addition, these studies indicate that risk factors for developing colorectal cancer in Crohn's disease may be similar to that seen in ulcerative colitis (9). For example, there appears to be an important relationship between the risk of developing colorectal cancer and the duration of disease and extent of colonic involvement. Other features including the young age at cancer development, presence of dysplasia, and various other pathological features have also been found to be nearly identical to those found in patients with ulcerative colitis. Patients with Crohn's disease also appear to be at risk for development of small bowel cancer, particularly in patients with small bowel disease of long duration (10). There may also be an association between Crohn's disease and the risk of development of cholangiocarcinoma (11). The risk of other malignancies developing in Crohn's disease does not appear to be significantly elevated (7). With the better understanding of the risk and natural history of malignancies in Crohn's disease, more effective cancer prevention strategies and, thereby, an improved overall prognosis for affected patients may become possible.

I. CARCINOGENESIS

The exact cause of the increased risk of developing carcinoma in patients with inflammatory bowel disease is not known. Various factors that have been implicated include chronic inflammation, mucosal immunodeficiency, and genetic and dietary factors. Among them, chronic inflammation appears to have the most supporting evidence. The mechanism of the increased risk of cancer associated with chronic inflammation may be related to the local release of prostaglandins, nitrosamine, growth factors, and superoxide radicals because they are thought to be important in carcinogenesis (12–14). In addition, depletion of epithelial stem cells from the continuous proliferative response to chronic inflammation and associated tissue injury has been proposed as an alternative explanation for the frequent development of cancer associated with chronic inflammation (15).

There are many examples of malignancies thought to be causally related to chronic inflammation. They include malignancies in such diverse organ systems as dermatologic, genitourinary, ophthalmic, pulmonary, lymphoreticular, and gastrointestinal systems (14). For instance, malignancies in the gastrointestinal tract that are thought to be specifically associated with chronic inflammation include adenocarcinoma occurring in Barrett's esophagus from reflux esophagitis, gastric cancer associated with atrophic gastritis, gallbladder cancer related to chronic cholecystitis and cholelithiasis, cholangiocarcinoma associated with primary sclerosing cholangitis and Clonorchisis sinesis, and colorectal cancer related to inflammatory bowel disease. The striking similarity of carcinomas found in ulcerative colitis and Crohn's disease, two distinct chronic inflammatory conditions of the bowel, provides additional supporting evidence for the importance of chronic inflammation in carcinogenesis (9). A common underlying carcinogenic mechanism, such as the underlying chronic inflammation shared by both diseases, is much more likely to be the initiating cause rather than an undefined carcinogenic mechanism unique to either disease.

Recent studies on experimental colitis in animal models provide further evidence that chronic inflammation is critical in the development of colorectal cancer. In one study, colorectal cancer was shown to develop much more frequently in rats after an induction of chronic inflammation (16). Chalifoux and Bronson observed that spontaneous colitis of cotton top tamarins is associated with frequent development of colorectal cancer. They noted that these cancers "never occurred in the absence of diffuse colitis" and its incidence was dependent on the duration of colitis. Several researchers induced experimental colitis in various animal species with dextran sulfate sodium, an agent without known intrinsic carcinogenic property (18,19). Neoplastic changes, including precancerous dysplasia and carcinoma were found to develop in the colon of these animals after an induction of chronic colitis. Other noncarcinogenic irritants (amylopectin, capisacin, and carrageenan) can also induce nonspecific colonic inflammation as well as the neoplasm of the colon (20,21). These results suggest that it is the resultant chronic inflammation and not the specific carcinogenic effect of these compounds that are important in the development of cancer.

Further evidence supporting the importance of chronic inflammation in colon carcinogenesis comes from studies examining the effect of anti-inflammatory agents in affecting the development of colorectal cancer. For example, a variety of nonsteroidal anti-inflammatory agents, including aspirin, indomethacin, sulindac, and piroxicam, has been found to inhibit the growth of tumor in the colon of rodents treated with carcinogens. In addition, this effect appears to be dose related and reversible upon discontinuation of medications (22–25). Similarly, studies in humans have suggested that these anti-inflammatory agents can help regress neoplastic polyps in patients with familial polyposis (26,27). Epidemiological studies have provided supporting evidence that the risk of developing colorectal cancer may be reduced by a regular use of these medications (28,29). In addition, findings from recent studies in patients with ulcerative colitis indicate that the incidence of cancer associated with ulcerative colitis may be decreasing with the use of anti-inflammatory agents (30,31). The mechanisms underlying these empiric observations on the effect of anti-inflammatory agents, however, has not yet been fully explored.

II. COLON CANCER

A. Cancer Risk

Colorectal cancer is the most frequent malignant complication in patients with Crohn's disease. However, determining the exact magnitude of the risk is difficult. Studies indicate a wide variation in the estimated risk of development of colorectal cancer. The overall relative risk of colorectal cancer development in Crohn's disease when compared with the general population ranges from 1.1 to 26.6 (Table 1) (3–8,32–34). In general, larger studies with longer duration of follow-up indicate that the risk is high (3–8). However, some of these studies can be criticized for various potential biases such as selection and referral biases (35,36). Other studies suggest that the risk associated with Crohn's disease is lower or not increased at all (32–34). These studies, however, were performed mostly on a smaller cohort with a shorter duration of follow-up and probably suffered from a greater degree of sampling error (35,36). It is likely that the true risk associated with the cancer risk in Crohn's disease falls somewhere within reported range. Prospective studies with longer follow-up and careful attention to various important cancer risk factors would be helpful in better defining the true risk of development of colorectal cancer in Crohn's disease.

The absolute number of cancer cases reported in association with Crohn's disease, nevertheless, remains less than that seen with ulcerative colitis (3–9,32–34,37–55). For example, in my experience with a study involving 6217 patients with inflammatory bowel disease, there were nearly twice as many patients with ulcerative colitis who developed colorectal cancer even though there were more patients with Crohn's disease (9). One possible explanation for these findings is that the true risk of developing colorectal cancer in Crohn's disease is less than that in ulcerative colitis. An alternative explanation is the possibility that cancer cases in Crohn's disease were underreported because the diagnosis of Crohn's colitis was not established until the late 1960s and many researchers previously believed that the development of cancer in inflammatory bowel disease was diagnostic of ulcerative colitis (58). A more likely explanation, however, is that the absolute area of colonic mucosa affected by the disease and, therefore, at risk is less in Crohn's

TABLE 1 Relative Risk of Developing Colorectal Cancer in Patients with Crohn's Disease

Author (ref.)	Study size	Cancer cases	Follow-up (years)	Relative risk
Fireman et al. (32)[a]	365	1	9.9	1.1
Kvist et al. (33)	473	3	9.0	1.3
Munkholm et al. (34)[a]	373	2	8.5	1.7
Gollop et al. (5)[a]	103	1	9.0	2.0
Ekbom et al. (3)[a]	1655	12	11.5	2.5
Gillen et al. (4)	281	8	20.0	3.4
Gyde et al. (7)	513	9	14.5	4.3
Greenstein et al. (6)	579	7	11.0	6.9
Weedon et al. (8)	449	8	N/A	26.6

[a]Population-based studies

N/A = information not available in the original study.

disease. Because Crohn's disease is limited to the small bowel in up to one-third of cases, there is smaller proportion of patients with Crohn's disease with colonic mucosa at risk (56,57). In addition, because Crohn's disease typically affects bowel mucosa discontinuously with a skipped pattern, the absolute area affected by the disease is probably less in patients with Crohn's colitis. Moreover, there may be fewer patients with Crohn's disease whose colon is at risk because patients with Crohn's colitis frequently undergo surgical resection. A similar mechanism may also be playing a role in the probable lower risk of cancer in left-sided ulcerative colitis in which less bowel is at risk (6). In patients with ulcerative proctitis with a minimal area of affected bowel, the cancer risk is thought to be negligible.

B. Risk Factors

Colonic involvement is one of the most important risk factors in the development of cancer complications in patients with Crohn's disease (Table 2) (3,4,9,37,38). Ekbom et al. found that the risk of colorectal cancer developing in patients with Crohn's disease is significantly increased only in patients with colonic involvement (3). Thus, patients with ileal disease were found to have relative risk of 1.0, and patients with ileocolitis and colitis had relative risks of 3.2 and 5.6, respectively (Fig. 1) (3). Among patients with colitis, Crohn's patients with extensive colonic involvement may be at the highest risk. For example, Gillen et al. (4) found that all patients with colorectal cancer and Crohn's disease in their series had either extensive or total colonic disease. In addition, their review of the literature indicated that up to 73% of colorectal cancer in Crohn's disease was associated with extensive or total colonic disease (4). This finding is somewhat reminiscent of cancer risk in ulcerative colitis, in which extensive colonic involvement has been found to be one of most important risk factors in the development of cancer (6). On the contrary, it is unusual for patients with Crohn's disease limited to the small bowel to develop colorectal cancer (3,4,9). Because rare patients with small bowel disease and colorectal cancer are not routinely analyzed for pathological evidence of subclinical colitis, it is not yet known whether ileitis alone can predispose patients to development of colorectal carcinoma (61,62).

The duration of disease is another important contributing factor in the development of cancer in patients with Crohn's disease (4,9,37). Most cancer cases develop after a long

TABLE 2 Importance of Various Risk Factors in the Development of Cancer in Crohn's Disease

Risk factors	Colorectal cancer	Small bowel cancer
Long disease duration	+++	++++
Disease involvement		
Colon	++++	–
Small bowel	–	++++
Young age at disease onset	+	N/A
Presence of stricture	+	+
Presence of fistula	+	+
Bypassed loops of bowel	+	+++

N/A = data not available.

Relative Risk

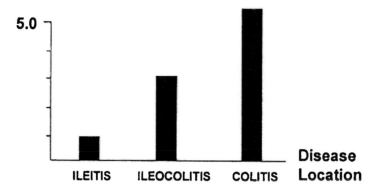

FIG. 1 The relative risk of developing colorectal cancer as a function of the extent of Crohn's disease. (From Ref 3.)

disease duration (approximately 20 years), although cancer can develop around the time of diagnosis of Crohn's disease in a minority of cases (Fig. 2). Thus, a review of reports indicates that greater than 75% of all patients with Crohn's disease who developed colorectal cancer had disease duration of greater than 8 years (9,37–55). Paradoxically, a minority of patients (25%) with short disease duration at the time of cancer diagnosis were often much older than patients with long duration of disease (9). A chance occurrence of sporadic colorectal cancer related to age, therefore, may partly account for the short duration of disease in these older patients because colorectal cancer is one the most common tumors affecting this age group (63). In addition, patients with short disease

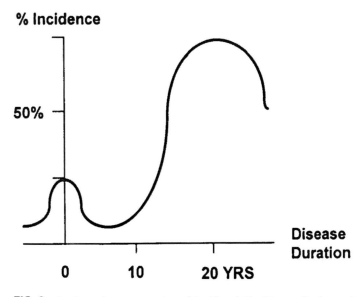

FIG. 2 A schematic representation of the bimodal incidence of colorectal cancer in Crohn's disease patients with cancer. (From Ref 9.)

duration frequently have a history of poorly characterized bowel symptoms, such as frequent loose bowel movements and vague abdominal pain, or a diagnosis of irritable bowel syndrome (9,37). Because it is difficult to define the time of onset of Crohn's disease, it is possible that these patients with cancer had previously undiagnosed Crohn's disease (4,9,37).

An additional risk factor thought to be important in the development of cancer in patients with Crohn's disease is the early age at onset of disease (3,4,8). One study found that patients whose disease was diagnosed before 30 years of age had nearly 10 times the risk compared with those diagnosed at older ages (3). Others have found that the presence of colonic stricture, particularly in patients with long-standing disease, is also associated with a high risk of developing carcinoma (64). Other risk factors thought to be important in the development of colorectal cancer include concomitant presence of fistula and bypassed segment of colorectum (37,38,65–70).

C. Clinicopathological Features

Clinicopathological features of carcinoma seen in patients with Crohn's disease are distinct from those of sporadic colorectal carcinoma but similar to those seen in ulcerative colitis (Table 3) (9,37). Similar to colorectal cancer in patients with ulcerative colitis, colorectal cancer in patients with Crohn's disease develops at a younger age (approximately 10 years) than in the general population (4,9,37,55). As discussed, the risk of developing colorectal cancer increases after a disease duration of 8 years or greater in most patients with Crohn's disease. The duration of disease to the diagnosis of cancer is approximately 20 years for most patients with Crohn's disease (4,9,37,55).

Carcinoma in Crohn's disease tends to develop in the region of diseased bowel (4,9,37,55). In up to 85% of cases, carcinomas have been found to develop near the region of grossly diseased segment of the colon (9). Predilection for cancer to develop at the site of disease activity probably accounts for the predominance of cancer in the right and rectosigmoid colon in Crohn's disease (4,9,37). This is in contrast to the dominance of

TABLE 3   Similarity of Clinical and Pathological Features of
Carcinoma in Inflammatory Bowel Disease

	Crohn's disease	Ulcerative Colitis
Clinical Features		
Age at cancer (median)	54.5 yr	43.0 yr
Duration of disease (median)	15 yr	18 yr
Disease of more than 8 years	75%	90%
Colonic involvement	100%	100%
5-Year survival	46%	50%
Pathological Features		
Cancer in diseased bowel	85%	100%
Synchronous cancer	11%	12%
Mucinous carcinoma	22%	15%
Signet-cell carcinoma	7%	6%
Presence of dysplasia	73%	79%
Duke's C carcinoma	52%	53%

Source: Ref. 9.

rectosigmoid carcinoma in patients with ulcerative colitis whose disease invariably involves the distal colon (71). As is the case in ulcerative colitis, patients with multiple carcinomas at diagnosis (synchronous cancer) are common in approximately 10% of patients with colorectal cancer related to Crohn's disease (9,39,43,55,65). Mucinous and signet-ring tumor types tend to comprise approximately 25% of all tumors seen in the setting of Crohn's disease (9,37,41,54). Among Crohn's disease patients with tumor, dysplasia can be found in approximately 75% to 80% of cases (9,37,41,54). The overall 5-years survival rate of patients with colorectal cancer related to Crohn's disease is similar to that found in ulcerative colitis at approximately 50% (9,55,72–74).

D. Dysplasia

Precancerous marker, dysplasia, is defined as an unequivocal neoplastic transformation of the epithelium. It is often accompanied by genetic abnormalities on flow cytometric and molecular biological analyses (75). Although most clinical information is based on studies in patients with ulcerative colitis, dysplasia found in patients with Crohn's disease indicates a high likelihood of concomitant presence of carcinoma (9,37,41,54,76–79). Dysplasia is classified as negative, indefinite, or positive (79). The diagnosis of dysplasia is further subdivided into low-grade and high-grade dysplasia. In low-grade dysplasia, the mucosal crypts are enlarged, with decreased mucin production, nuclear enlargement, hyperchromasia, cellular crowding, and abnormal nuclear stratification. Dysplasia may also be associated with certain architectural changes, including the branching of crypts and back-to-back glandular formation, suggestive of adenomatous or villous transformation. An important feature of low-grade dysplasia is that the nuclear changes are confined to the basal portion of the epithelial crypt. In high-grade dysplasia, the nuclear changes are more extreme, with pronounced nuclear pleomorphism and hyperchromasia. In addition, nuclear changes often extend beyond the basal portion of the epithelium.

Recent evidence suggests that dysplasia in Crohn's disease may have similar important clinical implications as those of ulcerative colitis (9,37,41,54,80–84). Dysplastic changes seen in patients with Crohn's disease have pathological features indistinguishable from those seen in ulcerative colitis (37,41,54,81). Dysplasia can be found near the area of tumor in 83% to 100% of cases and distant from the tumor in 23% to 70% of cases (9,37,39,41,54). The incidence of dysplasia in Crohn's disease patients without carcinoma, on the other hand, is low, at approximately 2% (40). A report of development of carcinoma in a subset of patients who were initially found to have dysplasia provides additional evidence that the dysplasia–carcinoma sequence is important in the development of cancer in Crohn's disease (84).

The clinical application of dysplasia as a precancerous marker in patients with inflammatory bowel disease has been limited mainly to patients with ulcerative colitis. Even in patients with ulcerative colitis, however, its use can be difficult due to the variability in its interpretation. The interobserver agreement for the diagnosis of dysplasia can range from 66% to 96% (76–78). Intraobserver disparities in the interpretation of the same specimen can also occur. It appears likely that any cancer surveillance program in Crohn's disease would also encounter similar difficulty with the usage of this cancer marker.

E. Biomarkers of Cancer Other than Dysplasia

There is a need to develop a better marker of malignancy in inflammatory bowel disease. One of the main difficulties in using dysplasia as a precancerous marker is that it can be difficult to distinguish from reactive changes. In addition, focal dysplastic lesions can be missed during random biopsy sampling and there is a well-described intraobserver and interobserver variation in the diagnosis of dysplasia. As a result, recent efforts have been directed at the search for more sensitive and specific biomarkers of neoplasia associated with inflammatory bowel disease (85,86).

Flow cytometric analysis allows an objective quantitation of abnormal amount of cellular DNA. Several investigators have found that the aneuploidy detected by flow cytometry in patients with inflammatory bowel disease correlates well with the presence of dysplasia or carcinoma (75,87–91). These studies suggest that flow cytometry may be useful in following patients at increased risk of developing carcinoma. Whether use of flow cytometry will enhance or supplement the histological analysis of tissue obtained from endoscopic biopsies remains to be seen, particularly because of its high cost and the lack of widespread experience with this technique.

Several other potential markers of malignancy are under investigation. They include abnormal binding of lectin to the colonic epithelium and specific antibodies directed against oncofetal and tumor-associated antigens such as sialosyl-Tn, TAG-72, CEA, CA 19-9, and CA 50 (87,92–98). Recent studies have also examined mutational events associated with neoplastic progression in inflammatory bowel disease. These investigations include analysis of mutation in oncogenes such as K-ras and allelic deletion of tumor suppressor genes including p53, DCC, APC, and Rb (75,99–101). These investigations suggest that more objective markers of malignancy should be available soon for clinical application.

F. Cancer Prevention

1. Primary Chemoprevention

An ideal approach to the management of the cancer risk in patients with Crohn's disease involves blocking steps important in carcinogenesis before the actual initiation and progression of neoplastic transformation. Recent studies suggesting the efficacy of anti-inflammatory agents such as sulfasalazine in the prevention of cancer development in patients with ulcerative colitis provide an intriguing primary cancer preventive strategy (9,30,31). If a pathogenic mechanism underlying the risk of developing cancer in Crohn's disease is similar to that in ulcerative colitis, then a similar preventive strategy may be applicable. Since these agents are being prescribed also for the maintenance of remission in patients with Crohn's disease, this approach has an added appeal of not requiring additional intervention. Nevertheless, further studies confirming their efficacy in patients with inflammatory bowel disease are necessary before they can be recommended for this indication.

2. Prophylactic Colectomy

As in ulcerative colitis, prophylactic colectomy may be considered for patients with Crohn's disease at the highest risk. This would include patients with extensive colitis of long duration, particularly if the disease is refractory or if there are significant associated complications. Indiscriminate resective surgery, however, cannot be recommended because most patients do not go on to develop carcinoma and there is a high recurrence rate of the disease following surgery (3–9,103,104).

3. Colonoscopic Surveillance

Periodic colonoscopy with biopsy for the detection of dysplasia is an alternative potential cancer preventive strategy. This approach, however, remains controversial because establishing a beneficial effect of cancer surveillance can be difficult (35,36,105). One of the main reasons for this difficulty is the large number of patients and long duration of study (15 to 20 years) required to demonstrate its impact on cancer stage and survival (35,36,106). In addition, it is difficult to conduct controlled studies because of the ethical issues involved in the prospective randomization of patients at high risk of cancer development to a control arm. Furthermore, patient compliance can be a problem because not all patients would accept colectomy if dysplasia is detected, and multiple procedures can pose logistical difficulty and inconvenience, particularly for patients who are young and mobile. Finally, the potential cost of performing regular colonoscopies in a large number of patients with Crohn's disease has an enormous economic implication. It is likely that any future attempt to examine the impact of cancer surveillance in patients with Crohn's disease would have to carefully address these issues if they are to conclusively establish its role in the management cancer risk in patients with Crohn's disease.

a. Potential Surveillance Strategy. Despite difficulties in demonstrating the beneficial effect of cancer surveillance, there are many supporting arguments for instituting colonoscopic surveillance in patients with Crohn's disease. One important argument is that a growing number of studies are indicating that the risk of developing cancer in patients with Crohn's disease is significantly increased (3–8). In addition, studies demonstrating a rising incidence of Crohn's disease in the general population suggest that a greater number of patients are becoming at risk of development of carcinoma (59,60). Moreover, because cancer in Crohn's disease tends to develop at a relatively younger age, there is a greater urgency in attempting to prevent this complication (4,9,37,55). In addition, pathological studies have suggested that dysplasia found in patients with Crohn's disease has similar ominous clinical implication and is likely to be useful in detecting patients at increased risk (37,41,81–84). Furthermore, early detection of cancer followed by a surgical resection is the only effective curative treatment available (107,108). Finally, it is encouraging that cancer surveillance programs in patients with ulcerative colitis have been recently shown to help detect cancer at an earlier stage and improve the mortality rate related to cancer (109,110).

Thus, it appears both timely and appropriate to initiate cancer surveillance research program in patients with Crohn's disease (9,37,65,84). To be cost-effective, such a program should probably be limited to a well-defined high-risk group of patients with extensive Crohn's colitis of long duration. Because there is no evidence to suggest that patients with noncolonic disease are at a risk, patients whose Crohn's disease is confined to the small bowel can probably be excluded (3,9). In such a program, periodic surveillance should probably begin after 8 to 10 years of disease when the risk appears to rise significantly (9,37). It may also be sensible to gradually decrease the screening interval as disease duration increases because evidence suggests a duration-dependent increase in the cancer risk (4,9,37,55). For patients who present with Crohn's colitis after 50 years of age, surveillance starting at the time of diagnosis may be appropriate because carcinoma is frequently seen after a short disease duration in older patients. This is particularly true if there is a history consistent with subclinical Crohn's disease before the time of diagnosis (4,9,37).

During colonoscopy, a full examination of the colon should be performed when possible, although this may be technically difficult and hazardous in patients with severe stricture (111). After intubation, random biopsy samples taken at fixed intervals from the entire length of the colon help maximize sampling of affected mucosa. Because of predilection for cancer to develop in the region of diseased bowel, the diagnostic yield may be enhanced if biopsy sampling emphasized grossly diseased areas (45,9,37,71). Additional biopsies or brushing should be obtained also from the area of stricture and fistula. Biopsy samples from each segment of the colon should then be placed in separately labeled containers to facilitate a repeat biopsy of the area if needed.

When high-grade dysplasia is found, affected individuals should probably be advised to undergo surgical resection if the finding is confirmed by an independent experienced pathologist. Total colectomy should be also considered in patients with low-grade dysplasia found on successive biopsy studies. In contrast, the risk of carcinoma in patients with isolated low-grade dysplasia is likely to be low. These patients can probably be followed up successfully with careful serial biopsy studies.

III. SMALL BOWEL CANCER

Small bowel cancer is a rare disease with an incidence of 0.1 per 100,000 persons per year in the general population (112). Because of the relative rarity of Crohn's disease, Darke and colleagues have estimated that the probability of Crohn's disease and small bowel cancer occurring independently in a given patient is less than one in 1 billion (112). The approximately 100 cases of small bowel cancer reported in patients with Crohn's disease, therefore, suggests a likely association (10,55,112–119).

Nevertheless, the exact risk of developing small bowel cancer in patients with Crohn's disease is not well known. Some studies have estimated that the relative risk may be as high as 115 times that of the general population (6). However, the relative rarity of both small bowel cancer and Crohn's disease makes it difficult to assess the exact magnitude of the risk (6,120,121).

The risk of developing small bowel cancer in patients with Crohn's disease appears to be the highest among patients with small bowel involvement (see Table 2) (6,9,10). In the largest series to date, Rebeiro et al. found evidence for small bowel Crohn's disease in all cancer patients examined (10). On the other hand, it is rare to find cases of small bowel cancer in patients with the disease limited to the colon (9). Long duration of disease appears to be another determinant important in the development of cancer (10,114). There also appears to be an increased risk of developing cancer in patients who have undergone bypass surgery rather than resection of the small bowel. Nearly one third of small bowel cancer reported in Crohn's disease has developed in patients who had undergone this type of surgery (113,122). Because most of these cancers occurred long after diversionary surgery, it is not clear whether the development of carcinoma was related to the bypass surgery or long disease duration. If chronic unresected disease is associated with an increased risk of developing carcinoma, then extra caution may be necessary when performing strictureplasty that leaves the disease bowel in situ (121). When performing this type of surgery, therefore, it is probably advisable to perform a careful biopsy study to rule out dysplasia or unsuspected carcinoma at the time of surgery (55). Other factors thought to play a role in the development of small bowel cancer include male sex, hazardous occupation, presence of fistula and stricture, and the chronic use of 6-mercaptopurine (10,41,119,121).

Clinical and pathological features of small bowel cancer in Crohn's disease are distinct from de novo carcinoma. It tends to develop at a young age of approximately 46 years compared with 61 years for sporadic cases (10,114,118,119). The median disease duration at diagnosis of small bowel carcinoma is typically long, at approximately 25 years (10,118). Because carcinoma tends to develop in the diseased segment of small bowel and the distal small bowel is the most frequently involved site in Crohn's disease, small bowel carcinoma is usually found in the distal small bowel in patients with Crohn's disease (10,37,38,115,117). In contrast, de novo small bowel cancer is typically found in the proximal small bowel (10,115). Multifocal tumors (synchronous cancer) can be seen in up to 22% of cancer cases related to Crohn's disease (123). Similar to colorectal cancer in Crohn's disease and ulcerative colitis, dysplasia can be found in the area adjacent to as well as distant from the carcinoma (41,50,83,124,125).

Intestinal obstruction is the most common symptom (119). Other frequent complaints include perforation, abdominal abscess, fistula formation, and bleeding (118). As a result, symptoms associated with small bowel cancer are often difficult to distinguish from those associated with active disease, and there is often a delay in the diagnosis of cancer. Thus, small bowel cancer in Crohn's disease is often diagnosed at a more advanced stage, with attendant poor prognosis (10,115,118,119). It is, therefore, important to have a high awareness of this possibility in following up patients with Crohn's disease.

Because of the extreme rarity of patients with this complication, however, it is doubtful that any cost-effective preventive strategy can soon be implemented. The technical difficulty of examining the small bowel with the endoscope, the frequent presence of narrow strictures, and the relative insensitivity of barium studies further limit the options in effectively surveying these patients. Patients who have sudden changes in symptoms, such as complete obstruction that fails to respond to conservative medical management, however, should be carefully assessed for the possibility of carcinoma.

IV. CHOLANGIOCARCINOMA

Although the association of cholangiocarcinoma with ulcerative colitis, particularly in the setting of primary sclerosing cholangitis, is well established, this association is not as well determined in patients with Crohn's disease (126–129). There has been a total of nine patients reported with such complication (11,130–133). Because there is a limited number of cases of cholangiocarcinoma associated with Crohn's disease, it is not yet certain whether this association is real. Gyde et al. could not demonstrate an association from an analysis of 513 patients with Crohn's disease (7). This difficulty is somewhat reminiscent of the earlier controversy regarding the association between colorectal carcinoma and Crohn's disease. Recently, this association has become better appreciated, as the clinical experience with Crohn's colitis has accumulated since the 1960's when it became widely accepted as a distinct clinical entity (3–8,32–34,58). It may be that both Crohn's disease and cholangiocarcinoma are so rare that an extensive number of patients and follow-up years is required before an association can be established with certainty.

In our recent review of cholangiocarcinoma associated with inflammatory bowel disease over a 34-years period, we identified five cases among 3093 patients with ulcerative colitis, but only one case among 3124 patients with Crohn's disease (11). In comparison, the reported incidence of cholangiocarcinoma in the general population is up to 4.5 cases per 100,000 (127). Although it is difficult to estimate the cancer risk on the basis of few patients, the observed rate is clearly higher in patients with ulcerative colitis and Crohn's disease (observed to expected ratio: 35.8 to 7.1, respectively). If an increased risk for cholangiocarcinoma exists for Crohn's disease, it appears that the risk is less than that seen with ulcerative colitis.

A careful review of reported cases reveals many similarities of cholangiocarcinoma seen in Crohn's disease to that seen in ulcerative colitis. In general, cholangiocarcinoma in ulcerative colitis occurs at a younger age than in sporadic cases (42 versus 66 years), after long disease duration (more than 10 years), and colectomy does not appear to protect against the development of carcinoma (126–129). Cholangiocarcinoma in patients with Crohn's disease also tends to occur in younger patients (mean 49 years) and after long disease duration (mean 14 years). Bowel surgery does not appear to be protective against development of cholangiocarcinoma. Similar to cholangiocarcinoma occurring in ulcerative colitis, in which up to 20% of cases may have concomitant colorectal carcinoma or dysplasia, concomitant colorectal carcinoma may also be seen (126). Finally, the location of the carcinoma is hilar in most cases, as is usually the case in ulcerative colitis (127,128,132).

There are some dissimilarities as well. Unlike the male predominance of approximately 63% seen with cholangiocarcinoma occurring in ulcerative colitis, there is a female predominance (88%) (126–129, 132). The colonic involvement by inflammatory bowel disease is infrequent (25%), whereas the ileal involvement is common (100%). The presence of documented primary sclerosing cholangitis (28%) is less frequent compared with cholangiocarcinoma occurring in ulcerative colitis in which up to 60% of cases may have concomitant sclerosing cholangitis (126–129,132). In fact, a lower rate of cholangiocarcinoma complicating Crohn's disease may be explained by the lower rate of primary sclerosing cholangitis seen with Crohn's disease, particularly because primary sclerosing cholangitis is thought to predispose the patient to malignant transformation (126,132,134,135).

V. OTHER MALIGNANCIES

A. Intestinal Tumors

There have been isolated reports of adenocarcinoma involving stomach and proximal small intestine in patients with Crohn's disease (7,39,51,136–138). Similarly, rare cases of carcinoid tumors of the ileum have been described (33,55,139). In addition, squamous carcinoma of the intestinal tract has been reported in the setting of perianal Crohn's disease (38). These cases are uncommon but notable because of the rarity of these types of cancer.

Intestinal lymphoma is another rare entity that has been described sporadically in patients with Crohn's disease (139–142). These cases are predominantly associated with fistulous and perianal disease and tumors are usually found in areas of active disease. Symptoms associated with colorectal lymphoma are usually indistinguishable from those of colorectal carcinoma, and preoperative diagnosis is often difficult. Pathological analysis usually reveals a predominance of B-cell type lymphomas. In addition, primary intestinal Hodgkin's disease complicating Crohn's disease has been reported (142).

B. Extraintestinal Tumors

A number of extraintestinal malignancies have been described in the setting of Crohn's disease. They include tumors of skin, breast, lung, genitourinary tract, cervix, thyroid, and pancreatic islet cell (7,136,143,144). In addition, soft-tissue sarcomas, osteogenic sarcomas, and desmoid tumors have been reported. In general, there are no statistically significant increases in the overall risk of extraintestinal malignancies in Crohn's disease with the possible exception of lymphoma (6,7,33,144,145). The implication of rare reports of histiocytic lymphoma of the brain that may be possibly related to the use of 6-mercaptopurine deserves further analysis (145).

REFERENCES

1. Crohn BB, Ginzburg L, Oppenheimer GO. Regional ileitis: a pathologic and clinical entity. JAMA 1932; 99:1323–1329.
2. Warren S, Sommers SC. Cicatrizing enteritis (regional enteritis) as a pathological entity. Am J Pathol 1948; 24:475–501.
3. Ekbom A, Helmick C, Zack M, et al. Increased risk of large bowel cancer in Crohn's disease with colonic involvement. Lancet 1990; 336:357–359.
4. Gillen CD, Andrews HA, Prior P, et al. Crohn's idsease and colorectal cancer. Gut 1994; 35:651–655.
5. Gollop JH, Phillips SF, Melton LJ, et al. Epidemiological aspects of Crohn's disease: a population based study in Olmsted County, Minnesota, 1943–1982. Gut 1988; 29:49–56.
6. Greenstein A, Sachar D, Smith H, et al. A comparison of cancer risk in Crohn's disease and ulcerative colitis. Cancer 1981; 48:2742–2745.
7. Gyde SN, Prior P, Maccartney JC, et al. Malignancy in Crohn's disease. Gut 1980; 21:1024–1029.
8. Weedon DD, Shorter RG, Ilstrup DM, et al. Crohn's disease and cancer. N Engl J Med 1973; 289:1099–1103.
9. Choi PM, Zelig MP. Similarity of colorectal cancer in Crohn's disease and ulcerative colitis: implications for carcinogenesis and prevention. Gut 1994; 35:950–954.
10. Ribeiro MB, Greenstein AJ, Heimann TM, et al. Adenocarcinoma of the small intestine in Crohn's disease. Surg Gynecol Obstet 1991; 173:343–349.
11. Choi PM, Nugent FW, Zelig MP, et al. Cholangiocarcinoma and Crohn's disease. Dig Dis Sci 1994; 39:667–670.
12. Sporn MB, Roberts AB. Peptide growth factors and inflammation, tissue repair, and cancer. J Clin Invest 1986; 78:329–332.
13. Lupulescu A. Enhancement of carcinogenesis by prostaglandins. Nature 1978; 272:634–636.
14. Weitzman SA, Gordon LI. Inflammation and cancer: role of phagocyte-generated oxidants in carcinogenesis. Blood 1990; 76:655–663.
15. Zajicek G. Inflammation initiates cancer by depleting stem cells. Med Hypothesis 1985; 18:207–219.
16. Pozharisski KM. The significance of nonspecific injury for colon carcinogenesis in rats. Cancer Res 1975; 35:3824–3830.
17. Chalifoux LV, Bronson RT. Colonic adenocarcinoma associated with chronic colitis in the cotton top marmoset, *Saguinus oedipus*. Gastroneterology 1981; 80:942–946.
18. Yamada M, Ohkusa T, Okayasu I. Occurrence of dysplasia and adenocarcinoma after experimental chronic ulcerative colitis in hamsters induced by dextran sulfate sodium. Gut 1992; 33:1521–1527.
19. Tamaru T, Kobayashi H, Kishimoto S, et al. Histochemical study of colonic cancer in experimental colitis of rats. Dig Dis Sci 1993; 38:529–537.
20. Kitano A, Takayasu M, Hiki M, et al. Epithelial dysplasia of the rabbit colon induced by degraded carrageenan. Cancer Res 1986; 46:1374–1376.
21. Shioda Y, Brown W, Ahnen DJ. Serial observations of colonic carcinogenesis in the rat. Gastroenterology 1987; 92:1–12.
22. Pollard M, Luckert PH. Treatment of chemically-induced intestinal cancers with indomethacin. Proc Soc Exp Biol Med 1981; 167:161–164.
23. Reddy BS, Maruyama H, Kelloff G. Dose-related inhibition of colon carcinogenesis by dietary piroxicam, a nonsteroidal antiinflammatory drug, during different stages of rat colon tumor development. Cancer Res 1987; 47:5340–5346.
24. Reddy BS, Nayini J, Tokumo K, et al. Chemoprevention of colon carcinogenesis by concurrent administration of piroxicam, a nonsteroidal antiinflammatory drug with difluoromethylornithine, an ornithine decarboxylase inhibitor, in diet. Cancer Res 1990; 50:2562–2568.

25. Narisawa T, Satoh M, Sano M, et al. Inhibition of initiation and promotion by *N*-methylnitrosurea–induced colon carcinogenesis in rats by non-steroid anti-inflammatory agent indomethacin. Carcinogenesis 1983; 4:1225–1227.

26. Rigau J, Pique JM, Rubio E, et al. Effects of long-term sulindac therapy on colonic polyposis. Ann Intern Med 1991; 115:952–954.

27. Labayle D, Fischer D, Vielh P, et al. Sulindac causes regression of rectal polyps in familial adenomatous polyposis. Gastroenterology 1991; 101:635–639.

28. Rosenberg L, Palmer JR, Zauber AG, et al. A hypothesis: nonsteroidal anti-inflammatory drugs reduce the incidence of large-bowel cancer. JNCI 1991; 83:355–358.

29. Thun MJ, Namboodiri MM, Heath CW. Aspirin use and reduced risk of fatal colon cancer. N Engl J Med 1991; 325:1593–1596.

30. Langholz E, Munkholm P, Davidsen M, et al. Colorectal cancer risk and mortality in patients with ulcerative colitis. Gastroenterology 1992; 103:1444–1451.

31. Pinczowski D, Ekbom A, Baron J, et al. Risk factors for colorectal cancer in patients with ulcerative colitis: A case-control study. Gastroenterology 1994; 107:117–120.

32. Fireman Z, Grossman A, Lilos P, et al. Intestinal cancer in patients with Crohn's disease: a population study in central Israel. Scand J Gastroenterol 1989; 24:346–350.

33. Kvist N, Jacobsen O, Norgaard P, et al. Malignancy in Crohn's disease. Scand J Gastroenterol 1986; 21:82–86.

34. Munkholm P, Langholz E, Davidsen M, et al. Intestinal cancer risk and mortality in patients with Crohn's disease. Gastroneterology 1993; 105:1716–1723.

35. Collins RH, Feldman M, Fordtran JS. Colon cancer, dysplasia, and surveillance in patients with ulcerative colitis: a critical review. N Engl J Med 1987; 316:1654–1658.

36. Sackett DL, Whelan G. Cancer risk in ulcerative colitis: scientific requirements for the study of prognosis. Gastroneterology 1980; 78:1632–1635.

37. Hamilton SR. Colorectal carcinoma in patients with Crohn's disease. Gastroneterology 1985; 89:398–407.

38. Connell WR, Sheffield JP, Kamm MA, et al. Lower gastrointestinal malignancy in Crohn's disease. Gut 1994; 35:347–352.

39. Keighley MRB, Thompson H, Alexander-Williams J. Multifocal colonic carcinoma and Crohn's disease. Surgery 1975; 78:534–537.

40. Warren R, Barwick K. Crohn's colitis with carcinoma and dysplasia—report of a case and review of 100 small and large bowel resections for Crohn's disease to detect incidence of dysplasia. Am J Surg Pathol 1983; 7:151–159.

41. Petras RE, Mir-Madjlessi SH, Farmer RG. Crohn's disease and intestinal carcinoma. Gastroenterology 1987; 93:1307–1314.

42. Martinelli V, Bellucci M. Terminal ileitis and cancer of the right colon. Ann Ital Chir 1959; 36:557–572.

43. Wein MA, Spector N. Regional ileitis complicated by adenocarcinoma: report of a case. Am J Gastroenterol 1964; 41:58–63.

44. Atwell JD, Duthie HL, Goligher JC. The outcome of Crohn's disease. Br J Surg 1965; 52:966–972.

45. Perrett AD, Truelove SC, Massarella GR. Crohn's disease and carcinoma of colon. BMJ 1968; 2:466–468.

46. Hywel-Jones J. Colonic cancer and Crohn's disease. Gut 1969; 10:651–654.

47. Kipping RA. Crohn's disease of the colon with carcinoma of the rectum. Proc R Soc Med 1970; 63:753.

48. Hardy DG, Youngs GR. Crohn's disease and carcinoma of the rectum. Int Surg 1972; 57:504–506.

49. Darke SG, Parks AG, Grogono JL, et al. Adenocarcinoma and Crohn's disease—a report of 2 cases and analysis of the literature. Br J Surg 1973; 60:169–175.

50. Simpson S, Traube J, Riddell RH. The histologic appearance of dysplasia (precarcinoma-

tous change) in Crohn's disease of the small and large intestine. Gastroenterology 1981; 81:492–501.

51. Cooper DJ, Weinstein MA, Korelitz BI. Complications of Crohns' disease predisposing to dysplasia and cancer of the intestinal tract: considerations of a surveillance program. J Clin Gastroenterol 1984; 6:217–224.

52. Kvist N, Jacobsen O, Norgaard P, et al. Malignancy in Crohn's disease. Scand J Gastroenterol 1986; 21:82–86.

53. Wyatt MG, Houghton PW, McCmortensen NJ, et al. The malignant potential of colorectal Crohn's disease. Ann R Coll Surg Engl 1987; 69:196–198.

54. Richards ME, Rickert RR, Nance FC. Crohn's disease–asociated carcinoma—a poorly recognized complication of inflammatory bowel disease. Ann Surg 1989; 209:764–773.

55. Savoca PE, Ballantyne GH, Cahow CE. Gastrointestianl malignancies in Crohn's disease—a 20 year experience. Dis Colon Rectum 1990; 33:7–11.

56. Both H, Torp-Pederson K, Kreiner S, et al. Clinical appearance at diagnosis of ulcerative colitis and Crohn's disease in a regional patient group. Scand J Gastroenterol 1983; 18:987–991.

57. Farmer RG, Whelan G, Fazio VW. Long-term follow-up of patients with Crohn's disease. Gastroenterology 1985; 88:1818–1825.

58. Thayer WR. Crohn's disease (regional enteritis): a look at the last 4 years. Scand J Gastroenterol Suppl 1970; 6:165–185.

59. Binder V. Epidemiology, course and socio-economic influence of inflammatory bowel disease. Schweiz Med Wochenschr 1988; 118:738–742.

60. Mayberry JF. Recent epidemiology of ulcerative colitis and Crohn's disease. Int J Colorect Dis 1989; 4:59–66.

61. Gomes P, Boulay CD, Smith CL, et al. Relationship between disease activity indices and colonscopic findings in patients with colonic inflammatory bowel disease. Gut 1986; 27:92–95.

62. Camilleri M, Proano M. Advances in the assessment of disease activity in inflammatory bowel disease. Mayo Clin Proc 1989; 64:800–807.

63. Silverberg E. Cancer statistics, 1984. CA 1984; 34:7–23.

64. Yamazaki Y, Ribeiro MB, Sachar DB, et al. Malignancy colorectal strictures in Crohn's disease. Am J Gastroneterol 1991; 86:882–885.

65. Korelitz B. Carcinoma of the intestinal tract in Crohn's disease: results of a survey conducted by National Foundation of Ileitis and Colitis. Am J Gastroneterol 1983; 78:44–46.

66. Church JM, Weakley FL, Fazio VW, et al. The relationship between fistulas in Crohn's disease and associated carcinoma. Dis Colon Rectum 1985; 26:361–366.

67. Victor DW Jr, Thompson H, Allan RN, et al. Cancer complicating defunctioned Crohn's disease. Clin Oncol 1982; 8:163–165.

68. Traube S, Simpson S, Riddell RH, et al. Crohn's disease and adenocarcinoma of the bowel. Dig Dis Sci 1980; 25:939–944.

69. Lavery IC, Jagelman DG. Cancer in the excluded rectum following surgery for inflammatory bowel disease. Dis Colon Rectum 1982; 25:522–524.

70. Shorter RG. Risks of intestinal cancer in Crohn's disease. Dis Colon Rectum 1983; 26:686–689.

71. Choi PM. Predominance of rectosigmoid neoplasia in ulcerative colitis and its implication on cancer surveillance. Gastroenterology 1993; 104:666–667.

72. Hughes RG, Hall JI, Block GE, et al. The prognosis of colorectal cancer complicating ulcerative colitis. Surg Gynecol Obstet 1978; 146:46–48.

73. Prior P, Gyde SN, MacCarthy JC, et al. Cancer morbidity in ulcerative coltis. Gut 1982; 23:490–497.

74. Ritchie JK, Howley PR, Lennard-Jones JE. Prognosis of carcinoma in ulcerative colitis. Gut 1981; 22:752–755.

75. Burmer GC, Rabinovitch PS, Haggitt RC, et al. Neoplastic progression in ulcerative coltiis: histology, DNAcontent, and loss of a p53 allele. Gastroenterology 1991; 103:1602–1610.

76. Butt JH, Jonishi F, Morson PC, et al. Macroscopic lesions in dysplasia and carcinoma complicating ulcerative colitis. Dig Dis Sci 1983; 28:18–26.

77. Ransohoff D, Riddell R, Levin B. Ulcerative colitis and colonic cancer: problems in assessing the diagnostic usefulness of mucosal dysplasia. Dis Colon Rectum 1985; 28:383–388.

78. Rosenstock E, Farmer RG, Petras R, et al. Surveillance for colonic carcinoma in ulcerative colitis. Gastroenterology 1985; 89:1342–1346.

79. Riddell R, Goldman H, Ransohoff D, et al. Dysplasia in inflammatory bowel disease: standard classification with provisional clinical applications. Hum Pathol 1983; 14:931–966.

80. Shamsuddin AKM, Phillips RM. Preneoplastic and neoplastic changes in colonic mucosa in Crohn's disease. Arch Pathol Lab Med 1981; 105:283–286.

81. Craft CF, Mendelsohn G, Cooper HS, et al. Colonic "precancer" in Crohn's disease. Gastroenterology 1977; 73:1431–1433.

82. Simpson S, Traube J, Riddell R. The histologic appearance of dysplasia (precancerous change) in Crohn's disease of the small and large intestine. Gastroenterology 1981; 81:492–501.

83. Cuvelier C, Bekaert E, DePotter C, et al. Crohn's disease with adenocarcinoma and dysplasia. Am J Surg Pathol 1989; 13:187–196.

84. Korelitz BI, Lauwers GY, Sommers SC. Rectal mucosal dysplasia in Crohn's disease. Gut 1990; 31:1382–1386.

85. Biasco G, Paganelli GM, Miglioli M, et al. Cell proliferation biomarkers in the gastrointestinal tract. J Cell Biochem Suppl 1992; 16G:73–78.

86. Levin B. Ulcerative colitis and colon cancer: biology and surveillance. J Cell Biochem Suppl 1992; 16G:47–50.

87. Fischbach W, Mossner J, Seyschab H, et al. Tissue carcinoembryonic antigen and DNA aneuploidy in precancerous and cancerous colorectal lesions. Cancer 1990; 65:1920–1824.

88. Levine DS, Rabinovitch PS, Haggitt RC, et al. Distribution of aneuploid cell populations in ulcerative colitis with dysplasia or cancer. Gastroenterology 1991; 101:1198–1210.

89. McKinley MJ, Budman DR, Kahn E. High grade dysplasia in Crohn's colitis characterized by flow cytometry. J Clin Gastroenterol 1987; 9:452–455.

90. Löfberg R, Broström O, Karlen P, et al. Carcinoma and DNA aneuploidy in Crohn's colitis—a histological and flow cytometric study. Gut 1991; 32:900–904.

91. Porschen R, Robin U, Schumacher A, et al. DNA aneuploidy in Crohn's disease and ulcerative colitis: results of a comparative flow cytometric study. Gut 1992; 33:663–667.

92. Boland CR, Lance P, Levin B, et al. Abnormal goblet cell glycoconjugates in rectal biopsies associated with an increased risk of neoplasia in patients with ulcerative colitis: early results of a prospective study. Gut 1984; 25:1364–1371.

93. Fozard JB, Dixon MF, Axon AT. Lectin and mucin histochemistry as an aid to cancer surveillance in ulcerative colitis. Histopathology 1987; 11:385–394.

94. Ahnen DJ, Warren GH, Greene LJ, et al. Search for a specific marker of mucosal dysplasia in chronic ulcerative colitis. Gastroneterology 1987; 93:1346–1355.

95. Allen DC, Foster H, Orchin JC, et al. Immunohistochemnical staining of colorectal tissues with monoclonal antibodies to ras oncogene p21 product and carbohydrate determinant antigen 19-9. J Clin Pathol 1987; 40:157-162.

96. Frykholm G, Enbled P, Pahlman L, et al. Expression of the carcinoma associated antigen CA 19-9 and CA50 in inflammatory bowel disease. Dis Colon Rectum 1987; 30:545.

97. Kornbluth A, Present D, Rubin P, et al. Sialosyl-Tn antigen (s-Tn) in non-dysplastic biopsies may predict development of cancer or dysplasia in ulcerative colitis (abstr). Gastroenterology 1991; 100:A221.

98. Thor A, Itzkowitz SH, Schlom J, et al. Tumor associated glycoprotein (TAG-72) expression in ulcerative colitis. Int J Cancer 1989; 43:810-815.

99. Meltzer SJ, Mane SM, Wood PK, et al. Activation of c-Ki-ras in human gastrointestinal dysplasias determined by polymerase chain reaction products. Cancer Res 1990; 50:3727-3730.

100. Greenwald BD, Harpaz N, Yin J, et al. Loss of heterozygosity affecting the p53, Rb2 and mcc/apc tumor suppressor gene loci in dysplastic and cancerous ulcerative colitis. Cancer Res 1992; 52:741-745.

101. Yin J, Harpaz N, Tong Y, et al. p53 point mutation in dysplastic and cancerous ulcerative colitis lesions. Gastroneterology 1993; 104:1633-1639.

102. Prantera C, Pallone F, Brunetti G, et al. Oral 5-aminosalicyclic acid (Asacol) in the maintenance treatment of Crohn's disease. Gastroenterology 1992; 103:363-368.

103. deDombal FT, Burton I, Goligher JC. Recurrence of Crohn's disease after primary excisional surgery. Gut 1971; 12:519-527.

104. Lee ECG, Papaioannou N. Recurrences following surgery for Crohn's disease. Clin Gastroenterol 1980; 9:419-438.

105. Gyde S. Screening for colorectal cancer in ulcerative colitis: dubious benefits and high costs. Gut 1990; 31:1089-1092.

106. Lashner BA, Hanauer SB, Silverstein MD. Optimal timing of colonoscopy to screen for cancer in ulcerative colitis. Ann Intern Med 1988; 108:274-278.

107. Fazio VW, Tjandra JJ. Primary therapy of carcinoma of the large bowel. World J Surg 1991; 15:568-575.

108. Schofield PF, Jones DJ. Colorectal neoplasia—III: Treatment and prevention. BMJ 1992; 304:1624-1627.

109. Choi PM, Nugent FW, Schoetz DJ Jr, et al. Colonoscopic surveillance reduces mortality from colorectal cancer in ulcerative colitis. Gastroneterology 1993; 105:418-424.

110. Lennard-Jones JE, Melville DM, Morson BC, et al. Precancer and cancer in extensive ulcerative colitis: findings among 401 patients over 22 years. Gut 1990; 31:800-806.

111. Koobatian GJ, Choi PM. Safety of surveillance colonoscopy in long-standing ulcerative colitis. Am J Gastroneterol 1994; 89:1472-1475.

112. Darke SG, Parks AG, Grogano SL, et al. Adenocarcinoma and Crohn's disease. A report of two cases and analysis of the literature. Br J Surg 1973; 60:169-175.

113. Greenstein AJ. Cancer in Crohn's disease after diversionary surgery. A report of seven carcinomas occurring in excluded bowel. Am J Surg 1978; 135:86-90.

114. Lightdale CJ, Sternberg SS, Posner G et al. Carcinoma complicating Crohn's disease. Report of seven cases and review of the literature. Am J Med 1975; 59:262-268.

115. Fresko D, Lazarus SS, Dotan J, et al. Early presentation of carcinoma of the small bowel in Crohn's disease ("Crohn's Carcinoma"). Case reports and review of the literature. Gastroenterology 1982; 82:783-789.

116. Savage RA, Farmer RG, Hawk WA. Carcinoma of the small intestine associated with transmural ileitis (Crohn's disease). Am J Clin Pathol 1975; 63:168-178.

117. Collier PE, Turowski P, Diamond DL. Small intestinal adenocarcinoma complicating regional enteritis. Cancer 1985; 55:516-521.

118. Hawker P, Gyde SN, Thompson H et al. Adenocarcinoma of the small intestine complicating Crohn's disease. Gut 1982; 23:188-193.

119. Senay E, Sachar DB, Keohane M, et al. Small bowel carcinoma in Crohn's disease. Cancer 1989; 63:360-363.

120. Sachar DB. New concepts of cancer. Mt Sinai J Med 1983; 50:133-137.

121. Lashner BA. Risk factors for small bowel cancer in Crohn's disease. Dig Dis Sci 1992; 37:1179-1184.

122. Faintuch J, Levin B, Kirsner JB. Inflammatory bowel disease and their relationship to malignancy. Crit Rev Oncol hematol 1985; 2:323.

123. Nesbit RR, Elbadawi NA, Morton JH, et al. Carcinoma of the small bowel: a complication of regional enteritis. Cancer 1976; 37:2948-2959.

124. Fleming KA, Pollock AC. A case of Crohn's carcinoma. Gut 1975; 16:533-537.

125. Newman RD, Bennett SJ, Pascal RR. Adenocarcinoma of the small intestine arising in Crohn's disease, demonstration of a tumor-associated antigen in invasive and intraepithelial components. Cancer 1975; 36:2016–2019.

126. Mir-Madjlessi SH, Farmer RG, Sivak MV. Bile duct carcinoma in patients with ulcerative colitis. Dig Dis Sci 1987; 32:145–154.

127. Ritchie JK, Allan RN, Macartney J, et al. Biliary tract carcinoma associated with ulcerative colitis. Q J Med 1974; 43:263–279.

128. Akwari O, van Heerden JA, Foulk WT, et al. Carcinoma of bile ducts associated with ulcerative colitis. Rev Surg 1976; 33:289–293.

129. Schrumpf E, Fausa O. The frequency of cholangiocarcinoma in primary sclerosing cholangitis. J Hepatol 1989; 9:83.

130. Berman MD, Falchuk KR, Trey C. Carcinoma of the biliary tree complicating Crohn's disease. Dig Dis Sci 1980; 25:795–797.

131. Legge DA, Carlson HC. Cholangiographic appearance of primary carcinoma of the bile ducts. Radiology 1980; 102:259–266.

132. Altaee MY, Johnson PJ, Farrant JM, et al. Etiologic and clinical characteristics of peripheral and hilar cholangiocarcinoma. Cancer 1991; 68:2051–2055.

133. Krause JR, Ayuyang HQ, Ellis LD. Occurrence of three cases of carcinoma in individuals with Crohn's disease treated with metronidazole. Am J Gastroenterol 1985; 80:978–982.

134. Martin FM, Rossi RL, Nugent FW, et al. Surgical aspects of sclerosing cholangitis. Ann Surg 1990; 212:551–558.

135. Rosen CB, Nagorney DM, Wiesner RH, et al. Cholangiocarcinoma complicating primary sclerosing cholangitis. Ann Surg 1990; 213:21–25.

136. Greenstein AJ, Sachar DB, Smith H, et al. Patterns of neoplasia in Crohn's disease and ulcerative colitis. Cancer 1980; 46:403–407.

137. Meiselman MS, Ghahremani CG, Kaufman MW. Crohn's disease of the duodenum complicated by adenocarcinoma. Gastrointest Radiol 1987; 12:333–336.

138. Van Landingham SB, Kluppel S, Symmonds R, et al. Coexisting carcinoid tumor and Crohn's disease. J Surg Ocnol 1983; 24:310.

139. Lee GB, Smith PM, Seal RME. Lymphosarcoma in Crohn's disease: report of a case. Dis Colon Rectum 1977; 20:351.

140. Collins WJ. Malignant lymphoma complicating regional enteritis: case report and review of literature. Am J Gastroenterol 1977; 68:177–181.

141. Shepherd NA, Hall PA, William GT, et al. Primary malignant lymphoma of the large intestine complicating chronic inflammatory bowel disease. Histopathology 1989; 15:325–337.

142. Codling BW, Keighley MRB, Slaney G. Hodgkin's disease complicating Crohn's disease. Surg 1977; 82:625–628.

143. Storgaard L, Bischoff N, Henriksen FW, et al. Survival rate in Crohn's disease and ulcerative colitis. Sand J Gastroenterol 1979; 14:225–230.

144. Greenstein AJ, Gennuso R, Sachar DB, et al. Extra intestinal cancers in inflammatory bowel disease. Cancer 1985; 56:2914–2921.

145. Present DH, Meltzer SJ, Krumholz MP, et al. 6-Mercaptopurine in the management of inflammatory bowel disease: short and long term toxicity. Ann Intern Med 1989; 111:641–649.

COMMENTARY

Burton I. Korelitz   *Lenox Hill Hospital and New York University School of Medicine, New York, New York*

This is a fine review and analysis on what is known about the relationship between Crohn's disease and carcinoma. The most compelling relationship is between carcinoma of the colon and Crohn's colitis. Dr. Choi has been at the forefront in providing data that show a similar predisposition of patients with Crohn's colitis and with ulcerative colitis to development of such disease. Furthermore, the proportion of cases with colon cancer preceded by dysplasia is more clearly the same or almost the same as with ulcerative colitis. Perhaps the fewer resections performed in Crohn's disease is in proportion to a wide armamentarium of effective drugs and postponement of the need for surgery. Given the circumstances, a strong case is made for surveillance in long-standing Crohn's disease involving the colon, despite the greater challenge to successfully perform colonoscopy in the presence of multiple pseudopolyps, nodules, strictures, and abscesses. Dr. Choi and his colleagues have also shown that such surveillance is not merely an academic exercise, but does lead to saving lives.

29
Ileal Pouch in Crohn's Disease

R. John Nicholls   *St. Mark's Hospital, Harrow, England*

Ileal pouches originated from the researches of Kock who, in the 1960s, developed the continent ileostomy, followed in the 1970s by the ileoanal procedure of Parks. Both operations revolutionized the surgical management of ulcerative colitis, and, to a lesser extent, familial adenomatous polyposis and certain functional disorders, for example, megarectum. The indications for pouch procedures have centered around the pathological appearance of the disease in question. Essentially, pouch procedures have been applied to disorders that affect the large bowel and the mucosa in particular, allowing a complete removal of the large bowel mucosa through a combination of conventional excision of the colon and rectum with a mucosectomy in the distal anorectal stump.

Crohn's disease, therefore, is unsuitable in light of the scope of procedures resulting in an ileal reservoir. The disease can affect any part of the gastrointestinal tract and is transmural in its distribution within an affected segment. There is a high incidence of anal disease and of recurrence after abdominal surgery. For these reasons, Crohn's disease has been regarded a priori as a contraindication to pouch operations. This has been especially true of the ileoanal procedure, but, other than Kock, most surgeons have also been reluctant to use the continent ileostomy operation in patients with Crohn's disease.

Nevertheless, some patients with Crohn's disease have had pouch operations and the outcome is reviewed in this chapter. The reasons for this are either not deliberate, owing to mistaken diagnosis, or deliberate, with full knowledge of the presence of Crohn's disease. In this latter circumstance, patient preference is the usual reason that the procedure is performed.

I. INDICATIONS

A. Mistaken Diagnosis

The distinction between Crohn's disease and ulcerative colitis can be difficult. Pathological criteria for each may overlap at both the macroscopic and microscopic levels. In a proportion of patients undergoing surgery for inflammatory bowel disease, the pathologist is unable to make a confident diagnosis of either ulcerative colitis or Crohn's disease on biopsy material. In such cases, clinical and radiological features taken with histological evidence can result in patients being allocated to one or the other type of inflammatory bowel disease group. There is still a small number of patients in whom a definitive diagnosis cannot be reached. These cases are best described as "indeterminate colitis."

The diagnostic difficulty between the two forms of inflammatory bowel disease has been recognized for many years (1). The pathological criteria for distinguishing between them have been clearly defined by Lockhart-Mummery and Morson, Cook and Dixon, and Schachter and Kirsner (2–4). The macroscopic and microscopic features have been summarized by Lennard-Jones et al. (5). Confusion can arise if there are insufficient numbers of characteristic attributes of either disorder or if there is considerable over-lapping of features of either. In addition, atypical appearances can be seen, making it impossible to arrive at a confident diagnosis. Histologically, these patients have been labeled as having "colitis unclassified" or "colitis unclassified possibly/probably Crohn's disease or ulcerative colitis."

The term "indeterminate colitis" was introduced by Price to describe operation specimens from patients with inflammatory bowel disease in which histological appearances were typical neither of ulcerative colitis nor Crohn's disease (6). The diagnostic label is essentially histopathological. It has no further meaning than that the histopathologist cannot distinguish between the two. Approximately 10% to 15% of all resection specimens fall into this category. Usually, the dilemma arises in specimens removed during an acute phase of the disease. In Price's original series of 30 operative specimens, 27 were from patients with severe acute colitis, often with megacolon. This may lead to the occurrence of features atypical of ulcerative colitis. For example, the severity of inflammation may be most marked in the transverse colon where maximal dilatation has occurred. Previous treatment of the rectum by local steroids may give the impression of rectal sparing. Severe ulceration may be irregular in distribution, spuriously suggesting skip lesions. At a microscopic level, the severity of acute inflammation may obscure histological features more specific for either condition. Fissuring can occur in acute severe ulcerative colitis and transmural inflammation may even be present. Thus, the diagnosis of indeterminate colitis is more likely to follow examination of a severely diseased operative specimen.

The diagnostic error in patients having pouch surgery has been responsible for the majority of patients whose Crohn's disease was treated by this procedure. In a series of 272 patients having ileoanal procedures, nine (3.5%) had Crohn's disease. A similar rate of six (3%) of 210 patients who underwent operation at St. Mark's Hospital was found to have Crohn's disease (7). Fleshman et al. reported that five (3%) of 179 patients had Crohn's disease, and Hyman et al. observed a somewhat higher incidence of 25 (7%) of 362 patients (8,9). In these series Crohn's disease was, in most cases, not suspected before the pouch operation.

How can the diagnostic accuracy become more refined? Furthermore, what is the fate of patients with a histological diagnosis of indeterminate colitis? In both circumstances, the combination of clinical and radiological features along with the histopathological findings is essential. The cardinal feature of Crohn's disease is patchiness. This word implies disconnected lesions and is applicable both macroscopically and microscopically. Endoscopic features that show areas of vascular pattern separated by areas of inflammation or radiological evidence of skip lesions are almost diagnostic of Crohn's disease. The presence of small bowel disease should exclude ulcerative colitis. An anal lesion is less diagnostic. Approximately 10% of patients with ulcerative colitis who have a proctocolec-tomy have an anal lesion. Of 112 such patients with ulcerative colitis proven histologically at one hospital, 12 (10%) had an anal lesion (10). These were, however, minor, including low fistula in ano and fissure. Although rectovaginal fistula does occur in ulcerative colitis, its presence is more likely to indicate Crohn's disease (11). High or complex fistula in ano or anal ulceration should be regarded to be more likely in Crohn's disease than in ulcerative colitis (12).

The most reliable histological features that distinguish the two diseases include crypt distortion and the distribution of inflammatory cells within a biopsy sample. Crypt distortion is characteristic of ulcerative colitis and much less common in Crohn's disease. Within the lamina propria, inflammatory cell infiltrate is diffuse in ulcerative colitis; in Crohn's disease it is patchy within an individual biopsy specimen and often varies markedly from specimen to specimen. Indeed, single crypts can have surrounding inflammation adjacent to normal crypts. Granulomas are less specific; they can occur in ulcerative colitis in response to mucin release from ruptured crypts, and they may be seen in mucosa from ileal reservoirs in cases unequivocally having originally had ulcerative colitis. Their presence may sway the diagnosis toward Crohn's disease, but they are not necessarily diagnostic (13).

The pathological features of Crohn's or ulcerative colitis are more usually seen in the chronic stages of disease. This is typified by the granulomas in up to 60% of cases with chronic Crohn's colitis, but in only 25% of those in the acute phase (6,14). The features of monocytolysis, capillary engorgement, and acute V-shaped clefts described by Price in many of his cases of indeterminate colitis are merely indicators of fulminant disease (6). The same can be said of the presence of muscle dissolution and disintegration in which toxic dilatation is present, whatever the cause (15,16).

There are ample radiological descriptions of Crohn's disease and ulcerative colitis (17). Double-contrast enema examination offers a specific diagnosis in approximately 90% of cases (17,18). Thus, there is a group of 10% of the patients in whom the condition is radiologically indeterminate. Computed tomography is of some value. Gore et al. studied a series of patients with Crohn's disease, ulcerative colitis, or indeterminate colitis (19). Abdominal and pelvic scans were assessed for bowel wall thickness and homogeneity; mesenteric, retroperitoneal, and extraperitoneal fat homogeneity and Houncefield number; the width of the presacral space; presence of mesentery; and presence of extraluminal contrast material (fistulas, sinus tracks, and mesenteric lymph node size). In some cases, this examination distinguished between Crohn's disease and ulcerative colitis, but in those with indeterminate colitis, no further useful information came from the investigation (20).

In clinical practice, the clinician relies mostly on histopathological diagnosis. This is available through formal examination of an already excised colectomy specimen in patients having an initial colectomy with ileostomy and preservation of the rectal stump. These cases form a large proportion of those referred for potential pouch surgery. In patients with an intact large bowel, the source of histopathological diagnosis comes from endoscopic colorectal biopsies. A report of uncertainty or indeterminate colitis by the histopathologist simply expresses an inability to commit judgment to a specific diagnosis. On receiving such a report, the clinician must place it within the general context of the case, including clinical and radiological factors. Wells et al. reported a series of 46 such patients in whom it was possible by such an analysis to reclassify 30 (66%) into either "probable Crohn's disease" or "probable ulcerative colitis." Nineteen were placed in the Crohn's disease group on the basis of a history of anal disease including fissure, fistula, abscess, stenosis, or edematous skin tag. One patient had a rectal stricture, one a rectovaginal fistula, and one a sinus from the rectum to the skin over the sacrum. Of the 14 patients who had satisfactory radiological studies, 13 showed a distribution of abnormalities suggesting Crohn's disease rather than ulcerative colitis. Of the 11 patients in whom the diagnosis was thought to be in the ulcerative colitis group, one had a preoperative barium enema with features showing diffuse inflammation consistent with ulcerative colitis. Two patients gave a history of successfully treated anal fistula; in both, however, the radiological features strongly favored ulcerative colitis. Thus, of 46 patients with histological uncertainty, only 16 remained in this state after consideration of clinical and radiological factors (21). In these cases, it is also essential to take further endoscopic biopsies to establish the true diagnosis as far as possible. Changes of diversion proctitis in a defunctioned rectum, however, can add to confusion.

The longterm natural history of patients with indeterminate colitis, in whom further histologic study combined with radiological and clinical assessment still leave the question unresolved, is of considerable importance when selecting patients for pouch surgery. There is some clinical information on this question. Pezim et al. reported the outcome of restorative proctocolectomy in 25 patients with indeterminate colitis out of 514 consecutive patients having the operation for inflammatory bowel disease during the same period (1981–1986) (22). All were believed to have ulcerative colitis preoperatively; however, the histopathological report showed features that were indeterminate. The patients were followed up for a mean of 35 months (range 1–74 months) following closure of the defunctioning ileostomy. Pelvic sepsis occurred in 8% of patients and a subsequent pouchitis also in 8%. Overall failure, defined by excision of the pouch, was 8%. The respective rates in the group of 489 patients with undisputed ulcerative colitis were 4%, 18%, and 4%, respectively. These data suggest that, in the short term, there is no evidence that indeterminate colitis confers a worse prognosis than ulcerative colitis in patients having restorative proctocolectomy. In the group of 46 patients reported by Wells et al., the 16 with "true" indeterminate colitis were followed up for a median period of 10 years (range 2.5–28 years) (21). During this period, three were subsequently classified as having ulcerative colitis and only one as having Crohn's disease. These data also suggest that it is reasonable to perform pouch surgery in patients with indeterminate colitis after taking clinical, radiological, and histopathological evidence into consideration.

B. Patient Preference

There has been no objective statement on the influence of the patient's wishes in choosing a pouch operation when the diagnosis is known to be Crohn's disease. Anecdotal examples abound. Myrvold and Kock, in reporting their 52 cases of Crohn's disease having the Kock ileostomy procedure, do not specify how many were carried out through mistaken diagnosis and how many by patient desire (23). They do say, however, that such patients should have Crohn's disease confined to the large bowel who would otherwise not be suitable for colectomy with ileorectal anastomosis. A high proportion of these patients encounter complications that may lead to failure, and careful case selection, is essential. With regard to ileoanal reservoir operations, the only indication is when the patient refuses a permanent ileostomy. Even in this circumstance, the clinician is unable to comply when there is a significant anal sepsis or sphincter incompetence. Here, neither the clinician nor the patient has a choice. Given the greater risk of failure of restorative proctocolectomy in Crohn's disease, it is unwise to encourage surgeons to offer the procedure. Complications, treatment time, and ultimate failure are frequent enough in patients with ulcerative colitis so that it would risk bringing the procedure into some disrepute by extending the indications to Crohn's disease. Good surgery is mostly due to good case selection.

II. RESULTS

There are several although not many publications reporting the outcome of pouch surgery in patients with Crohn's disease.

A. Kock Ileostomy

Myrvold and Kock reported a series of 52 patients with Crohn's disease having a continent ileostomy (24). Of these, 36 had a preoperative diagnosis of ulcerative colitis, and 16 were known to have Crohn's disease. There was one (1.9%) operative death and 14 (27%) major complications. These included nipple subluxation (10), intestinal fistula (8), and prolapse and stricture (2). Crohn's disease recurred in 26 patients (53%). There were two deaths during the follow-up period and eight patients had the pouch removed. Of the 41 remaining patients with an intact pouch, 37 were continent, and 35 of these were continent and healthy. Myrvold, in referring to this series, observes that the incidence of postoperative complications requiring surgery was twice as high in patients with Crohn's disease (26%) as in those with ulcerative colitis (13%) (24). The incidence of reservoir removal was five times the rate in the Crohn's disease group. Valve slippage was no different than in patients with ulcerative colitis, but the occurrence of fistula was greater. The crude recurrence rate of Crohn's disease at 35% was comparable to that in patients with Crohn's disease having a conventional proctocolectomy for Crohn's disease (25). Bloom et al. reported eight patients with Crohn's disease out of a total of 95 having a Kock ileostomy (26). Of these, seven had been free of disease for 5 years before the operation. At a mean follow-up of 27.4 months (4–50 months), revision was required in two patients, one patient died of dehydration with no evidence of Crohn's disease, one patient developed recurrence with aphthous ulceration in the pouch, and one patient developed a perianal fistula. At the time of the review, all patients were continent and pleased with the result. With a revision rate of 28% at a follow-up of 2.5 years, these results are encouraging. Gerber et al. reported on the outcome of 16 patients with Crohn's disease out of a total of 100 undergoing the continent ileostomy procedure (27). Of the 16, the diagnosis was known preoperatively in 15. In these cases, five had small intestinal involvement and 11 large intestinal. There was a suggestion that operative complications were different in each group. Enteric fistulation occurred in all five patients with small intestinal involvement requiring surgical closure in three and excision of the pouch in one. In contrast, fistula developed in only one of the 11 patients with large bowel involvement, requiring a surgical closure. The follow-up, ranging from 4 to 54 months, was too short to allow comment on long-term outcome (27,28).

Other researchers have reported a poor outcome after the Kock ileostomy procedure in Crohn's disease (29). In a consecutive series of 100 patients with Kock pouch constructions, seven patients were judged histologically to have Crohn's disease. An eighth patient developed severe ileal disease 13 years postoperatively raising the possibility of Crohn's disease in this patient. There was some histological evidence to support the diagnosis. All seven patients known to have Crohn's disease at the time of the pouch construction experienced serious complications within the first year. These included fistulization in two, obstruction and leakage due to transmural disease of the stoma in three, and diarrhea with excessive mucous secretion in two. Of the whole group of eight patients, four required removal of the pouch and four continued medical treatment for ileitis. This complication rate was significantly higher than that occurring in the 87 patients having the operation for ulcerative colitis. Of these, six patients underwent excision of the pouch, and, overall, 17 (20%) required treatment for complications (which were minor in six). These authors felt strongly that Crohn's disease is a contraindication to the Kock reservoir procedure.

B. Ileoanal Reconstruction

In a large retrospective review of 179 patients undergoing restorative proctocolectomy, there were five patients with Crohn's disease. Most patients (163) had ulcerative colitis and 11 familial adenomatous polyposis. Crohn's disease was diagnosed postoperatively in all 5 cases. Two patients with Crohn's disease developed ileoanal anastomotic leakage postoperatively and one was found to have Crohn's disease after the ileal reservoir was removed after attempts to repair a delayed fistula in ano. The authors state that late fistulization occurred in five (2.8%) patients of the total series, including two patients with Crohn's disease (8). Of seven patients with Crohn's disease reported up to that time, six had required removal (30–33). Cohen regarded Crohn's disease as an absolute contra-indication to an ileoanal pouch procedure (34). Galandiuk et al. reported the Mayo Clinic experience of reoperation for pouch-related complications of 982 patients who underwent surgery between 1981 and 1989. Of the total, 114 (12%) required reoperation, excluding surgery for small bowel obstruction. Of these, 20% ultimately required excision of the pouch. There were 16 patients diagnosed as having Crohn's disease, 14 of whom had complications requiring further surgery. All had diarrhea and the incidence of septic complications in the region of the ileoanal anastomosis was 44%. At the time of assess-ment, nine patients had a diverting ileostomy, and there were four ultimate failures requiring excision with end ileostomy.

In focusing specifically on the fate of patients with Crohn's disease having restorative proctocolectomy, the result from three large North American clinics are not promising. Deutsch et al., in following the expanded series of Fleshman et al., reported the outcome in nine patients with Crohn's disease of a total of 272 patients who underwent surgery between 1982 and 1989 (8,36). The diagnosis was recognized in five patients immediately postoperatively, and, in four it developed after a mean interval of 2.5 years. These patients included five females and four males with a mean age of 29 years. Interestingly, seven patients had had an initial colectomy for severe acute disease, and, although, the diagnosis of Crohn's disease was suspected in three, it was not confirmed. In the group of five patients known to have Crohn's disease immediately postoperatively, three were well with a functioning pouch at a mean follow-up of 33 months; the other two had the pouch removed for anal fistulation. In the other four patients, the diagnosis was made an average of 17 months after closure of the ileostomy following the appearance of a pouch-vaginal fistula in three and anal fissures and stenosis in one patient. Two patients required excision of the reservoir, one had a functioning ileal pouch with a persistent fistula, and the patient with stenosis was functioning with intubation to empty the pouch. In this group of four patients, Crohn's disease was confirmed histologically in the two requiring excision of the pouch; in the other two, it had not been. In a report from the Lahey Clinic, Koltun et al. studied retrospectively 288 patients having restorative proctocolectomy (37). Of these, 18 (6%) had indeterminate colitis, six (2%) Crohn's disease, and 29 (10%) familial adenoma-tous polyposis. The remaining 235 (82%) had ulcerative colitis. There was a significant difference in the complication and late failure rate in the indeterminate and Crohn's disease group compared with patients with ulcerative colitis. Nine patients (50%) in the indeter-minate colitis group, and four (67%) of the Crohn's disease patients developed a perineal complication. These high rates compared with eight (3%) cases of perineal complications in the ulcerative colitis group. None of the polyposis patients developed a perineal complication. Five (28%) patients of the indeterminate colitis group required a permanent stoma compared with one (0.4%) patient with ulcerative colitis. In the four patients with Crohn's disease who developed fistula, all were managed by simple laying open and none required an ileostomy. This study included only patients with fistula occurring at 6 or more months after closure of the ileostomy. The median follow-up time was 40 months (range 6–109 months) from closure of the stoma. Thus, it is possible that further complications may have occurred in the Crohn's disease patients. In contrast with the report of Pezim et al., indeterminate colitis was found to have a poor prognosis in this study (22). In another large series from the Cleveland Clinic reported by Hyman et al., there were 25 patients with Crohn's disease of a total of 362 patients who underwent ileoanal pouch procedures (9). Of these, the diagnosis was considered preoperatively in nine patients, and, in the remaining 16, it was diagnosed after removal of the rectum. There was one postoperative death, and, of the remaining 24 patients, seven have required removal of the pouch. Six of these seven are in the group of nine patients with a preoperative feature suggesting Crohn's disease. This group included the first operative death and in another patient, the pouch was defunctioned. Thus, only one of the nine had a functioning pouch at the time of assessment. This is in marked contrast to the 16 patients who did not have clinical features suggesting possible Crohn's disease preoperatively. Of these, only one had the pouch removed, and the remaining 15 had satisfactory function. Removal of the pouch in this group was for anorectal sepsis. The clinical features suggesting Crohn's disease in the nine patients included an anal lesion (fissure, fistula, stricture) in five patients, rectovaginal fistula in one, and Crohn's type distribution of inflammation in the large bowel in three. This emphasizes the need for caution in case selection in patients with anal disease. Grobler et al. reported 20 cases of Crohn's disease or indeterminate colitis of a total of 80 patients having restorative proctocolectomy for inflammatory bowel disease (38). Eight (40%) of these proctocolectomies failed within 18 months. Nicholls reported five (2.5%) patients with Crohn's disease of 210 restorative proctocolectomies; all of these failed (7).

The conclusion from these reports is that patients with Crohn's disease have a high complication rate and high failure rate after restorative proctocolectomy. Particular risk factors appear to be the presence of clinical or radiological lesions suggesting Crohn's disease and small intestinal involvement. The incidence of failure is a function of the duration in follow-up. It will be interesting to see the outcome after a longer period of assessment. Patients requiring restorative proctocolectomy are usually young. The operation should be durable if it is to be effective.

C. Anorectal Sepsis

Anorectal sepsis is the most common complication of Crohn's disease after restorative proctocolectomy, and is the most important cause of failure. Of the nine patients with Crohn's disease suspected preoperatively reported by Hyman et al., five of the six who had excision of the pouch had a septic complication at the ileoanal anastomosis (9). This was also the reason for excision in the eighth case requiring excision. Anal lesions do occur in patients with extensive ulcerative colitis, but they are usually minor. Fissure and low anal fistula were found in 12 of a series of 112 patients undergoing proctocolectomy for ulcerative colitis (39). Nevertheless, when an anal lesion is present, all efforts must be made to exclude Crohn's disease preoperatively. Here, the clinician relies essentially on the histopathological evaluation, and multiple biopsies may be required. In a series of 168 restorative proctocolectomies reported by Keighley and Grobler, there were 10 with indeterminate colitis and 10 with Crohn's disease (40). Of the total group, fistula developed in 27 (16%); fistulization was from the ileoanal anastomosis in 16 (9.5%), two of the 10 patients with Crohn's disease, developed in enterocutaneous fistula and pouch excision was required in both. Of 10 patients with pouch-vaginal fistula, four had Crohn's disease and one indeterminate colitis. Of the 10, two required exicision of the pouch, including one case with Crohn's disease and one case with indeterminate colitis. Thus, of the 10 patients with Crohn's disease, fistula developed in six and 3 required exicision. This was in contrast to an incidence of pouch-vaginal fistula in the 103 patients with ulcerative colitis of 5%, none of which cases required excision of the pouch. This emphasizes, once again, the increased risk of septic complications with Crohn's disease; it also shows that not all fistulas from the reservoir or ileoanal anastomosis are based on this diagnosis (40). Groom et al. had previously made a similar observation in their report of 17 pouch-vaginal fistulas in 161 female patients (41). Among these, there was not one case of Crohn's disease. This was verified by a review of the histological sections in all cases. The condition was almost always associated with a septic complication at the ileoanal anastomosis, however. O'Kelly et al. reported six (12%) cases in a series of 50 female patients (42). The underlying lesion was sepsis at the ileoanal anastomosis. Five patients presented early and two late (more than 6 months from closure of the ileostomy). Repair in the early cases was successful, but it failed in the two presenting late, both of whom were subsequently judged to have Crohn's disease and both needed removal of the reservoir. Groom et al. had previously distinguished between fistulization appearing early and late (41). The prognosis of the former is good, that of the latter much poorer, even the absence of Crohn's disease.

D. Pouchitis

Inflammation of the mucosa in ileal pouches was first recognized in continent ileostomies by Kock (43). Handelsman et al. subsequently reported it in ileoanal reservoirs (44). Histological changes following reservoir construction of a chronic inflammatory or atrophic type had been reported previously in both Kock and ileoanal reservoirs by Philipson et al. and Nicholls et al. (45,46). Pouchitis is a clinical condition that must be associated with histological inflammation of the ileal reservoir to make the diagnosis (47). It occurs predominantly in ulcerative colitis and only rarely familial adenomatous polyposis. A subgroup of patients with pouchitis includes those with Crohn's disease. In most series, these patients formed a small fraction of the total number of patients having pouchitis (48–52). Careful review of the original colectomy specimen in patients with pouchitis has supported the concept that the condition is an entity in its own right and not a manifestation of Crohn's disease (53). This view was supported by Tytgat and van Deventer and Moskowitz et al. (54,55). The diagnosis of Crohn's disease from biopsies of ileal reservoir mucosa can be difficult because granulomas may be present in patients with an incontestable diagnosis of ulcerative colitis (56). Granulomas may be caused by foreign body reaction around particulate matter derived from the lumen or by mucin released within the mucosa as a result of damage a reaction of the inflammatory process. Fissures also may be nonspecific. The patient with a biopsy showing granuloma formation should not be given a diagnosis of Crohn's disease without very careful review of the histological section from the original operative specimen (13). This situation may account for the case described by Handelsman et al. in which severe inflammation developed, requiring removal of the pouch 13 years after the original construction (29). The authors state that there was some ileal inflammation with granulomatous characteristics at the time of original resection, but repeated reviews of the colectomy specimen confirmed ulcerative colitis with backwash ileitis. Examination of the resected pouch showed ileitis of indeterminate type, raising the possibility of coexistence of ulcerative colitis with Crohn's disease. Alternatively, this may have been a case of nonspecific pouchitis. In their remaining seven patients with Crohn's disease, at least two appeared to have symptoms due to ileitis. Of the eight failures reported by Hyman et al., there was pouch inflammation in four (9). Myrvold reported a crude recurrence rate for Crohn's disease in the 52 Kock reservoirs originally described by Myrvold and Kock to be 35% over a period of 10 or more years (23,26).

The diagnosis of Crohn's ileitis in an ileal reservoir should be made after an assessment of all histopathological and clinical evidence, including a review of any previous histological condition of the large bowel, any anal lesion past or present, and a review of radiographs.

III. CONCLUSION

This chapter emphasizes the avoidance of reservoir procedures in patients with Crohn's disease; thus, careful preoperative case selection is essential. When a patient with Crohn's disease inadvertently has the operation, then complications are likely and failure is significantly greater than in patients with ulcerative colitis. Some procedures, however, appear to have a good long-term result. These patients often form a small fraction of the total, or, at best, no more than 60%.

REFERENCES

1. Kent TH, Ammon RK, DenBesten L. Differentiation of ulcerative colitis and regional enterities of colon. Arch Pathol 1970; 89:20–29.
2. Lockhart-Mummery HE, Morson BC. Crohn's disease (regional enteritis) of the large intestine and its distribution from ulcerative colitis. Gut 1960; 1:87–105.
3. Cook MG, Dixon MF. An analysis of the reliability of detection and diagnostic value of various pathological features in Crohn's disease and ulcerative colitis. Gut 1973; 14:255–262.
4. Schacter H, Kirsner JB. Definition of inflammatory bowel disease of unkown aetiology. Gastroenterology 1975; 68:591–600.
5. Lennard-Jones JE, Lockhart-Mummery HE, Morson BC. Clinical and pathological differentiation of Crohn's disease and proctocolitis. Gastroenterology 1968; 54:1162–1170.
6. Price AB. Overlap in the spectrum of non-spectrum inflammatory bowel disease—"colitis-indeterminate." J Clin Pathol 1978; 31:567–577.
7. Nicholls RJ. Restorative proctocolectomy with various types of reservoir. World J Surg 1987; 11:751–762.
8. Fleshman JW, Cohen Z, McLeod RS, Stern H, Blair J. The ileal reservoir and ileoanal anastomotic procedure: factors affecting technical and functional outcome. Dis Colon Rectum 1988; 31:10–16.
9. Hyman NH, Fazio VW, Tuckson WB, Lavery IC. The consequence of ileal pouch-anal-anastomosis for Crohn's colitis. Dis Colon Rectum 1991; 34:653–657.
10. Mortensen NJMcC. In: Nicholls RJ, Bartolo DCC, Mortensen NJMcC, eds. Restorative proctocolectomy. Oxford, England: Blackwell Scientific, 1992:11.
11. Radcliffe AG, Ritchie JK, Hawley PR, Lennard-Jones JE, Northover JMA. Anovaginal and rectovaginal fistula in Crohn's disease. Dis Colon Rectum 1988;31:94–99.

12. Morson BC, Dawson IMP. In: Morson BC, Dawson IMP, eds. Morson and Dawson's Gastrointestinal Pathology, ed. Oxford, England: Blackwell Scientific, 265–266.

13. Warren BF, Shepherd NA. The role of pathology in pelvic ileal reservoir surgery. Int J Colorect Dis 1992; 7:68–75.

14. Lennard-Jones JE. Definition and diagnosis. In: Engel A, Larsson T, Regional Enteritis (Crohn's disease). Skandia International Symposia 1992; 5:105–112, Stockholm: Nordiska Bokhandelns Forlag.

15. Roth JCA, Valdes Dapena A, Stein GN, Bockus HL. Toxic megacolon in ulcerative colitis. Gastroenterology 1959; 37:239–255.

16. Lumb G, Protheroe RHB, Ramsey GS. Ulcerative colitis with dilatation of the colon. Br J Surg 1975; 43:182–188.

17. Caroline DF, Evers K. Colitis: radiographic features and differentiation of idiopathic inflammatory bowel disease. Radiol Clin North Am 1987; 25:47–66.

18. Laufer J, Hamilton J. The aradiological differentiation between ulcerative colitis and granulomatous colitis by double contrast radiology. Am J Gastroenterol 1976; 66:259–269.

19. Gore RM, Marn CS, Kirby DF, Vogelzand RL, Neiman HL. CT findings in ulcerative, granulomatous and indeterminate colitis. ASR Am J Radiol 1984; 143:279–284.

20. Lee KS, Medline A, Shockey S. Indeterminate colitis in the spectrum of inflammatory bowel disease. Arch Pathol Lab Med 1979; 193:173–176.

21. Wells AD, McMillan I, Price AB, Ritchie JK, Nicholls RJ. Natural history of indeterminate colitis. BR J Surg 1991; 78:179–181.

22. Pezim ME, Pemberton JH, Beart RW, et al. Outcome of indeterminate colitis following ileal pouch–anal anastomosis. Dis Colon Rectum 1989; 32:653–658.

23. Myrvold HE, Kock NG. Continent ileostomy in patients with Crohn's disease. Gastroenterology 1981; 80:1237.

24. Myrvold HE. The continent ileostomy. World J Surg 1987; 11:720–726.

25. Hellberg R, Hulten L, Rosengren C, Ahren C. The recurrence rate after primary excisional surgery for Crohn's disease. Acta Chir Scand 1980; 146:435–443.

26. Bloom RJ, Larsen CP, Watt R. Oberhelman HA. A reappraisal of the Kock continent ileostomy in patients with Crohn's disease. Surg Gynecol Obstet 1986; 162:105–108.

27. Gerber A, Apt MH, Craig PH. The Kock continent ileostomy. Surg Gynecol Obstet 1983; 156:345–350.

28. Goldman SC, Rombeau JL. The continent ileostomy: a collective review. Dis Colon Rectum 1978; 21:594–599.

29. Handlesman JC, Gottlieb LM, Hamilton SR. Crohn's disease as a contraindication to Kock pouch (continent ileostomy). Dis Colon Rectum 1993; 36:840–843.

30. Dozois RR. Ileal "J" pouch-anal anastomosis. Br J Surg 1985; 72(suppl):S80–82.

31. Nicholls RJ, Moskowitz RL, Shepherd NA. Restorative proctocolectomy with ileal reservoir. BR J Surg 1985; 72(suppl):S76–79.

32. Becker JM, Raymond JL. Ileal pouch–anal anastomosis: a single surgeon's experience with 100 consecutive cases. Ann Surg 1986; 204:375–381.

33. Rothenberger DA, Wong WD, Buls JG, Goldberg SM. The S ileal pouch–anal anastomosis. In: Dozois RR, ed. Alternatives to Conventional Ileostomy. Chicago: Yearbook Medical, 1985:345–362.

34. Cohen Z. Anastomose ileo-anale: contreindications operatoires. Ann Chir 1993; 47:946–947.

35. Galandiuk S, Scott NA, Dozois RR, Kelly KA. Ileal pouch–anal anastomosis. Reoperation for pouch-related complications. Ann Surg 1990; 212:446–454.

36. Deutsch AA, McLeod RS, Cullen J, Cohen Z. Results of the pelvic pouch procedure in patients with Crohn's disease. Dis Colon Rectum 1991; 34:475–477.

37. Koltum WA, Schoetz DJ, Roberts PL, Murray JL, Coller JA, Veidenheimer MC. Indeterminate colitis predisposes to perineal complications after ileal pouch–anal anastomosis. Dis Colon Rectum 1991; 34:857–860.

38. Grobler S, Hosie KB, Affice E, Keighley MRB, Thompson H. Outcome of restorative proctocolectomy in patients when the diagnosis is suggestive of Crohn's disease. Gut 1993; 34:1384–1388.

39. Hunt T, Talbot IC, Nicholls RJ. Unpublished observation.

40. Keighley MRB, Grobler SP. Fistula complicating restorative proctocolectomy. Br J Surg 1993; 80:1065–1067.

41. Groom JS, Nicholls RJ, Hawley PR, Phillips RKS. Pouch-vaginal fistula. Br J Surg 1993; 80:936–940.

42. O'Kelly TJ, Merrett M, Mortensen NJMcC, Dehn TCB, Kettlewell M. Pouch-vaginal fistula after restorative proctocolectomy: aetiology and management. Br J Surg 1994; 81:1374–1375.

43. Kock NG, Darle N, Hulten L, Kewenter J, Myrvold H, Phillipson B. Ileostomy. Curr Probl Surg 1977; 14:36–38.

44. Handelsman JC, Fishbein Rh, Hoover HE, Smith GW, Haller JA. Endorectal pull-through operation in adults after colectomy and excision of rectal mucosa. Surgery 1983; 93:247–253.

45. Philipson B, Brandberg A, Jagenburg R, Kock NG, Lager I, Ahren C. Mucosal morphology, bacteriology and absorption in intraabdominal ileostomy reservoir. Scand J Gastroenterol 1975; 10:145–153.

46. Nicholls RJ, Belleveau P, Neill M, Wilks M, Tabaqchali S. Restorative proctocolectomy with ileal reservoir: a pathophysiological assessment. Gut 1981; 22:462–468.

47. Madden MV, Farthing MJG, Nicholls RJ. Inflammation in ileal reservoirs: pouchitis. Gut 1990; 31:247–249.

48. Nicholls RJ, Pezim ME. Restorative proctocolectomy with ileal reservoir for ulcerative colitis and familial adenomatous polyposis: a comparison of three reservoir designs. Br J Surg 1985; 72:470–474.

49. Pemberton JH, Kelly KA, Beart RW, Dozois RR, Wolff BG, Ilstrup DM. Ileal pouch–anal anastomosis for chronic ulcerative colitis. Long term results. Ann Surg 1987; 206:504–513.

50. Everett WG. Experience of restorative proctocolectomy with ileal reservoir. Br J Surg 1989; 76:77–81.

51. Wexner SD, Jenson L, Rothenberger DA, Wong WD, Goldberg SM. Long term functional analysis of the ileoanal reservoir. Dis Colon Rectum 1989; 32:275–281.

52. Zuccaro G, Fazio VW, Church JM, Lavery IC, Ruderman WB, Farmer RG. Pouch ileitis. Dig Dis Sci 1989; 34:1505–1510.

53. Subramani K, Sachar DB, Harpaz N, Bilotta J, Rubin PH, Janowitz HB. Resistant pouchitis: does it reflect underlying Crohn's disease? Gastroenterology 1990; 98:A205.

54. Tytgat GNJ, van Deventer SJH. Pouchitis. Int J Colorectal Dis 1988; 3:226–228.

55. Moskowitz RL, Shepherd NA, Nicholls RJ. An assessment of inflammation in the reservoir after restorative proctocolectomy with ileoanal ileal reservoir. Int J Colorectal Dis 1986; 1:167–174.

56. Shepherd NA. The pathology of the ileal reservoir. Int J Colorectal Dis 1989; 4:206–208.

30
The Effects of Nonsteroidal Anti-Inflammatory Drugs on Crohn's Disease

Joseph B. Felder   *Lenox Hill Hospital, New York, New York*

The group of agents known as nonsteroidal anti-inflammatory drugs (NSAIDs) can have deleterious effects on small bowel and colonic mucosa as well as the upper gastrointestinal tract (1–11). NSAIDs specifically cause ulceration of the jejunum and ileum (12–14). The clinical manifestations of NSAID-associated gastrointestinal tract toxicity are extensive and include diarrhea, abdominal discomfort, strictures, ulceration, and blood and protein loss (15).

Specific reference to the effects of NSAIDs in Crohn's disease has also been reported. Bjarnason et al. demonstrated a Crohn's disease–like ileitis with ileocecal inflammation (16,17). Four other cases with exacerbations of Crohn's disease after taking NSAIDs have been published (9,18,19). Schwartz (9) reported a case of a 49-year-old man using ibuprofen for 6 weeks who developed an exacerbation of Crohn's colitis. Ritschard and Fillipini (18) reported the case of a 26-year-old women with Crohn's ileocolitis who developed acute disease after 2 weeks of diclofenac therapy. In two of the four cases reported by Kaufmann and Taubin, a 58-year-old man and a 46-year-old man, both with Crohn's disease of the colon in remission, were treated briefly with phenylbutazone and indomenthacin and both developed active colitis (19).

I. PERSONAL OBSERVATIONS

On the inflammatory bowel disease service at Lenox Hill Hospital in New York City, we encountered patients with onset of Crohn's disease and exacerbation of Crohn's disease after their use of NSAIDs. We studied all patients with ulcerative colitis and Crohn's disease who experienced a severe enough exacerbation or onset of disease to require admission to the IBD service within a 14-month period (20). We compared the IBD patients with a control population with irritable bowel syndrome (IBS). The charts were reviewed and we interviewed 100 patients, 60 with IBD and 40 with IBS. Thirty-six had Crohn's disease and 24 had ulcerative colitis. Of 20 patients with Crohn's disease who used NSAIDs, a correlation between the two could be reasonably ascertained in 14. In four additional patients without a history of Crohn's disease, onset of the illness followed the use of NSAIDs (Table 1).

TABLE 1 NSAIDs and Crohn's Disease

	Number of patients (%)	
	Crohn's Disease	Irritable Bowel Syndrome
Never used NSAIDs	7	0
Used NSAIDs but not enough information to correlate with disease	5	2
Used NSAIDs but no correlation to exacerbation or onset of disease	6 (25%)	35 (92%)
NSAIDs correlated with exacerbation or onset of disease	18 (75%)	3 (8%)

Source: Ref. 20.

In this study, 75% of all the Crohn's disease patients who used NSAIDs and provided an adequate history displayed new onset or an exacerbation of their Crohn's disease, whereas 92% of the IBS control population used NSAIDs without apparent provocation of their disease. This was statistically significant (see Table 1).

The length of time that NSAIDs were used before the onset of illness ranged from 2 days to 10 years. The most common NSAIDs taken by patients in both the Crohn's disease and IBS groups included ibuprofen, aspirin, naproxen, and indomethacin.

II. MECHANISM OF ACTION

The mechanism by which NSAIDs provoke Crohn's disease has not been clarified, but it is probably by the same mechanism that has been proposed for NSAID-induced enterocolitis that is not related to Crohn's disease (17,21,22) and probably involves the arachidonic acid metabolism pathways shown in Figure 1 (23). Membrane phospholipids found in the colon are catalyzed by phospholipases to arachidonic acid. The arachidonic acid is then further metabolized either via the cyclooxygenase pathway into different prostaglandins or via the lipoxygenase pathway, which results in the formation of leukotrienes, especially LTB4, an active mediator in many inflammatory processes. The prostaglandins and leukotrienes (PGI2, PGE2, PGD2, PGF2, TXB2, 12 HETE, LTB4, SRSA) are the end products of arachidonic acid metabolism that are synthesized in the bowel and are collectively referred to as eicosanoids.

Intestinal prostaglandins have cytoprotective abilities (1,24). Leukotrienes, on the other hand, have deleterious effects on the colonic mucosa. The use of NSAIDs has been associated with increased gut permeability (16,25). The increased permeability is probably mediated by an inhibition of the cyclooxygenase pathway. NSAIDs interfere with the cyclooxygenase pathway, thereby causing a decrease in prostaglandin production and ultimately causing a disruption in the cytroprotective mucosal barrier that the prostaglandins provide. It has been suggested that when the cyclooxygenase pathway is blocked, arachidonic acid is preferentially metabolized via the lipoxygenase pathway, causing increased amounts of leukotrienes to be formed (26).

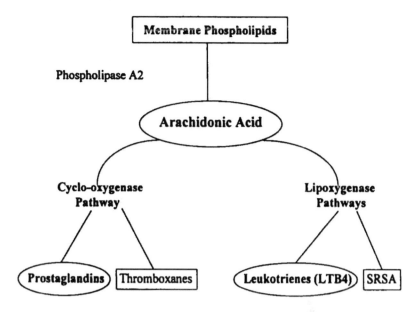

FIG. 1 Arachidonic acid metabolism. (From Ref. 23.)

III. CLINICAL CONSIDERATIONS

Approximately 30 million patients around the world take NSAIDs regularly (27). A large percentage of IBD patients use NSAIDs including 70% of those patients with Crohn's disease in our study.

Side effects of medications used for the treatment of Crohn's disease may include headaches, arthralgias, or myalgias. The extraintestinal manifestations of IBD include problems like ankylosing spondylitis and arthritis. An uneducated patient invariably reaches for the common over-the-counter NSAID preparation that is easily available, or the physician may prescribe it without realizing the potential danger of exacerbating the underlying Crohn's disease. This has been particularly common in orthopedic practices.

When symptoms warrant the use of NSAIDs, non-NSAID analgesics such as acetaminophen should be used first as an alternative. If non-NSAID–type therapies are not helpful or adequate, consideration should be given to changing the patient's drug treatment for Crohn's disease. Only as a last resort should NSAIDs be considered for treatment, and then, only under extreme scrutiny.

When an extraintestinal manifestation such as arthritis is the presenting problem, it should be considered that, as the underlying bowel disease is controlled, so will the arthritis. Therefore, treatment should be directed at the underlying Crohn's disease. Patients with osteoarthritis or rheumatoid arthritis and Crohn's disease pose a particularly difficult dilemma.

Although Crohn's disease has been provoked with as little as one pill, NSAID-induced Crohn's disease appears to be dose related. Therefore, if no alternative exists, NSAIDs should be used at the lowest possible dose necessary for an adequate response (9,28). Consideration should be given to combining low-dose NSAIDs with other medications, which, on their own, would not be adequate.

NSAID-induced reactivation of Crohn's disease or NSAID-induced new onset of Crohn's disease should be treated the same way that an exacerbation or onset of Crohn's disease is treated. Steroids and 5-aminosalicylic acid compounds should be used for acute-phase therapy, and the NSAIDs should be withdrawn.

IV. CONCLUSION

A large percentage of the general population as well as a large percentage of the Crohn's disease population use NSAIDs. When these medications are used, there appears to be a correlation between them and onset or exacerbations of Crohn's disease. The mechanism by which this occurs is most likely the same as the mechanism by which NSAIDs induce enterocolitis not related to Crohn's disease. Based on these findings, it is recommended that patients with a history of Crohn's disease avoid using NSAIDs.

REFERENCES

1. Bjarnason I, Smethurst P, Fenn CG, et al. NSAID small bowel injury and cytoprotection. Gastroenterology 1989; 97(5):1344–1345.
2. Day TK. Intestinal perforation associated with osmotic slow release indomethacin capsules. BMJ 1983; 287:1671–1672.
3. Debenham GP. Ulcer of the cecum during oxyphenbutazone (Tandearil) therapy. Can Med Assoc J 1966; 94:1182–1184.
4. Gould SR, Brash AR, Connelly ME. Increased protaglandin production in ulcerative colitis. Lancet 1977; 2:98.
5. Kornbluth A, Gupta R, Gerson CD. Life threatening diarrhea after short term misoprostol use in a patient with Crohn's ileocolitis. Ann Intern Med 1990; 113:474–475.
6. O'Brien WM, Bagby GF. Rare adverse reactions to nonsteroidal antiinflammatory drugs. J Rheumatol 1984; 12(3)562–567.
7. Phillips MS, et al. Enteritis and colitis associated with mefenamic acid. BMJ 1983; 287–162.
8. Ravi S, Keat AC, Keat ECB. Colitis caused by nonsteroidal antiinflammatory drugs. Postgrad Med J 1986; 62:773–776.
9. Schwartz HA. Lower gastrointestinal side effects of nonsteroidal antiinflammatory drugs. J Rheumatol 1981; 8:952–954.
10. Mendelsohn RA. Non-steroidal anti-inflammatory drugs and inflammatory bowel disease. In: Korelitz BI, Sohn N, eds. Management of Inflammatory Bowel Disease. St. Louis: Mosby-Year Book, 1992; 45–52.
11. Gibson GR, Whitacre EB, Ricotti CA. Colitis induced by non-steroidal anti-inflammatory drugs. Arch Intern Med 1992; 152:625–632.
12. Sturges HF, Krone CL. Ulceration and stricture of the jejunum in a patient on longer term indomethacin therapy. Am J Gastroenterol 1973; 59:162–169.
13. Venturatos SG, Hines C, Blalock JB. Ulceration of the small intestine in a patient with celiac disease. South Med J 1984; 77:520–522.
14. Shack ME. Drug induced ulceration and perforation of the small bowel. Ariz Med 1966; 23:517–523.
15. Aabakken L, Osnes M. Nonsteroidal antiinflammatory drug induced disease in the distal ileum and large bowel. Scand J Gastroenterol 1989; 24(suppl 163):48–55.
16. Bjarnason I, So A, Levi AJ, Peters TJ, Williams P, Zanelli GD, Gumpel JM, Ansell B. Intestinal permeability and inflammation in rheumatoid arthritis: effects of nonsteroidal antiinflammatory drugs. Lancet 1984; 2:1171–1174.
17. Bjarnason I, Zanelli G, Smith T, Prouse P, Williams P, Smethurst P, Delacey G, Gumpel MJ,

Levi AL. Nonsteroidal antiinflammatory drug induced intestinal inflammation in humans. Gastroenterology 1987; 93:480–489.

18. Ritschard T, Fillipini L. Nebenwirkungen nicht steroidaler antirheumtika auf den unteren intestinaltrakt. Dtsch Med Wochenschr 1986; 111:1561–1564.

19. Kaufmann HJ, Taubin HL. Nonsteroidal antiinflammatory drugs activate quiescent inflammatory bowel disease. Ann Intern Med 1987; 107:513–516.

20. Felder JB, Korelitz BI. The influence of non-steroidal antiinflammatory drugs on inflammatory bowel disease. Am J Gastroenterol 1992; 87:316.

21. Madhock R, MacKenzie JA, Lee FD, Bruckner FE, Terry TR, Sturrock RD. Small bowel ulceration in patients receiving nonsteroidal antiinflammatory drugs for rheumatoid arthritis. QJ Med 1986; 255:53–58.

22. Banerjee AK, Peters TJ. Experimental nonsteroidal antiinflammatory drug induced enteropathy in the rat: similarities to inflammatory bowel disease and effect of thromboxane synthetase inhibitors. Gut 1990; 31:1358–1364.

23. Rampton DS, Hawkey CJ. Prostaglandins and ulcerative colitis. Gut 1984; 25:1399–1413.

24. Robert A. Cytoproduction by prostaglandins. Gastroenterology 1979; 77:761–767.

25. Jenkins RT, Rooney PJ, Jones DB, et al. Increased intestinal permeability in patients with rheumatoid arthritis: a side effect of oral nonsteroidal antiinflammatory drug therapy. Br J Rheumatol 1987; 26:103.

26. Semble EL, Wu WC. Prostaglandins in the gut and their relationship to nonsteroidal antiinflammatory drugs. Baillieres Clin Rheumatol 1989; 3:247–269.

27. Banerjee AK. Enteropathy induced by nonsteroidal antiinflammatory drugs. BMJ 1989; 298:1539–1540.

28. Rampton DS, McNeil NI, Sarner M. Analgesic ingestion and other factors preceding relapse in ulcerative colitis. Gut 1983; 24:187–189.

COMMENTARY

Burton I. Korelitz, M.D.   *Lenox Hill Hospital and New York University School of Medicine, New York, New York*

Nonsteroidal antiinflammatory drugs play a large role in the course of Crohn's disease. Just as a careful history of using NSAIDs is essential in exacerbation of upper gastro-intestinal disease, so it is for inflammatory bowel disease. The influence of NSAIDs in provoking activity—even fulminating activity—in Crohn's disease (and ulcerative colitis) is obvious. Whether this relationship between disease process and the drug will provide any clue regarding etiology remains to be determined. Perhaps the reaction in IBD is the same as that of the NSAIDs colitis unrelated to IBD but exaggerated by the predisposition. Nevertheless, the potential clues here should not be neglected,

Meanwhile, NSAIDs should be contraindicated in patients with Crohn's disease and ulcerative colitis.

31
Medical Therapy of Crohn's Disease: Obsolete or Unproven Approaches

Samuel Meyers   *Mount Sinai School of Medicine and Mount Sinai Hospital, New York, New York*

Despite recent advances and the introduction of new drugs, no cure for Crohn's disease exists. This goal must await better understanding of the cause or pathogenesis of this complex, mysterious disorder. Medical therapy, however, may help control the disease and improve the patient's quality of life. In the years since the description of Crohn's disease, many agents have been postulated to have therapeutic potential. Some have been forgotten and others were found to have little or no benefit after controlled trials were completed. Still others await validation. This chapter provides an overview of these intriguing ideas.

I. IMMUNOMODULATING THERAPY

In earlier years, no medical treatment of Crohn's disease aroused more controversy than therapy with azathioprine and 6-mercaptpurine (1). By now, though, a much clearer picture has emerged concerning their risks, benefits, and indications. Cyclosporin also has a potential role as a treatment for patients with Crohn's disease (2,3).

A variety of other immunomodulating agents and approaches have been proposed to have hypothetical efficacy. Fourteen patients with refractory Crohn's disease received parenteral methotrexate therapy (4). Eleven (78%) had an objective response as measured by disease activity indices. Five with colitis had healing as seen by colonoscopy, and four had normal histological appearance at 12 weeks. Controlled studies of methotrexate are in progress.

Colibiogen is a protein-and bacteria-free peptide extract of *E-scherichia coli* that has immunomodulatory effects. Nine patients with active Crohn's disease were treated exclusively with this material for at least 16 weeks. All showed improvement in disease activity; however, the only immune parameters to improve were those associated with clinical improvement, no matter how improvement was achieved (5).

Fusidic acid is an antibiotic that possesses a T-cell–specific immunosuppressive effect similar to that of cyclosporin, but without the potential for severe, side effects. A pilot study of eight patients treated for 8 weeks suggested a benefit (6). Another pilot study tested the role of the immunosuppressant razoxane in Crohn's colitis (7). Razoxane alone was given in nine patients for 3 to 18 months. It brought active refractory disease into remission in all of the patients. Acute leukemia may occur after therapy using high doses of razoxane. This was not seen after a median of 6 years of observation in this study in which lower doses were used. Cyclophosphamide has been used to treat a few Crohn's disease patients who developed azathioprine-induced pancreatitis, but the results were inferior (8). These potentially beneficial agents need careful study, so that their possible roles can be decided.

Crude indications of impaired cell-mediated immunity in many patients with Crohn's disease, at one time, suggested a rationale for the therapeutic use of immunostimulants (9). Oral administration of bacillus Calmette-Guérin (BCG) vaccine has been used to stimulate the immune response, but controlled trials have shown no benefit of this agent in the therapy of Crohn's disease (10,11).

Levamisole and transfer factor also are capable of stimulating immunity, but controlled trials have shown no evidence of their therapeutic efficacy in Crohn's disease (12–15). The proposed role of levamisole in maintaining a remission attained by other conventional medical therapies has not been confirmed in controlled trials (16). Furthermore, a severe, acute polyarthropathy has been reported in a patient with Crohn's disease receiving levamisole (17). The lack of proven efficacy and the potential for side effects should eliminate this drug as treatment for Crohn's disease. Interferon is another agent with an immune stimulatory activity; preliminary trials have suggested that it is beneficial for patients with Crohn's disease (18,19). However, there is insufficient evidence to define its exact therapeutic role.

Intravenous immunoglobulin preparations have been used in the treatment of a small number of patients with Crohn's disease (20–23). The rationale for this therapy is based on the hypothesis that Crohn's disease is caused by an abnormal immune response to gut-associated antigens, an autoimmune response, or an infectious agent. Any apparent efficacy of the immunoglobulins may be due to their immunomodulating or antimicrobial properties as demonstrated in other diseases (24,25). Clinical benefits with no side effects were noted. However, controlled studies are necessary before this agent can be recommended for the therapy in Crohn's disease.

Lymphoplasmapheresis was initially reported in a clinical study of six patients with Crohn's disease (26). The symptoms of one patient were controlled by this therapy alone. In the other five, corticosteroid requirements were reduced. Clinical relapses were managed in these patients by lymphoplasmapheresis, without increasing their corticosteroid dose. The experiment was repeated among seven additional patients. Five achieved prolonged remissions, from 18 to 32 months, but two had prompt relapses (27). The protocol was then altered so that only T lymphocytes were removed. Twenty of 21 patients undergoing T-cell apheresis achieved remission for more than 1 year. The experience was then expanded to 54 patients, among whom 51 had a significant remission lasting at least 1 year. When parenteral nutrition was used to elevate the lymphocyte count so that more cells could be removed, the remissions lasted 2 years (27). Twelve additional patients who had been unresponsive to prednisone for 2 years underwent T-cell apheresis therapy, which resulted in clinical improvement in all cases (28). However, the remissions were short-lived. A reduction in circulating soluble immune complexes or T cells may be a possible basis for the benefit of these therapeutic approaches. This idea was supported by an assessment of 46 plasmapheresis treatments in 17 patients with circulating immune complexes and/or extraintestinal manifestations of Crohn's disease. There was a reduction of the circulating immune complexes in 85% of patients, and clinical remission was achieved in 71% (29). However, there was no correlation noted between the efficacy of lymphoplasmapheresis therapy and the number of lymphocytes and/or monocytes removed

(28). Perhaps other soluble or cellular immune alterations are involved in the mechanisms of action. Further study of these approaches may show them to be useful in a select group of patients. However, these procedures are too cumbersome and expensive to treat ordinary groups of patients with Crohn's disease.

Preoperative blood transfusion has been associated with a decreased postoperative recurrence rate of ileitis and ileocolitis (30,31). A possible explanation is an immuno-modulating effect of the blood transfusion, which may include an increase in specific and nonspecific suppressor T cells, increased suppressor cell activity, reduced natural killer cell activity, or increased numbers of immunoglobulin-secreting cells in the circulation. Furthermore, phagocytic cell activity is reduced because of the ingestion of the altered transfused blood cells. Not all observers, however, have confirmed the association of transfusion with reduced postoperative recurrence rates (32–34).

II. MISCELLANEOUS AGENTS AND APPROACHES

Disodium cromoglycate, a mast cell stabilizer, has been suggested to have a beneficial effect in the therapy of ulcerative colitis. In Crohn's disease, however, controlled trials show no benefit over placebo (35–37).

The effects of vitamin A in supporting normal intestinal epithelium and mucus production provided the rationale for a therapeutic trail in Crohn's disease (38). It was reported to improve clinical symptoms and to reverse impaired intestinal permeability in one patient but not in others (39,40). A long-term, double-blind study found no significant effect of vitamin A in preventing relapse of Crohn's disease (41).

Gut irrigation effects a simultaneous reduction in the bacterial microflora of the bowel and removal of bacterial antigens (42,43). Through a tube positioned in the jejunum, 18 L of normal saline were infused over 2 hours in groups of patients with Crohn's disease. Improvement in symptoms and laboratory data were reported from these small, un-controlled reports. This therapy is unconventional and may theoretically be associated with significant fluid and electrolyte changes. In cases with partial intestinal obstruction, there are potential complications. Based on current information, I do not support this therapeutic approach.

Superoxide Dismutase (SOD) has been used for the therapy of Crohn's disease. The assumed mechanism of action of SOD is the protection of tissue from the direct cytotoxicity of superoxide radicals generated by the respiratory burst of activated neutro-phils. SOD packaged in liposomes was given subcutaneously to seven patients and applied locally to skin lesions in two others with Crohn's disease (44,45). Brief beneficial results were reported. This approach was further studied during an 8-year period in 26 patients (46). Four received oral therapy, whereas the others received intramuscular injections. SOD was not used in combination with corticosteroids or sulfasalazine; however, the simultaneous use of metronidazole was frequent. The acceptability of treatment was good and no adverse effects were seen. There was a satisfactory clinical response after short-term therapy in 73% of the patients. Also impressive was the 82% occurrence of satisfactory long-term results. Relapses promptly responded to the resumption of therapy. In some patients, concomitant subcutaneous desferrioxamine treatment was used for 15 days. The chelation of free iron may help reduce tissue damage caused by polymorpho-nuclear cells. These results are preliminary and have to be confirmed by controlled trials.

There is evidence in inflammatory bowel disease for a pathogenic role of inflamma-tory mediators, especially leukotriene B_4. This is generated via the 5'-lipoxygenase pathway of arachidonic acid metabolism. Dietary supplementation with fish oils, rich in long-chain n-3 polyunsaturated fatty acids, provides an alternative substrate for 5'-lipoxygenase. This alternative pathway reduces the arachidonic acid–derived production of leukotriene B_4 in favor of the relatively inactive luekotriene B_5. In addition, fish oils reduce the synthesis of lipoxygenase products derived from arachidonic acid. However, any clinical benefit seen in Crohn's disease should not necessarily be attributed to inhibition of leukotriene synthesis. There are a number of other anti-inflammatory actions of fish oils, including suppression of interleukin-1 synthesis, inhibition of platelet-activating factor and aggregation, scavenging of free radicals, and alteration of membrane fluidity. Despite the theoretical basis for therapy with fish oil, a 7-month controlled trial in 39 Crohn's disease patients showed no benefit of dietary supplementation (47). Another study evaluated supplemental fish oil in patients receiving treatment with an elemental diet. No incremental benefit was detected with the addition of the fish oil (48).

Hypoproteinemia is commonly due to malnutrition or protein loss through the diseased gut. However, albumin or amino acid replacement therapy is not helpful for the patient with protein-losing enteropathy. The administered protein is rapidly lost through the inflamed, leaky gut. Corticosteroid therapy quickly improves the protein loss and is the preferred therapy for this complication.

Crohn's disease is often accompanied by subnormal concentrations of the trace element zinc. Because zinc plays a variable role in the development and maintenance of the cellular immune reponse, a possible role of supplementation in Crohn's disease was considered. Mesalamine, with and without zinc supplements, was studied in a controlled trial (49). Six patients with mild to moderately active Crohn's disease were included in the study group (49). All patients had low plasma zinc concentrations. Zinc supplementation resulted in a decrease in their natural killer cell activity. However, there was no effect on the clinical disease.

Saccharomyces boulardii has several effects that might make it an attractive therapeutic agent against Crohn's disease. It has an inhibitory effect on the growth of intestinal bacteria, neutralizes bacterial toxins, increases the activity of brush boarder disaccharidases, and increases the release of secretory IgA into the intestinal lumen. The efficiency of *S. boulardii* was studied in a controlled trial of 20 patients with moderately active Crohn's disease (50). The concomitant administration of *S. boulardii* and other basic therapies significantly reduced the disease activity. The reduction of diarrhea was especially impressive. It remains to be determined whether the course of Crohn's disease will be influenced by the *S. boulardii* or if it is just symptomatic therapy.

III. THE PLACEBO LESSON

For a disease with such a variable and protracted course as Crohn's disease, a great deal about its natural history must be known if any standard or proposed therapy is to be properly evaluated. Unfortunately, such information is not available. Patients do not go untreated with current drugs or surgery to allow evaluation of their course. The only exceptions, I believe, are the placebo groups of clinical trials. Despite the many limitations inherent in the study of these patients, information of value can be learned (51).

A patient sick enough to require treatment for Crohn's disease can get better with no specific "active" drug therapy. When patients are observed for approximately 4 months, between 19% and 50% improve enough so they can, by the definition of these studies, be considered to have gone into remission. Even after long periods of observation, approximately 20% remain well at 1 year and 10% at 2 years. Maintenance studies of patients already in remission, regardless of the method by which they came into remission, show that up to 75% of the patients continue in remission at the end of 1 year and up to 62% by 2 years. Thus, sick patients with Crohn's disease may get better with a variety of medical or surgical approaches, or even by themselves. Having gotten better, they may continue to be well for a year or longer.

IV. CONCLUSION

The history of the medical therapy for Crohn's disease is strewn with ideas that seemed initially to have great promise, only later to be proven to have little or no use. Some approaches may have benefit, but, in their current form, they are too cumbersome for routine use. Still others remain to be formally studied in controlled trials. The therapeutic history outlined and the lessons learned from examining the placebo information should be a reminder to temper enthusiasm. New ideas for therapy of this devastating disease are exciting. However, to make real advances, we must insist on thorough efficacy and safety studies before accepting the proposed therapy.

REFERENCES

1. Korelitz B. Immunosuppressives. In: Peppercorn M, ed. Therapy of Inflammatory Bowel Disease. New York: Marcel Dekker, 1990:103–133, and Mt Sinai J Med 1983; 50:144–147.
2. Brynskov J, Freund L, Rasmussen SN, et al. A placebo-controlled, double-blind, randomized trial of cyclosporine therapy in active chronic Crohn's disease. N Engl J Med 1989; 321:845–850.
3. Brynskov J, Freund L, Norby Rasmussen S, et al. Final report on a placebo-controlled, double-blind, randomized, multicentre trial of cyclosporine treatment in active Crohn's disease. Scand J Gastroenterol 1991; 26:689–695.
4. Kozarek RA, Patterson DJ, Gelfend MD, Botsman VA, Ball TJ, Wilshe KR. Methotrexate induces clinical and histologic remission in patients with refractory inflammatory bowel disease. Ann Intern Med 1989; 110:353–356.
5. Auer VIO, Roder A, Mittelstaedt A. Treatment of Crohn's disease with colibiogen. Cellular reactions of the immune system in patients with Crohn's disease. Fortschr Med 1985; 46:1076–1080.
6. Langholz E, Brynskov J, Bendtzen K, Vilien M, Binder V. Treatment of Crohn's disease with fusidic acid: an antibiotic with immunosuppressive properties similar to cyclosporine. Aliment Pharmacol Ther 1992; 6:495–502.
7. Kingston RD, Hellman K. Razoxane for Crohn's disease and non-specific proctitis. Br J Clin Pract 1992; 46:252–255.
8. Nyman M, Hansson I, Eriksson S. Long-term immunosuppressant treatment in Crohn's disease. Scand J Gastroenterol 1985; 20:1197–1203.
9. Meyers S, Sachar DB, Taub RN, Janowitz HD. Significance of anergy to dinitrochlorobenzene (DNCB) in inflammatory bowel disease: family and postoperative studies. Gut 1978; 19:249–252.
10. Burnham WR, Lennard-Jones JE, Heckeltsweiler P, Colin R, Geffroy Y. Oral BCG vaccine in Crohn's disease. Gut 1979; 20:299–333.
11. Rahban S, Sherman JH, Opeiz G, et al. BCG treatment of Crohn's disease. Am J Gastroenterol 1979; 71:196–201.
12. Segal AW, Levi AJ, Loewi G. Levamisole in the treatment of Crohn's disease. Lancet 1977; 2:382–384.

13. Wesdorp E, Schellenkens PTA, Weening RS, et al. Levamisole in Crohn's disease. A double-blind controlled trial. Digestion 1978; 18:186–191.

14. Sachar DB, Rubin KP, Gumaste V. Levamisole in Crohn's disease: a randomized, double-blind, placebo-controlled clinical trial. Am J Gastroenterol 1987; 82:536–539.

15. Vicary FR, Chambers JD, Dhillon P. Double-blind trial of the use of transfer factor in the treatment of Crohn's disease. Gut 1979; 20:408–413.

16. Modigliani R, Pieddeloup C, Hecketsweiler P, et al. Effect of levamisole on the prevention of developmental flare-ups in quiescent Crohn's disease: a prospective multicenter controlled trial in 155 patients. Gastroenterol Clin Biol 1983; 7:683–692.

17. Benfield GFA, Felix-Davies DD, Thompson RA, Asquith P. Severe acute polyarthropathy associated with levamisole therapy in a patient with Crohn's disease. Eur J Rheumatol Inflamm 1984; 7:63–65.

18. Vantrappen G, Coremans G, Billiau A, DeSomer P. Treatment of Crohn's disease with interferon. A preliminary clinical trial. Acta Clin Belg 1980; 35:238–242.

19. Wirth HP, Zala G, Meyenberger C, et al. Alpha-interferon therapy of Crohn's disease: initial clinical results. Schweiz Med Wochenschr 1993; 123:1384–1388.

20. Cottier H, Hassia A. Immunoglobulins in chronic inflammatory diseases. Vox Sang 1986; 51(suppl 2)39–43.

21. Wolf A, Gaedicke G, Leupold D, Kohne E. Treatment of morbus Crohn with intravenous immunoglobulin. Monatsschr Kinderheilkd 1988; 136:101–103.

22. Knoflach P, Muller C, Eibl MM. Crohn disease and intravenous immunoglobulin (letter). Ann Intern Med 1990; 112:385–386.

23. Levine DS, Fischer SH, Christie DL, Haggitt RC, Ochs HD. Intravenous immunoglobulin therapy for active, extensive, and medically refractory idiopathic ulcerative or Crohn's colitis. Am J Gastroenterol 1992; 87:91–100.

24. Berkman SA, Lee ML, Gale RP. Clinical uses of intravenous immunoglobulins. Ann Intern Med 1990; 112:278–292.

25. Yocum MW, Kelso JM. Common variable immunodeficiency: the disorder and treatment. Mayo Clin Proc 1991; 323:705–712.

26. Bicks RO, Groshart KD, Mercaso S. Lymphoplasmapheresis in Crohn's disease, a pilot study (abstr). Gastroenterology 1984; 88(part II):1027.

27. Bicks RO, Groshart KD. The current status of T-lymphocyte aphereses (TLA) treatment of Crohn's disease. J Clin Gastroenterol 1989; 11:136–138.

28. Faradji A, Duclos B, Bohbot A, et al. Treatment of severe Crohn's disease by lymphocyte apheresis. Ann Med Interne (Paris) 1988; 139(Suppl 1):55–59.

29. Dittrich C, Granger W, Lenzhofer R, Lochs H, Abel-Telkes B. Plasmapheresis in extra-intestinal manifestations of Crohn's disease. Wien Klin Wochenschr 1984; 96:679–684.

30. Williams JG, Hughes LE. Effect of perioperative blood transfusion on recurrence of Crohn's disease. Lancet 1989; 2:131–133.

31. Peters WR, Fry RD, Fleshman JW, Kodner IJ. Multiple blood transfusions reduce the recurrence rate of Crohn's disease. Dis Colon Rectum 1989; 32:749–753.

32. Scott AD, Ritchie JK, Phillips RK. Blood transfusion and recurrent Crohn's disease. Br J Surg 1991; 78:455–458.

33. Post S, Kunhardt M, Sido B, Schurman G, Herfarth C. Effect of blood transfusions on the rate of recurrence of Crohn's disease. Chirurg 1992; 63:35–38.

34. Makowiec F, Loble M, Jenss H, Starlinger M. Do perioperative blood transfusions affect the postoperative recurrence rate in Crohn's disease? Z Gastroenterol 1992; 30:20–30.

35. Williams SE, Grundman MJ, Baker RD, Turnberg LA. A controlled trial of disodium cromoglycate in the treatment of Crohn's disease. Digestion 1980; 20:395–398.

36. Binder V, Elsborg L, Greibe J, et al. Disodium cromoglycate in the treatment of ulcerative colitis and Crohn's disease. Gut 1981; 22:55–60.

37. Franchi F, Meneghelli M, Seminara P, Spadini M, Bonomo R. Failure of disodium cromoglycate

in the treatment of 17 patients with chronic inflammatory diseases of the intestine. Minerva Gastroenterol Dietol 1982; 28:285–291.

38. Dvorak AM. Vitamin A in Crohn's disease (letter). Lancet 1980; 1:1303–1304.

39. Kogh M, Sundquist T, Tagesson C. Vitamin A in Crohn's disease (letter). Lancet 1980; 1:766.

40. Norrby S, Sgodahl R, Tagesson C. Ineffectiveness of vitamin A therapy in severe Crohn's disease. Acta Chir Scand 1985; 151:465–468.

41. Wright JP, Mee AS, Parfitt A, Marks IN, et al. Vitamin A therapy in patients with Crohn's disease. Gastroenterology 1985; 88:512–514.

42. Wellman W, Schmidt FW. Intestinal lavage in the treatment of Crohn's disease. A pilot study. Klin Wochenschr 1982; 60:371–373.

43. Wellman W, Fink PC, Schmidt FW. Whole-gut irrigation as antiendotoxinaemic therapy in inflammatory bowel disease. Hepatogastroenterology 1984; 31:91–93.

44. Emerit J, Loeper J, Chomette G. Superoxide dismutase in the treatment of post-radiotherapeutic necrosis and of Crohn's disease. Bull Eur Physiopathol Respir 1981; 17(suppl) 287–288.

45. Niwa Y, Somiya K, Michelson AM, Puget K. Effect of liposomal-encapsulated superoxide dismutase on active oxygen-related human disorders. A preliminary study. Free Radic Res Comms 1985; 1:137–153.

46. Emerit J, Pelletier S, Tosoni-Verlignue MM. Phase II trial of copper zinc superoxide dismutase (CuZnSOD) in treatment of Crohn's disease. Free Radic Biol Med 1989; 7:145–149.

47. Lorenz RL, Weber PC, Szimnau P, Heldwein W, Strasser T, Loeschke K. Supplementation with n-3 fatty acids from fish oil in chronic inflammatory bowel disease—a randomized, placebo-controlled, double-blind cross over trial. J Intern Med 1989; 255(suppl 1):225–232.

48. Scheurlen M, Steinhilber D, Daiss W, Clemens M, Schmidt H, Jaschonek K. Effects of an elemental diet containing fish oil on neutrophil LBT$_4$ synthesis and membrane lipid composition. Prog Clin Biol Res 1989; 301:505–509.

49. Van De Wal Y, Van Der Sluys A, Verspaget HW, et al. Effect of zinc therapy on natural killer cell activity in inflammatory bowel disease. Aliment Pharmacol Ther 1993; 7:281–286.

50. Pein K, Holz J. Therapeutic effects of *Saccharomyces boulardii* on mild residual symptoms in a stable phase of Crohn's disease with special respect to chronic diarrhea—a pilot study. Z Gastroenterol 1993; 31:129–134.

51. Meyers S, Janowitz HD. "Natural history" of Crohn's disease. An analytic review of the placebo lesson. Gastroenterology 1984; 87:1189–1192.

32

The Experience of Crohn's Disease: Is the Bed Now a Table?

Howard M. Spiro   *Yale University School of Medicine, New Haven, Connecticut*

A clergyman, reflecting on his experience when he was sick with pneumonia told how he had shrunk away from the healthy doctors towering over him. They were strong and he was weak. They were full of energy, and he was too tired to turn over. They were confident, optimistic even, but he was lost in fear and trembling. Weakness and pessimism are emotions that physicians rarely consider. Optimists by nature, victors in education and training, sworn enemies of death, physicians prefer the triumphs of Handel's *Messiah* to the sorrows of Mahler's *Kindertotenliede*. Physicians strive for empathy, but prefer the isolation of equanimity; they want to feel compassion, but their training wrings it out of them.

I. THE IMPORTANCE OF NARRATIVE

It is only when physicians become patients that the wide gulf between care giver and patient is recognized. So-called "pathography" tells the tale of illness, narrates what the patient fears and not what the physician finds, and gives the history of the disease, letting the physician know the anguish that disease brings. Physicians identify with doctor-patients better than others. The stories of physicians who have fallen sick are the ones that physicians understand the best.

More than ever, physicians can do so much for patients, but, more than ever, in the United States at least, patients complain that their physicians are aloof, interested only in technology, cool, and impersonal. Communication may be the watchword, but it is by computer and Internet and not so much by voice and ear. The treatment of inflammatory bowel disease (IBD) involves words as well as drugs and the comforting power of what physicians can say almost as much as what they can do. Communication goes both ways and physicians should consider what the patients should tell us.

II. PHYSICIANS AS PATIENTS

A few years ago, as a colleague and I collected the accounts of physicians who had been sick, we looked for clues as to how we might come to terms with illness, disability, death and, I suspect worst of all, retirement (1). In physicians, the fear of death is stronger than in most other people, but that fear is repressed, thanks to training. What my colleague and I quickly found in most stories was that physicians cannot express their feelings and are skilled at denying that they are sick. They are not very introspective.

Medical students are chosen for achievement and energy, for interest in science not in humanities, for action and not for contemplation. The pace in professional life leaves little time for brooding. Medical students may turn hypochondriac with each new disease they study, but practicing physicians believe that they are invulnerable, almost as if they have made a pact with the Creator: "I will take care of the sick, but you will keep me well." When physicians get sick, they are usually lonely patients, always on the watch, vigilant for what they know can go wrong. Still, they try to be the good patients that tradition depicts, suffering but not complaining. When, finally, sick physicians accept disability, they want reassurance, even at the expense of truth, and they want the compassion that they might not always have shown their own patients.

It is not easy for one physician to take care of another, because physicians identify with their colleagues so readily. Physicians in charge of another physician who is sick may even feel angry because sick physicians expose their human vulnerability. But that anger remains subconscious and merges with a special empathy for the colleague who becomes ill, in such reversal of what has come to seem the "natural" order of things.

For such reasons, reading about a physician's travails with IBD has more impact on physicians than reading about other kinds of patients. For other people who get sick, feelings of anxiety and fear are mixed, but they have no special knowledge. Physicians who get sick find themselves on the other side of the desk, or lying in bed, not standing beside it. The familiar aspects of the hospital change: physicians know their way around when they are vertical, but the physician–patient on a stretcher finds familiar routes suddenly full of disorienting obstacles. Most important, control is lost even as physicians try to remain in charge of their own care, forgetting that the judgement of the sick is clouded. Guilt looms large in physician–patients who must rest when work has been light and life, for most of us physicians define ourselves by our work; when things are not going right, we try to work harder than ever.

With this prologue, my comments are not so much focused on the problems of sick physicians in general but on some experience of IBD, particularly Crohn's disease, in which a cure endlessly recedes on the horizon. And, the message that I read from the accounts of sick physicians is that we physicians should take more time to listen to what our patients say. Gastroenterologists spend too much time at the endoscopy table and not enough time at the bedside.

Crohn's disease is a transfiguring disease of uncertain cause with humiliating symptoms whose therapy has changed little in 40 years despite the triumphs described in other chapters of this book. A person can persevere with abdominal pain, grimacing or hiding the pain. Inescapable, uncontrollable diarrhea, is another matter. Theologians and philosophers have written much about pain and found lessons in chronic pain, but none have written of the affirmative quality of diarrhea. To my knowledge, no one has found lessons for life in having to rush off to the toilet or dirtying one's pants. Patients should be asked what Crohn's disease has done to them and how it has affected their lives in every way and every day.

One of the problems in current management of IBD is the emphasis on the objective model of science, the visual images, that is, management by colonoscopy. The following example is common. A patient who receives a diagnosis of IBD, returns to the physician's office pleased with improvement and reports that everything is going well. Too often, the physician responds "Hold on. Let's see if you are right. I'll look in your rectum to find out." Only after the patient has been duly inverted and the rectum inspected with sigmoidoscopy does the physician agree, "Yes, you are feeling very much better." Physicians prefer the seeming accuracy of the eye to the real truth of the ear. What they see, they believe. As Elaine Scarry remarks, "To have pain is to know, to hear about pain is to be in doubt" (2).

Disease is what the doctor can find, but *illness* is what the patient feels. If IBD is looked at as a disease, then its extent is scrutinized, its duration is contemplated, and nomenclature for dysplasia is standardized. Recurrences are treated with steroids and diarrhea with opiates, and the amount of inflammation reduced by therapy is measured. At conferences on the pathological distinctions between Crohn's disease and ulcerative colitis, experts classify and quantify in a scientific way, and each new drug is praised. But, physicians rarely listen to what the patient has to say in meetings held by such organizations as the Crohn's and Colitis Foundation.

But, when the illness of IBD is regarded, patients have quite different questions and concerns: (a) disability ("Where is the toilet? Can I give that lecture? Can I play tennis?"), (b) anxiety ("Why another sigmoidoscopy? What is eating at me?"), (c) foreboding ("Do I have cancer? Do I need an ileostomy?"), and (d) suffering ("I am so sick of my troubles and the doctors.")

Crohn's disease often seems to me like cancer, or what is still called "mental illness," because it transforms life. Once a person has cancer, physician-patients point out, that person is never the same again and is never free from the fear of its recurrence. A person who has had cancer is always a "cancer patient," even after "recovery." Patients with peptic ulcer rarely join together in groups, because, however serious, peptic ulcer can be dealt with. Crohn's disease is another matter. Diarrhea remains an ever-present threat, cancer a long-term concern, and loneliness, anxiety, dependency, depression, and guilt must be integrated into daily life.

A few years ago, I gathered together from our larger collection the accounts of physicians who were sick with IBD (3). These experiences make clear what it is like to be a patient with that disease. Writing their accounts proved to be a welcome catharsis for all six physicians. Two of the six became gastroenterologists, the two women became psychiatrists. IBD had developed in three before they attended medical school and in the other three during medical school, but all were young when they got sick. By stressing the unpleasant or unusual aspects of physician's encounters with IBD, I illuminate for the physicians and nurses who care for them the troubles that IBD brings to patients. I admire the physical and emotional resiliency of most physician–patients who keep going with a fierce, almost heroic, determination to resist. Physician–patients over again tell how they continue to work.

Several characteristics stand out, as quotations from some accounts show.

III. DENIAL

In physician–patients, denial of disease and disability often leads to steroid-induced complications. It is hard to separate denial from secrecy, a desire for privacy; in general, as long as possible, physicians try to hide from others that they have IBD. I have known some physicians, especially those with Crohn's disease, to go to extraordinary lengths to keep their disability hidden. I have wondered whether the literal loss of control that the diarrhea brings has anything to do with that attempt.

When he began his gastrointestinal fellowship, Maurice tried to continue "to function as if everything were normal." He had learned that he had the disease as a medical student when, apparently, he was a good patient. During his fellowship, he began to treat himself with high-dose steroids, despite weight loss.

> High-dose oral steroids seemed . . . of no benefit . . . I lost over 20 pounds, going from a lean baseline to a walking skeleton.
>
> Still I resisted seeking medical help . . . . Meanwhile I continued to work . . . . I had to plan my day carefully around irregular bathroom breaks. I stuffed bathroom tissue in my pockets . . . had a roll of paper towels under the front seat of my car (less obvious than a roll of toilet paper), and cursed the lack of restrooms in the hospital parking garage. I often could barely make it from home to the hospital lobby.
>
> I took to coming late every day to conserve my limited energies. I made believe I was somewhere in the hospital if paged while still at home . . . . I became progressively weaker. I began waiting for elevators, even to go down one flight, leaning against walls to rest whenever I could do so without being seen. I also sat on patients beds whenever feasible . . . . I often experienced lightheadedness, but I concluded that it was not due to anemia because the hematocrits I checked on myself were always normal. I did consider that they might be falsely elevated because of dehydration, but I rejected that interpretation because I thought I was drinking plenty.

For Maurice, only the organic counted. By taking steroids, he thought he was doing everything his physician would do and resolutely avoided the comfort that comes from letting someone else take over.

An intern, Mallory had involuntary diarrhea as the first sign of his IBD.

> All interns at the hospital where I worked wore high-collared white shirts, white pants, and . . . white coats. One day . . . while riding up the elevator, I felt a voilent cramp . . . and the urge to move my bowels . . . . The old elevator with at least half dozen other people in it moved slowly upwards . . . . To my surprise and chagrin, I felt a bowel movement being propelled down the back of my left leg. Immediately, the odor of stool appeared and my face flushed . . . .
>
> As the elevator finally came to a stop, I rushed to the nearest bathroom to find the seat and the back of my left pants leg bright red . . . . I cleaned my clothing as much as possible, put them on again in their wet condition, walked like a whipped pup to the ward . . . .
>
> I was relieved when I got past the first few nurses, interns, and patients without any of them expressing surprise or scorn. As the afternoon progressed, my ever-perceptive resident asked me if I was all right, and I assured him and myself that this was just a case of acute gastroenteritis.

Mallory managed to get through his residency hiding the disease from his fellows as well as from himself. Twenty-five years after the onset of his troubles, he welcomed the development of a stricture in his rectum as helping to control his diarrhea. Only later could he accept an operation.

David developed IBD in high school where he took the hazing that was necessary to join a fraternity.

It was important for me to get my share of physical hazing with my peers during pledgeship and initiation into high school and college fraternities. Paddling the buttocks was a significant part of this hazing . . . . frequently I simply "took my share" of the paddle and ignored or "forgot" that I had been warned not to allow such to happen to me.

Later, David learned, despite massive steatorrhea, how to hide his disease as best he could.

My weight began to fall despite a voracious appetite . . . . I became defensive about my weight loss and general appearance. I detested being told how thin I was. Among my friends and acquaintances, my failure to gain weight despite my huge appetite was frequently mentioned and discussed. I became self-conscious about my diarrhea and steatorrhea. Not only was I constrained to know where the toilet was located—especially at restaurants—but I had to devise methods of disguising . . . the terrible odor that emanated from the stool. I would light matches or cigars, or on occasion would burn paper in attempting to eliminate the smell in the restroom.

It is one thing to live with a disease, it is another to hide it.

IV. GUILT

The stigma of Crohn's disease and ulcerative colitis may have its origin in the psychosomatic formulations of the 1940s when patients were said to be responsible for their disease. These ideas have largely been discarded, but the hints of contempt that are so easy to find in the early literature are reminders of how much physicians, even in the 1990s, hold patients responsible for how they fare.

The . . . stigma associated with certain medical conditions . . . never occurred to me until I learned that ulcerative colitis, in classical psychosomatic theory, belongs to a group of chronic diseases whose etiology may be rooted in personality. Though modern psychiatry largely rejects this "illness as metaphor" interpretation, I've heard faculty refer to ulcerative colitis in the context of psychogenic illness and have since been especially reulctant to disclose my condition.

Physicians still generalize, even if subconsciously, about the psyche of patients with IBD.

I was especially sensitive to the generalizations that seemed prevalent among fellow physicians about patients with ulcerative colitis . . . . I recall in particular my personal physician during medical school taking me with him to see a patient in the emergency room: a young woman with inflammatory bowel disease.

The patient was lying on a stretcher, crying uncontrollably and complaining of abdominal pain . . . . My physician tried to calm her by revealing in a voice loud enough to be heard through the sobs, "See this young doctor here? He has colitis, too!"

I felt my face redden. I wanted to look behind me to see whether anyone had heard him. Could I be compared to a patient who shared only a disease process with me? I felt, "Certainly not," and proceeded to make that clear.

Illness is equated with weakness.

Doctors, by and large, associated illness with weakness .... The dependent, complaining patient is considered weak, stupid, and generally less worthy than the independent patient. The Puritan ethic clearly prevails among U.S. physicians. Patients earn the respect of their caretakers when they are stoical—the "silent sufferers." I recall being complimented by my attending and others when I withstood the obvious pain of incision and drainage of a small peristomal infection without flinching.

V. HOSTILITY

The uneasy civil war between physician–patient and physician–care giver is especially striking in cases of IBD. Patients live in the domain of perpetual colonoscopy, and it is not difficult to sympathize with the anger of young people away at college trying to establish independence but suddenly reliant upon authority figures.

"Well, Judy, you've got what you've been working on." With that cryptic statement my gastroenterologist, aware of my dread of ulcerative colitis, walked out of the room .... Suddenly, with my doctor's stark pronouncement ... my fate had been sealed.

My surgeon's soul could not reach back. Frequently, when he came to see me, he would not look at me. His gaze would often avoid mine to wander toward the window or the television. I yearned for him to sit for a minute, hold my hand, give me some reassurance. He never did. He checked the NG tube and noted it was draining copious amounts of fluid. He checked out my ileostomy bag and noted the absence of any output .... The sicker I became, the colder he became, and the more death loomed .... He was taking my failure to recover as a personal failure.

VI. CONCLUSION

The Ds of chronic disease offer a convenient mnemonic to remind physicians about such matters: (a) disability, (b) dependency, (c) depression, (d) doctors, (e) diagnostic tests, and (f) drugs. When I think about those Ds, I think of illness and not simply of Crohn's disease.

In treating patients with Crohn's disease, physicians should ask not only, "What can I do?" but also, "Who is my patient?" There are tests and procedures, but, however important they are, physicians should also take time to listen to what their patients want to tell them. Sometimes, the healing power of listening may prove almost as strong as that which comes as immunosuppressives or 5-aminosalicylic acid derivatives. Words can comfort and words can afflict. Physicians should use words almost as much as drugs.

REFERENCES*

1. Mandell H, Spiro H. When Doctors Get Sick. New York: Plenum, 1987.
2. Scarry E. The Body in Pain. New York: Oxford University Press, 1985.
3. Spiro HM. Six physicians with inflammatory bowel disease. J Clin Gastroenterol 1990; 12:636–642.

---

*All quotations in this chapter are reproduced from reference 3, which was extracted from reference 1.

33

The Future of Crohn's Disease: New Developments in Etiopathogenesis and Therapeutics

Maria T. Abreu   *Cedars–Sinai Medical Center, Los Angeles, California*

Stephan R. Targan   *Cedars–Sinai Medical Center and UCLA School of Medicine, Los Angeles, California*

In this chapter, we speculate about fertile areas of research in Crohn's disease. The first section focuses on the etiopathogenesis of Crohn's disease, reflecting on old work in the field and how it can be placed in a modern immunological context. The remainder of the chapter bridges bench research in inflammatory bowel disease with strategies to treat patients. Special attention is paid to ways in which patients can be stratified to predict natural history of disease and response to treatment based on genetic and biochemical data. Figure 1 is an overview of these strategies.

I. ETIOPATHOGENESIS

The cause of Crohn's disease has been elusive from the first description of the disease. In all likelihood, the difficulty lies in the fact that "one cause" does not exist. Rather, distinct combinations of genetic and environmental factors lead to clinical disease. Originally, investigators explored infectious agents such as mycobacteria to explain the granulomatous inflammation that characterizes Crohn's disease. This topic is addressed in Chapter 2. In this section, we incorporate theories of autoimmunity with classical and nonclassical views of bacterial causes.

A. Lessons from Animal Models of Intestinal Inflammation

Even though it is difficult to demonstrate infection in most patients with Crohn's disease, the idea that an infection can trigger chronic inflammation is not unreasonable. Perhaps the most revealing studies of the potential role of bacteria in initiation of chronic inflammation come from genetically engineered mouse models (Table 1). Investigators have developed at least three types of genetically engineered mice that develop intestinal inflammation as a result of disrupting cytokine genes, the interleukin (IL)-2 gene, the IL-10 gene, or T-cell receptor genes. Although, chronic enterocolitis or colitis develops in these models, they do not exactly reproduce human ulcerative colitis or Crohn's disease. Relevant to these animal models is the concept that two general types of T helper cells are recognized by the pattern of cytokines they produce. T helper 1 (Th1) cells secrete IL-2, interferon (IFN)-γ, and tumor necrosis factor (TNF), whereas T helper 2 (Th2) cells

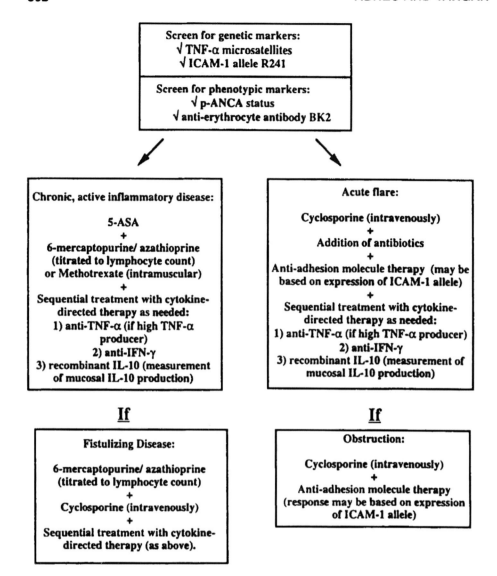

FIG. 1 Algorithm for managing patients with Crohn's disease.

produce IL-4, IL-5, IL-6, and IL-10 (1). These cytokines, in turn, are an important signal in the differentiation and class-switching of B cells. For example, IFN-γ leads to the production of IgG2 and IgG3 by B cells, whereas IL-4 is integral to IgE secretion.

1. The IL-2 Knockout Mouse

Disease similar to ulcerative colitis with colonic bleeding and ulceration develops in Knockout mice with a disruption in the IL-2 gene (2). Mice with an inability to produce IL-2 are said to have a Th2 predominance. These mice have increased numbers of activated B cells, both in peripheral blood and the intestinal mucosa, and, not surprisingly, increased numbers of IgG1 and IgE-secreting cells. In addition to histological colitis, these animals produce anticolon antibodies. It is unclear whether these antibodies develop in the late

TABLE 1 Animal Models of Inflammatory Bowel Disease

Murine Model	Clinical Features	Immunological Features	Requirement for Intestinal Bacteria	Reference
IL-2 Knockout Mouse	Colonic bleeding, ulceration	↑B cells, ↑IgG1, ↑IgE; anticolon antibodies	Yes. Animals in germ-free environment do not develop disease.	2
T cell Receptor Mutant	Diarrhea, colonic thickening	↓αβ T cells, esp. CD4+	Not addressed.	3
IL-10 Knockout Mouse	Mucosal inflammation involving entire intestinal tract.	Normal B cell and T cell functions; ↑IFN-γ in response to nematode infection.	Yes. Animals in pathogen-free environment have only proximal colon disease.	4
SCID Mouse reconstituted with CD45RBʰⁱ CD4+ T cells	Inflammation of colon extending to muscularis, deep fissuring ulcers	CD4 T cells produce ↑IFN-γ, ↓IL-10 and IL-4	Not addressed.	111

stages of colitis or occur prior to overt disease. The other unexplored possibility is that these anticolon antibodies cross-react with antigens on lumenal bacteria similar to epithelial cell antigens.

The IL-2 deficient mice are not only informative with respect to the idea of T helper cell shifts influencing the development of colitis but also with regard to the effect of lumenal bacteria on initiation of inflammation. Colitis develops spontaneously in these mice when they are bred under standard pathogen-free conditions. Intestinal inflammation does not develop in the same animals bred in a completely germ-free facility, and, only mild histological colitis without clinical disease develops in animals bred in a facility with limited bacterial contamination. This study does not address the effect of decontamination on intestinal inflammation.

2. T Cell Receptor Mutant Mice

Mice with mutations in the T-cell receptor (TCR) genes or the class II (MHC) major histocompatibility complex genes are deficient in both αβ and γδ T cells and develop a disease like ulcerative colitis. By contrast, mice with mutations in the recombination-activating gene (RAG-1), which renders them deficient in mature T and B lymphocytes, do not have development of intestinal inflammation (3). Both types of mice, TCR mutants and RAG mutants, are bred under the same pathogen-free conditions. The investigators did not study the effect of a germ-free environment on the colitis. The TCR mutant mice corroborate the idea that T helper cells are necessary to regulate an overzealous immune response to ubiquitous lumenal antigens in the colon.

3. The IL-10 Knockout Mouse

Interleukin-10 is a cytokine produced by Th2 cells and macrophages; it inhibits Th1 cell development and downregulates Th1 cytokine responses. Chronic enterocolitis involving the gut from the duodenum to colon develops in genetically engineered mice that are deficient in IL-10 cytokine (4). Even though their levels of immunoglobulins are normal, they have an inability to suppress Th1 immune responses. Their enterocolitis is thought to be from overproduction of cytokines by antigenically stimulated Th1 cells and macrophages as a result of disruption of Th2 signals, that is, IL-10. Presumably, the reason for inflammation localized to the intestine is the exposure to food and bacterial antigens. Animals kept in a specific pathogen-free environment have inflammation limited to their proximal colon. These animal models support the hypothesis that commensal bacteria play an important role in the initiation and perpetuation of chronic intestinal inflammation when there is an appropriate alteration in host immune response.

There are two themes that have emerged from the serendipitous finding of spontaneous intestinal inflammation in these mice. First, there exists a balance of T helper cell populations in the intestinal tract that limit each others function, especially with respect to cytokine secretion. In the abscence of this balance, unregulated Th1 or Th2 activity leads to pathological chronic inflammation. Second, the inciting event leading to deregulated inflammation is most likely lumenal antigens. Bacterial antigens are implicated specifically because of the absence of inflammation when animals are kept in germ-free conditions.

B. Blending Bacterial and Autoimmune Theories of Crohn's Disease

Some researchers have argued that conditions that are attributed to autoimmunity such as rheumatoid arthritis, sarcoidosis, and inflammatory bowel disease are caused by extremely slow-growing bacteria (5). In inflammatory bowel disease, this theory is supported by the isolation of mycobacteria from the intestines and mesenteric lymph nodes of patients with Crohn's disease (6,7). More recently, the polymerase chain reaction has been used to amplify mycobacterial DNA from tissue affected by Crohn's disease (8–10). This view is not widely held because of the difficulty in reproducibly culturing these organisms and the failure of conventional antimycobacterial drugs to treat Crohn's disease (11–14). In the following sections, we explore other human diseases caused by infectious agents for which more information is known.

1. Slow-Growing Bacteria and the Host Response

Rather than an all or nothing view of infection versus autoimmunity, for certain types of infection, the host immune response and not the inherent virulence of the organism is responsible for the severity of clinical disease. The ability to effectively eradicate specific infectious agents such as *Leishmania* and *Mycobacterium leprae* depends on the specific pattern of immune response. *Leishmania* are protozoan parasites that replicate in macrophages. These parasites cause a clinical spectrum of disease ranging from a self-limited cutaneous infection to disseminated systemic disease (15). Inbred strains of mice inoculated with *Leishmania major* have development of a spectrum of disease similar to that in humans. Studies of responding T-cell populations and their cytokine patterns in the draining lymph nodes of these mice have revealed distinct differences between mice able to control the infection and those with fatal disease. Production of IFN-γ by Th1-type T cells is associated with the ability to heal lesions, whereas production of IL-4 by Th2-type T cells is associated with hypergammaglobulinemia and disseminated disease (16). Indeed, treatment with anti–IL-4 antibodies permits control of *Leishmania* infection in susceptible BALB/c mice (17). Tumor nectosis factor-α is also involved in clearance of *Leishmania* in vivo as evidenced by the inability to clear infection if TNF-α is neutralized (18).

In humans, *M. leprae* causes clinical disease analogous to leishmaniasis. Patients with lepromatous leprosy have large numbers of the *M. leprae* bacilli infecting dermal macrophages and neuronal Schwamm cells throughout their body surface (19,20). By contrast, patients with tuberculoid leprosy have a relative paucity of bacilli infecting dermal macrophages and have discrete cutaneous lesions, but have prominent nerve damage. These diverse clinical manifestations are due to the ability or inability of the host to mount an effective cell-mediated immune response. The ability to mount an effective cell-mediated response is, in turn, related to the responding T cells and their cytokine patterns. As in leishmaniasis, a Th1 response characterized by production of IFN-γ and IL-2 is associated with preferential activation of macrophages and containment of the bacilli, that is, tuberculoid leprosy (21,22). A Th2 response characterized by production of IL-4, IL-5, and IL-10 leads to production of antibodies to the organism, which are ineffective in controlling disease, and leads to the clinical manifestations of lepromatous leprosy. Interleukin-4 also facilitates development of CD8+ T-suppressor clones, which further downregulate CD4+ T-cell responses (23).

But what determines the predilection for a Th1 versus Th2 response in the lesions of leprosy or leishmaniasis? This question is the subject of intense investigation. Interleukin-12 is a cytokine produced by infected macrophages, which leads to secretion of IFN-γ by natural killer cells (24). The IFN-γ, in turn, causes differentiation of T helper cells toward the Th1 pathway. Indeed, susceptible mice given recombinant IL-12 at the time of infection with *L. major* are cured of disease because of this shift away from Th2 development and toward Th1 (25). Likewise, if Crohn's disease can be attributed to chronic infection, such as mycobacterial infection, it is more likely to occur as a result of the host response than to the inherent virulence of the organism. Genetic factors are most likely at the root of Th1 versus Th2 shifts in response to infecting microorganisms, but the genes responsible for this have not yet been identified.

2. New Evidence for an Inappropriate Response to Common Bacterial Antigens in Crohn's Disease

Alternatively, common pathogenic or nonpathogenic intestinal bacteria may trigger chronic inflammation in the absence of persistent infection. This tenet is difficult to prove because of the need to identify patients prospectively with a particular infection in whom inflammatory bowel disease goes on to develop. Recently, a novel autoantibody to an erythrocyte antigen was identified in the sera of patients with Crohn's disease and ulcerative colitis (26). Investigators, using anti-idiotypic monoclonal antibodies to specific heavy chain, variable (V_H) segments of immunoglobulins, identified V_H 3-15-type antibodies bound to erythrocytes in submucosal vessels of intestinal biopsy specimens from patients with ulcerative colitis and Crohn's disease. These anti-erythrocyte antibodies (AEAs) were not found in healthy control subjects (0%) but were found in patients with *Campylobacter jejuni* enterocolitis (70%). The AEA were found at a high titer in 100% of Crohn's disease patients and a much lower titer in 90% of ulcerative colitis patients. This study has clinical relevance because it introduces an autoantibody that can be used to distinguish idiopathic inflammatory bowel disease and *C. jejuni* enterocolitis from other colitides. These findings support the theory of molecular mimicry in autoimmunity and raise the possibility that *C. jejuni* infection serves as a trigger for inflammatory bowel disease in the genetically susceptible host. The prevalence of prior *C. jejuni* infection is not higher in patients with inflammatory bowel disease compared with control subjects (27). There is no evidence that this autoantibody is directly pathogenic or that patients with Crohn's disease have ongoing *C. jejuni* infection. Thus, the presence of these autoantibodies suggests an ongoing B-cell response to a presumably eradicated organism in patients with Crohn's disease and failure of the host immune response to develop tolerance to this antigen.

C.   Recent Insights in the Immunology of Crohn's Disease

1.   Th1 Predominance in Crohn's Disease

Unlike for leprosy and leishmaniasis, no organism has been conclusively demonstrated to cause Crohn's disease. Investigators have attempted to characterize the immune response by studying cellular and soluble mediators of inflammation. Most recently, cytokines secreted by peripheral blood and lamina propria lymphocytes have received attention in light of the importance of the Th1/Th2 dichotomy in cell-mediated immune responses in animal and human models of disease. Several laboratories have described an increase in IL-2 and IFN-γ production by lamina propria mononuclear cells from patients with Crohn's disease but not patients with ulcerative colitis (28–30). On this basis, T helper cells in the lamina propria of Crohn's disease are said to have a Th1 predominance compared with those in ulcerative colitis and control lamina propria, which have a Th2 predominance. It is unclear whether these differences in cytokine patterns of Crohn's patients versus control patients and ulcerative colitis patients are a primary cause of disease rather than an effort of other factors. For example, genetic predisposition for IL-2 or IFN-γ overproduction has not been described as a cause of autoimmunity. In light of the models of leishmaniasis and leprosy, a Th1 predominance would predict a more vigorous cell-mediated immune response, especially to mycobacterial pathogens. Indeed, Crohn's disease can be viewed as being similar to tuberculoid leprosy, which is characterized by an intense cellular response to *M. leprae* and a low bacillary load. In this scenario, Crohn's disease may be an overzealous cell-mediated response to a bacterial or self antigen. Teleologically, the intestinal immune response seen in Crohn's disease may have been advantageous under specific circumstances such as poor sanitation but may be disadvantageous, especially in first world countries with improved hygiene (31).

2.   TNF-α: Too Much or Too Little of a Good Thing

Finally, the cytokine that has received the most attention recently for its potential pathogenic role in inflammatory bowel disease is TNF-α. Tumor recrosis factor is a pleiotropic cytokine produced by macrophages and activated lymphocytes that is responsible for activation of macrophages and polymorphonuclear neutrophils PMNs, and systemic effects such as cachexia and hypotension (32–34). The gene for TNF-α is located within the major histocompatibility complex (MHC) and has been implicated in states of autoimmunity (35). Two conditions for which TNF-α underproduction is thought to have a causal role are systemic lupus erythematosus (SLE) and type 1 diabetes mellitus (36). In murine models of both diseases, administration of TNF-α delays or prevents the onset of lupus nephritis or insulitis, respectively (37). Exploiting genetic engineering technology, Probert et al. generated transgenic mice whose T cells constitutively express TNF (38). These mice showed abnormalities in their lymphoid tissues consisting of depletion of lymphocytes in the thymus and lymph nodes. Most dramatic is the development of a wasting syndrome, widespread vascular thrombosis, and necrosis of liver and pancreas.

This study did not examine pathology in the gastrointestinal tract as a possible explanation for the wasting syndrome. Future investigations may include these observations.

Similar reasoning has prompted investigation of TNF-α in inflammatory bowel disease. Differences in methodology and site of sampling has led to controversies over the level of TNF-α production in Crohn's disease (39). In general, TNF-α–secreting mononuclear cells are increased in the lamina propria of active Crohn's disease, and stimulated TNF-α production by peripheral blood mononuclear cells is also elevated in Crohn's disease patients (40–42). The reason for individual variation in the level of TNF-α production is probably immunogenetic. For example, differences in the promoter regions of certain TNF alleles lead to increased or decreased transcription of the gene (43,44). Most recently, analysis of polymorphisms within five microsatellite regions of the TNF gene has revealed a distinct haplotype that is present in approximately 25% of Crohn's disease patients (45). Although, the TNF-α secreting phenotype corresponding to this particular haplotype is yet to be defined, it may be a marker for TNF-α overproduction and/or a clinically distinct subset of patients.

D. Summary

In summary, all these studies of cellular subsets and individual cytokines provide more questions than answers about the etiopathogenesis of Crohn's disease. Reflecting on the genetically engineered mouse models of intestinal inflammation it is not farfetched to imagine that a genetic predisposition to over production or underproduction of certain critical cytokines, in the presence of concomitant bacterial infection, may lead to the phenotypic expression of Crohn's disease. The next step in research is more difficult and requires going beyond measuring individual cytokines to linking the network of interacting cells. The observed differences in Crohn's disease presentation may, thus, be related to the particular genetic and environmental factors leading to chronic intestinal inflammation in a given individual. The next two sections discuss known genetic and phenotypic markers associated with Crohn's disease and how that knowledge may be applied to therapy for the disease.

Possible causes of chronic intestinal inflammation in Crohn's disease are as follows:

1. Shift of T helper cells toward Th1 development; manifested by increased presence of IL-2, IFN-γ, and TNF-α.
2. Chronic infection with slow growing organism such as mycobacteria combined with an exuberant Th1 (granulomatous) response.
3. Relative deficiency of Th2 cytokines such as IL-10 and IL-4.
4. Persistent T-cell activation of common bacterial antigens.
5. Molecular mimicry between bacterial antigen and self-antigen combined with an inability to develop immunologic tolerance.

II.   STRATIFICATION OF CROHN'S DISEASE: GENETIC AND PHENOTYPIC MARKERS

A. Using the Model of Rheumatoid Arthritis

The rheumatologists have led gastroenterologists in the quest to identify genetic markers of disease that predict natural history of disease and response to therapy. Genotyping of patients with rheumatoid arthritis has revealed distinct clinical correlations associated with

HLA alleles (46). Seropositive rheumatoid arthritis is associated with a short sequence within the HLA-DRB1 gene located in the HLA-DR4 region (47,48). Weyand et al. conducted a study of 102 rheumatoid arthritis patients in which both HLA-DRB1 alleles were examined for the presence of this disease-linked sequence (46). Patients with a "double-dose" of specific HLA-DRB1 alleles containing this disease-linked sequence had more severe clinical disease. Nodular disease was present in 100% of these patients compared with 59% in patients with only a single dose of the disease-linked sequence. Joint surgery was performed in 60% of the double-dose rheumatoid patients compared with 25% of the single-dose patients. Because the methodology used to determine the HLA-DRB1 status of the individual patient is relatively simple, namely polymerase chain reaction followed by oligonucleotide hybridization, this test can be applied outside of a research setting. Rather than waiting for severe, morbid disease to manifest itself, rheumatologists may now use HLA-typing to plan immunomodulatory therapy (49).

B. Genetic Markers of Crohn's Disease

The inherent difficulty of the search for the genes involved in inflammatory bowel disease relates to the complexity of the pattern of inheritance. Complex segregation analysis predicts that an autosomal recessive mode of inheritance is operative in approximately 7% of families (50). It is more likely that multiple genes interact to produce a single disease. This prediction compounded by the intricacy of the human genome is analogous to the search for a needle in a haystack. Even so, several genetic associations have been described for both ulcerative colitis and Crohn's disease. These have been discussed in Chapter 2. The next important step is to relate these genotypes to clinical phenotypes. In this way, genetic analyses may someday be used to prognosticate the course of an individual's disease and provide specialized therapy or avoid ineffectual therapy. Ultimately, prevention may be feasible.

The majority of the genetic associations that have been sought in Crohn's disease and ulcerative colitis are related to MHC antigens, specifically HLA class II associations. The MHC region is an obvious place to begin the search for genetic markers in autoimmunity. MHC molecules define the repertoire of T-cell receptors in a given individual by participating in positive and negative selection of T cells in the thymus. Subsequently, antigen-presenting cells expressing membrane MHC present peptide antigens to T cells in an MHC-restricted fashion, that is, the T-cell receptor must recognize the peptide antigen/MHC complex (51). The theoretical prediction of HLA class II associations in autoimmune diseases is corroborated by several autoimmune diseases such as insulin-dependent diabetes mellitus, multiple sclerosis, and rheumatoid arthritis for which these associations have been confirmed (48,52).

With respect to inflammatory bowel disease, there is debate over the HLA-specificities in ulcerative colitis and Crohn's disease. Much of the debate arises because of attempts to compare HLA associations across ethnic groups, which is not statistically valid (53). In a large study of carefully ethnically matched cases and controls, Toyoda et al. identified a positive association with the combination of DR1 and DQw5 alleles in Crohn's disease (Table 2) (54). This study did not address clinical correlates with genetic markers. Studies in ulcerative colitis have suggested that the association of DR2 is most significant in patients with total colonic involvement (55–57).

Most studies have analyzed HLA genes, but other immune-related genes are being examined for their role in inflammatory bowel disease. These include the TNF genes,

TABLE 2 Stratification of Patients with Crohn's Disease

Genetic Markers (Reference)	Clinical/Therapeutic Implications	Phenotypic Markers (Reference)	Clinical/Therapeutic Implications
DR1/DQw5 (54)	Unclear. May predict development of Crohn's disease in first-degree relatives.	p-ANCA (+) subset (approx. 20%)	Ulcerative colitis features (left-sided disease, bleeding) (74).
TNF microsatellite haplotype: a2b1c2d4e1 (45)	Unclear but possible link to TNF-α production and response to anti-TNF-α treatment.	Antierythrocyte antibodies (BK2) (26)	Ability to discriminate between ulcerative colitis and Crohn's disease by serologic test.
ICAM-1 gene allele R241 (73)	Association with p-ANCA positivity.		

interleukin-1 receptor antagonist (IL-1RA) gene, and intercellular adhesion molecule (ICAM) genes. It seems that a particular haplotype consisting of polymorphic variants within five microsatellite regions of the TNF genes is associated with Crohn's disease (45). It is possible that this haplotype is linked to a particular polymorphism within the TNF gene, or its promoter, or to another nearby gene that subsequently contributes to the development of Crohn's disease. Mansfield et al. studied the allelic frequency of a polymorphism within the TNF-α gene promoter and found no differences between Crohn's disease patients, ulcerative colitis patients, and a control population (58). This study is limited because it only examines one polymorphic variant within the TNF-α promoter. Measurements of TNF-α production and clinical correlations will help to apply these genetic findings to the care of patients. The Mansfield et al. study also examined the frequency of three IL-1RA alleles and found an overrepresentation of allele 2 in patients with ulcerative colitis, especially those with total colonic involvement, compared with Crohn's disease patients and a control population. The association of ICAM genes and Crohn's disease is discussed in the next section.

Genetic markers cannot be used to predict first-degree relatives who will develop inflammatory bowel disease. The risk of inflammatory bowel disease developing in first-degree relatives of Crohn's disease patients ranges from 13% to 35% (53,59). Perhaps the most accurate assessment of the risk comes from a study by Yang et al., which analyzed the lifetime risk of inflammatory bowel disease developing in first-degree relatives of Jewish patients with Crohn's disease compared with non-Jewish patients (60). The estimated risk for Jewish versus non-Jewish families was 7.8% and 5.2%, respectively. Thus, although 27% of Crohn's disease patients would be predicted to have the DR1/DQw5 haplotype, which is heritable, the disease would develop in a much smaller percentage to their first-degree relatives (54). The genetic association of affected first-degree relatives is being studied.

C. Phenotypic Markers of Crohn's Disease

For more than 20 years, subtypes of Crohn's disease have been recognized based on clinical course of disease (61–64). The patient must already have manifested complications of their disease, such as fistulas or obstruction, to be properly classified. More importantly, these general categories (e.g., perforating versus cicatrizing) do not dictate distinct therapeutic options. Similar to the use of genetic associations to predict natural history of disease and the development of disease in yet unaffected relatives, subclinical disease markers such as autoantibodies are being studied for the same reasons. Because they are "subclinical," patients may be spared complications of their disease. The best studied subclinical marker in inflammatory bowel disease is the antineutrophil cytoplasmic antibody (ANCA). The present of ANCA in patients with inflammatory bowel disease was first described by Saxon et al. (65). Distinct from the ANCA found in vasculitides, the immunofluorescent staining pattern in inflammatory bowel disease is perinuclear, not cytoplasmic, and is referred to as p-ANCA. The prevalence of p-ANCA is higher for ulcerative colitis than Crohn's disease, 50% to 86% versus 15% (66,67). P-ANCA is not associated with disease activity or extent of colitis but has most recently defined other important clinical subsets of ulcerative colitis (65,66). Approximately 5% of patients with ulcerative colitis who undergo ileal pouch–anal anastomosis (IPAA) develop chronic pouchitis, that is, recurrent inflammation of the ileal pouch requiring therapy (68). The frequency of p-ANCA positivity in ulcerative colitis patients with chronic pouchitis compared with ulcerative colitis patients without pouchitis is 100% versus 50% (69). If patients with left-sided ulcerative colitis are divided into those who are treatment-resistant (failure to respond to topical therapy and oral 5-aminosalicylic acid (5-ASA) within 6 to 8 weeks) and treatment-responsive, treatment-resistant patients have a higher frequency of p-ANCA positivity, 87% versus 62% (70).

Unfortunately, the overlap in p-ANCA positivity in these two examples still does not permit a prediction of who will develop treatment-resistant ulcerative colitis or chronic pouchitis. P-ANCA is useful in the preoperative evaluation of patients undergoing IPAA. Although IPAA is contraindicated in patients with Crohn's disease, as many as 10% of patients can only be categorized as having indeterminate colitis (71). In one study of patients who underwent total colectomy for indeterminate colitis, none developed subsequent small bowel disease requiring surgery (72). The natural history of indeterminate colitis following IPAA is unclear, however. Confirmed p-ANCA positivity in some of these patients would support a diagnosis of ulcerative colitis rather than Crohn's disease. Conversely, a low positive ANCA titer or a cytoplasmic staining ANCA pattern by immunofluorescence would support a diagnosis of Crohn's disease and alert the clinician to potential postoperative complications of IPAA.

Despite the low prevalence of ANCA in Crohn's disease patients, an interesting genetic correlation was recently identified between ANCA-positive Crohn's disease patients and ANCA-negative ulcerative colitis patients (73). Intercellular adhesion molecules (ICAM) are cellular receptors that mediate transendothelial migration of leukocytes as well as facilitate B-cell–T-cell interactions. Based on the hypothesis that polymorphisms in these ICAM genes can affect the level of inflammation in the host, investigators have sought an association between ICAM genes and phenotypic markers of inflammatory bowel disease. A particular ICAM-1 allele, R241, is present in 8% of control subjects, ANCA(+) ulcerative colitis, and ANCA(–) Crohn's disease. By contrast, this allele was present in 19.6% of ANCA(+) Crohn's disease patients and 16% of ANCA(–) ulcerative colitis patients. These results not only suggest a role for ICAM genes in the pathogenesis of inflammatory bowel disease but also support a distinction for an overlap group of ulcerative colitis and Crohn's disease patients based on ANCA status that is, ANCA(+) Crohn's disease/ANCA(–) ulcerative colitis.

This study done on ICAM genes and ANCA highlights the possibility that there exists a clinically distinct group of Crohn's disease patients definable by their ANCA status. Vasiliauskas et al. examined the clinical characteristics of 22 ANCA(+) Crohn's disease patients compared with 14 matched ANCA(–) Crohn's disease control subjects. Crohn's disease patients with a high ANCA titer were more likely to exhibit features similar to those of ulcerative colitis such as rectal bleeding, left-sided colon involvement by endoscopy, and histopathological features of crypt abscesses without granulomas than were Crohn's disease patients with a low ANCA titer or ANCA(–) (74). If these findings are corroborated in a larger study, ANCA may be useful in predicting the natural history of a subset of Crohn's disease patients.

III. TREATMENT—IS A CURE IN SIGHT?

As more sophisticated, specific therapies emerge for the treatment of inflammatory bowel disease, patient selection will be critical to reduce potential toxicities and cost of these therapies while maximizing benefits. As discussed in the preceding section, rheumatologists are successfully using HLA-typing to treat particular rheumatoid arthritis patients with immunomodulatory therapy. This section forecasts ways in which conventional Crohn's disease therapy may be used more safely and effectively. Future avenues of treatment based on bench research and ongoing clinical trials are also discussed.

A. Conventional Therapy: Is It Time to Start Over or Start Sooner?

Most clinicians who care for patients with Crohn's disease agree that short bowel is the most ominous complication of this disease. In most cases, this relatively uncommon but morbid condition arises from undertreatment of disease, especially early in its course. For this reason, a low threshold for using maintenance therapy should be advocated. This maintenance therapy, as discussed in Chapters 6 and 9, currently consists of 5-ASA products and/or immunosuppressive medications.

1. Antimetabolite Therapy

Even though many studies have documented the long-term benefits of 6-mercaptopurine (6-MP) or azathioprine therapy and few long-term toxicities, many physicians are still reluctant to choose it for maintenance (75,76). Several parameters would make these immunosuppressive drugs more appealing. One limitation is the fundamental lack of understanding of how these drugs work. The ability to easily measure a drug level or other surrogate marker that would help to predict bone marrow toxicity and establish a therapeutic index more accurately would be helpful. At present, we are left to increase the drug until a salutary effect or dangerous leukopenia occurs. Studies examining the metabolites of 6-MP have not elucidated relevant measurements that can be used prospectively to predict a response (77). Finally, the protracted length of time before the onset of therapeutic benefit is often too long for many sick patients to wait without an intervening complication. There is some evidence in children with acute lymphoblastic leukemia that suggests a cumulative amount of 6-MP is necessary for a therapeutic effect to occur (78). This cumulative dose has not been calculated for patients with inflammatory bowel disease. For this reason, clinical trials are exploring "loading" patients with 6-MP to shorten the initial lag phase. Induction of leukopenia by 6-MP has shortened the time to remission from 14.3 weeks to 8.8 weeks (79). In this study, leukopenia was defined as a leukocyte count of less than 5000. It is important to determine whether lymphopenia rather than general leukopenia is associated with response to the drug. Once established, a favorable lymphocyte range may be used by clinicians to guide dosing.

Methotrexate has emerged as another important alternative to 6-MP and azathioprine, especially in patients who have not improved on these drugs or have had toxicity to these drugs. Kozarek et al. originally published the results of an open-label trial of methotrexate given intramuscularly at a dose of 25 mg per week to patients with Crohn's disease or ulcerative colitis who were steroid dependent or had failed 6-MP and azathioprine therapy (80). The results were encouraging, with 11 of 14 patients with Crohn's disease responding to the drug. More recently, Feagan et al. published the results of a double-blind, placebo-controlled multicenter study of methotrexate in Crohn's disease patients who had been unable to discontinue steroids for the preceding 3 months (81). Patients were randomized to receive weekly methotrexate, 25 mg intramuscularly or placebo, during the 16 week trial. Remission, defined as a reduction in Crohn's Disease Activity Index (CDAI) score to less than 150 and discontinuation of prednisone, was achieved in 39% of the treated group compared with 19% of the placebo group. Reduction in CDAI scores and quality of life scores was evident by approximately 4 weeks. At this juncture, it is unclear how best to maintain remission in these patients, whether it be by continued intramuscular methotrexate at a lower dose or by change to oral therapy. This question is currently being evaluated by the same group of researchers. A significant number of patients in the treated group, 17% versus 2% in the placebo group withdrew from the study because of drug toxicities. Concurrent administration of folate at a dose of 5 to 27.5 mg per week has reduced the side effects from methotrexate in patients with rheumatoid arthritis without reducing the efficacy of the drug (82). As gastroenterologists add methotrexate to their armamentarium of inflammatory bowel disease drugs, it will be important to reduce drug toxicities to improve patient compliance.

2. Antibiotic Therapy

Antibiotics have received mixed publicity in the primary treatment of inflammatory bowel disease. The few randomized, controlled trials of antibiotics that have been accomplished have failed to show a statistical benefit (83,84). Several reasons exist for these lukewarm results. As stated previously, Crohn's disease exists in many (poorly characterized) forms. Crohn's disease patients are sometimes given common antibiotics, usually for an unrelated condition, and they have a dramatic, albeit ephemeral, effect on their disease activity. It is not possible to predict which patients will react this way. The vague theory is that antibiotics cause a reduction in antigenic load, that is, bacteria, which reduces the level of intestinal inflammation. It can be presumed that antibiotic nonresponders are patients in whom bacteria are not involved in perpetuation of inflammation or the inciting organism is resistant to the chosen antibiotic. In the provocative animal models of inflammatory bowel disease discussed earlier, most of the mice models did not develop gut inflammation without both a particular immunological defect and environmental bacteria. These animal studies do not address the effect of bowel decontamination once inflammation has begun. It is likely that bacteria are necessary for the initiation of the inflammatory process but the perpetuation of inflammation results from the failure of the host immune system to downregulate the cycle of cytokine and cell-mediated destruction.

Although gut microorganisms are legion, it may be that a single type of bacteria is responsible for triggering chronic inflammation. For example, one plausible hypothesis is that bacterial wall antigens mimic self-antigens such as intestinal epithelial cell wall components. Antiepithelial cell antibodies have commonly been described in inflammatory bowel disease (85–87), but whether these are pathogenic or a secondary manifestation of epithelial cell destruction is unclear. For this reason, simply eradicating the microorganism may be insufficient to stop continued epithelial cell damage. In a competent immune system, however, these autoreactive lymphocytes directed at both self and foreign bacteria should be deleted or rendered anergic, regardless of whether molecular mimicry is the culprit.

There may yet be another role for antibodies in Crohn's disease—prevention. If a proband is identified with Crohn's disease or ulcerative colitis, unaffected family members can be studied genetically and phenotypically, and their likelihood for disease development can be predicted. If the likelihood of developing the disease is high, prophylactic antibiotics may someday be recommended during travel or exposure to foreign pathogens or eradication of a particular causative organism.

B. What Is New on the Treatment Horizon

Treatment for inflammatory bowel disease generally reduces the function of several arms of the immune system (e.g., corticosteroids) or reduces the extent of damage caused by inflammatory mediators (e.g., 5-ASA products). As the pathophysiology of Crohn's disease and ulcerative colitis is better understood, the individual cells of the immune system, cytokines, and/or bacteria that can be selectively eliminated or attenuated to control disease activity will be identified.

1. T Cell–Directed Immunosupressants

a. Cyclosporin. Cyclosporin is a drug originally designed for use as an immunosuppressant in patients undergoing organ transplantation (88). This drug inhibits the ability of T cells to produce interleukin-2 (IL-2), which, in turn, prevents activation and proliferation of T cells. In inflammatory bowel disease treatment, cyclosporin is commonly used in severe ulcerative colitis that is refractory to intravenous steroid therapy (89,90). Institution of intravenous cyclosporin can prevent acute colectomy in more than 80% of patients. Although the exact pathophysiology is not completely understood, cyclosporin is not ideal as a maintenance drug for ulcerative colitis. In large part, this may be due to fluctuations in cyclosporin levels when oral dosing is used, especially in patients with rapid gut transit times, or to development of tolerance to the drug (91). The percentage of ulcerative colitis patients who continue to be in remission 6 months after treatment with intravenous cyclosporin followed by oral cyclosporin is decreased to 50% to 63% (92,93). The rapid action of cyclosporin combined with its relatively brief maintenance effect in inflammatory bowel disease makes it a useful bridge to chronic immunosuppressive therapy, such as 6-MP, with its long lag time of action. Clinical trials are not yet available to support this concept, but many centers are already using this approach.

Two randomized, controlled clinical trials have been published using cyclosporin in Crohn's disease (94,95). The results in Crohn's disease have not been as encouraging as those in ulcerative colitis, but patient selection and dosing are probably the reasons for these less impressive findings. Brynskov et al. selected patients with chronically active Crohn's disease whose disease was "unresponsive" to corticosteroid treatment and who were not on 6-MP concurrently. Cyclosporin was administered twice a day, orally, to achieve a level of 400 to 800 ng/ml of whole blood for a total of 3 months. The response rate for those receiving drug was 59% compared with 32% in the placebo group. The clinical improvement in the group of responders, however, was modest and ability to discontinue steroids was not part of the study design. The more recent trial by Feagan et al. examined the benefit of low-dose cyclosporin (goal level 200 ng/ml of whole blood) in maintaining remission in Crohn's disease patients whose disease had been active within the preceding 2 years. This study found a trend toward a shorter relapse time in patients receiving cyclosporin compared with placebo. Based on these results, it is safe to conclude that oral cyclosporin, especially at levels less than 400 to 800 ng/ml of whole blood, is ineffective at maintaining remission in Crohn's disease.

Even less is known about cyclosporin in the treatment of acute Crohn's disease. There are several scenarios in which cyclosporin may soon prove to play an important role. The first is severe Crohn's colitis with features similar to severe ulcerative colitis. Patients who fail to respond to intravenous steroids would receive intravenous cyclosporin in an effort to prevent urgent surgery. A second common situation is when the patient with Crohn's disease presents with an intestinal obstruction that is relatively resistant to steroids and it is unclear whether the obstruction is due largely to inflammation or fibrosis. In this case, a trial of intravenous cyclosporin would discern the need for surgery versus more aggressive medical therapy. Third, intravenous cyclosporin has been successfully used to achieve rapid closure of fistulas in patients with Crohn's disease. Hanauer et al. treated a total of 12 fistulas in five patients with intravenous cyclosporin for 6 to 10 days followed by oral cyclosporin (135). Complete cessation of drainage was seen in 10 fistulas in a mean time of 8 days. Of these 10 closures, five fistulas had recurrent drainage between 3 weeks and 7 months of oral cyclosporin. Three of the five patients were given 6-MP or azathioprine concurrently with cyclosporin. Although many of the patients in this small case series had recurrence of their drainage, the rapid effect of cyclosporin is encouraging. Present and Lichtiger found similar results in 16 patients with Crohn's disease complicated by fistulas (96). Acute response to cyclosporin resulted in seven fistula closures and seven patients with decreased fistula output. Five patients had a relapse when they were switched to oral therapy. It is likely that early institution of conventional immunosuppressive drugs, such as 6-MP or azathioprine, in combination with the rapid, short-term effect of cyclosporin will lead to decreased patient morbidity from fistulous complications.

b. FK 506. FK 506 is a macrolide antibiotic with immunomodulatory properties similar to those of cyclosporin (97). It also inhibits IL-2 production by T cells, thereby inhibiting T-cell proliferation. In many transplantation centers, it is used as primary immunosuppression after solid organ transplantation. There does not seem to be an improved therapeutic index with FK 506 compared with cyclosporin with respect to neurotoxicity and nephrotoxicity (98). There is insufficient evidence that blood levels attained with oral dosing of FK 506 are more stable than those with cyclosporin. Thus, a course of FK 506 in a patient with Crohn's disease should be reserved for those patients who have had an adverse reaction to cyclosporin, especially if it is idiosyncratic, or who initially responded to a course of cyclosporin but have since become resistant to it.

c. Lymphocyte Apheresis and Anti-CD4 Antibody Treatment. T-cell subsets play a central role in the initiation and perpetuation of chronic intestinal inflammation. Without lymphocytes, inflammation from many causes, and in many places, would be attenuated. Several uncontrolled trials have suggested lymphocyte apheresis is beneficial in achieving remission of Crohn's disease and discontinuation of steroids (99–102). On this premise, French investigators completed a randomized controlled trial of lymphocyte apheresis to assess the efficacy of this therapy in maintaining Crohn's disease remission (103). Patients were subjected to nine sessions of lymphocyte apheresis over a 4- 5-week period in which

3.5×109 lymphocytes were removed per session. Although patients randomized to apheresis were able to discontinue steroids, their relapse rate was higher than in the placebo group. These results are not surprising in that the activated lymphocytes responsible for the perpetuation of gut inflammation have already homed to the lamina propria and are no longer in the peripheral circulation. Moreover, newly replenished lymphoctes would respond in a similar fashion as those removed. It is likely that, if the sessions of lymphocyte apheresis had been continued for a longer period of time, infectious complications would have arisen. Finally, the morbidity, time, and expense of this kind of therapy make it impractical even if it were more effective.

Similar reasoning to lymphocyteapheresis has led several groups to investigate the use of monoclonal antibodies directed against the CD4 molecule in the treatment of Crohn's disease (104). CD4 is expressed on the surface of all T helper cells. Tangential evidence that a depetion of $CD4^+$ cells may lead to a remission in Crohn's disease comes from case reports of patients with Crohn's disease who became infected with human immunodeficiency virus (HIV) and subsequently went into remission from their Crohn's disease (105). There have been at least two subsequent reports of patients with concurrent active inflammatory bowel disease and HIV-related immunosuppression (28,84,106,107). One case report describes the use of anti-CD4 antibodies in three patients, one with Crohn's disease and two with ulcerative colitis (108). Only one patient with ulcerative colitis had a response lasting more than 1 month. There is little doubt that activation of $CD4^+$ T cells is involved in the pathophysiology of Crohn's disease, but targeting such a broad arm of the immune system is likely to have other harmful ramifications.

2. Cytokine-Directed Therapy

Cytokines are soluble mediators secreted by immune cells, epithelial cells, endothelial cells, and fibroblasts, which are capable of recruiting and activating cells of the immune system. They can also be directly cytotoxic to other cells. Almost all known cytokines have been studied for their role in inflammatory bowel disease. Many cytokines have been demonstrated to be elevated in the serum and lamina propria of patients with inflammatory bowel disease. Not all of these, however, merit investigational therapy, and it is unclear which cytokines are central to the inflammatory process or are merely an epiphenomenon of inflammation. Human diseases such as leishmaniasis and animal models using genetic engineering to overexpress or underexpress specific cytokine genes have suggested some answers and provoked ideas for current and future therapeutic trials.

a. Anti–TNFα Therapy. One of the most exciting areas of bench and bedside research in Crohn's disease is the role of TNF-α in chronic inflammation. TNF-α is a pleiotropic cytokine with actions ranging from septic shock and cachexia to protection from viral and parasitic infections (32,34). Because TNF-α alone can mediate hypotension, anti–TNF-α therapy was originally sought to decrease circulating TNF-α in patients with gramnegative sepsis. The two principal ways in which this was accomplished were soluble TNF receptors or monoclonal antibodies to TNF-α itself. The monoclonal antibodies to TNF-α have been developed in mice but are "humanized," such that the antigen-recognizing portion is murine and the remainder of the antibody is human. Several clinical trials concluded that this anti–TNF-α was not efficacious in septic shock (109). The same strategy was then used to treat patients with rheumatoid arthritis. Twenty patients with active rheumatoid arthritis were treated with a chimeric monoclonal anitbody to TNF-α.

Overall, these patients had a significant reduction in their swollen joint count and felt clinically improved (110).

Powrie et al. recently reported an animal model in which severe combined immunodeficiency (SCID) mice reconstituted with CD45RB^{high} CD4$^+$ T cells develop severe colonic inflammation (111). This inflammation can be abrogated by the administration of monoclonal antibodies to TNF-α or monoclonal antibodies to IFN-γ.

Trials are ongoing to study the effect of soluble TNF receptors and anti-TNF antibodies in Crohn's disease. Interest in TNF-α–lowering strategies for the treatment of Crohn's disease has arisen out of observations that TNF-α levels are high in the mucosa of patients with Crohn's disease (30,38,40,105,112,113). A pilot study from the Netherlands reports the treatment of five patients with steroid-dependent Crohn's disease who were given chimeric monoclonal antibody to TNF-α (114). All five patients normalized their CDAI scores and showed endoscopic healing of their disease. Although the pilot results are encouraging, it is probable that larger patient studies will reveal some nonresponders. The biological determinants for response or lack of response are under investigation. Specifically, the basal and stimulated levels of TNF-α production differ between individuals. It is thus possible that low TNF-α producers may not benefit from further TNF-α–lowering measures. Identifying the subset of patients who will benefit from this therapy is the next focus of research.

Foreseeable problems with the use of monoclonal antibodies to treat disease include development of host antibodies to the mouse portion of the monoclonal antibody and allergic reactions once the person has been sensitized to the chimeric antibody. Drugs that prevent the synthesis and secretion of endogenous TNF-α may be forthcoming. TNF-α is translated in a 26-kD proform that is processed intracellularly and secreted as a 17-kD active form. Metalloproteinase enzyme inhibitors have been developed that can inhibit this processing and, thus, may be used to lower systemic TNF-α more effectively (115,116).

b. Anti-IFN-γ Therapy. Interferon gamma is an important immunoregulatory cytokine that is elevated in the mucosa of patients with Crohn's disease (55,88,117,118). One important effect of IFN-γ is thought to be its ability to induce expression of HLA class II molecules on the surface of colonic epithelial cells (119). This would permit epithelial cells to act as antigen-presenting cells and lead to epithelial cell destruction. The combination of IFN-γ and TNF-α has also been shown to be cytotoxic to certain colonic epithelial cell lines (120). IFN-γ–lowering therapies have not been used to treat Crohn's or other human diseases. The Powrie et al. study highlights the importance of the Th1 cytokines, IFN-γ and TNF-α, in mediating colonic inflammation in the CD45RB^{high} SCID mouse model. Monoclonal antibodies to IFN-γ prevented development of colitis in these mice for up to 12 weeks, whereas anti-TNF antibodies could only prevent severe disease but continued to permit mild disease. This study is supportive evidence that anti–IFN-γ therapy may be rational to attempt in inflammatory bowel disease.

c. IL-1 and the IL-1 Receptor Antagonist. Interleukin-1a and IL-1b are related polypeptides with a broad range of effects, including activation of B cells and T cells, osteoblast activation, induction of IL-8 secretion, and initiation of fever (121). These cytokines have a naturally occurring antagonist, IL-1 receptor antagonist (IL-1RA), which blocks the binding of IL-1 to its receptor. The major source of IL-1 and IL-1RA is mononuclear cells. Evidence that IL-1 is involved in the pathological condition of inflammatory bowel disease consists of reports of enhanced IL-1 production by inflamed mucosa (122). More compelling evidence that IL-1 is an important inflammatory cytokine is studies in rabbits with immune complex colitis whose disease can be ameliorated with administration of IL-1RA (123). IL-1RA is being investigated as a treatment for ulcerative colitis but no reports have yet been published. Its effects in Crohn's disease are less clear.

d. *The Ying and Yang of IL-2.* Interleukin-2 is an essential cytokine in lymphocyte activation and proliferation and is associated with Th1 type responses. Measurements of IL-2 production by lamina propria mononuclear cells (LPMCs) from patients with Crohn's disease and ulcerative colitis have revealed differences both in spontaneous and stimulated IL-2 production. Namely, LPMCs from ulcerative colitis have significantly lower IL-2 production than control subjects, whereas LPMCs from Crohn's disease patients have significantly greater IL-2 production than control subjects (28,124). A disease that is more similar to ulcerative colitis than Crohn's disease develops in the IL-2 Knockout mouse (2). Supportive evidence of a harmful role for IL-2 in Crohn's disease comes from a case report of two patients with Crohn's disease who received IL-2 for treatment of renal cell carcinoma and their Crohn's disease flared (125). Cyclosporin and FK 506 are potent inhibitors of IL-2 transcription. Monoclonal antibodies that block the interaction of IL-2 with its receptor have been used in animal models to inhibit graft-versus-host disease and allograft rejection. Thus far, this treatment has not been used in human inflammatory bowel disease. Anti–IL-2 therapy is sufficiently broad immunologically to predict that a subset of patients will respond.

e. *Il-4 and IL-10: More of a Good Thing May Be Better.* Interleukin-4 and IL-10 are both cytokines secreted by Th2-type T cells. The best studied function for IL-4 is as a growth and differentiation factor for B cells (126). IL-4 is a critical cytokine in class switching of B cells to produce IgE and, thus, has been implicated in the pathophysiology of hypersensitivity. IL-10 is an immunoregulatory cytokine that can downregulate expression of Th1-type cytokines such as IL-2 and IFN-γ (127). Of these two cytokines, IL-10 is the most promising in the treatment of inflammatory bowel disease. Therapy with IL-4 may reasonably be expected to exacerbate allergic symptoms.

Rationale for the use of IL-10 in inflammatory bowel disease comes from two murine models of intestinal inflammation that have already been described in this chapter. The first is the IL-10 knockout mouse, which develops mucosal inflammation involving the entire intestinal tract, reminiscent of Crohn's disease (4). The other is the SCID mice reconstitued with CD45RB^{high} T cells, which develop colitis (111). This colitis can be prevented by cotransfer of CD45RB^{lo} T cells or by systemic administration of recombinant IL-10. The implication is that the CD45RB^{high} T cells represent the Th1 compartment of T helper cells, exemplified by an overproduction of IFN-γ and TNF-α, whereas the CD45RB^{lo} T cells represent the Th2 compartment. Mice reconstituted with CD45RB^{high} T cells alone produce very low levels of the Th2 cytokines IL-4 and IL-10. However, only administration of IL-10, and not IL-4, is able to prevent the colitis and downregulate production of IFN-γ and TNF-α. Information is not available on the role of IL-10 in inflammatory bowel disease, but this seems to be a fruitful therapeutic arena for many autoimmune diseases.

3. *Stopping Neutrophil Traffic with Adhesion Molecule Antagonists*

It is tempting to consider inhibiting the migration of effector cells to the intestinal mucosa as a means of blocking inflammation. Ligands on lymphocytes and neutrophils interact with receptors on venular endothelial cells to transmigrate into tissues at sites of inflammation. Because particular adhesion molecules are expressed by subsets of inflammatory cells, these adhesion molecules can be targeted individually to prevent homing of lymphocytes to Peyer's patches in the gut (128). The particular ligand-receptor pairs involved in homing lymphocytes to the intestinal mucosa are endothelial leukocyte adhesion molecule-1 (ELAM-1), ICAM-1/lymphocyte functional antigen (LFA-1), and vascular cell adhesion molecule-1 (VCAM-1)/very late antigen (VLA-4). Immunohistochemical studies of intestinal tissue from Crohn's disease patients, ulcerative colitis patients, and colon cancer control patients have revealed a correlation between the degree of inflammation and the expression of ELAM-1 and ICAM-1 by endothelial cells lining venules (118,54,66,129–131). Using the cotton-top tamarin model of acute and chronic colitis, Podolsky et al. studied the effect of antibodies against ELAM-1 and VLA-4 (found predominantly on lymphocytes and monocytes) on the histological activity of colitis (132). Antibodies to VLA-4 were much more effective in attenuating inflammation. This blockade may affect not only lymphocytes migration but also lymphocyte–lymphocyte interactions. Inhibiting leukocyte migration into areas of inflammation reduces the manifestations of disease activity in inflammatory bowel disease as well as other rheumatic conditions. Corticosteroids, for example, reduce the expression of E-selectin and ICAM-1 by endothelial cells (133). Ultimately, corticosteroids are not able to change the natural history of inflammatory bowel disease. We predict that therapy directed at inhibiting leukocyte transmigration into the gut will be effective in treating acute flares of inflammatory bowel disease but it is doubtful that their effect will be long-lasting.

C. Combination Therapy

Combining chemotherapeutic drugs directed at different points of the cell cycle is more effective than using a toxic dose of one drug. With a greater variety of anti-inflammatory medicines available for the treatment of inflammatory bowel disease, gastroenterologists have the opportunity to choose additive, or potentially, synergistic, combinations of immunomodulatory drugs. Few studies examine combination therapies prospectively, however. It is likely, for example, that maintenance therapy with 5-ASA drugs, which are directed at inflammatory mediators, combined with 6-MP, directed at cell-mediated signals, may be more effective than either alone. Soon, drugs or antibodies directed at cellular subsets and cytokines may act synergistically. In the murine model of collagen-induced arthritis, mice exposed to the combination of anti-CD4 and anti–TNF-α antibodies achieved significantly greater reductions in paw-swelling, limb involvement, and joint erosion than with either treatment alone (134). In addition, the anti-CD4 treatment diminished the antibody response to hamster anti-TNF.

Monoclonal antibody therapy is the most accessible way of interfering with soluble and cellular mediators of inflammation. These antibodies can be predicted to have a finite usefulness because of the development of host anti-monoclonal antibodies. Concurrent use of long-term immunosupressants such as 6-MP might lessen the development of these host antibodies and maintain a remission achieved by monoclonal antibody therapy. As with TNF metalloproteinase inhibitors, the next step is to develop drugs that interrupt the synthesis and secretion of specific cytokines without causing significant toxicity. The goal of therapy in inflammatory bowel disease is to target a few critical points in the inflammatory cascade that will be sufficient to control pathological intestinal inflammation without perturbing host immunity to a dangerous extent.

D. Custom-Fitting Therapy for Individual Patients

Now that we have the ideas and the technology to develop new treatments for patients with inflammatory bowel disease, can we predict who will respond? Can we predict who will need these medicines before complications develop? The answer is no—but soon. Information that is being collected prospectively in the form of genotypic analyses will be correlated to clinical variables of disease activity and phenotypic markers such as cytokine and autoantibody production to plan appropriate intervention. For example, the over-representation of allel 2 of the IL-1RA gene may predict a more severe course of ulcerative colitis characterized by decreased secretion of IL-1RA and responsiveness to anti-IL-1 therapy (58). It is easy to see why a trial of anti–IL-1 monoclonal antibodies might fail if given to all patients with ulcerative colitis. Only approximately 35% of patients studied had this allele and might be expected to respond to IL-1–directed therapy. Biochemical information will also be helpful. Peripheral blood lymphocytes or lamina propria lymphocytes obtained from mucosal biopsies can be studied for their spontaneous and induced production of key cytokines such as IFN-γ and TNF-α. Knowledge of abnormal secretory patterns may be used during a flare to choose the appropriate anticytokine therapy. Modern molecular techniques will make it relatively easy to screen for a panel of Crohn's disease and ulcerative colitis–associated genes. This genetic information combined with a panel of autoantibody measurements, such as p-ANCA, AEAs and biochemical data will provide a rational basis for the medical management of inflammatory bowel disease.

REFERENCES

1. Parker DC. T cell dependent B cell activation. Ann Rev Immunol 1993; 11:331–360.
2. Sadlack B, Merz H, Schorle H, Schimpl A, Feller Ac, Horak I. Ulcerative colitis–like disease in mice with a disrupted interleukin-2 gene. Cell 1993; 75:253–261.
3. Mombaerts P, Mizoguchi E, Grusby MJ, Glimcher LH, Bhan AK, Tonegawa S. Spontaneous development of inflammatory bowel disease in T cell receptor mutant mice. Cell 1993; 75:274–282.
4. Kuhn R, Lohler J, Rennick D, Rajewsky K, Muller W. Interleukin-10–deficient mice develop chronic entercolitis. Cell 1993; 75:263–274.
5. Rook GA, Stanford JL. Slow bacterial infections or autoimmunity? (Review) Immunology Today 1992; 13:160–164.
6. Burnham WR, Lennard-Jones JE, Sandford JL. Mycobacteria as a possible cause of inflammatory bowel disease. Lancet 1978; 2:693–696.
7. Chiodini RJ, Van Kruiningen HJ, Thayer WR, Coutu JA. Spheroplastic phase of mycobacteria isolated from patients with Crohn's disease. J Clin Microbio 1986; 24:357–363.
8. Tsianos EV, Masalas CN, Merkouropoulos M, Dalekos GN, Logan RF. Incidence of inflammatory bowel disease in north west Greece: rarity of Crohn's disease in an area where ulcerative colitis is common. Gut 1994; 35:369–372.
9. Chadwick VS. Lymphocyte apheresis in Crohn's disease (editorial; comment). Gastroenterology 1994; 107:579–581.
10. Cambridge G, Rampton DS, Stevens TR, McCarthy DA, Kamm M, Leaker B. Anti-neutrophil antibodies in inflammatory bowel disease: prevalence and diagnostic role. Gut 1992; 33:668–674.
11. Whorewell PH, Davidson IW, Beeken WL, Wright R. Search by immunofluorescence for antigens of tota virus, *Pseudomonas maltophila* and *Mycobacterium kansasii* in Crohn's disease. Lancet 1978; 2:697–698.

12. Rosenberg WMC, Bell JI, Jewell DP. *Mycobacterium paratuberculosis* DNA cannot be detected in Crohn's disease tissues (abstract). Gastroenterology 1991; 100:A247.

13. Rutgeerts P, Geboes K, Vantrappen G, et al. Rifabutin and ethambutol do not help recurrent Crohn's disease in the neoterminal ileum. J Clin Gastroenterol 1992; 15:24–28.

14. Shaffer JL, Turnberg LA. Does antituberculous chemotherapy for Crohn's disease provide long term benefit? A five year follow-up study (abstract). Gut 1989; 30:A458.

15. Reed SG, Scott P. T-cell and cytokine responses in leishmaniasis (review). Curr Opin Immunol 1993; 5:524–531.

16. Heinzel FP, Sadick MD, Mutha SS, Locksley RM. Production of interferon gamma, interleukin 2, interleukin 4, and interleukin 10 by $CD4^+$ lymphocytes in vivo during healing and progressive murine leishmaniasis. Proc Natl Acad Sci U S A 1991; 88:7011–7015.

17. Sadick MD, Heinzel FP, Holaday BJ, Pu RT, Dawkins RS, Locksley RM. Cure of murine leishmaniasis with anti–interleukin 4 monoclonal antibody. Evidence for a T cell–dependent, interferon gamma–independent mechanism. J Exp Med 1990; 171:115–127.

18. Titus RG, Sherry B, Cerami A. Tumour necrosis factor plays a protective role in experimental murine cutaneous leishmaniasis. J Exp Med 1989; 170:2097–2104.

19. Kaplan G, Cohn ZA. Leprosy and cell-mediated immunity (review). Curr Opin Immunol 1991; 3:91–96.

20. Modlin RL. Th1-Th2 paradigm: insights from leprosy (review). J Invest Dermatol 1994; 102:828–832.

21. Cooper CL, Mueller C, Sinchaisri T-A, et al. Analysis of naturally occurring delayed-type hypersensitivity reactions in leprosy by in situ hybridization. J Exp Med 1989; 169:1565–1581.

22. Yamamura M, Uyemura K, Deans RJ, et al. Defining protective responses to pathogens: cytokine profiles in leprosy lesions. Science 1991;254:277–279.

23. Sieling PA, Abrams JS, Yamamura M, Salgame P, Bloom BR, Rea TH. Immunosuppressive roles for IL-10 and IL-4 in human infection. In vitro modulation of T cell responses in leprosy. J Immunol 1993; 150:5501–5510.

24. Scharton TM, Scott P. Natural killer cells are a source of interferon gamma that drives differentiation of CD4+ T cell subsets and induces early resistance to *Leishmania major* in mice. J Expe Med 1993; 178:567–577.

25. Heinzel FP, Schoenhaut DS, Rerko RM, Rosser LE, Gately MK. Recombinant interleukin 12 cures mice infected with *Leishmania major*. J Exp Med 1993; 177:1505–1509.

26. Berberian LS, Valles-Ayoub Y, Gordon LK, Targan SR, Braun J. Expression of a novel autoantibody defined by the VH3-15 gene in inflammatory bowel disease and *Campylobacter jejuni* enterocolitis. J Immunol 1994; 153:3756–3763.

27. Blaser MJ, Hoverson D, Ely IG, Juncan DJ, Wang WL, Brown WR. Studies of *Campylobacter jejuni* in patients with inflammatory bowel disease. Gastroenterology 1984; 86:33.

28. Mullin GE, Lazenby AJ, Harris ML, Bayless TM, James SP. Increased interleukin-2 messenger RNA in the intestinal mucosal lesions of Crohn's disease but not ulcerative colitis. Gastroenterology 1992; 102:1620–1627.

29. Gurbino C, Sabbah S, Menezes J, Justinich C, Marchand R, Seidman EG. Interleukin-2 production in pediatric inflammatory bowel disease: evidence for dissimilar mononuclear cell function in Crohn's disease and ulcerative colitis. J Pediatr Gastroenterol Nutri 1993; 17:247–254.

30. Breese E, Braegger CP, Corrigan CJ, Walker-Smith JA, MacDonald TT. Interleukin-2 and interferon-gamma–secreting T cells in normal and diseased human intestinal mucosa. Immunology 1993; 78:127–131.

31. Gent AE, Hellier MD, Grace RH, Swarbrick ET, Coggon D. Inflammatory bowel disease and domestic hygiene in infancy (see comments). Lancet 1994; 343:766–767.

32. Tracey KJ, Cerami A. Tumor necrosis factor: an updated review of its biology (review). Crit Care Med 1993; 21:S415–S422.

33. Molloy RG, Mannick JA, Rodrick ML. Cytokines, sepsis and immunomodulation. (Review). Br J Surg 1993; 80:289–297.

34. Dinarello CA. Interleukin-1 and tumor necrosis factor: effector cytokines in autoimmune diseases (review). Semin Immunol 1992; 4:133–145.

35. Dunham I, Sargent CA, Trowsdale J, Campbell DR. Molecular mapping of the human major histocompatibility complex by pulse field gel electrophoresis. Proc Nat Acad Sci U S A 1987; 84:7237–7241.

36. Jacob CO, Fronek Z, Lewis GD, Koo M, Hansen JA, McDevitt HO. Heritable major histocompatability complex class-II associated differences in production of tumor necrosis factor alpha: relevance to genetic predisposition to systemic lupus erythematosus. Proc Natl Acad Sci U S A 1990; 87:1233–1237.

37. Jacob CO. Tumor necrosis factor and interferon gamma: relevance for immune regulation and genetic predisposition to autoimmune disease (review). Semin Immunol 1992; 4:147–154.

38. Probert L, Keffer J, Corbella P, et al. Wasting, ischemia, and lymphoid abnormalities in mice expressing T cell–targeted human tumor necrosis factor transgenes. J Immunol 1993; 151:1894–1906.

39. Stevens C, Walz G, Singaram C, et al. Tumor necrosis factor-alpha, interleukin-1 beta, and interleukin-6 expression in inflammatory bowel disease. Dig Dis Sci 1992; 37:818–826.

40. Breese EJ, Michie CA, Nicholls SW, et al. Tumor necrosis factor alpha–producing cells in the intestinal mucosa of children with inflammatory bowel disease. Gastroenterology 1994; 106:1455–1466.

41. Plevy SE, Targan SR, Deem RL, Toyoda H. Increased mucosal TNF-alpha mRNA levels and numbers of TNF-alpha producing cells are unique to Crohn's disease mucosal inflammation (abstr). Gastroenterology 1994; 104:A754.

42. Bouma G. Oudkerk Pool M, v Blomberg BME, Meuwissen SGM, Pena AS. Different spontaneous and stimulated TNF production in patients with Crohn's disease and ulcerative colitis (abstr). Gastroenterology 1994;

43. McGuire W, Hill AVS, Allsopp CEM, Greenwood BM, Kwiatkowski D. Variation in the TNF-alpha promoter region associated with susceptibility to cerebral malaria. Nature 1994; 371:508–511.

44. Wilson AG, Symons JA, McDowell TL, DiGiovine FS, Duff GW. Effects of tumor necrosis factor (TNF alpha) promoter base transition on transcriptional activity. Br J Rheumatol 1994; 33:89.

45. Plevy SE, Targan SR, Rotter JI, Toyoda H. Tumor necrosis factor (TNF) microsatellite associations within HLA-DR2+ patients define Crohn's disease (CD) and ulcerative colitis (UC)-specific genotypes (abst). Gastroenterology 1994; 106:A754.

46. Weyand CM, Hicok KC, Conn DL, Goronzy JJ. The influence of HLA-DRB1 genes on disease severity in rheumatoid arthritis. Ann Intern Med 1992; 117:801–806.

47. Wallin J, Hillert J, Olerup O, Carlsson B, Strom H. Association of rheumatoid arthritis with a dominant DR1/Dw4/Dw14 sequence motif, but not with T cell receptor beta chain gene alleles or haplotypes (see comments). Arthritis Rheum 1991; 34:1416–1424.

48. Goronzy JJ, Weyand CM. Interplay of T lymphocytes and HLA-DR molecules in rheumatoid arthritis (review). Curr Opin Rheumatol 1993; 5:169–177.

49. Gough A, Faint J, Salmon M, et al. Genetic typing of patients with inflammatory arthritis at presentation can be used to predict outcome. Arthritis Rheuma 1994; 37:1166–1170.

50. Orholm M, Iselius L, Sorensen TI, Munkholm P, Langholz E, Binder V. Investigation of inheritance of chronic inflammatory bowel diseases by complex segregation analysis (see comments). BMJ 1993; 306:20–24.

51. Abbas A KJ S 1991 General properties of immune responses in: Cellular and Molecular, Lichtman A H, Pober JS. The Major Histocompatability Complex. In: Abbas AK, Lichtman

AH, Pober JS, eds. Cellular and Molecular Immunology. Philadelphia: WB Saunders, 1991:99–114.

52. Ryder LP, Svejgaard A. Genetics of HLA disease association. Annu Rev Genet 1981; 15:169–187.

53. Satsangi J, Jewell DP, Rosenberg WM, Bell JI. Genetics of inflammatory bowel disease. Gut 1994; 35:696–700.

54. Toyoda H, Wang SJ, Yang HY, et al. Distinct associations of HLA class II genes with inflammatory bowel disease. Gastroenterology 1993; 104:741–748.

55. Asakura H, Tsuchiya M, Aiso S, et al. Association of human lymphocyte-DR2 antigen with Japanese ulcerative colitis. Gastroenterology 1982; 82:413–418.

56. McConnell RB. Ulcerative colitis—genetic features. Scand J Gastroenterol 1982; 18(suppl 88):14.1.

57. Masuda H, Nakamura Y, Tanaka T, Hayakawa S. Distinct relationship between HLA-DR genes and intractability of ulcerative colitis. Am J Gastroenterol 1994; 89:1957–1962.

58. Mansfield JC, Holden H, Tarlow JK, et al. Novel genetic association between ulcerative colitis and the anti-inflammatory cytokine interleukin-1 receptor antagonist. Gastroenterology 1994; 106:637–642.

59. Farmer RG, Michener WM, Mortimer EA. Studies of family history among patients with inflammatory bowel disease. Clin Gastroenterol 1980;9:271–277.

60. Yang H, McElree C, Roth MP, Shanahan F, Targan SR, Rotter JI. Familial empirical risks for inflammatory bowel disease: differences between Jews and non-Jews. Gut 1993; 34:517–524.

61. DeDombal FT, Burton I, Goligher JC. Recurrence of Crohn's disease after primary excisional surgery. Gut 1971; 12:519–527.

62. Greenstein AJ, Sachar DB, Pasternack BS, Janowitz HD. Reoperation and recurrence in Crohn's colitis and ileocolitis. N Engl J Med 1975; 293:685–690.

63. Sachar DB, Wolfson DM, Greenstein AJ, Goldberg J, Styc-Zynski R, Janowitz HD. Risk factors for postoperative recurrence of Crohn's disease. Gastroenterology 1983; 85:917–921.

64. Prantera C, Levenstein S, Capoccia R, et al. Prediction of surgery for obstruction in Crohn's ileitis. Dig Dis Sci 1987; 32:1363–1369.

65. Saxon A, Shanahan F, Landers C, Ganz T, Targan S. A distinct subset of antineutrophil cytoplasmic antibodies is associated with inflammatory bowel disease. J Allergy Clin Immunol 1990; 86:202–210.

66. Duerr RH, Targan SR, Landers CJ, Sutherland LR, Shanahan F. Anti-neutrophil cytoplasmic antibodies in ulcerative colitis: comparison with other colitides/diarrheal illnesses. Gastroenterology 1991; 100:1590–1596.

67. Shanahan F, Duerr RH, Rotter JI, et al. Neutrophil autoantibodies in ulcerative colitis: familial aggregation and genetic heterogeneity. Gastroenterology 1992; 103:456–461.

68. Sandborn WJ. Pouchitis following ileal pouch–anal anastomosis: definition; pathogenesis; and treatment. Gastroenterology. In press.

69. Sandborn WJ, Landers CJ, Tremaine WJ, Targan SR. Antineutrophil cytoplasmic antibody correlates with chronic pouchitis after ileal pouch–anal anastomosis. Am J Gastroenterol. In press.

70. Sandborn WJ, Landers CJ, Tremaine WJ, Targan SR. Unexpectedly high frequency of antineutrophil cytoplasmic antibody in treatment-resistant left-sided ulcerative colitis. Dig Dis Sci. In press.

71. Lee KS, Medline A, Shockey S. Indeterminate colitis in the spectrum of inflammatory bowel disease. Arch Pathol Lab Med 1979; 103:173–176.

72. Wells AD, McMillan I, Price AB, Ritchie JK, Nicholls RJ. Natural history of indeterminate colitis. Br J Surg 1991; 78:179–181.

73. Yang H, Vora DK, Targan SR, Toyoda H, Beaudet AL, Rotter JI. Association of intercellular

adhesion molecule-1 (ICAM-1) polymorphisms with subsets of inflammatory bowel disease (IBD) stratified by antineutrophil cytoplasmic antibodies (ANCAs). J Clin Invest. In press.

74. Vasiliauskas EA, Plevy SE, Ferguson DM, Vidrich A, Landers C, Targan SR. Perinuclear antineutrophil cytoplasmic antibodies (pANCA) in patients with Crohn's disease (CD) define a clinical subgroup (abstr). Gastroenterology 1995;

75. Korelitz BI, Adler DJ, Mendelsohn RA, Sacknoff AL. Long-term experience with 6-mercaptopurine in the treatment of Crohn's disease. Am J Gastroenterol 1993; 88:1198–1205.

76. Present DH, Meltzer SJ, Krumholz MP, Wolke A, Korelitz BI. 6-Mercaptopurine in the management of inflammatory bowel disease: short- and long-term toxicity. Ann Intern Med 1989; 111:641–649.

77. Cuffari C, Theoret Y, Duhaime A, Seidman E. Measurement of erythrocyte 6-mercaptopurine (6-MP) metabolites in IBD patients: correlation with efficacy and toxicity (abstr). Gastroenterology 1994; 106:A1021.

78. Dibenedetto SP, Guardabasso V, Ragusa R, DiCataldo A, Miraglia V, Ippolito AM. 6-Mercaptopurine cumulative dose: a critical factor of maintenance therapy in average risk childhood acute lymphoblastic leukemia. Pediatr Hematol Oncol 1994; 11:251–258.

79. Colonna T, Korelitz BI. The role of leukopenia in the 6-mercaptopurine-induced remission of refractory Crohn's disease. Am J Gastroenterol 1994; 89:362–366.

80. Kozarek RA, Patterson DJ, Gelfand MD, Botoman VA, Ball TJ, Wilske KR. Methotrexate induces clinical and histologic remission in patients with refractory inflammatory bowel disease. Ann Intern Med 1989; 110:353–356.

81. Feagan BG, Rochon J, Fedorak RN, et al. Methotrexate for the treatment of Crohn's Disease. N Eng J Med 1995; 332:292–297.

82. Morgan SL, Baggott JE, Vaughn WH, et al. Supplementation with folic acid during methotrexate therapy for rheumatoid arthritis. Ann Intern Med 1994; 121:833–841.

83. Ambrose NS, Allan RN, Keighley MR, Burdon DW, Youngs D, Barnes P. Antibiotic therapy for treatment in relapse of intestinal Crohn's disease. A prospective randomized study. Dis Colon Rectum 1985; 28:81–85.

84. Sutherland L, Singleton J, Sessions J, et al. Double blind, placebo controlled trial of metronidazole in Crohn's disease. Gut 1991; 32:1071–1075.

85. Broberger O, Perlmann P. Autoantibodies in human ulcerative colitis. J Exp Med 1959; 110:657–673.

86. Das KM, Dubin R, Nagai T. Isolation and characterization of colonic tissue-bound antibodies from patients with idiopathic ulcerative colitis. Pro Nat Acad Sci U S A 1978; 75:4528–4532.

87. Snook JA, Lowes JR, Wu KC, Priddle JD, Jewell DP. Serum and tissue autoantibodies to colonic epithelium in ulcerative colitis. Gut 1991; 32:163–166.

88. Kahan BD. Role of cyclosporine: present and future (review). Transplant Proc 1994; 26:3082–3087.

89. Lichtiger S, Present DH. Preliminary report: cyclosporin in treatment of severe active ulcerative colitis. Lancet 1990; 336:16–19.

90. Lichtiger S, Present DH, Kornbluth A, et al. Cyclosporine in severe ulcerative colitis refractory to steroid therapy. N Engl J Med 1994; 330:1841–1845.

91. Brynskov J, Freund L, Campanini MC, Kampmann JP. Cyclosporin pharmacokinetics after intravenous and oral adminstration in patients with Crohn's disease. Scand J Gastroenterol 1992; 27:961–967.

92. Prokupek DA, Kashyap PK, Targan SR, Plevy SE, Choi P. Cyclosporin in the treatment of refractory UC: clinical determinants of a successful outcome at 6 months (abstract). Gastroenterology 1994; 106:A756.

93. Kornbluth A, Lichtiger S, Present D, Hanauer S. Long-term results of oral cyclosporin in patients with severe ulcerative colitis: a double-blind, randomized, multicenter trial (abstract). Gastroenterology 1994; 106:A714.

94. Brynskov J, Freund L, Rasmussen SN, et al.. A placebo-controlled, double-blind, randomized trial of cyclosporine therapy in active chronic Crohn's disease. N Engl J Med 1989; 321:845–850.

95. Feagan BG, McDonald JWD, Rochon J, et al. Low-dose cylosporine for the treatment of Crohn's disease. N Engl J Med 1994; 330:1846–1851.

96. Present DH, Lichtiger S. Efficacy of cyclosporine in treatment of fistula of Crohn's disease. Dig Dis Sci 1994; 39:374–380.

97. Fung JJ, Starzl TE. FK 506 in solid organ transplantation (review). Transplant Proc 1994; 26:3017–3020.

98. Fung JJ, Alessiani M, Abu-Elmagd K, et al. Adverse effects associated with the use of FK 506 (review). Transplant Proc 1991; 23:3105–3108.

99. Bicks RO, Groshart KD, Mercado S. Lymphoplasmapheresis in Crohn's disease: a pilot study (abstract). Gastroenterology 1984; 88:A1027.

100. Bicks RO, Groshart KD, Chandler RW. T-lymphocyte apheresis in the treatment of Crohn's disease. Gastroenterology 1995; 90:A1140.

101. Bicks RO, Groshart KD, Luther RW. Total parenteral nutrition (TPN) plus T-lymphocyte apheresis (TLA) in the treatment of severe chronic active Crohn's disease (abstract). Gastroenterology 1988; 94:A34.

102. Bicks RO, Groshart KD. T-lymphocyte apheresis in the treatment of chronic active Crohn's disease (abstract). Gastroenterology 1991; 100:A197.

103. Lerebours E, Bussel A, Modigliani R, et al. Treatment of Crohn's disease by lymphocyte apheresis: a randomized controlled trial. Groupe d'Etudes Therapeutiques des Affections Inflammatoires Digestives (see comments). Gastroenterology 1994; 107:357–361.

104. Stronkhorst A, Tytgat GN, van Deventer SJ. CD4 antibody treatment in Crohn's disease. Scand J Gastroenterol Suppl 1992; 194:61–65.

105. James SP. Remission of Crohn's disease after human immunodeficiency virus infection. Gastroenterology 1988; 95:1667–1669.

106. Bernstein BB, Gelb A, Tabanda-Lichauco R. Crohn's ileitis in a patient with longstanding HIV infection. Am J Gastroenterol 1994; 89:937–939.

107. Bernstein CN, Snape WJ Jr. Active idiopathic ulcerative colitis in a patient with ongoing HIV-related immunodepression. Am J Gastroenterol 1991; 86:907–909.

108. Emmrich J, Seyfarth M, Fleig WE, Emmrich F. Treatment of inflammatory bowel disease with anit-CD4 monoclonal antibody (letter). Lancet 1991; 338:570–571.

109. Natanson C, Hoffman WD, Suffredini AF, Eichacker PQ, Danner RL. Selected treatment strategies for septic shock based on proposed mechanisms of pathogenesis (review). Ann Intern Med 1994; 120:771–783.

110. Elliott MJ, Maini RN, Feldmann M, et al. Treatment of rheumatoid arthritis with chimeric monoclonal antibodies to tumor necrosis factor alpha. Arthritis Rheum 1993; 36:1681–1690.

111. Powrie F, Leach MW, Mauze S, Menon S, Barcomb Caddle L, Coffman RL. Inhibition of Th1 responses prevents inflammatory bowel disease in SCID mice reconstituted with CD45RBhi CD4+ T cells. Immunity 1994; 1:553–562.

112. Plevy SE, Targan SR, Deem RL, Toyoda H. Increased mucosal TNF-alpha mRNA levels and numbers of TNF-alpha producing cells are unique to Crohn's disease mucosal inflammation (abstract). Gastroenterology 1994; 104:A754.

113. Reinecker HC, Steffen M, Witthoeft T, Pflueger I, Schreiber S, Raedler A. Enhanced secretion of tumour necrosis factor–alpha, IL-6, and IL-1 beta by isolated lamina propria mononuclear cells from patients with ulcerative colitis and Crohn's disease. Clin Exp Immunol 1993; 94:174–181.

114. van Dullemen HM, Hommes DW, Meenan J, et al. Complete remissions of steroid-refractory Crohn's disease after administration of monoclonal anti-TNF antibody cA2 (abstract). Gastroenterology 1994; 106:A1054.

115. McGeehan GM, Becherer JD, Bast RC, et al. Regulation of tumour necrosis factor-alpha processing by a metalloproteinase inhibitor. Nature 1994; 370:558–561.

116. Gearing AJH, Beckett P, Christodoulou M, et al. Processing of tumour necrosis factor-alpha precursor by metalloproteinases. Nature 1994; 370:555-557.

117. Breese E, Braegger CP, Corrigan CJ, Walker-Smith JA, MacDonald TT. Interleukin-2– and interferon-gamma–secreting T cells in normal and diseased human intestinal mucosa. Immunology 1993; 78:127–131.

118. Fais S, Capobianchi MR, Pallone F, et al. Spontaneous release of interferon gamma by intestinal lamina propria lymphocytes in Crohn's disease. Kinetics of in vitro response to interferon gamma inducers. Gut 1991; 32:403–407.

119. Salomon P, Pizzimenti A, Panja A, Reisman A, Mayer L. The expression and regulation of class II antigens in normal and inflammatory bowel disease peripheral blood monocytes and intestinal epithelium. Autoimmunity 1991; 9:141–149.

120. Abreu-Martin MT, Vidrich A, Lynch DH, Targan SR. Divergent induction of apoptosis and IL-8 secretion in HT-29 cells in response to TNF-alpha and ligation of Fas antigen. J Immunol 1995; (submitted)

121. Dinarello CA, Wolff SM. The role of interleukin-1 in disease. N Engl J Med 1995; 328:106–113.

122. Mahida YR, Wu K, Jewell DP. Enhanced production of interleukin 1–beta by mononuclear cells isolated from mucosa with active ulcerative colitis and Crohn's disease. Gut 1989; 30:835–838.

123. Cominelli F, Nast CC, Clark BD, et al. Interleukin-1 (IL-1) gene expression, synthesis, and effect of specific IL-1 receptor blockade in rabbit immune complex colitis. J Clin Invest 1990; 86:972–980.

124. Gurbindo C, Sabbah S, Menezes J, Justinich C, Marchand R, Seidman EG. Interleukin-2 production in pediatric inflammatory bowel disease: evidence for dissimilar mononuclear cell function in Crohn's disease and ulcerative colitis. J Pediatr Gastroenterol Nutri 1993; 17:247–254.

125. Sparano JA, Brandt LF, Dutcher JP, DuBois JS, Atkins MB. Symptomatic exacerbation of Crohn disease after treatment with high-dose interleukin-2. Ann Intern Med 1993; 118:617–618.

126. Snapper CM, Finkelman FD, Paul WE. Regulation of IgG1 and IgE production by IL-4. Immunol Rev 1988; 102:51–75.

127. Malefyt RDW, Abrams J, Bennett B, Figdor CG, Vries JED. Interleukin 10 (IL-10) inhibits cytokine synthesis by human monocytes: an autoregulatory role of IL-10 produced by monocytes. J Exp Med 1991; 174:1209–1220.

128. Salmi M, Jalkanen S. Regulation of lymphocyte traffic to mucosa-associated lymphatic tissues (review). Gastroenterol Clin North Am 1991; 20:495–510.

129. Ohtani H, Nakamura S, Watanabe Y, et al. Light and electron microscopic immunolocalization of endothelial leucocyte adhesion molecule-1 in inflammatory bowel disease. Morphological evidence of active synthesis and secretion into vascular lumen. Virchows Archiv A Pathol Anat 1992; 420:403–409.

130. Nakamura S, Ohtani H, Watanabe Y, et al. In situ expression of the cell adhesion molecules in inflammatory bowel disease. Evidence of immunologic activation of vascular endothelial cells. Lab Invest 1993; 69:77–85.

131. Koizumi M, King N, Lobb R, Benjamin C, Podolsky DK. Expression of vascular adhesion molecules in inflammatory bowel disease. Gastroenterology 1992; 103:840–847.

132. Podolsky DK, Lobb R, King N, Benjamin CD, Pepinsky B, Sehgal P. Attenuation of colitis in the cotton-top tamarin by anti–alpha 4 integrin monoclonal antibody. J Clin Invest 1993; 92:372–380.

133. Cronstein BN, Weissman G. The adhesion molecules of inflammation (review). Arthritis Rheum 1993; 36:147–157.
134. Williams RO, Mason LJ, Feldmann M, Maini RN. Synergy between anti-CD4 and anti-tumor necrosis factor in the amelioration of established collagen-induced arthritis. Pro Nat Acad Sci U S A 1994; 91:2762–2766.
135. Hanauer SB, Smith MB. Rapid closure of Crohn's disease fistulas with continuous intravenous cyclosporin A (see comments). Am J Gastroenterol 1993; 88:646–649.

Index

Printed in the United States
93368LV00001B/5/A

9 780824 794101

T - #1071 - 101024 - C0 - 254/178/28 [30] - CB - 9780824794101 - Gloss Lamination